I0489486

THE UNIQUE HERBAL

NEW INSIGHTS INTO ANCIENT MEDICINES

VOLUME TWO (D-H)

ROBERT DALE ROGERS (RH) AHG

Copyright © Prairie Deva Press 2017 by Robert Dale Rogers.

ALL RIGHTS RESERVED.

ISBN: 978-1-5485-2166-0

No portion of this book, except for a brief review, may be reproduced, or copied and transmitted,
without the permission of the author.

All photos are by the author (who holds the copyright)
or are in the public domain, except where noted.

This book is for educational purposes only.
The suggestions, recipes and historical information are not meant to replace a medical advisor.
The author assumes no liability for unwise or unsafe usage by readers of this book.

For those interested in using herbal medicine, seek the advice of a professional.

CONTENTS

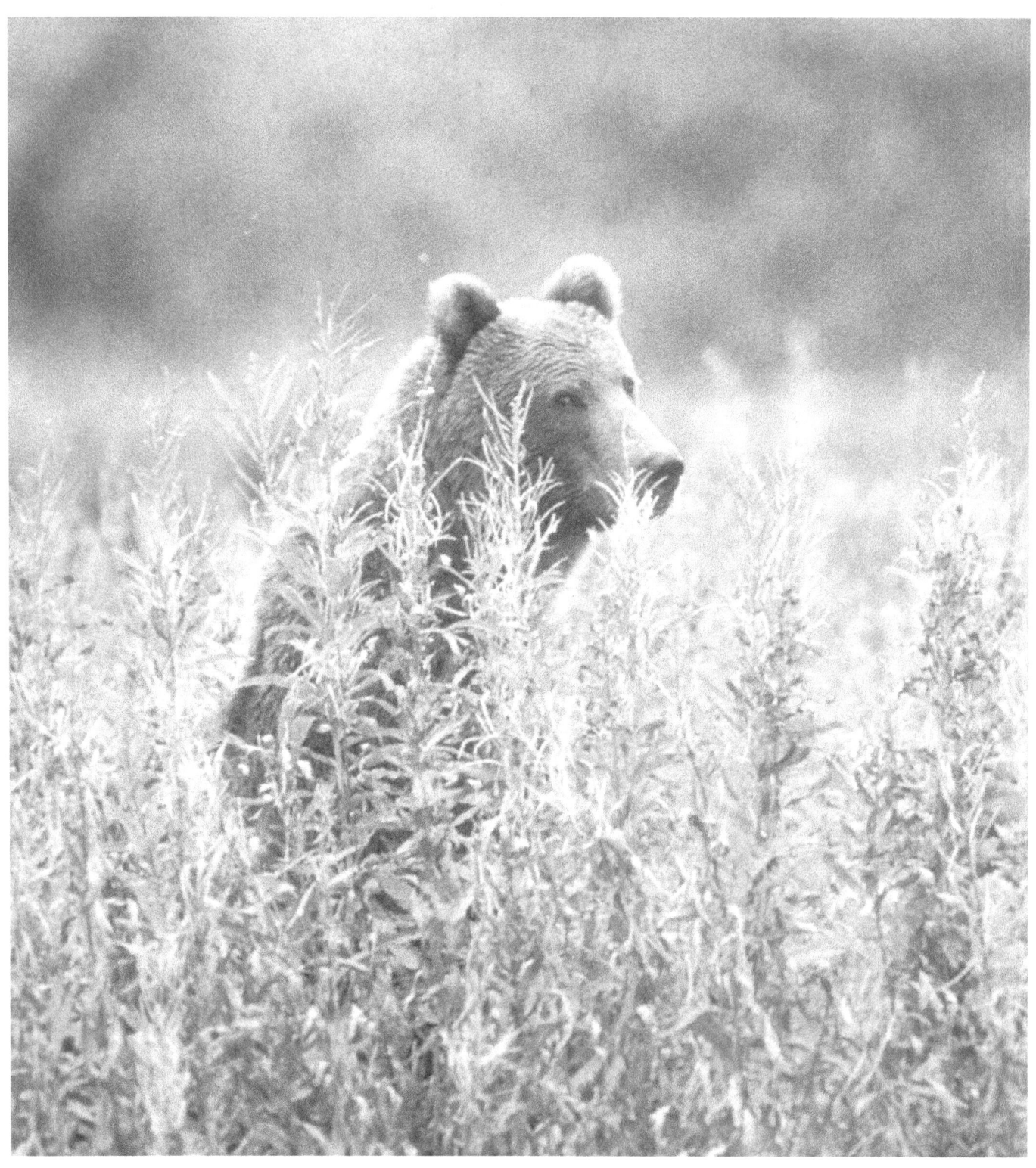

Tall grass provides perfect cover for a curious bear!

INTRODUCTION

Over the years,I have accumulated some information, a bit of knowledge and even a little wisdom about medicinal plants.

Many of the healing herbs in this volume set are relatively unknown; and some are little used in day-to-day clinical practice. Some are well known, but not utilized to their full extent of possibilities.

It is my hope that these pages may lead to a new and expanded materia medica, and a wider appreciation of many, often neglected, overlooked, and useful medicinal plants.

North American herbals tend to repeat, with increasingly useful additions, the same hundred or so plant medicines. The purpose of this book is to expand that awareness and hope that other herbalists will begin to look at the plants in their backyard and explore, observe and experience for themselves.

In turn, we could reconnect and continue the work begun in past centuries by the Eclectics and other plant people.

Like some of my previous publications, this book records indigenous use of medicinal herbs, garnered respectfully from the oral tradition, as well as work by various cultures around the world, the Eclectic physicians, modern herbalists, and recent scientific findings on various plant constituents.

It also includes homeopathic usage, essential oils, hydrosols, gemmotherapy, flower essences, personality traits, spiritual properties and astrological correspondences.

Please contact me if you wish to contribute;I am always learning.

Some Other Books by Robert Dale Rogers - www.amazon.com/author/robertdalerogers

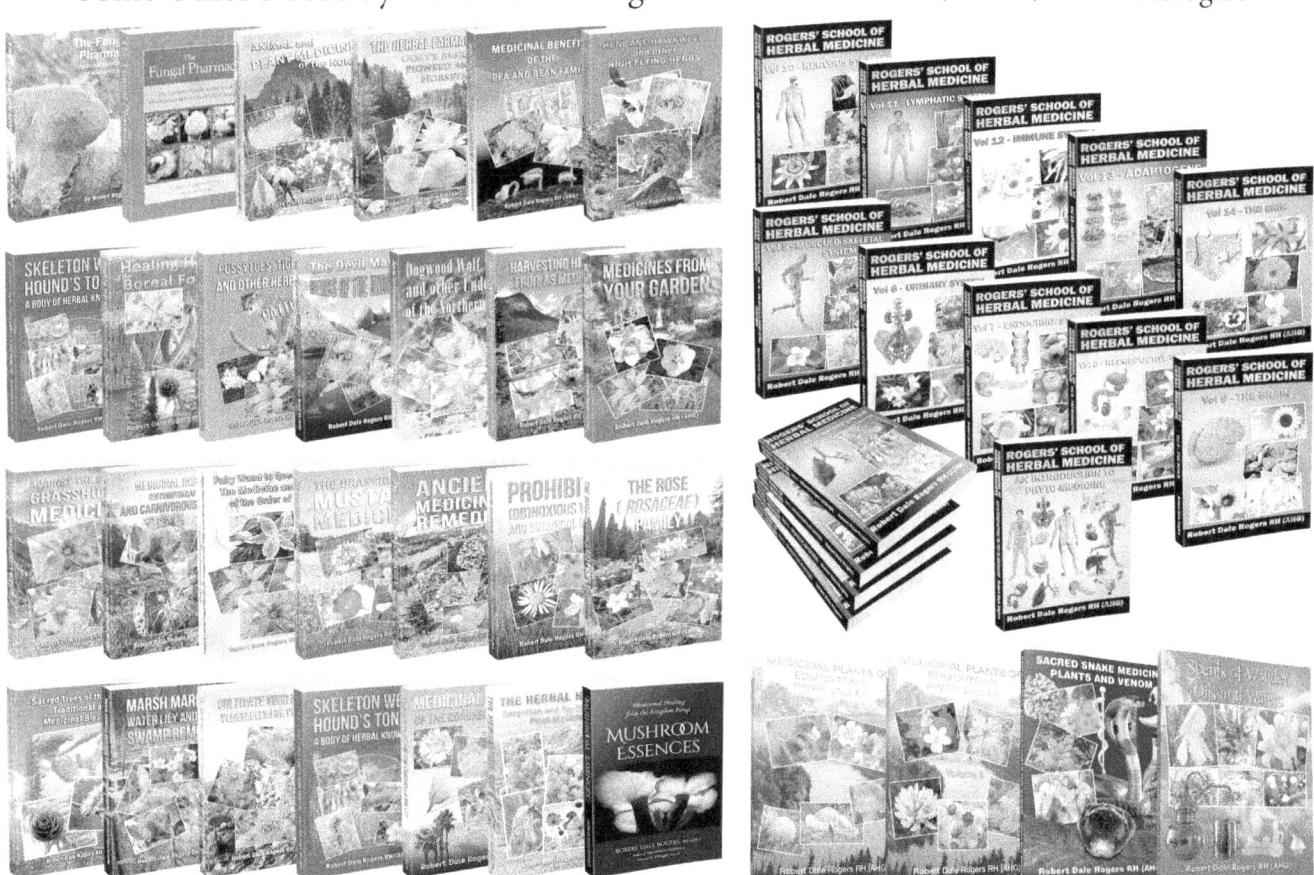

www.selfhealdistributing.com or www.scentsofwonder.ca - email: scents@telusplanet.net - Fax: 1 780-439-9540

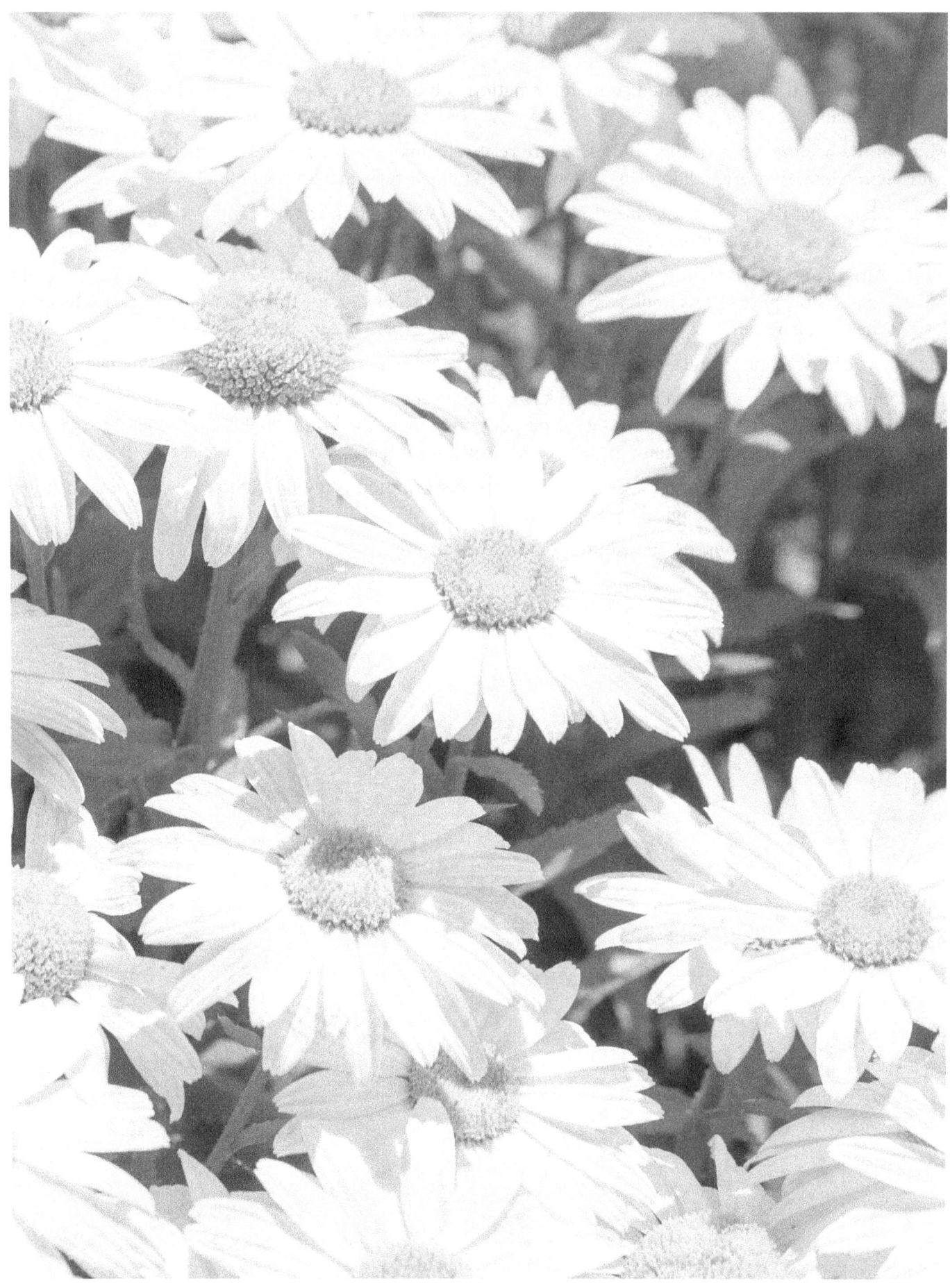

OX-EYE DAISY
MOON FLOWER
(*Chrysanthemum leucanthemum* L.) no longer accepted
(*Leucanthemum vulgare* Lam.)
PARTS USED- flowers, stems and leaves

Ten thousand ox-eyes watch the vroom of traffic. British daisies open skyward, cheerfully gormless, but these bend their gaze to the ground because they are a Balkan subspecies of the vulgar *Leucanthemum* picked for the lycanthrope: white flowers for Olga the Werewolf.
PAUL EVANS

Right up in the Bossy's eyes, looked the daisy boldly, But, alas! To his surprise,
Bossy ate him, coldly.
Listen! daisies in the fields, hide away from Bossy! Daisies make the milk she yields and her coat grow glossy!
So, each day, she tried to find, Daisies nodding sweetly, and, although it's most unkind, bites their heads off neatly!
M. DELAND

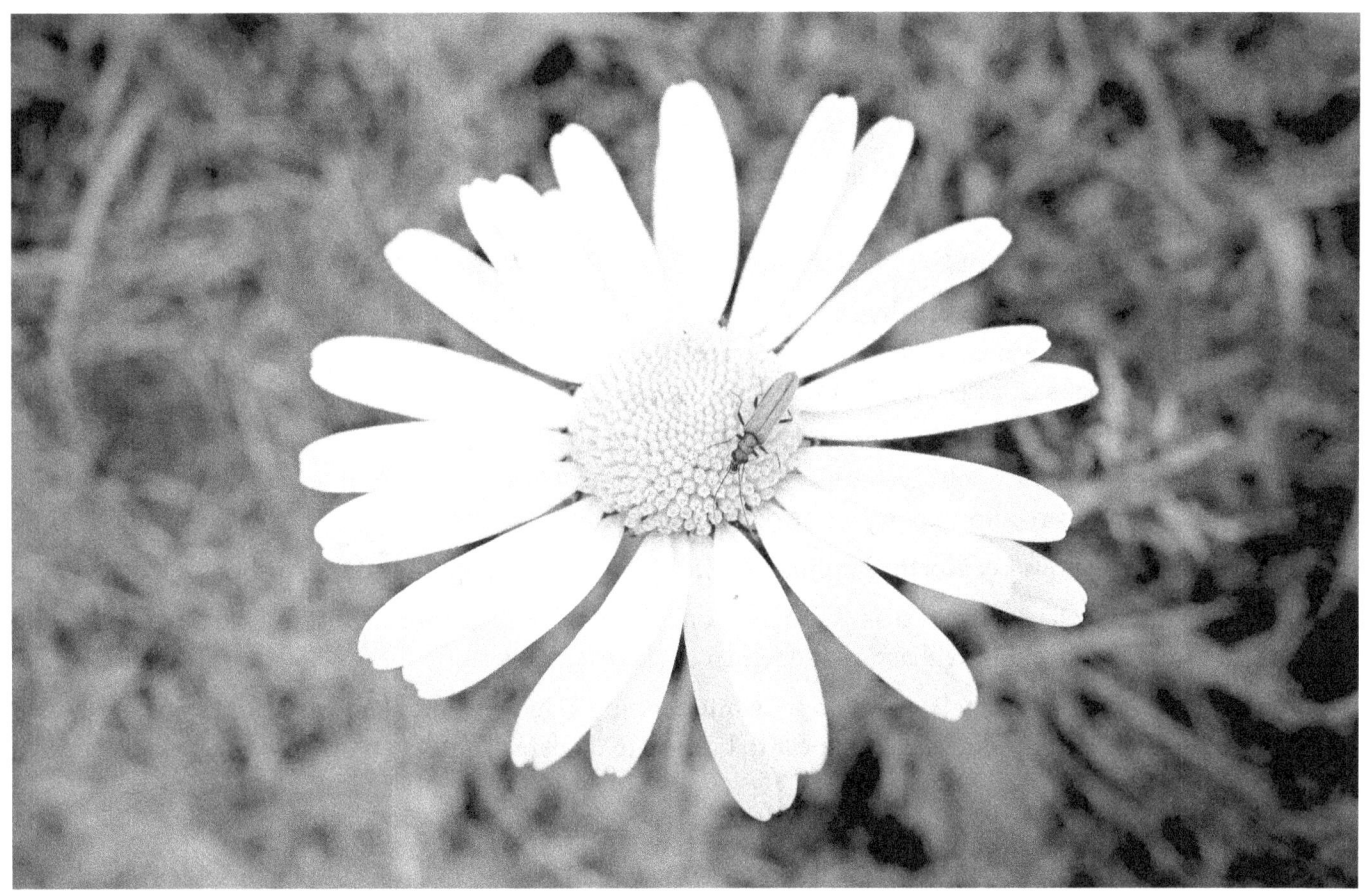

OX EYE DAISY

Daisy is from the English "day's eye" and in turn from the Anglo Saxon ***DAEGES EYE***. The genus is from the Greek ***KHRUSANTHEMON*** meaning golden flower, while leucanthenum means, white flower. Pyrethrum is from the ancient Greek **PYRETHRON**.

The daisy is a familiar and welcome flower in the Prairies. The Daisy is not one flower as each white "petal" is an individual flower. Or more accurately, the 20-30 white "petals" are not individual at all, but composed of 5 false petals fused together. The golden centre or eye is composed of tubular flowers, complete with pistils, stamens and sepals. A magnifying glass helps.

According to Roman myth, the daisy originated when the meadow nymph Belides changed herself into a daisy to avoid the amorous attentions of Vertumnus, the God of the Orchards.

During Greek times, it was considered a plant of the moon, and sacred to the goddess Artemis, due in large part to its therapeutic use with menstruation. Marguerite of Anjou, France, loved the plant and embroidered it on her robes before sailing to England to marry Henry VI. He fought the War of the Roses, and the daisy joined the banners, gaining the name Marquerite. In Spanish, this became Margarita. Marguerite means pearl in French.

Much later, the Catholic Church usurped and dedicated the plant to St. Margaret and Saint Mary Magdalene. The Moon daisy was then called maudlin or maudelyn, in her honour.

In Flanders, it is called Madeliefie or Meizoetje, derived from Maghet lieve, meaning beloved virgin, or Maghet suete, for sweet virgin.

There is much speculation as to which St. Margaret it is. St. Margaret of Antioch is unlikely, as is St. Margaret of Valois. The best guess is St. Margaret of Cortona whose birth date of February 22 used to be considered the first day of spring.

The Old English Herbarium, translated into Anglo-Saxon over a millennium ago, says that ox-eye daisy is "for damage to the body coming from an overabundance of bile. Take the juice of this plant and give it to drink.

It will restore the natural color, and the person will look as though coming from a hot bath".

It means "innocence" in the language of flowers, and is the national flower of Latvia, and state flower of North Carolina.

Ox eye Daisy is the star flower of Gretchen in Goethe's *Faust*: "He love me, he loves me not".

The similar looking Shasta Daisy is a hybrid of Luther Burbank, who crossed ox-eye with a Japanese daisy in 1890. He described the flower as "a plant at once graceful enough to please the eye and hardy enough to grow in any soil…a daisy that surpasses any dreams".

In Scotland, the Oxeye was called the "moon daisy", or "thunder daisy", for it's power against thunderstorms. It was also known as Gool, and goolriders were appointed to remove the "weed" from fields of grain. The farmer with the largest crop was required to pay a fine of a castrated ram.

It was the official state flower of North Carolina until 1941, when "weedophobics" took action to change it.

It is said that whoever picks the first daisy of the season will be possessed with a spirit of flirting; and sleeping with the root under your pillow will assure the return of an absent lover.

Even today, the plucking of petals one by one, while reciting "He loves me, he loves me not", is a popular superstition. Incidentally, the flower may appear to have 20 to 30 petals, but if you look closely you will see five distinct groupings.

The flowers release compounds that attract carrion and dung flies for pollination. This is not obvious at first, but a bouquet of daisies in a closed room will soon remind you of sweet cow pies. Despite this, the fresh flower was spread on floors in medieval Europe to discourage fleas.

Natives including the Mohegans used infusions for spring tonics or fever.

There is no recorded history of Ox Eye Daisy use by the Cree or Blackfoot because it is naturalized from Europe. However, the Northern Cree of Alberta have named daisy as **WAPIKWAN**.

Another Cree name in some regions is **ISKWEW OWEHOWINA**.

Métis in northern Alberta use the leaves and flowers in a tea for soothing the nerves of adults and reducing hyperactivity in children.

The Fox tribe used the plant tea as an antispasmodic, in small doses.

The daisy was long esteemed for medicinal properties. Associated with Artemis, it was considered specific for female ailments. It was also a wound healer; the leaves combined with wax and oils for this purpose.

Linnaeus noted that horses, sheep and goats eat it, but not cows and pigs.

The fresh juice was used for ruptures, and other inflammations. An old remedy for broken ribs was to drink the juice and apply a poultice of the juice mixed with milk and wheat flour. The flowers were prepared as a soothing tea for coughing or wheezing of asthma; or added as a decoction to ale to treat liver ailments like jaundice. Some people use the fresh flowers like dandelion for wine making.

The roots help check the night sweats associated with pulmonary disorders.

The fresh, young leaves and white petals can be added to salads, or thrown into the bath. Lumiere, an upscale Vancouver restaurant, is a regular buyer of the plant for salad mixes.

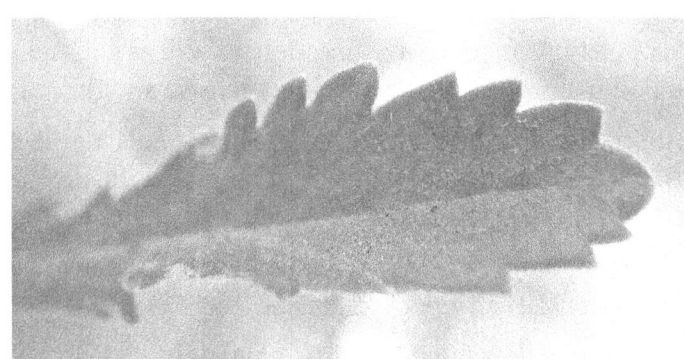

OX EYE DAISY LEAF

Dried, the flowers are a great addition to potpourri mixtures, or burned as incense for lightening the atmosphere.

The flowers repel fleas; the powdered flowers can be sprinkled on pet's fur for this purpose. It is a fairly weak insecticide, but easy to collect. The US Dept of Agriculture has found scabrin effective against armyworms, flies, etc.

The polyacetylenes are phototoxic to mosquito larvae.

The crab spider, colored yellow and white, sets her web in the ox-eye daisy.

When the plant withers by mid summer, she moves to the Black-eyed Susan, which blooms in fall and she changes her colors to deep yellow and brown.

The plant roots, colonized with mycorrhizae, will grow under crude oil exposure, and reduce concentrations in soil. Noori A et al, *Int J Phytoremediation* 2015 June 29.

MEDICINAL

CONSTITUENTS- ox-eye daisy- various polyacetylenes, pyrethrins (scabrin), hydrocyanic acid, inulin, and essential oil containing chrysanthenone and verbenone.
The ligulate flowers contain vitexin, apigenin, umbelliferone, scopoletin and cosmosin; The tubular flowers contain two phenolic carboxylic aicds and seven flavonoids, including chlorogenic acid, caffeic acid, rutin, hyperin, chrysin 7-glucuronide, quercitin, luteolin, isorhamnetin, chrysin, and apiin (3%); as well as platiphylline and senecionine.
Also found are acacetin, scopoletin, 1,7-hexadecadien-10, 12, 14-triyne; 1,8-tridecen-11,13,15-triyne; 4-tridecen-7,9,11-triyn-1-ol; 1,8-hexadecadien-10,12,14-triyn-(6,7)-oxirane; 3,5-tri-decadien-7,9,11-triyn-1-yl-3-methyl-2-butenoate; and trideca-3,5,7,9,11-pentain-1-ol and its acetate.
Also includes cyclitols including meso-inositol, L(-)quercitol and a C-glycosyl flavone, containing cyclitol instead of a sugar.
Leaves- 500 IU vitamin A/100 grams

Oxeye Daisy herb decreases secretions when taken warm or at room temperature. For bronchitis, asthma or whooping cough where mucous membranes are red, inflamed and excessively moist, use warm infusions of the leaves and flowers.

When used as a tonic, it acts similar to Chamomile, calming night sweats and nightmares.

It is related to Feverfew (*C. parthenium*) and possesses some anti-inflammatory properties, but is much milder. It relieves night sweats or secretions, such as vaginal discharges, or runny eyes and nose. These conditions respond to the mildly astringent Oxeye Daisy, by slowing the body's over-reaction to allergens, and reducing excessive secretion of mucous. Seasonal allergies are also relieved, if one does not have allergies to the sunflower family.

In cases of acidic, concentrated urine, it is a reasonable diuretic, helping dilute strong smelling urine. The mild astringent and anti-bacterial compounds help soothe inflamed urinary epithelial tissue.

It is a reasonably effective hemostat, although not in the league of Fleabane or Shepherd's Purse. In regions of the former USSR, it is a household remedy for internal hemorrhages, including uterine and gastrointestinal.

For gastritis, with hyper-secretions of the mouth and stomach, or a gastric ulcer that lingers, and won't fully heal, Daisy comes into good service.

Scopoletin is hypotensive in action, as well as anti-spasmodic, anti-bacterial and anti-fungal; apigenin is anti-inflammatory, antispasmodic, hypotensive and diuretic, and acacetin inhibits histamine release activity.

Apiin, also found in parsley and celery, is a flavonoid with *in vitro*, and *in vivo* antioxidant activity. Li P et al, *Food Function* 2014 5(1):50-6. Apiin is a powerful anti-inflammatory compound. In one study it showed potency seven times lower than indomethacin. Mencherini T et al, *J Pharm Pharmacol* 2007 59)6):891-7.

The compound appears to induce TNF (tumor necrosis factor) suggesting benefit in activating phagocytosis. Kunizane H et al, *Yakugaku Zasshi* 1995 115(9):749-55.

William Cook, a famed Eclectic physician wrote in 1869: "The flower heads of this plant are almost the same qualities as *Anthemis nobilis*. I have not used them extensively, but am satisfied they will make a remedy similar to the chamomile as a tonic and antispasmodic…a warm infusion will secure a full perspiration, with capillary stimulation. As a tonic, it seems best suited for nervous disposition and hysteria."

Work by Sardari et al, at the University of Alberta, and Faculty of Pharmacy, showed anti-fungal activity in 9 of 12 species from *Aspergillus, Candida,* and *Cryptococcus* tested. Full report is available in *Pharmaceutical Biology* 1998 36(2):180-88.

Terry Willard considers Oxeye Daisy a specific for bleeding in the splenic or sigmoid flexure; and an effective douche for cervical ulceration.

As it is anti-fungal and anti-bacterial, Oxeye makes an acceptable douche, as well as a cleansing, disinfecting wash. Use as a hair and beard rinse for scalp and skin fungal infections. Be careful as it can stain clothing!

Fluid extracts of the root possess similar properties.

Oxeye Daisy pollen is one of the eight plant pollens that constitute Cernilton, a previous available herb formulation for treating benign prostatic hypertrophy and prostate cancers.

HOMEOPATHY

Chrysanthemum leucanthemum–Oxeye Daisy has specific action on the sweat producing glands. At the same time, it quiets the nervous system like lady slipper root. Specifically, it alleviates right-sided tearing pain in the bones of the jaw and temple.

Pain in the teeth and gums, made worse by touch and better by heat, is also helped. The patients are irritable and tearful.

Night sweats and overly excited nervous systems also helped.

DOSE- Use mother tincture- 20 drops up to three times daily. The 12th potency may be used for mental and emotional agitation. Boericke.

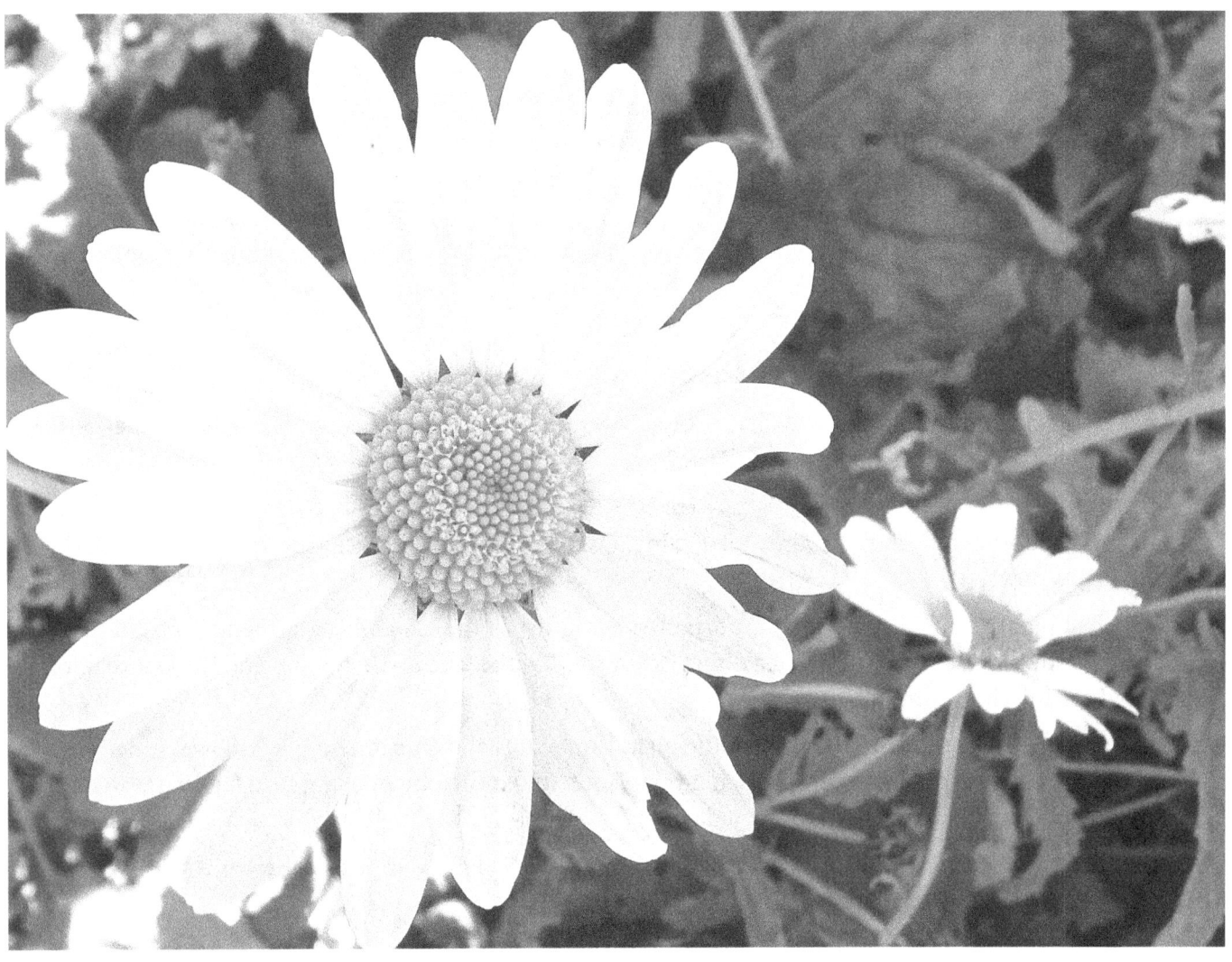

OX EYE DAISY

ESSENTIAL OILS

Ox Eye Daisy yields from 0.4-0.5% of a thin, light yellow oil that unfortunately darkens with age, as well as thickens.

It contains nine components with farnesene (38.3%), alpha bisabolol (15.5%), farnesol (4.2%) and nerolidol 4.9% the most plentiful identified components, as well as chrysanthenone and verbenone.

FLOWER ESSENCES

Oxeye daisy flower essence is the twin, the shadow or the opposite of Bach's White Chestnut. Whereas Bach's remedy was for the " gramophone of the mind", where there is a need to stop the repetitive chatter in the mind; Oxeye is for the individual who has difficulty opening up.

Some of the most difficult transitory states involve an immediate emotional gushing; but a reflective time of thought and contemplation. This flower essence allows one to stay in that mental mantra state; to wrestle with those moralistic and ethical questions where both sides of the question and answer ring true.

PRAIRIE DEVA

Ox-eye daisy flower essence is useful for obtaining the whole perspective; and for being centered. It helps to move out of positions of being over focused and allows us to tune into a larger perspective. Ox-eye Daisy helps us to synthesize the elements of our lives in new and creative ways. **PACIFIC**

Oxeye daisy flower essence helps develop positive attitude; and help dispel negative thoughts; it quiets the mind allowing for better concentration on task at hand. It also increases the ability to feel love; become a better listener; and promotes a feeling of happiness. It repels negative psychic attack; is a good anti-depressant; and controller of quick outbursts of anger, and those easily annoyed. It also is good for coordinating individuals in group activity. **MT. JULIUS**

FLORACHOLOGY®

Daisy has a plant sound melody of C, D, E, F, G, A, B, a Soul Tone of B and auric colour of dark blue.

SPIRITUAL PROPERTIES

Spontaneous aspiration of Nature towards the Divine. Oxeye Daisy is wide open, spontaneous, irrevocable in its spontaneous power. **THE MOTHER**

This universal plant is one of the most important species. It has the capability of opening up the wisdom chakra at the crown of the head, allowing a direct "knowing " of the truth. The colours and the fact that it is so widespread are the clue to this quality.

Often thought of as the "humble" daisy, this little plant is in reality the Queen of the wildflower kingdom. It is to be prized for the gift which it offers to each human soul. Make a tea by pouring near-boiling water on the petals of only one flower. Drink three times a day. **HILARION**

Daisies help accentuate and enhance solitary child-like states. It is a place in which there is a sense of self, but his self is closer to the life-force incarnating motivation.

Primarily it allows an individual a sense of aloneness that is not lonely.

The emotions associated with this state of being are joy, peace, and a greater sense of overall well-being.

The reduction of stiffness occurs not only on the medicinal level. It is vibrational, and when one is troubled in movement and flexibility, a childlike state is of great benefit.

Daisy enhances the ability to ask a question over and over in the mind, like a mantra. The energy in the shoulder areas becomes more relaxed. There is a strengthening of the emotional body, the soul body is stimulated and the TB miasm is eased. Use daisy when Venus and the moon are in conjunction; or when Venus moves into Aries. **GURUDAS**

The effervescent open-armed joy and bliss of the Ox Eye Daisy spirit brings a sense of completion. **ECLARE**

Many times the spirit of the plant comes in some kind of a personification like the Celtic-looking priestess of Eyebright or the playful sprite of Daisy; other times, it is an animal-like creature like the giant pink-purple butterfly of Red Clover. It can also be an energy essence, like the brightly shining star of Borage or the large oval yellowish-white energy field of St. John's Wort, or even an energy pattern like the cross-stitch of cedar. **MONTGOMERY**

PERSONALITY TRAITS

In the end, of course, when a flower cannot co-opt or avoid or out-strategize an enemy, it may have to destroy him.

The armyworm feeds on daisies. The daisy's defense is to produce a chemical mildly toxic in the dark and highly toxic in ultraviolet light. As the worm eats the plant, it absorbs this chemical which eventually moves through its circulation system to the surface of its skin. On a nice spring day, the sun shines warmly. First the armyworm glows florescent blue. Then it shrivels up and turns black.   **RUSSELL**

This remedy [Ox-eye daisy] work(s) constitutionally in women torn between what they feel in their heart and what their head tells them. They dream of romantic, perfect love and complete happiness, which, however, clashes with everyday life. At the same time real closeness is avoided, insofar they have not noted some imperfections already, for fear of falling flat on their face in a relationship or more literally translated, 'to end up with a bloody nose', an allusion to the tendency to epistasis. Cutting the umbilical cord with the parents was difficult. Like other Asteraceae resembling Arnica, Chrysanthemum is a good remedy for hemorrhages, particularly in relation to metrorrhagia since abortion, for dysmenorrheal or for allergy-induced epistaxis. There is a tendency for bruising and wounds to heal slowly.   **MÜLLER**

DOCTRINE OF SIGNATURES

Ox-eye Daisy's solitary nature is a signature of simplicity and individualism. It represents a safe, comfortable feeling of being alone without feeling lonely.

It has characteristic mandala patterns that magnetically attract us to its yellow centre, the colour of which relates to the third and seventh chakra.

The centre is like a golden yellow head with a white halo, giving a feeling of deep relaxation, peace, inner knowing and a deeper spiritual understanding.

The white ray flowers represent purification and cleansing, and with the yellow depressed disk, the flower offers a balance between intuition and intellectualism.

The pronounced saw tooth leaves are like a sharp knife, used externally to treat wounds and bruises.

The leaves and stems are very acrid, suggesting a cleansing of wounds on all levels, such as emotional bitterness, mental and emotional chaos, trying too hard to figure things out, or childhood or inner child wounds.
                                                                                       PALLASDOWNEY

RECIPES

TINCTURE- 20 drops 3X daily. Ox-eye daisy tincture is made from the fresh plant 1:4 at 50% alcohol.

INFUSION- 2-4 ounces three times daily

INSECTICIDE- The freshly dried flower heads can be powdered and sealed in airtight container until use.

Or use the fresh plant tincture and add one tbsp of dish detergent to each cup of water for spraying.

Another method is to take ten grams of powdered flowers to four ounces of denatured alcohol. Shake and let stand for 24 hours. Pour through a coffee filter, and pour into glass spray bottle. Dilute one ounce to one gallon of water.

Spray at dusk for maximum effect, as bright sunlight deactivates the insecticidal activity.

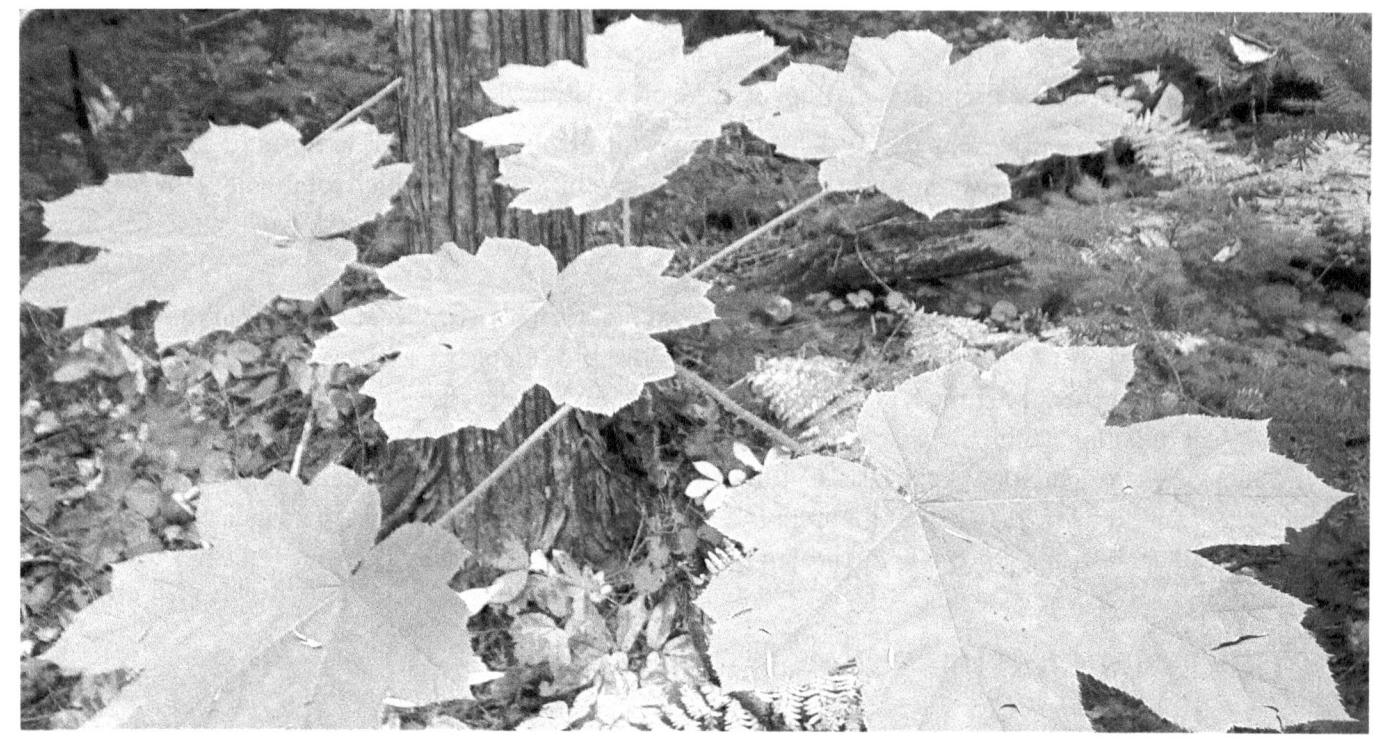

DEVIL'S CLUB

DEVIL'S CLUB
(***Oplopanax horridus*** [Sm.] Miq.)
PARTS USED- inner bark of trailing rhizomes, or recumbent stems.

Devil's Club confronts ill with a perspective of cohesion. It is a strongly adaptogenic herb having a modifying effect on the limbic system. It treats such conditions as schizophrenia… **CRUDEN**

Oplo is from the Greek **HOPLON** or weapon. Panax is from the Greek **PAN** meaning everything and **AKOS** for remedy. Horridum means bristly or wild. Names ending in panax are treated as masculine, thus horridus rather than the more commonly seen horridum, is the correct designation. But then again, is taxonomy a science? Or just another opinion?

Indeed, Devil's Club is an all remedy weapon against many ailments!

It is certain that settlers moving north from Edmonton to the Peace Country encountered this member of the ginseng family on wagon trails through the Swan Hills; where it still grows today. And the encounters would not have been pleasant- with the thorn-covered, sprawling bush tearing human and horse alike. The French-speaking settlers called it Bois Piquant.

The spines are very painful, and will often form *Staphylococcus* eruptions or boils within 36 hours of penetration. The cure is, of course, Devil's Club decoctions internally and externally applied. I can personally testify to their nastiness, suffering from a small needle for over a year that finally settled down to an enclosed scar tissue on side of left palm.

Like wild sarsaparilla, it has many adaptogenic properties related to the Ginseng family.

Both the standing and recumbent stems that have fallen and buried themselves are used for medicine. The actual root should be left for regeneration.

The recumbent stems have no thorns, and thus are easier to harvest, but both contain medicinal properties, almost exclusively in the green under the bark.

Traditionally, indigenous people would cut the recumbent stems into 1-3 feet lengths and bury them near their dwellings, for use when needed.

Coastal people like the Haida used tea infusions for general strength, colds, stomach ulcers, gallstones and constipation. They rubbed the scarlet berries on their head to treat lice, dandruff, and to make their hair gleam.

Pieces of the light wood were attached to fish lures to ensure good fishing, while the stems with their lethal thorns were dangled outside an octopus's den. The stems were placed under beds or above a doorway to protect the household and inhabitants.

The neighboring Aleuts drink the tea for cold and pain relief. They burn the bark to a white ash to apply to cuts. Many tribes made their sweat lodges of devil's club to keep out intruders.

Contemporary Tlingit have observed bears treating their battle wounds by eating Devil's Club! The Dena'ina of Alaska call it **HESHKEGHKA'A**, meaning "big, big prickle". Which it is!

Wet'suwet'en of north-central British Columbia call it Big Thorn or **WHISCO**. It was traditionally used for tuberculosis, colds, flu, and heart disease, often combined with subalpine fir, mountain ash or spruce bark.

The Thompson know the plant as /K'ETYE?. They would drink a tea of small pieces of the recumbent stem as a tonic, blood purifier, and heal ulcers.

Charcoal from the burned stems was mixed with animal or fish fat for blue face painting. The Crow of Montana used the aromatic recumbent root by combining it with tobacco as a smoke to relieve headaches.

Ashes from the leaves were dusted over burns. The heated inner bark was applied directly to injured areas and bandaged in place.

A piece of the recumbent stem was chewed well and applied to troublesome teeth. A teaspoon of root powder in a tablespoon of oil was taken internally as a pain reliever.

The same root powder makes a baby talc, or mild, perfumed deodorant powder. Or the root can be boiled and mashed into a paste; a very effective poultice for reducing swellings caused by insects, boils, or swollen glands.

The Dena'ina of Alaska bake the inner bark until dry and then rub until soft. This is applied to affected area for 3-4 hours before changing to help draw out the infection. One native Alaskan name **CUKILANARPAK** means "large plant with needles."

The root was used in steam baths for arthritis, rheumatism, body pain, stomach problems and as a skin tonic.

And the fresh, inner bark was rubbed on mother's breast to stop the flow of milk. Cree living near Lesser Slave Lake used the root to prevent premature birth, and to re-establish menstrual flow after childbirth.

My old friend and herbal buddy James Green shared his research on traditional use of Devil's Club, rated according to medicinal use.

Arthritis/rheumatism (13 groups); protection and purification (12); general tonic (10); skin- burns, cuts, infections (8); stomach and digestion (8); tuberculosis (8), coughs and colds (8), childbirth and postpartum care (4); diabetes (4); broken bones (3); internal hemorrhage (2); and analgesic (2).

Ryan Drum, who knows Devil's Club as intimately as anyone, cites the contemporary use by coastal people.

Headache relief, hangover cure, internally and externally for *Staphylococcus infections*, to treat and prevent blood poisonings, gallstone remediation, and to cure hyperactive thyroid are some of its modern uses.

Its nickname "Tlingit Aspirin" derives from its analgesic benefit.

An excellent ethnobotanical review is found in HerbalGram #62.

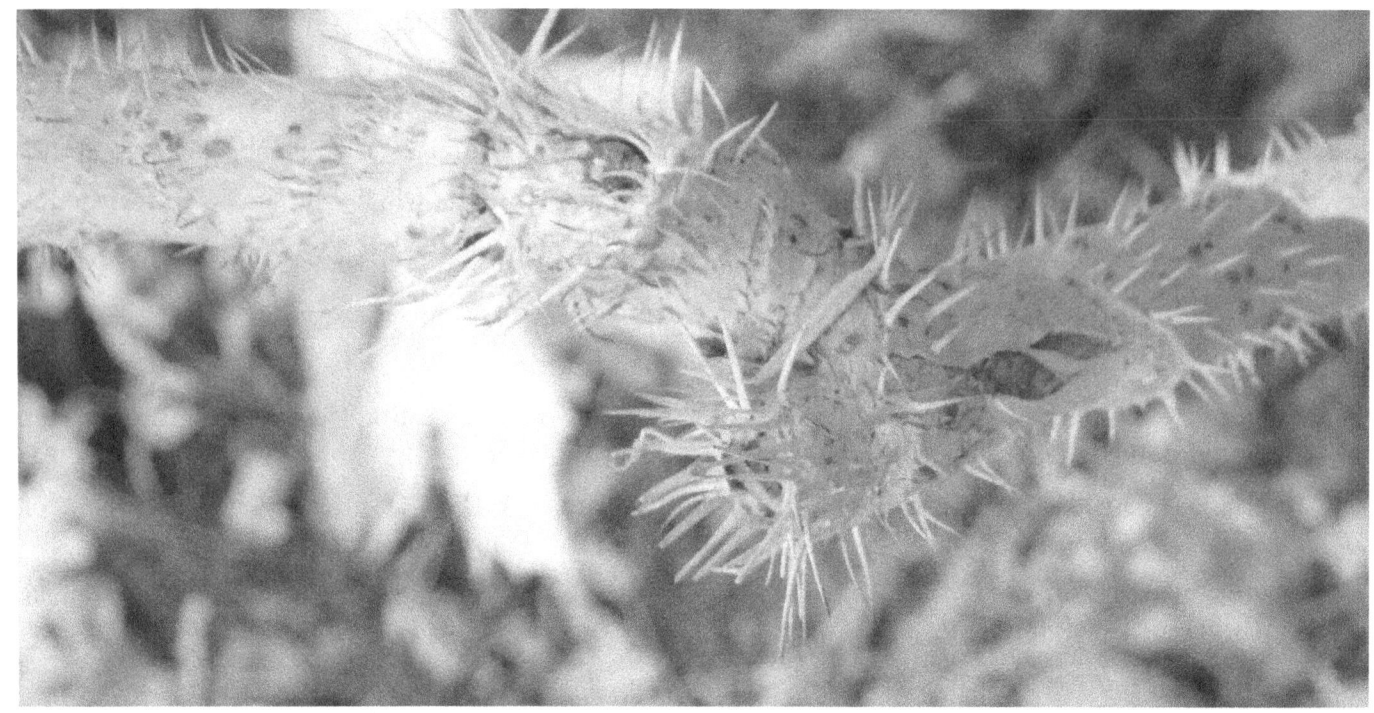

NASTY SPINES ON BRANCHES

MEDICINAL

CONSTITUENTS- fresh inner bark of recumbent stem- araliasides and pananosides, as well as an essential oil containing trans nerolidol, t-cadinol, torreyol, alpha cubebene, spathulenol, dodinene, bulnesol, dodecenol, cadenene, and cedrol; as well as various unsaturated fatty acids, polyynes (falcarinol, falcarindiol, oplopandiol, oplopantriol A, opladiol and oplopandiol acetate), oplopanone, 9,17-octadeca-diene-12,14-diyne-1,11,16-triol, 1-acetate-4, sesamin, neroplomacrol, neroplofurol; saponins, glycerides, stearic acid, stigmasterol, beta sitosterol, six lignan compounds, 1,3 benzodioxole, 5.5' tetrahydro-1H,3H-furo[3,4-c] furan 1,4-diyl) bis and tannins, seven phenylpropanoids including ferulic acid, 3-acetylcaffeic acid, caffeic acid, homovanillyl alcohol 4-O-beta-D-glucopyranoside, 3-hydroxyphenethyl alcohol 4-O-beta-D-glucopyranoside, 3,5-dimethoxycinnamyl alcohol 4-O-beta-4-glycopyranoside and 3-dimethoxycinnamyl alcohol 4-O-D-glucopyranoside; three coumarins scopoletin, esculetin and 3'-angeloyl-4'acetyl-cis-knellactone; 3,10,11-trihydroxy-3,7,11-trimethyl 1,6-dodecadiene, adenosine and adenine. Ether extracts of the root yield equinopanacene, a sesquiterpene, and equinopanacol, a sesquiterpene alcohol. Also present in root are oplopantriol A and B.

Devil's Club is an adaptogen, like its cousin Ginseng. The fresh root improves stamina and fatigue, without over stimulating. It is neutral and moistening in nature.

In order for a plant to be considered adaptogenic it must follow three criteria. It must be innocuous and cause minimal disorders in physiology, it must be non-specific in activity, and must exhibit amphoretic, or normalizing and balancing action. Roseroot, Schisandra berry, American Ginseng, Maral Root and Devil's Club are the most important plants native or hardy to our part of the world exhibiting adaptogenic influence.

The incumbent root bark enhances the Hypothalamus-Pituitary-Adrenal Axis (HPAA) and the central nervous system associated with depression and asthenia.

Devil's Club has been used historically for hypoglycemic effects. It is probably most advantageous to the late onset, over stressed, overweight, diabetic, that would use it on a regular basis. It seems to cut cravings for sugar and help lower elevated blood lipids and sugars. It works similar to cocklebur, but with no known side effects.

Devil's Club extracts may have their greatest role in reducing the serious implications from years of diabetes-kidney and heart diseases, blindness, and gangrene.

It is worth noting that water extracts do not seem to lower blood sugar. Instead, use a tincture for this purpose.

Work by Molokovsky et al, *Premlemy Endokronologii* 1989 35 found the root lowered blood sugar levels in diabetic rats. Early work by Large et al, *Can Med J Assoc* 1938 39 found hypoglycemic activity in rabbits.

A pilot study by Thommasen et al, *Can Fam Physician* 1990 36:62-65 found no significant hypoglycemic effect from water extracts at a very low dosage.

For weight loss, Devil's Club seems to work temporarily, by inducing loss of appetite. If taken continually, it stops working in 3-4 months and weight returns.

This may tie into the idea of Devil's Club having some thyroid influence, and thus its use to treat hyperthyroid conditions.

Certainly, the herb has some as yet not fully understood tonic effect on the pituitary and hypothalamus.

It does work wonders for some women suffering menopausal hot flashes, and postpartum exhaustion in new mothers. Some sources cite a diminishing effect on breast milk, but I have no personal record of this effect.

Cold infusions of the root are best for rheumatoid arthritis, another auto-immune situation, but taken during times of remission.

It is not for the acute stage but again an adaptogen that helps build body reserves of energy. It may be useful in impotence, physical and mental fatigue, various sexual dysfunction, or recuperation after an operation.

It is a respiratory stimulant and useful expectorant that helps thin mucous and remove it from congested lungs.

It possesses strong anti-bacterial action against staph infection- both external washes and internal cold infusions. In large amounts it can be a strong laxative.

Of interest to researchers is a study reported in *Endocrinology* 1955 56 by Graham and Noble showing the dried roots contained a drug that inhibited the effect of pregnant mare's serum on growth of rat's ovaries. Control ovaries enlarged eight times compared to the test sample. No follow up has been done!

There are some reports that, similar to Garden Sage (*Salvia officinalis*), herb infusions act as anti-galactagogue. That is, breast milk will dry up, helping the weaning process.

In 1995 at the University of British Columbia, a research team headed by Alison McCutcheon found inner bark extracts partially inhibited the bovine respiratory syncytial virus. *J Ethnopharm* 49:2.

Activity against Gram positive, Gram negative and Mycobacterium organisms was found, including *M. tuberculosis*, *M. avium* and MRSA, or methicillin-resistant *Staphylococcus aureus*.

Towers et al, at UBC, found one compound active against *S. aureus, B. subtilis, E. coli, Pseudomonas aeruginosa* and *Candida albicans*.

Kobaisey et al, *J Nat Prod* 1997 60 found two new polyynes, as well as three existing and known compounds. Laboratory studies showed significant anti-candida, anti-bacterial and anti-mycobacterium activity, with the ability to kill *Mycobacterium tuberculosis*, and isoniazid-resistant *M. avium*. This would appear to confirm some of the traditional uses of Devil's Club by various native tribes for tuberculosis. The inner bark was found to be the most active part.

Inui et al, *J Nat Prod* 2010 73:4 identified new polyynes that show antagonism to TB cells. Falcarindiol and to a lesser extent, oplopandiol, are the main effective anti-mycobacterial constituents.

Joseph Tai et al, *J Ethnopharm* 108:2 found 70% ethanol extracts active against a number of cancer cell lines including K562, MCF7 and MDA-MB-468.

The extracts, in very low dosage, were synergistic with camptothecin and paclitaxel. The latter drug is synthesized from taxol once derived from various Yew species.

Early work by Wattenberg, *Carcinogenesis* 1991 12:1 found nerolidol, from the root, inhibits large bowel neoplasia.

More recent work found inhibition of ovarian cancer cell lines, including those with cisplatin sensitive resistance. At low concentrations, Devil's Club induced apoptosis and at higher doses killed cancer cells by necrosis. This makes the herb a good adjunct therapy for a very difficult hormonal cancer. Tai et al, *J Ethnopharm* 2009 Oct 13.

Stem extracts at 0.1mg/ml arrest a number of cancer cell lines in S and G2/M phases, with significantly induced expression of cyclin A. Induction of apoptotic cells was 45.2% after 72 hours compared to control of 9.2%. Wang et al, *Fitoterapia* 2009 August 14.

Three colorectal cell lines, one breast cancer cell line (MCF-7), and non-small cell lung cancer cell line showed anti-proliferative activity. The berry extract showed activity against MCF-7 cancer cell lines, as well.

Sun et al, *Phytother Res* 2010 24:8 and *J Ethnopharm* 132:1 reported 70% and 100% ethanol extracts show anti-proliferative activity against human breast and non-small cell lung cancer lines. A more recent study found mice afflicted with acute myeloid leukemia survived longer when given water containing a 70% plant root tincture. McGill CM et al, *Phytotherapy Research* 2014 Feb 20.

The herb induces apoptosis and regulation of cell cycle transition in human colorectal cancer cells. Li et al, *Anticancer Res* 2010 30:2.

A 70% tincture showed efficacy in experimental models of acute myeloid leukemia. McGill CM et al, *Phytother Res* 2014 28(9):1308-14. Oplopantriol A, isolated from the herb, induced apoptosis in both HCT-116 and SW-480 cancer cell lines via several pathways including the tumor necrosis factor related route. Zhang Z et al, *Nutrients* 2014 6(7):2668-80.

The same compound may induce cancer cell death through inducing endoplasmic reticulum stress and BH3 proteins Noxa and Bim. Jin HR et al, *Cell Death Dis* 2014 24:5:e1190.

It may be a useful adjunct in the treatment of pancreatic cancer. When combined with paclitaxel as a 70% tincture it showed synergistic inhibition of pancreatic ductal carcinoma. Cheung SS et al, *Nutr Cancer* 2015 67(6):954-64. Or better yet, why not combine devil's club with natural paclitaxel from hazelnut hulls, stems and leaves?

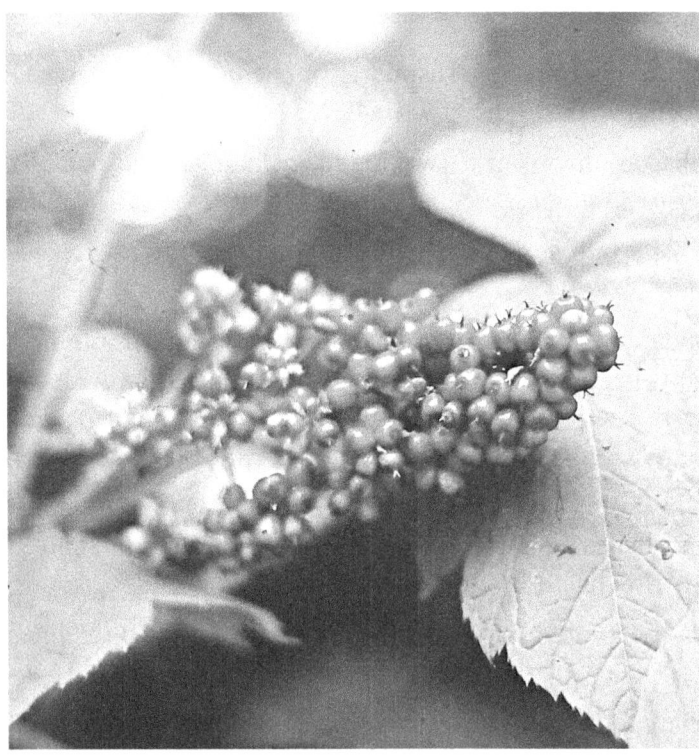

DEVIL'S CLUB BERRIES

Devil's Club has a number of compounds that produce significant synergy and potency from re-combined fractions, increasing by 108% the efficacy against tuberculin organisms. Invi et al, *J Chromatog A* 1151:1-2.

A sesquiterpene, as well as alcohol and ketone derivative, has been isolated from the related *O. japonicus*, and may be present in our own variety. The ketone is used commercially in Japan, to treat coughs and colds.

Oplopanone is anti-pyretic and anti-tussive agent; while the common stigmasterol and beta sitosterol possess anti-rheumatic and anti-cholesterol activity.

Adenosine is important in cellular metabolism and the formation of ATP and ADP. It possesses insulinic effects, stimulates respiration and is a vasodilator, with cardiac tonic effect. Adenine is a purine that helps form DNA, RNA, vitamins and coenzymes. It is anti-viral, vasodilator, and stimulates the central nervous system.

HOMEOPATHY

Devil's Club increases confidence, a calm mind, well-being and relaxation.

Delusions include weightlessness, being a fish or having fish eyes or being from a different world.

There is a desire for asparagus, raw mushrooms, garlic, honey, coffee and sweets. Sexual drive is increased in menopausal and post-menopausal women. Delusion of belonging to the opposite sex.

DOSE- 30C. Proving was done by Lucy De Pieri in Canada with nine provers in 2007.

ESSENTIAL OIL

The stem and roots contain 54.5% (E)-nerolidol. Garneau et al, *Flav & Frag* 2006 20:5.

Nerolidol inhibits large intestine carcinogenesis, reduces ulcer activity, inhibits *Microsporum gypseum*, is an anti-feedant to gypsy moths, and as a trans-dermal agent appears to increase permeability. It is one of the important pheromones that female mites use to attract males for mating. The leaves contain 34% 2-methyl-6-p-methylbenzene-2-heptene and 8% phytol along with 45 other peaks. Li M et al, *Zhongguo Xian Dai Zhong Yao* 2009 11.

Recent work found 48 volatiles in root bark, including 52.5% S, E-nerolidol, 21.6% gamma-cadinol, and 3.6% S-falcarinol. Shao L et al, *Molecules* 2014 19(12): 19708-17.

FLOWER ESSENCES

The green petals yield a flower essence that is powerful and gentle. It is for those on vision quests; or individuals who have difficulty with issues of personal protection.

It is different than yarrow- in that it is not a psychic shield, but rather a warrior's spear.

The two are complementary and may be used well in combination.

Devil's Club flower essence is most useful for those in puberty; when the desire to strike out and rebel is often strongest.

At this stage in spiritual development there may be carelessness in the manner of recognizing and respecting those who possess "true power".   **PRAIRIE DEVA**

Devil's Club flower essence clears ambivalence about being present on the earth; helps one express one's truth firmly and clearly from the heart.   **ALASKA (RESEARCH)**

Devil's Club essence lifts the weight of the world off of your shoulders and comforts your weary soul. It is often used by social workers, medical professionals, caregivers and healers.   **TREE FROG**

Devil's Club helps both women and men to connect with their feminine energies through experiencing deep interconnection with all life. Enhances deep communication. Can be used for life's moments which require profound interaction, for potentially volatile situations such as extreme anger or impasse, or to heal devastation.
NETTLES AND MORE

SPIRITUAL PROPERTIES

According to legend, use of this plant began with a shaman observing bears wallowing the roots to heal their wounds. There are many folk tales that record how the fleeting hero, threw behind him some prickly object, which by magic, changed into a clump of devil's club. The enemy became entangled and destroyed by the vicious thorns.

To this day, it is placed above doorways, and in fishing boats to ward off evil. Shamans often wear a necklace of the root laced with spruce.

In native cultures, health consists of two aspects- the physical (or medicinal preparation); and the spiritual (or supernatural practice of shaman).

These two are often combined in practice and certainly where the use of Devil's Club is concerned.

The "sharp" quality of Devil's Club seems associated with its ability to provide immunity against witchcraft and evil spirits; and to bring luck and power to the user. Other prickly plants like wild rose, thistle share this role.

It is not the prickles or spines that give protection, but some innate quality in the infusion or decoction of the plant. Internal and external cleansing is important in the native quest for spiritual guardian power; and ultimately, for some, shamanic power. **PRAIRIE DEVA**

A lovely structural feature of Devil's Club is the growth of small buds from recumbent stems; these small buds grow vertically from the horizontal stems; they grow both outward and inward from the thick bark, producing exquisite tillite totally enspined shoots outside the bark; and within, the base of the shoot grows up to ten long horizontal woody fingers which clasp the recumbent stem as if two hands in prayer.

As the sprout ages and becomes a large stem, the subtending supine stem changes morphologically from a stem to a root, looses its spine sheath, and grows root on the earth side and slowly disappears as duff covers it. The long woody fingers grow into and fuse with the wood of the recumbent stem.

These sprout bases are sometimes found when stripping the bark and make beautiful reminders of Devil's Club's special powers. **RYAN DRUM**

Two of the most widespread spiritual uses are bathing with devil's club inner bark solution for personal protection and purification, and its use, particularly the spiny or de-spined aerial stems, as an amulet for protection against a variety of external influences. **LANTZ**

Devil's Club has the quality of being a chameleon. It is useful to pair it with another herb because it will enhance and augment the quality of any particular vibratory rate, colour or quality. In itself it is neither one nor another, but an enhancer of all.

Protection is what you see when you look at it on the outside but from the inside what you see is augmentation or enhancement as it functions as a magnifying glass. **EVELYN MULDERS**

The positive aspect of the warrior archetype enables us to stand for ourselves effectively, appropriately and even fiercely, whether the demons we face are within or without.

In working with Oplopanax I have come to understand its more specific use as an adaptogen, particularly with reference to its "warrior energy". Here is a plant who has softness and gentleness in the leaves, yet protects its gentleness well with its fierce spines. It is a good teacher for those too gentle souls who need to be a bit fiercer and stand their ground. **DEB FRANCES**

As a protective warrior herb, Oplopanax is well indicated for those weak, overly nice, timid souls who are easily overpowered in the face of adversity, or for those folks who express a desire to reclaim their power but cannot seem to do so, either from fear or the toxic overlay of family or cultural taboo. **DEBORAH FRANCES ND**

Dullness was a common sensation that the provers experienced, so it is not surprising that there was a need for stimulants. Provers had craving for beer and coffee even if they didn't usually drink coffee, or had aversion for coffee prior to the proving. **LUCY DE PIERI**

MYTHS AND LEGENDS

A man who had lost all his possessions gambling placed devil's club sticks all around him in a circle and ate the skin of each in turn, until they were all finished. Then he put the sticks under his head. Where he had defecated, there was lots of *Moneses uniflora*, all of which he ate. He then became sick and lost consciousness, but when he awakened, after eating still more of this plant, he got a powerful song and found a copper salmon and was able to regain his wealth.

SWANTON

A clean and pure prince, who was a great hunter, was able to get no game. After traveling all over his territory, he came to his hunting camp, tired and discouraged, and went to bed without eating.

While he was sleeping he had a vision of a beautiful woman. She showed him how to be successful, describing and demonstrating a common ritual of **SISATXW** which involves four nights of sex with one clean and industrious woman, one night in each corner of the house, followed by four nights of abstinence, accompanied by bathing in devil's club liquid and drinking the tea. This is to be followed by intercourse with the same woman and then again by bathing in devil's club. The woman then revealed that she was devil's club, and it is her bark that he was to use. The prince then proceeded to do as instructed in his vision, and in consequence he was so successful "it seemed as if the game ran towards him".

LESLIE JOHNSON

A supernatural wood-being, or "fairy" called **SKIL** in Haida…These names go back to one of his ancestors, who travelling far away from his village, came across a gigantic devil's club (*Oplopanax horridum*), which was like a tree, with leaves more than a metre across. The ancestor scraped off the bark and chewed the inner bark of this giant **TS'IIHLANJAAW** plant, then fell into a kind of trance. At this time a wood-being came to him and endowed him with exceptional spiritual powers. To this day, descendants of this man have inherited names that commemorate this special encounter.

TURNER

BOTANICA POETICA

Devil's Club to cleanse the blood
It's a bonus to the health
Rejuvenate and stimulate
Endurance you will have in wealth
In a case of Rheumatoid
Arthritic joints that are aflame
A cold poultice you'd apply
Inflammation you will tame
Oplopanax Horridum
For diabetes might have a role
The Native folk recommend it
Your sugar cravings to control
It's a very striking plant
Mucous it can stimulate
In the family of Ginseng
It can help expectorate
Devil's Club, a worthy tonic
Use the root bark for your tea
Adapt to life's ups and downs
Cope with stress more easily.

SYLVIA CHATROUX

RECIPES

COLD INFUSION- Take one heaping tbsp of bark or stems or root to one pint of water. Soak overnight and in morning gently warm. 1-3 ounces up to 3x daily. This is best for respiratory as the volatile oils are retained.

DECOCTION- 4-8 ounces 3x daily.

TINCTURE- 15-30 drops 3x daily. Begin with small doses and increase slowly.

Upright and recumbent stems for diabetes should be 25% alcohol; whereas 40% is better for the anti-microbial and anti-fungal activity. When available, a fresh root (decumbent stem) tincture at 1:2 and 60% alcohol is very good. The dried root and root bark is prepared at 1:5; at 25% for diabetic therapy; at 40% for infections.

CAUTION- Do not use in pregnancy.

Add a few drops of tincture to Five Flower Formula or Rescue remedy.

GATHERING THE BARK- Gather the recumbent stems after the leaves are yellowed. It is best gathered in fall, when the sterols and glycosides are most plentiful. Terry Willard prefers the spring bark tincture for adult onset diabetes. The spiny stem is also good, although less resinous than recumbent underground stem. Wear thick padded canvas jacket and protective gloves- hip waders are good!

The plant grows out from the centre, the overweighed stems falling and re-rooting. Gather from the older, central plants, and lay the stock in recovered pits to re-root. Wash the roots, and remove the outer bark. Dry carefully, at 70-80 degrees Fahrenheit, for 96 hours, or make a fresh tincture before mold sets in.

Ryan Drum notes that during the drying process, active constituents pass transdermally into those nearby. He notes contraindications for those individuals susceptible to drug flashbacks and PTS syndrome.

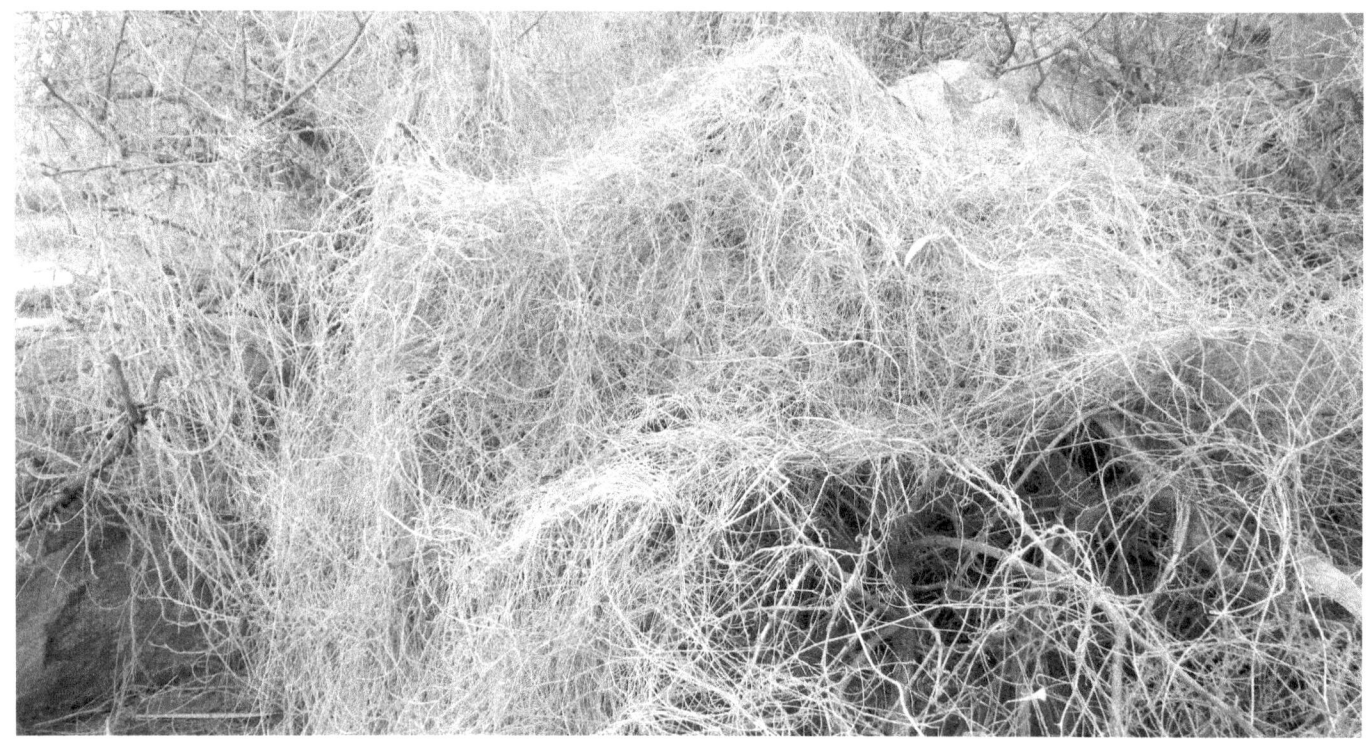

DODDER

DODDER
SCALDWEED
(***Cuscuta gronovii*** Willd. ex Schult)
BIG FRUIT DODDER
(***C. umbrosa*** Beyr. ex Hook.)
ALFALFA DODDER
(***C. epithymum*** [L.] L.)
PART USED- whole plant, seed

The liver and the spleen most faithfully
Of all oppressions she does ease and free.
Where has so small a plant such strength and store of virtues...?   **A. COWLEY**

The vine that keeps on winding and winding up the old post of a fence

Like the one that turned the curling stem and grew the flower the thing the mind knew once on the edge of the wild the vines entangled where those twisting tendrils joint the earth to the sky.   **REAUME**

It is Kushut: no root, no leaves, no fruit, no breeze, no shade. Unknown Arabian poet

Cuscuta is from the Arabic **KUSHKUT** meaning to dodder or bend. Or it may be from the Greek **KASSUO** meaning "to sew together".

Dodder is derived from the Frisian **DODD**, a bunch; and the Dutch **DOT**, raveled thread. Dodder is the plural of dodd, a bunch-dot or a hampered thread.

Dodder may come from the Old English, **DADIREN** to tremble, or more obscurely from the German **DOTTER** meaning "yolk of an egg", in reference to the yellow colour of the flower cluster.

From the dictionary dodder means to tremble or quiver from weakness or old age- as in doddering old fool! Doddered, the adjective, originally meant deprived of branches. Gronovii is named in honor of Jan F. Gronov, an 18th century Dutch botanist and teacher of Linnaeus. Epithymum means, upon Thymus.

Dodder is a parasitic, twining plant often seen growing on barbwire fences without any seeming root system. In fact, it has no real leaves, no chlorophyll, and difficult to spot. Worldwide there are nearly 200 species in the morning glory family. Costea M et al, *Botany* 2015 40:269-285. They propose new phylogenetic classification into four sub-genera and 18 sections. Only a taxonomist would care.

In early life, it has roots; but only until it finds a suitable host. It then attaches sucker-like "haustoria" and lives off the plants juices, the roots wither, their leaves reduce to scales, flowers and seeds form, and the cycle repeats.

The thread-like stems form large claustrophobic mats of waxy, glistening, yellow-orange "guts" that stifle, dehydrate and eventually kill their host. Artemisia, nettle and clover are amongst its local favorites. There are ten species indigenous to Canada, each dependant upon a specific host. *Cuscuta arvensis* is common to clover, *C. epithymum* to alfalfa, and *C. epilinum* to fields of flax.

Cuscuta reflexa, from the Indian subcontinent, and *C. chinensis* (*C. japonica*) are the most well-studied species.

When joined with alfalfa, the tiny flowers have a remarkably sweet perfume that is most pronounced towards evening.

Joined is not quite right, as the parasitic dodder produces haustoria that insert themselves into the host's vascular system to start drinking.

"It's probably one of the creepiest plants I know," says Dr. Colin Purrington, of Swarthmore College. "It's a horrible existence for the host plant. If plants could scream, they'd have the loudest screams when they have dodder attached.

Scent helps the dodder find its victim, for without deriving sustenance from a neighboring plant within six weeks, it would not survive.

Dr. De Moraes, *Science* 2006 Sept 29 looked at how dodder takes advantage of volatiles to target prey. Rick Karban, a University of California, Davis insect ecologist comments. "The significance of this study to me is that it indicates that without a central nervous system, plants are capable of behaving in ways that appear fairly sophisticated."

They twine counterclockwise, similar to Bindweed and opposite to most plants.

Susan Dudley and team at McMaster University found that plants have a secret social life.

They time-lapsed dodder sprouts and found them moving in a circular fashion, similar to a dog sniffing around a dinner buffet. This sense of smell led them to move towards their preferred victim.

A dodder sprout can lie on damp earth for four or five weeks waiting for something to turn up.

Michael Moore suggests that from a passing car "one might think Dodder to be some exotic recording tape tossed from a thoughtless, passing car."

Vermeulen is a bit more poetic, and suggests they resemble "spaghetti with a light coating of orange tomato sauce."

It symbolizes baseness and is ruled by Saturn. Helvetius, in his Doctrine of Signatures, placed dodder as ruling the intestine.

Dioscorides, in the 1st century AD, suggested dodder be combined with honey and salt to purge black bile, and lift melancholy.

In Persian traditional medicine, clover dodder was cathartic for melancholy and phlegm.

Avicenna (980-1037) wrote. "it fortifies the stomach, especially if boiled. If drank with vinegar, it eases the hiccup. Its fresh juice, or if ground and added to any kind of drink, fortifies the weak stomach, cleans the fetus abdomen from the dirtiness by cleaning the veins. It eases the urine, the menstruation, colic and decreases the hemorrhage. If boiled, it restrains the stomach and holds the discharge of the uterus."

Ibn-Masah added. "Cuscuta is good for the stomach specially if conserved adding to it seeds of anise, celery or fennel."

Culpepper tells us: "for it draws nourishment from what it grows upon, as well as from the earth where its root is, and thus you can see old Saturn is wise enough to have two strings to his bow.

This is accounted the most effectual for melancholy diseases, and the purge black or burnt colour, which is the cause of many diseases of the head and brains. as also for the trembling of the heart, faintings and swoonings. It is helpful in all diseases and grieves of the spleen."

Confusion over its energetics is due to the character of its host. Fuchs (1542:349) wrote the powers depend upon the "character of the parent (host): if it invades a warm plant, it strengthens its heating nature, and if it clings to a cold one, it will acquire the cold strength."

One magical use is to pick dodder and throw it over the shoulder. Return the next day; and if the dodder has attached itself to the plant again, the person loves you, if not- better luck next time. Thus it's alternate name, Love-Vine.

Guernsey farmers named it **HERBE D'EMEUTE** and so named for its powerful properties in the treatment of horned cattle. A handful of the fresh plant was placed on a cabbage leaf, rolled up and given to the cow to eat.

In parts of eastern England, it was known as Hairweed, and added to nettle tea in the fens of East Anglia for children with signs of scurvy between their fingers.

The string is used like twine in knot magic, and in the Bahamas the vine is tied around the waist to relieve backache.

Several native tribes used dodder. The Navaho used it as a ceremonial emetic; while the Paiute used "woman without children". California indigenous healers used Dodder as a hemostat, chewing the stem juice or sniffing the dry, powdered plant for nosebleeds.

The Pawnee used *C. gronovii* to determine the seriousness of a suitor. After plucking the vine, with thoughts of a specific young man in mind, she tosses it into weeds of host species. The second day after she returned to see if it had attached, and if so, she felt secure in the sincerity and faithfulness of her suitor.

The Cherokee poultice the roots of *C. gronovii* to treat bruises, and as part of a skin protection formula for cuts and bruises.

The Mayans called it ***X-KAN-LE-CAY***, meaing a little yellow fish snare, for its net-like appearance. Decoctions in a bath were used for tuberculosis or lice infestations; while infusions were given internally for fever, jaundice or biliousness. The use of the yellow threads for diseases of the liver, is yet another example of the doctrine of signatures.

Yerba sin raiz, or herb without root, is decocted and drank at Santa Domingo Pueblo to reduce the swelling from spider, and other insect bites.

In Chile, dodder is used as a love potion, and in the treatment of inflammatory tumours and for abortion.

It is often used in long-term tonic formulas to strengthen the uro-genital system.

The Chinese call it ***TU SI ZI*** or Bunny's Seed. It is so named due to the discovery of dodder's medicinal values, by watching a rabbit with an injured spine seek out the dodder seeds. The use of *C. chinensis* was first recorded in *Shen Nong Ben Cao Jing* about two millennium ago, especially indicated for kidney and liver deficiency.

The flavour is acrid and sweet, with neutral properties, useful in blurred vision, and liver/kidney insufficiency.

In Japanese Kampo medicine, dodder seed is known as **TOSHISHI**, and is sometimes pressed into a food bar.

It has a special effect on hair, and is used to treat premature graying of the hair in both men and women.

Dodder (*C. reflexa*) is employed in Ayurvedic medicine for difficulty in urinating, jaundice, muscle pain and coughs. It is known as Amarvalli or Amarvela.

It would be fair to say that farmers place dodder on the top ten list of noxious weeds.

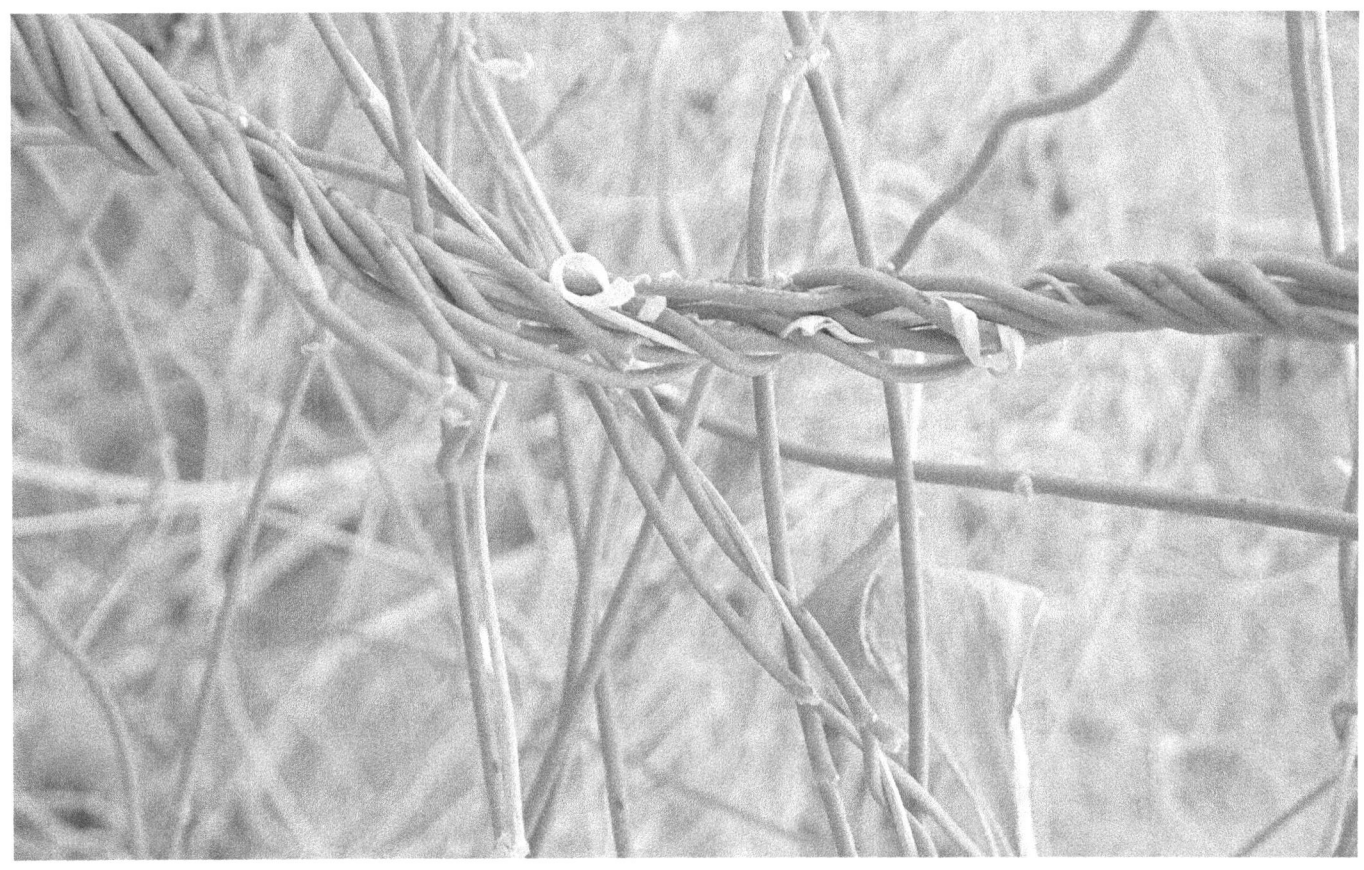

TWISTED DODDER VINES

MEDICINAL

CONSTITUENTS-whole plant- various species- bergegin (cuscutin), a resinous glycoside is considered the active ingredient. Cusculatin, a lactone, mannitol, and beta-sitosterol have also been isolated. A new tryptophan derivative alkaloid, cuscutamine has recently been isolated. Flavonoids such as kaempferol, quercitin and its 3-glycoside; as well as substituted p-hydroxycinnamic acids. They also contain purgative principles similar to bindweed. The yellow colour is due to yellow and orange carotenoids. Work by Loffler et al, *Biochem System Ecol* 1997(25):297-303 found all species of Cuscuta contain similar phenolics, including chlorogenic acid, 3,5-dicaffeoylquinic acid, 4,5-dicaffeoylquinic acid, hyperoside, quercitin, astragalin, kaempferol-3-O-galactoside and querctin-3-O-glycoside in various quantities.

C. reflexa aerial parts contain 5,6,7-trimethoxy-coumarin, swanalin and cis-swanalin.

Stem- cuscutin, cuscutalin, beta sitosterol, luteolin, berginin and kaempferol; as well as scoparone, p-coumaric acid, stigmasta-3,5-diene and 1-O-p-hydroxycinnamoylglucose.

seed- various flavonoids including quercitin, quercitin-3-0-galactoside, quercitin-3-0-apiosyl-(1»2)galactoside, quercitin-3-0-beta-galactosyl-7-0-beta-glucoside, kaempferol, astragalin, and hyperin; lignans cuscutosides A&B, pinoresinol, epipinoresiol, and pinoresinol 4-0-glucoside; cuscutamine (tryptophan alkaloid); amarbelin, arbutin, chlorogenic acid, caffeic acid and p-coumaric acid; as well as newly discovered acylated tri-saccharides.

C. chinensis- aerial and seed- flavonoids (3%) including kaempferol, quercitin, hyperoside, astragalin and lignans; phenolics including above and high content of kaempferol-3-O-glucoside; cuscutamine (tryptophan derivative alkaloid), cuscutosides A-D, pinoresinol, arbutin, beta sitosterol, d-sesamin, 9(R)-hydroxy-d-sesamin, D-pinoresinol, daucosterol.

Dodder is a good laxative-cathartic, and in small doses aids spleen inflammation, swollen lymph nodes and liver distress. For these purposes, it combines well with cleavers, another great climber. The plants are bitter and acidic

The threads may be gathered fresh and decocted with ginger for urinary complaints, kidney, spleen and liver, including jaundice.

Fresh juice from two related Brazilian dodders are used for throat hoarseness and spitting of blood.

Alfalfa dodder is one with which I am most familiar. Extracts of *C. epithymum* significantly reduce viability of cervical HeLa, colorectal HT29 and breast MDA-MB-468 cancer cell lines. Jafarian A et al, *Res Pharm Sci* 2014 9(2):115-22.

The Chinese use dodder seeds (*C. japonica*) for treating impotence, bedwetting due to kidney weakness, premature ejaculation, spermatorrhea, inflamed prostate and nerve pain. It is a nutrient to bone, sinew and cartilage.

The seed is used for both male and female infertility.

It is known as **TU SI ZI**, and used with either yin or yang tonic herbs depending upon the specifics. The name means either rabbit string seed or hare silk seed.

Cuscuta seed helps consolidate the Essence (Yin Jing) and thus slows down aging and prevents loss of body fluids.

A recent study found *C. japonica* extracts enhance hippocampal neurogenesis in mice, by stimulating neuronal cell proliferation, differentiation and maturation. Moon M et al, *Behav Brain Res* 2016 311:173-82.

A triple blind, randomized controlled trial found *C. planiflora* herb capsules, with conventional drugs, decreased depression in 43 patients.

Scores on the Beck Depression Inventory and Hamilton Depression Inventory showed better results than conventional drug alone. Firoozabadi A et al, *J Evid Based Complement Altern Med* 2015 20(2): 94-7.

In Iraq, dodder seed extract has been used to treat acne and dandruff; while the whole plant reduces inflammation, depresses the CNS, and has an anti-tumour effect. This may be due to the interferon inducing and antioxidant properties of the seed.

In Ayurvedic medicine, dodder is called *akasbel* (sky twiner), and used in several ways. Cold infusions of the seed are used for stomachaches and pains. Poultices are applied locally. The stem is decocted for constipation, flatulence, and bilious affections. Externally, the tea is used against itch and skin diseases.

Field Dodder (*C. campestris*) seed and whey may be useful for moderate to severe atopic dermatitis in adults. A randomized, DB, PC trial of 42 patients over 30 days found the formula helped skin barrier reconstruction and accelerated skin healing. Mehrbani M et al, *J Ethnopharm* 2015 172:325-32.

Oral doses of water extracts to rat, gave 70% inhibition of inflammation, possible due to sterol activity. Recent studies suggest it may be beneficial for treating sore knees and kidney problems. Niazi SG et al, *Pharm Biol* 2017 55(1):792-798.

Ethanol extracts given to mice with burn injury, increased serum hemolysin levels and the phagocytosis of peritoneal macrophages, indicative of immune stimulating effect.

Work by Yen et al, *Food Chem Tox* 2008 Jan 20 suggests that ethanol extracts are five times more potent than water extracts for antioxidant and liver protection against acetaminophen toxicity.

Herb decoctions of 5g/kg to rats also delayed the formation of cataracts due to galactose; indicating the elevated aldose reductase activity in galactose induced cataract lens was suppressed.

Cuscuta reflexa alcohol and water extracts show significant reduction in blood glucose in diabetic rats, similar to metformin. Repair of beta cells was also observed. Rath D et al, *J Ethnopharm* 2016 193:442-9.

A compound from this species showed anti-proliferative activity on HCT116 colorectal cancer cell lines. Riaz M et al, *Nat Prod Res* 2017 31(5):583-7.

Today, the dodder is being investigated for modern virus research. The plant serves as a "virus bridge" for immune research. Water extracts of *C. reflexa* have been shown to contain several flavonones, aromadendrin, and taxifolin, with anti-HIV activity. Mahmood et al, *Antiviral Chemistry and Chemotherapy* 1997 8:1.

Dodder has been shown in Traditional Chinese Medicine, to improve both immune response and the manner in which blood sugar is used in the body.

Further research is needed, as the plant shows useful hypotensive properties.

Work by Pai et al, *Fitoterapia* 77:7-8 showed broad-spectrum anti-microbial activity.

Kim et al, *Biol Pharm Bull* 30:8 found cuscuta seed may prevent fibrogenesis after liver injury.

The seed has a sweet taste, and warm property that acts on the liver, kidney and spleen meridians.

It has been used to prevent abortion, as well as kidney and bladder weakness such as frequent urination, or dripping afterwards, aching of the loins and knees.

Work by Yen et al, *J Ethnopharm* 111:1 found ethanol extracts of the seed prevent acetone-induced hepatoxicity in animal studies.

The seed is used to improve eyesight, such as blurred vision, and tinnitus, or ringing of the ears, combining well with astragalus seed (*A. complanatus*).

It helps relieve diarrhea due to low function of the spleen and kidneys; and has been used externally as a wash for vitiligo, combined with UV exposure.

When the seeds are mix-fried, the energy is warm and saltier. This quality makes the seed more valuable for impotence, premature ejaculation, bedwetting, vaginal discharge, threatened miscarriage, or metorrhagia during pregnancy.

The ground seeds, mixed with sesame oil, show 100% effectiveness against herpes zoster in several studies. Pan WH et al, *Asia Pacific Trad Med* 2008 4(4):47-51.

Another study found cooled seed decoctions, applied to acne twice daily for a week, improved skin quality in 94% of fifty patients. Yu GT, *Zhejiang J Trad Chin Med* 4:179.

For impotence, combine with lycium berry, puncture vine seed and schisandra berry; for frequent urination with elk antler and schisandra berry.

It nourishes the sperm and bone marrow, and strengthens sexual organs.

If it is desired to supplement the kidneys with both yang and yin influence, the salt mix-fried seed is used. To strengthen the yang of kidneys, the wine processed dodder pancake is used. This is prepared by cooking the seeds as porridge, and then crushing and mixing with rice wine and wheat bran to make medicinal pancakes, or **BING**.

Cuscuta seed helps consolidate Essence, slows down aging, and prevents loss of body fluids.

Recent work by Yang et al, *J Ethnopharm* 2008 119:1 found seed flavones reverse kidney yang deficiency, and help restore testosterone and ARmRNA levels in kidney and testes of animals.

A dried seed decoction was taken for three months by 13 patients with glomerulonephritis. Good results were obtained in 12 patients, resulting in 92% effectiveness. Xia MM et al, *Zhejiang J Integ Trad West Med* 2000 10(7) 439.

The seed was included in a human study, with other herbs, for treatment of erectile dysfunction. Shah GR et al, *BMC Complement and Altern Med* 2012 12:155.

In one study, thirty grams of seeds, decocted in water was given to twenty to 120 days for male infertility, chronic prostatitis, and erectile dysfunction. Wang Q, *Jiangsu J of Trad Chin Medicine* 2000 21(12):43.

In another study of 19 cases of male infertility, a combination of lychee and dried seeds of *C. chinensis*, taken every day for two months, showed 89.5% efficiency. Wang JG, *Hebei J Trad Chin Med* 2001 23(1): 53.

It appears to ameliorate immune suppression and bladder damage associated with the cancer drug cyclophosphamide. Raju N et al, *Appl Biochem Biotechnol* 2015 176(3): 742-57.

Water extracts of seeds promote the proliferation and differentiation of osteoblasts, suggesting use in osteoporosis. Yao CH et al, *J Biomed Mat Res* part B *Apply Biomaterial* 75:277-88; Yang HM et al, *J Med Food* 2008 12:85-92.

An alcohol extract 1:4 at 95% was applied to vitiligo, resulting in 80% efficacy when applied 2-3 times daily. *J Xian Univ School of Medicine* 1959 6:88.

A good review on *C. chinensis* by Donnapee S et al is found in *Journal of Ethnopharmacology* 2014 157:292-308.

Water extracts appear immunosuppressive, and ethanol extracts are immune stimulating.

CAUTION- Dodder is ill-advised for those suffering from hemorrhoids, as it contains anthracenosides which can cause blood to converge in the abdominal region. It is a mild uterine stimulant that should be avoided during pregnancy.

Some Chinese herbals suggest its use be avoided whenever there are open sores, wounds or abscesses, as the herb may reduce healing time.

Dodder is also contraindicated for patients suffering constipation, or dark, scanty urine.

HOMEOPATHY

Mother tincture of the fresh plant is used as a laxative in homeopathic medicine.

There is a loss of appetite with thirst for cold water. Tired and weak in morning. Tingling sensation in mouth when drinking cold water or eating sweets. Electric-like pain in left side of chest.

Vertigo, headache, runny nose worse in rainy cold weather. Pain between shoulder blades.

DOSE- Mother tincture to 200c. 5-10 drops as needed. Proving by Central Council for Research in Homeopathy in India with thirteen provers with 6c, 30c and 200c in 2002-03.

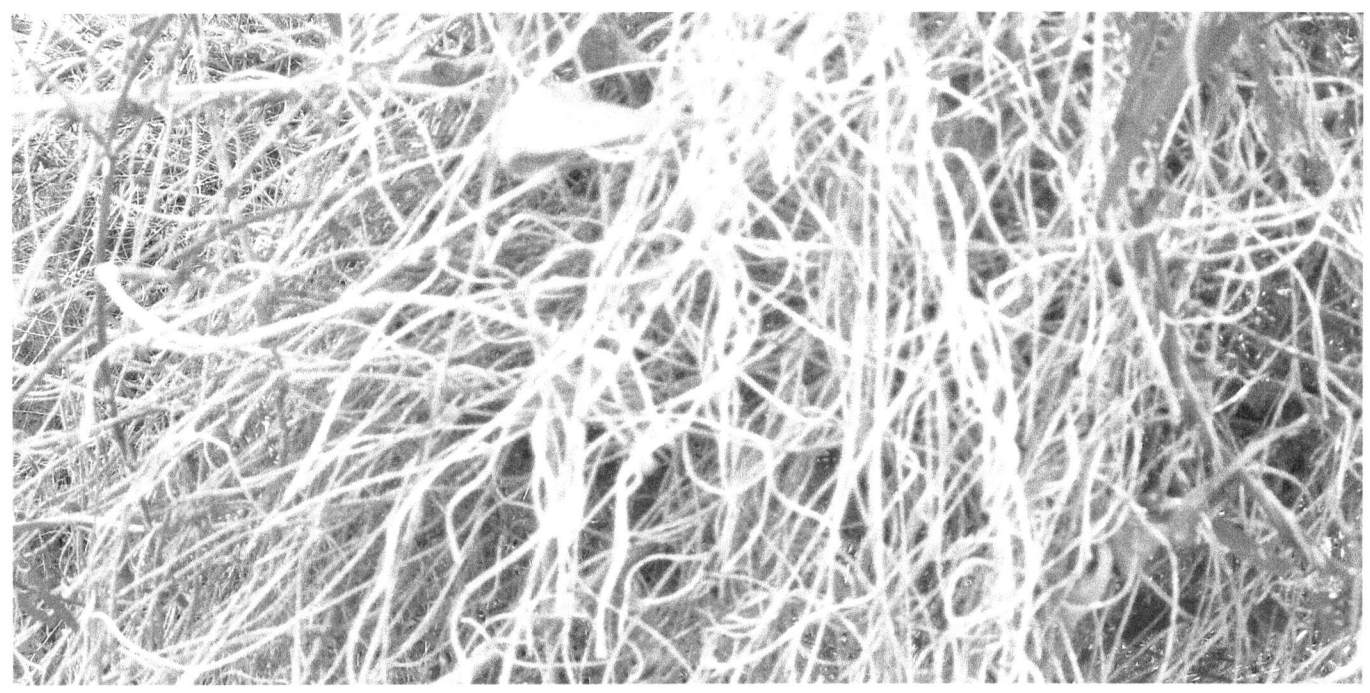

DODDER

SEED OIL

The seed oil of dodder is composed chiefly of linolenic acid (96%). It also has an interesting content of dipolyethenoid glycerides.

HYDROSOL

Dodder in seed is distilled and the water used for clarifying the eye, diseases of the liver, comforting the stomach and lungs, drives out stone and opens and cleanses the kidney through increased urination and bringing urine to passages. It also warms a cold womb, and brings on past due menstruation. Young children suffering ague or fever, even if breast feeding will benefit, according to Brunschwig, in *Book of Distillation*, 1530.

FLOWER ESSENCE

Dodder flower essence is for those individuals who have difficulty retaining their own sense of self. This is especially useful for teenagers who feel that being one of the crowd is all important; and that they will be judged for any displays of individual expression.

It is also useful for those who suffer from varying degrees of personality split; from early childhood traumas and abuse. The flower essence will help those who were abandoned, adopted, or orphaned at an early age; and who wonder what their genetic family is like and where they are. **PRAIRIE DEVA**

SPIRITUAL PROPERTIES

Dodder gives very good clues by its plant signature. At the first opportunity it will separate from its roots and become totally dependent on another plant; not only for nourishment, but for identity.

In some ways this is reminiscent of those who join religious cults or groups in the hope of "finding themselves". Too late, many find that their individualism or ego is discouraged in order to obtain "nirvana". Like the dodder, these individuals become dependent on others for support, leading to lack of judgment. **PRAIRIE DEVA**

A young man was hired by a farmer to look after his bunnies. The farmer warned him that the death of a bunny would cost him a quarter of his wages.

One day, the young man accidentally dropped a bamboo stick on a bunny, and broke its spine. The bunny lay on the ground unable to move. The young man was afraid the farmer would find out, so he took the bunny to a soybean field.

The farmer found that one bunny was missing, and sent the young man to the field to bring the bunny back. To his surprise, the bunny was running around the field. After a chase, he caught her and brought the bunny back to the cage.

Then, the young man intentionally broke another rabbit's back and took it to the same field. A few days later, it's back was completely healed.

"How could that have happened", he asked his father, who had suffered from backache for years.

"Maybe it's the soybean plants," mused his father.

The next day, the young man deliberately broke the back of another bunny and took her to the field. He watched what she ate, and saw it was the seeds of a parasitic plant growing amongst the soybeans.

The young man started to pick the seeds and decocted them for his father, who was cured of his backache.

The herb has been known as "bunny seed" ever since. **HENRY C. LU**

PERSONALITY TRAITS

The dodder personality is one defined by lack of roots. All effort to sever ties with the past has led to an individual lacking identity. These individuals have great difficulty being with themselves, and relating to others.

The negative Dodder is dependent on society for every need. They attract parasitic relationships, and yet, cannot seem to break this pattern. They are needy; and yet cold. In therapy, they are the so-called "energy-leeches", those requiring constant attention.

The positive Dodder takes time to be alone and reflect on their life. They make a conscientious effort to reconnect with family and loved ones because they have love to give. They make excellent therapists because of their ability to have healthy detachment from their clients. **PRAIRIE DEVA**

It (Dodder) lies in ambush like a pigmy field octopus, with deadly suckers for draining the sap of its victims. These it mats together in its wiry, sinuous coils, and chokes relentlessly by the acre. Nevertheless, the petty garrotter, like a toad "ugly and venomous, wears yet a precious jewel in its head". **DR. FERNIE**

MYTHS AND LEGENDS

Maidens of Pawnee Indians used Cuscuta gronovii to determine the seriousness and sincerity of a suitor. "A girl having plucked a vine, with the thought of the young man in mind tossed the vine over her shoulder, into the weeds of host species of this dodder…The second day after she would return to see whether the dodder had attached itself and was growing on the host. If so, she went away content with full assurance of her lover's sincerity and faithfulness. **GILMORE (1914)**

FLOWER TAROT

Dodder stands for ambition. Dodder is a grass with filiform stem which twine around other plants and attach themselves with their suckers, rapidly strangling the host plants.

The dodder symbolizes ambition, the compulsion to succeed with a negative side. Some would describe it as evil since this burning ambition is achieved at the cost of others, by destroying them. **GRIMAUD**

RECIPES

INFUSION- Hot infusions of the seed, as they are insoluble in cold water.

SEEDS- 7-15 grams.

TINCTURE- 5-10 drops up to three times daily for calming effect. High doses are laxative. The tincturing of seeds tends to bring out the warming potential, and is indicated in muscle and skeletal conditions. No health risks or side effects have been recorded when used as recommended. Do not use dodder seed with either constipation, or dark, scanty urine. The tincture is made with fresh plant at 1:4 and 40% alcohol.

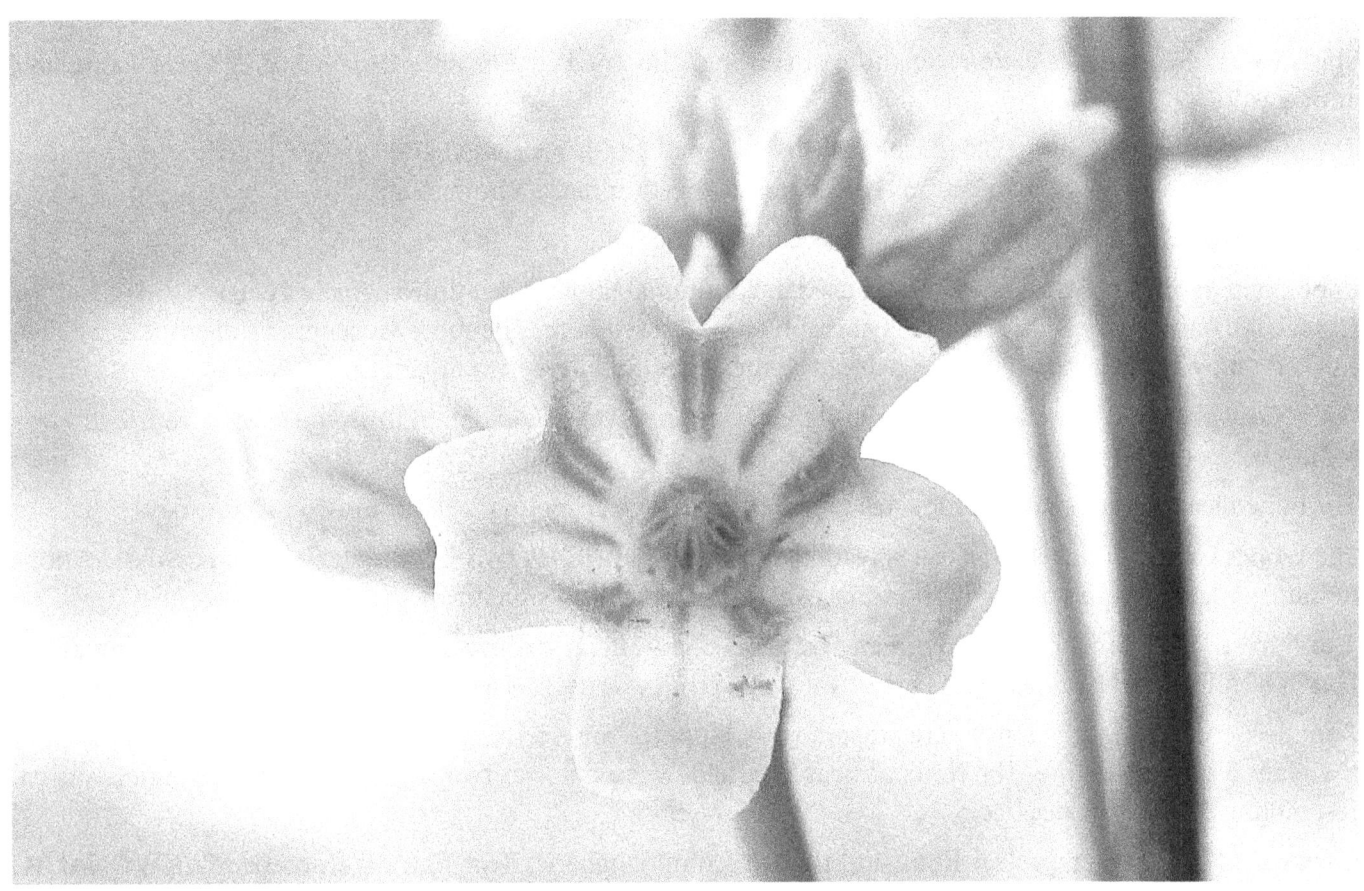

SPREADING DOGBANE FLOWER

SPREADING DOGBANE
BITTER ROOT
WEREWOLF ROOT
(*A. androsaemifolium* L.)
CANADIAN HEMP
INDIAN HEMP
NUNQUOT
(*Apocynum cannabinum* L.)
INTERMEDIATE DOGBANE
(*A. x floribundum* Greene [pro. sp.])
PARTS USED- creeping rootstock, and outer bark, flowers

Bird songs lessen after the dogbane leaves turned yellow in autumn.   **THOREAU**

Apocynum is derived from Greek **APO** meaning away, and **KUON** for dog.

Androsaemifolium is Latin meaning "man's blood-colored flower". *Cannibinum* means cannabis or Hemp.

Spreading dogbane is a tiny, inconspicuous shrub with beautiful, pink, fragrant flowers. All parts of the plant release a latex sap if bruised. This milky sap resembling mother's milk led to an early plant signature for promoting lactation.

Canadian Hemp has white flowers, with stems that become bright red in fall. Both plants initially look similar.

The flowers have been collected and used as part of love mixtures. They secrete a sweet liquid that is very attractive to flies.

The floss can be used as a cotton substitute or stuffing. The dried latex from the plant makes a very flammable gum elastic.

The outer bark is peeled just before the fruit has ripened and is processed and braided together to produce a thread finer and stronger than cotton. Three strands together make a bowstring.

Netting, twine, fishing line and even a coarse cloth can be made from the bark fibre.

Rabbit nets as long as 1.5 kilometers were used in communal hunts. A net drawstring has been found in Danger Cave, Utah dating over 5000 years old. One rabbit rope, stored in the Glenbow Museum in Calgary Alberta was worked on by many generations of Blackfoot. It measures 1.2 kilometers in length.

Peter Kalm observed that the Swedes around the Delaware River would obtain from the natives "fourteen yards (of dogbane rope) for a piece of bread."

The boiled leaves were rubbed over sores from poison ivy, clearing up the sores in two or three days.

The Woods Cree of Saskatchewan call Spreading Dogbane **TOTOSAPOWASK** or milk plant, and used decoctions to increase lactation in nursing mothers, based on the doctrine of signatures.

The Forest Potawtomi boiled the green fruit and drank it for dropsy and kidney problems. They call it **DODOCA'BOWÛNG** or, woman's breast weed. The root was used as a diuretic and urinary medicine.

Root decoctions (one inch long) were prepared by Chippewa, for external use in sore ears or eyes. They consider the plant a bear medicine. The roots of Bear Medicine were cut into two inch pieces and strung on a cord, resembling a bear claw necklace.

They called Indian Hemp, Bear Root; and the Spreading Dogbane, Bear Entrails Root, or **MAKWONAGIC ODJIBIK**. The former was used more for coughs, and the latter for heart palpitations, headaches, and as a very weak decoction for baby's colds.

The preferred part of dogbane is the elbow of the root. It is worth noting that just about all dogbane roots run true north and south.

Hemorrhage of the nose can be treated by inserted the plant floss moistened with the same decoction.

The Blackfoot call Canada Hemp, **NUXAPIST**, or Little Blanket as well as Many Spears. They used decoctions to prevent losing hair, smoked the leaves, and decocted the roots as a laxative.

Decoctions stimulate hair growth through vaso-dilation and mild irritation of the hair follicles. It was used as a final rinse after cleansing the scalp. The plant juice was a hair tonic, and a cleansing agent for buckskin.

The boiled root was taken once weekly as a temporary contraceptive, by both men and women, while the boiled green roots were used in heart and kidney ailments.

The dried and powdered roots were placed on hot rocks, and the fumes inhaled by headache sufferers.

The Cree poulticed the chewed leaves and bark, and applied it to wounds.

The Penobscot and Mi'kmaq call *A. cannabinum* "worm root", steeping that part in hot water and then drinking the tea to expel intestinal parasites.

Another variation for more serious headache, involved applying the powdered root moistened with water to new, incised temples.

A third method involved the snuffing of dried powder directly up the nostrils.

Heart palpitations were treated with an eight-inch root in one quart of water decocted for several minutes. Severe convulsions called for dogbane. About one foot of root was combined with one inch of Wild Pea root (*Lathyrus venosus*), decocted and then forced down the patient's mouth. It would be sprinkled on the chest or applied to palms of the hands, and soles of feet.

The fresh root was considered a specific for syphilis by several indigenous tribes in attempts to deal with this imported disease. Dr. Jones collected a mixture of the rind of spreading dogbane together with the wood of sugar maple, angelica stem, crab apple bark, swamp dock root, and the flower base of blue-eyed grass. The latter were used by Meskwaki women as a tea for injured womb.

The Cherokee used the roots of Indian Hemp, or Bowman's root, to treat uterine problems, female depression and nervousness. The Paiute used the fine, yellow stem silk for fiber. Long nets for rabbit drives were made from the twine. After rabbits were captured and skinned, the cordage was used to sew rabbit skin blankets.

It is said that in the northern Great Basin, the bark was mixed with tobacco for smoking.

The Shoshone name for the plant, **WANA**, is similar to **WASN**, their name for string or net. The Chumash of California used the thread for buckskin bags, bowstrings, and any kind of fishing equipment. The water apparently hardens it. Dragnets and river nets for catching salmon were made with the twine.

Algonquin women carried the seed with them upon marrying, to ensure plantings near their new residence.

The milky sap of both could well have been used as an arrow poison, due to cardiac glycoside content. The toxicity of the plant for horses and cows has been greatly exaggerated. A 1922 publication, from the New Mexico Agriculture Station, confused dogbane and the deadly oleander. Oops!

Although the monarch butterfly caterpillar prefers eating Milkweed, it will in some cases, resort to Dogbane foliage for sustenance. The Dogbane Leaf Beetle (*Chrysochus auratus*) spends most of its life on the plant, eating the leaves and laying its yellow eggs.

Flies are sometimes trapped in the flowers and held captive until death.

The two species sometimes interbreed and form a hybrid called *A. x floribundum*. It was formerly called *A. medium*, in the middle of the two species.

Research at University of Pennsylvania found *A. cannabium* plants, touched by humans were eaten by insects, while untouched plants remained healthy. They suspect the plant may release a chemical that protects it from humans (or browsers like deer), but attracts insects. Other plants, such as sulphur cinquefoil (*Potentilla recta*) and toadflax (*Linaria vulgaris*) have the opposite reaction and appear to thrive from human touch.

The leaves of the closely related *A. venetum (Trachomitum venetum)* are used in North China and Japan to make an herbal beverage. It is introduced and hardy to zone four.

A recent transgenic experiment found inserting a gene from this species into cotton increased yields and saline tolerance. Chen J et al, *Front Plant Sci* 2016 7:1041.

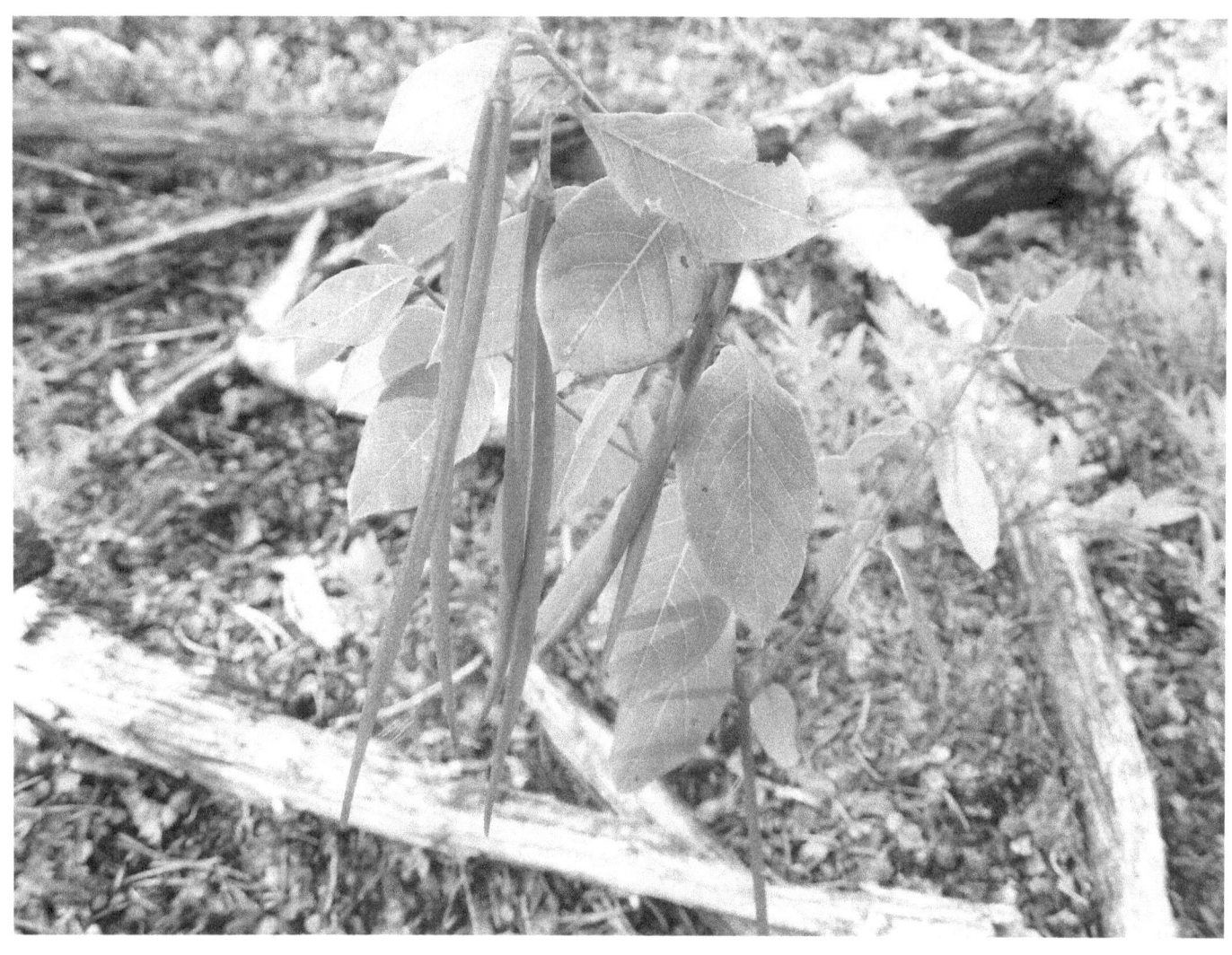

INDIAN HEMP SEED POD

MEDICINAL

CONSTITUENTS- *A. androsaemifolium* root- acetovanillone (apocynin), apocynein, apobioside, apocymarin(strophanthidin), K-strophanthoside, traces of ipuranil, and essential oil containing acetovanillin (160 ppm).
Aerial parts- androsterol, apocymamarin, caoutchouc, cymarin, homo-androsterol.
A. cannabinum- tannins, saponins, resins, cymarin, K-strophanthin, apocannoside, cynocannoside, alpha-amyrin, lupeol, oleanolic acid, androsterol, homo-androsterol, harmalol, 4-hydroxyacetophenone; acetovanillone (apocynin), p-hydroxyacetophenone, and an unidentified phenol.
seeds- 30% protein, 23% fat.
A. venetum leaf- various flavonoids including rutin, quercetin-3-O-sophoroside, isoquercitin, neoisorutin, hyperin, astragalin, kaempferol, plumbocatechin A, 8-O-methylretusin, kaempferol 3-O-(6"-O-acetyl)-beta-D-galactopyranoside, trifolin, isoquercitin-6'O-acetate, apocyanosides, triacontanol, beta-sitosterol, lupeol, scopoletin, isofraxidin, and hyperoside.
Root- cymarin, strophantidin, K-strophanthin-B.
Flower- kaempferol, quercitin, vanillic acid, baimaside, daucosterol, quercitin and kaempferol glucosides.

Spreading dogbane is good therapy for chronic constipation, where there is chronic liver disability.

It acts upon the gall duct, discharging bile and small gallstones. It combines well in decoctions with yellow dock root in 1:2 ratio, but in very small doses.

Nervous headaches, and other head pains due to sluggish venous capillary circulation in the brain indicate the use of dogbane. Facial neuralgia is relieved by fomentation of the decocted root, and combines well with cow parsnip seed for this purpose.

For edema and fluid retention, use a mild dried root infusion taken cold, or a tincture in water before meals. The powdered root is a sweat-inducing counter-irritant.

Grieve, in her book, called it a "Vegetable Tocar" or drainer, in reference to the plants ability to reduce fluid accumulation in liver cirrhosis.

Herbalists like Samuel Thomson used Dogbane as "one of the greatest correctors of the bile." Dr. Cook suggested it increases excretion of bile, not stimulates more manufacture.

"By its action on the biliary passages, it secures a free discharge of the bile, thus unloading the gall-cyst and relieving turgescence of the liver... It is best fitted for sluggish cases, where the pulse and the sensibilities are below normal.

Stools following the use are a trifle soft, and may even be made thin by large doses..\. It is best given in dry feces and muscular torpor, with bilious symptoms, when the system is sluggish; but is not suitable for sensitive and irritable conditions, nor is it best when piles are present."

The root is safe in proper dosage as Michael Moore explains. "Small doses of dogbane act as a vasoconstrictor, slowing and strengthening the heartbeat and raising the blood pressure. It is a strong diuretic, useful in cardiac dropsy and the like, but authorities differ whether it increases urine by irritation of the kidneys or dilation of the renal artery or both. In fact, one of the reasons preventing its more frequent use in medicine is the variability of absorption, metabolization, effects and pharmacology.

A safe and reliable dose is a single "0" capsule of the powdered root a day…One cardinal sign for the use of Dogbane is the adrenalin-stress individual who for years has had little daytime urination, instead urinating frequently in the evening and nighttime—the effect of daytime adrenergic stress constricting the renal artery and slowing down diuresis; this resumes when the person can relax.

This person, finally, usually in the fourth decade, starts to urinate less after relaxation and begins to notice water retention, poorly fitting shoes, and puffy ankles at night, perhaps first observed after a few very hot days or after flying to a very different climate. Dogbane capsules will relax the renal arteries and even postpone for a few years any potential kidney disease."

Both rhizome and leaf reduce inflammation, improve cardiovascular conditions, such as hardening of arteries, or atrial fibrillation, and may be useful in chronic conditions such as diabetes, and senile dementia.

Apocynin inhibited Nox2 expression and Nox (nicotinamide adenine dinucleotide phosphate or NADPH) oxidase, activity, reduced lipid peroxidation, suppressed the NFkappaB pathway and pro-inflammatory cytokines in lung tissue, during rat hemorrhagic shock study. Choi SH et al, *J Trauma Acute Care Surg* 2016 December 23.

Ochratoxin A (OTA) is a frequent contaminate of grain and pork products, as well as coffee, wine grapes and raisins. It is carcinogenic to humans and is related to kidney and urinary cancers. It also causes acute depletion of striatal dopamine, suggesting a role in Parkinson's disease, and due to its affinity for the hippocampus for Alzheimer's disease.

This toxin is also found in water damaged homes and heating ducts.

Post-operative cognitive decline is a common completion following anasethesia and surgery, especially in the elderly. Apocyinin reversed hippocampal parvalbumin interneuron loss in a mice study. Qiu LL et al, *Front Aging Neurosci* 2016 8:234.

Apocynin, an NADPH oxidase inhibitor, significantly attenuated OTA-induced apotosis, and inhibited calpain activity, suggesting benefit in protection of glomerulonephritis. Sheu ML et al, *Oncotarget* 2016 December 27. doi: 10.18632/oncotarget. 14270.

Apocynin attenuates elevated high mobility group box (HMGB)2 levels in myocardial infarction patients. In this clinical trial of 432 patients and 312 controls, apocynin reduced the hypoxic cell severity, and levels of HMGB2 that increase mycocardial infarction severity. Liu ZH et al, *Am J Physiol Heart Circ Physiol* 2016 Dec 23: ajpheart.00249.2016.

Apocynin, by inhibiting NADPH4 may modulate the effects of angiotensin, and benefit atrial fibrillation therapy. Lu G et al, *Biochem Biophys Res Commun* 2016 Dec 21.

It may help reduce vascular stiffness, structural elastin abnormalities and increased oxidative stress associated with hypertension. Martinez-Revelles S et al, *Antioxid Redox Signal* 2016 Dec 23. doi:10. 1089.

The compound may protect against vascular calcification by suppressing the ERK½ pathway. Feng W et al, *Oncotarget* 2016 7(750):83588-600.

Apocynin improved glucose tolerance and insulin sensitivity in older mice, as well as hepatic lipid deposition. This suggests a possible use of dogbane for non-alcoholic fatty liver disease, as well as metabolic syndrome. Nunes-Souza V et al, *Oxid Med Cell Longev* 2016;2016:1987960.

Apocynin may be useful in reducing inflammation associated with arthritis, via immune regulation. Pandey A et al, *Phytother Res* 2009 23(10):1462-8.

Strophanthidin is a cardenolide with action similar to digitoxin, specifically inhibiting the membrane protein Na+/K+ ATPase in heart muscle tissue that can lead to Ca2+ overload, diastolic dysfunction, arrythmia and heart failure.

Strophanthidin exhibits moderate cyctotoxicity against MCf-&, NCI and HepG2 cancer cell lines. Hsiao PY et al, *Phytochemistry* 2016 130:282-90.

Early studies in Germany gave eight healthy volunteers one milligram of K-strophanthoside rectally to evaluation cardiac influence. The benefit was equivalent to 0.50 milligrams of digoxin. Longhini C et al, *Arzneimittelforschung* 1979 29(5):827-9.

The root tea helps reduce the water retentive ascites associated with liver dysfunction including cases of hepatitis and cancer.

For alcohol withdrawal use dried root infusion and sip throughout day. Combine with the flower essence for maximum benefit.

Ether, acetone and benzene extracts of the plant show strong inhibition of *E. coli*. Bishop & MacDonald, *Can J Botany* 1951 29.

More recent work by Borchardt et al, *J Med Plants Res* 2008 2:5 found leaf and stem active against *Staphylococcus aureus*.

The leaf contains cymarin, also found in the root of Canadian Hemp and *A. venetum*. See below for medicinal application of cymarin.

The plant was officially listed in the *US Pharmacopoeia* until 1952.

Canadian Hemp root is used as a diuretic, kidney and cardiac tonic, but should not be used in cases of organic kidney damage. The Cherokee used it for kidney failure. At one time it was used externally for venereal warts and to promote hair growth.

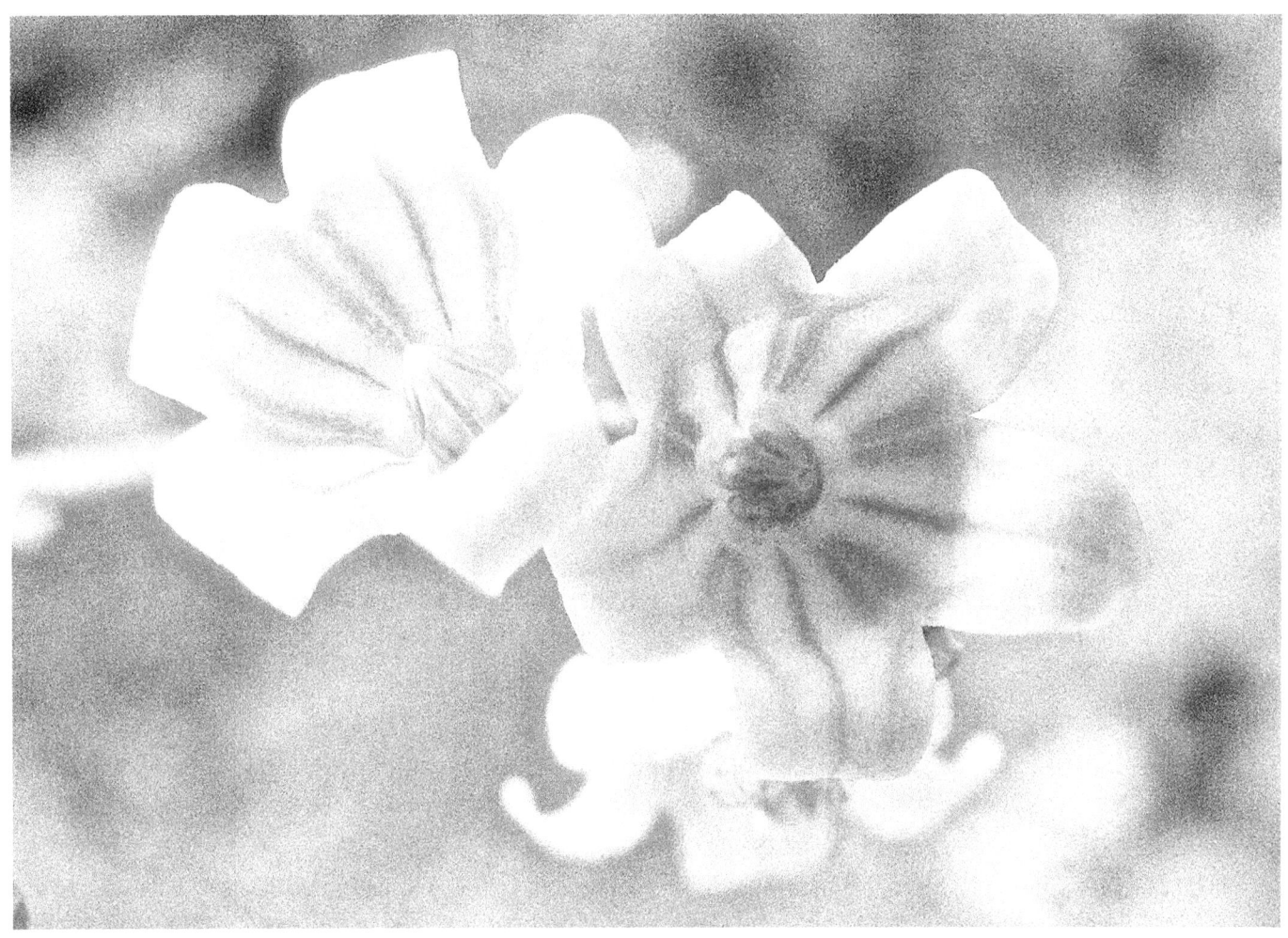

SPREADING DOGBANE FLOWERS

The root is a mild cardiac stimulant. In small doses, it acts as a vasoconstrictor, slowing and strengthening the heart, and raising blood pressure. Cymarin, one constituent, has the action of lowering pulse rate and increasing blood pressure.

It is a strong diuretic and is used for water retention. Authorities cannot agree whether this is due to kidney irritation, or dilation of the renal artery, or both. Urine output is greatly increased, but the solids in urine are not.

Small amounts, up to five drops at a time, help increase heart contractibility while decreasing the pulse rate.

When US President Benjamin Harrison had heart problems that would not respond to digitalis, his physicians gave him Canadian Hemp root and saved his life. He lived for many more years.

The fresh juice from Canadian Hemp is used in the external treatment of warts including genital and anal varieties.

Dr. Eli Jones, one of the great medical Eclectics, used Canadian Hemp root for growths in the breasts where there are small bunches, movable and hard like a rubber ball. Seven grams of powder are added to ounce of lanolin, and rubbed into the breast three times daily.

Cymarin shows significant cytotoxicity against six human cancer cell lines including HCT-116, HepG2, HeLa, SK-OV-3, SK-MEL-5 and SK-BR-3. Jung JW et al, *Molecules* 2015 20(11): 20823-31.

Other work found cymarin exhibits potent cytotoxicity against human solid tumor cell line A549 (lung carcinoma), but not active against leukemic cells (L1210). You YJ et al, *Phytother Res* 2003 17(5):568-70.

Apocynin is a powerful anti-inflammatory that reduces the production of superoxide from activated neutrophils and macrophages, while phagocytosis is unchanged. *Mediators Inflam* 2008 106507.

Harmalol is a beta carboline alkaloid, also found in buffalo berry (*Shepherdia canadensis*). Harmane alkaloids are MAO inhibitors used in various psychotrophic compounds such as ayahuasca. Harmala alkaloids are considered Schedule 9 prohibited substance under the Poisons Standard (October 2015).

P-hydroxyacetophenone inhibits activity of hepatitis B virus. Zhao Y et al, *Bioorg Med Chem Lett* 2015 25(7):1509-14.

Lupeol, a lupane type triterpene, inhibits melanoma cell lines. Hata K et al, *Biol Pharm Bull* 2000 23(8):962-7. It shows potential against prostate cancer and reduces skin cancer cell proliferation. Its great advantage is significant anti-inflammatory potential with no toxicity to normal cells.

Lupeol reduces oxalate kidney stone formation, inhibit cold sore (herpes simplex) replication, reduces inflammation and modulates immune function.

Lupeol shows remarkable activity against MRSA (methicillin-resistant *Staphylococcus aureus*). El Sayed AM et al, *Nat Prod Res* 2016 April 4:1-6.

Lupeol shows strong inhibition of osteoclast differentiation and bone loss. It may be useful for osteoporosis, Paget's disease, osteolysis associated with periodontal disease, as well as multiple myeloma. Im NK et al, *J Nat Prod* 2016 79(2):412-20.

Lupeol is compound found in birch bark.

Dr. William Cook recommended the fresh root be applied to rattlesnake bites, with a 1:16 infused tea drunk 2-3 ounces every hour. Maybe!I would probably also head to nearest source of anti-venom, if at all possible.

Chinese research into medical uses of dogbane (*A.venetum*) showed cardiac tonic benefit. The plant is known as **ZE QI MA**, for Mandarin, or **LO BOU MA YE**, in Cantonese. Other names include Marsh Lacquer Herb, **ZE QI CAO**, Lucky Lucky Hemp, **JI JI MA**, and **CHA YE HUA** meaning, Tea Leaf flower. The leaf tea has been used in Mongolia for centuries. Luoboma Tea is widely available in western China.

The plant leaf shows hypotensive activity and a good draining diuretic, useful in cardiac deficiency, heart disease, edema, hepatitis, and nephritis.

It appears to reduce oxidative stress and exerts cardio-protection against myocardial ischemia/reperfusion injury, in animal studies. Wang W et al, *Am J Chin Med* 2015 43(1):71-85.

Infusions of the plant leaf showed blood pressure lowering effect in humans of 10% when taken daily for four weeks, 13% when taken for eight weeks. The root is decocted as an 8% decoction, and 100 ml twice daily are taken until heart rate slows to 70-80 beats per minute. A daily maintenance of 50 ml leaf infusions has a similar benefit.

HDL, or "good cholesterol" as it is known, rose by 24% and heart performance was observed to improve. *Chinese J of Integrated Med* 1989 9:6.

The leaf tablet inhibits cardiac hypertrophy by suppressing phosphorylation of ERK½ and AKT. Qi J et al, *Evid Based Complement Alternat Med* 2014:769515.

The leaf extract, taken with GABA (100 mg), showed improvement by inducing deep sleep, in a human trial. Yamatsu A et al, *J Nutr Sci Vitaminol* (Tokyo) 2015 61(2): 182-7.

Posinol™, an extract from *A. venetum*, contains 4% flavonoid glycosides isoquercitrin and hypersoide; the latter shown to aid in mental relaxation. Marketed by Optipure, the product is said to be an alternative for those individuals concerned about the safety of St. John's Wort, and its content of hyperforin. One small animal study showed Posinol™ shortened immobility time, indicating possible anti-depressant activity similar to 20mg/kg of imipramine. More conclusive, human studies are needed.

A few case studies suggest 50 mg capsules helped patients with insomnia, improved concentration, stress reduction and decreased fatigue.

The studies varied from two weeks to 3.5 years, but not under very robust controls.

Hyperin and isofraxidin are effective sedative compounds. Chen M & Liu F, *Zhongguo Zhong Yao Za Zhi* 1991 16(10):609-11.

Isofraxidin is a major active compound of *Eleutherococcus senticosus*, commonly known as Siberian ginseng, and ash tree bark. It possesses anti-bacterial, anti-oxidant and anti-inflammatory activity. It appears to inhibit COX-2 protein expression, in the lungs, which regulates the production of PGE2 inflammation. Niu X et al, *Int Immunopharmacol* 2015 24(2):432-9.

A recent study by Kessler et al, *Arch Gen Psychiatry* 2005, which was double-blind, randomized, and parallel, involved men and women from 18-65 years of age with mild depression as rated by the Hamilton Rating Scale. Forty-seven patients were chosen, with 27 in the Posinol™ group for eight weeks.

An overall reduction in HAM-D score was 47.3 in the Posinol™ group. More than 50% of this group showed a score decrease of 50% or more. Blood analysis revealed that 50% of subjects in the Posinol™ group showed increased serotonin levels, and no adverse reactions were noted.

The leaf flavonoids produced significant anti-depressant effects, perhaps due to increased levels of noradrenaline and dopamine. Zheng M et al, *J Ethnopharm* 2013 147(1):108-13. Astragalin, also found in Astragalus root, possesses sedative and hypnotic effects, in a mouse study. Li X et al, *Nat Prod Res* 2016 26:1-5.

A recent female rat study suggests it may enhance ovarian function by increasing estrogen and progesterone levels, suggesting another approach to management of menopausal symptoms. At least in female rodents. Wei M et al, *Molecules* 2016 21:5.

Cymene has a similar effect to the glycoside strophantine, but is generally weaker. It has a stronger diuretic effect in edema, and is less cumulative.

Hyperoside may play a role in the prevention of cardiovascular disease. Hao XL et al, *Mol Med Rep* 2016 14(1):399-405. Hyperoside is more well-known as an important compound in Saint John's wort.

Hyperoside, derived from *A. venetum*, may protect the liver from toxicity related to acetominophen overdose, but accelerating harmless metabolism. Xie W et al, *Chem Biol Interact* 2016 246:11-19.

The leaves can be dried and rolled in a cigarette, to smoke in cases of chronic bronchitis with cough and wheezing. The dried leaves are made into an herbal beverage in North China and Japan. Studies by Xiong Quang Bo et al, *Planta Medica* 2000 66:2 indicate the leaf flavonoids have hepato-protective effects.

The leaf is sweet, bitter and cooling, and infused for daily use to clear heat, prevent dizziness and improve cardiac function. It helps lower blood pressure and reduce edema, and is highly regarded by the elderly for health maintenance. The leaves have little toxicity, and delay the aging process.

Based on clinical trials, the herb causes no severe side effect even when taken as a stable daily dose of 50mg/person for more than three years.

Corticosterone-induced neurotoxicity, commonly know as Roid Rage, is a predictable consequence of long-term cortisone drugs, both orally and externally. The herb appears to protect neurotoxicity in PC12 cells, possibly by decreasing Ca(2+) concentration, and up-regulating brain-derived neurotrophic factor and microtubular-associated protein 4 genes. Zheng M et al, *Cell Mol Neurobiol* 2011 31(3):421-8.

The modern Chinese physician, Wang Zhen-Qin noted the herb "is sweet, bland and slightly cold in nature, and prevents and treats hypertension in the elderly, the common cold, and bronchitis. It has a definite ability to enhance the immunity of the body, and is a herb that extends age and augments longevity."

Known as Luobuma Tea, the leaf infusions have been found to strongly inhibit glycation, a complication associated with diabetes and heart disease. Yokozawa et al, *Food Chem Tox* 2004:42. The leaf infusion inhibits renal oxidative stress in streptozotocin-induced diabetic rats. Chen HY et al, *Yao Xue Xue Bao* 2010 45(1):26-30.

For edema and reduced urination, combine the leaf with plantain seed, water plantain rhizome and umbrella polypore (*Polyporus umbellatus*) mushroom. The latter is one of my wife's favorite edible fungi, which I find in our river valley every summer.

It has been used in stubborn edema related to pregnancy, but attention to potassium levels is needed. The root contains cardiac glycosides and is a different medicine. Do not confuse the two.

The dried leaf may be combined with self heal or chrysanthemum flowers for hypertension or liver heat associated with headache, dizziness, restlessness and insomnia.

Extracts from all parts of the plant inhibit phosphodiesterase3, contributing to the cardiac tonic effect. Irie K et al, *J Nat Med* 2009 63(2):111-6.

Leaf extracts inhibit xanthine oxidase, suggesting benefit in gouty arthritis. Lau YS et al, *Nutrients* 2015 7(7):5239-53.

Research on Spreading Dogbane leaves may reveal similar profile of flavonoids.

Harmalol is an MAO-inhibiting beta carboline, as mentioned above, similar to compounds found in buffalo berry and wolf willow.

In studies involving the anti-viral activities of plants in North America, spreading dogbane showed inhibition of the polio, cowpox, measles and PRV virus.

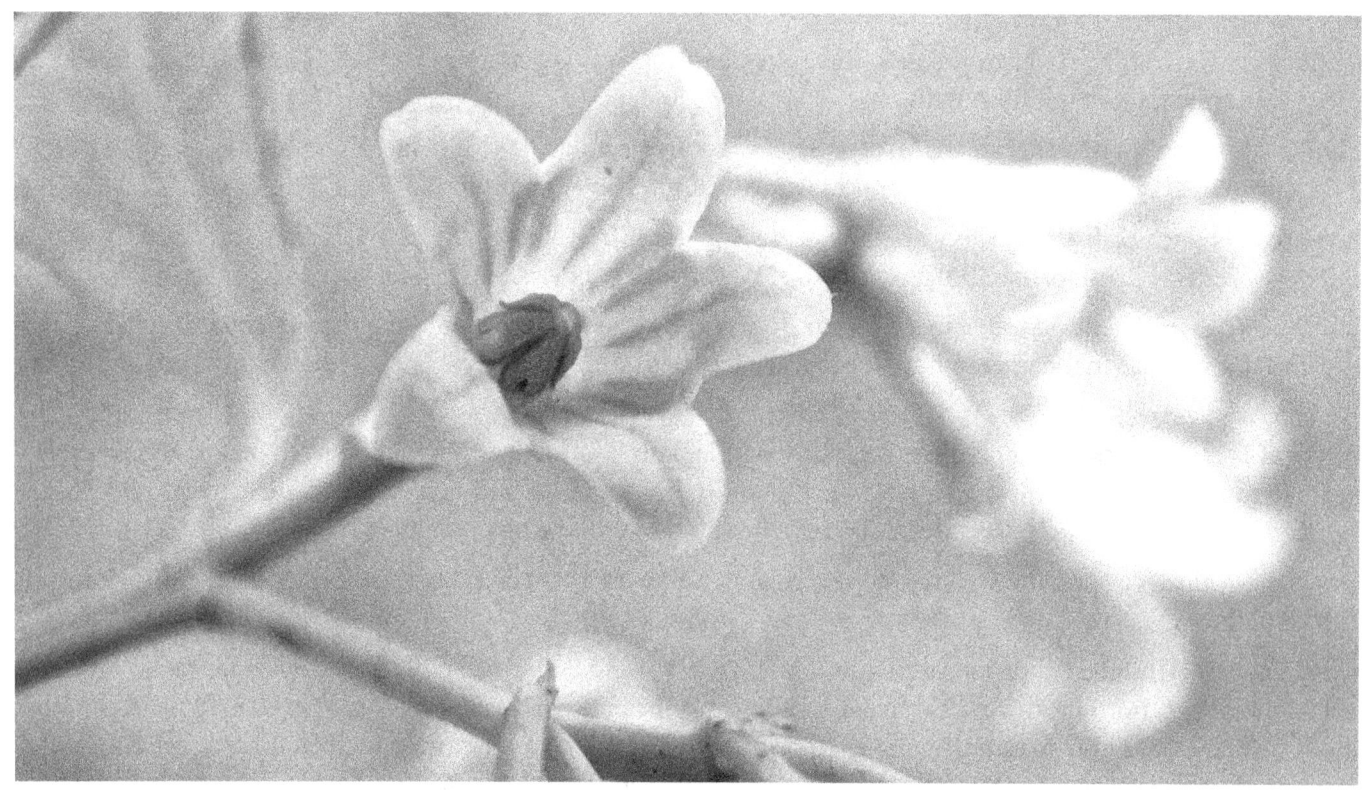

DOGBANE FLOWER

The fruit, flowers leaves, stems and roots have been investigated and found active against various gram-positive, gram-negative and mycobacterium.

Further research is warranted on our local plants. One patent exists from the former USSR with regards to apobioside from spreading dogbane for cardiovascular concerns.

Patents on *A. cannabinum* from the early 1900s exist for purified medicinal preparation. In 1965, a German patent for extraction of cymarin was granted. In 1979, a patent for the extraction of rubber and rubber-like substances from the latex was applied for and granted.

Early work by Belkin et al, *Journal of the National Cancer Institute* 1952 13 found that alcoholic extracts at sub-toxic doses showed damage to transplanted tumors in mice. Kupchan et al, *Journal Med Chem* 1964 7 803 found cymarin and apocannoside to possess anti-tumor activity.

Matthew Wood suggests that dogbane in flower essence or homeopathic form is helpful in a variety of cortisone dependence problems and collagen disease.

Dr. William Mitchell, Junior mentions its use in stubborn intractable cases of sciatica, a tip he learned from his mentor Dr. Bastyr.

HOMEOPATHY

Spreading Dogbane (*A. androsaemifolium*) symptoms for use include rheumatic pains that wander, with lots of tightening and stiffness. Swollen sensations are accompanied by trembling and fatigue.

There may be pain in all the joints, as well as the toes and soles of feet. There may be profuse sweating, excessive heat in feet, accompanied by tingling pain and cramping. It is used especially in cases of pains in all joints, pain in toes and soles, and swelling of hands and feet. Matthew Wood, in his foreword to *Healing Lyme Disease Naturally* by Wolf D. Storl writes, "I recommend *Apocynum androsaemifolium* homeopathic 6X for high impact cases that knock a person off the horse or the chair with their intensity."

A peculiar symptom that helps identify its use is that the patient thinks everything smells and tastes like honey.

DOSE- Tincture to the 6th potency. The mother tincture is made from the fresh rootstock.

Indian Hemp (*A. cannabinum*) is used for some of the above, but with exceptions. This Dogbane is one of the most efficient remedies in dropsy, liver ascites and various urinary problems including suppressed urination and strangury.

In Bright's disease, it helps the digestive complaints of nausea, vomiting, drowsiness and difficult breath. The dropsy is often accompanied by great thirst and gastric irritability.

Dogbane is used by homeopaths in the treatment of alcoholism. It greatly aids the withdrawal symptoms, but is recommended this not be used more than a week.

Dogbane also relieves long continued sneezing, and chronic nasal catarrh, dull headaches and poor memory.

The heartbeat is rapid and feeble, with low arterial tension, pulsating jugular vein, and irregularity. There is great restlessness and little sleep.

Symptoms are worse in cold weather and from cold drinks, better from warmth.

DOSE- Tincture (1-2 drops 3xdaily). In acute alcoholism take one dram of decoction in four ounces of water. The mother tincture is prepared from the fresh rootstock.

Cymarin- an active principle of dogbane- lowers pulse rate, and increases blood pressure.

ESSENTIAL OIL

The rhizome of dogbane (*Apocynum androsaemifolium*) yields about 0.016% of an essential oil. It contains furfurol, and aceto-vanillone, which results from the breakdown of a glucoside, androsin.

SEED OIL

Indian Hemp (*Acocynum cannabinum*) seeds contain up to 23% oil, the whole plant 4.5%, and the leaves and flowers 1.6%. Rubber latex of the whole plant is 1.16% of dry weight.

PERSONALITY TRAITS

Suppose a fly falls upon this innocent looking blossom. His short tongue, as well as the butterfly's, is guided into one of the V-shaped cavities after he has sipped; but getting wedged between the trap's horny teeth, the poor victim is held prisoner there until he slowly dies of starvation in the sight of plenty. The dogbane...ruthlessly destroys all poachers that are not big enough or strong enough to jerk away from its vice-like grasp. To be killed by slow torture and dangled like a scarecrow simply for pilfering a drop of nectar is surely an execution of justice medieval in its severity.
NELTJE BLANCHAN

[Apocynum] are waterlogged and overweight, swollen with water everywhere, especially swollen pitting ankles, and urinary troubles. They have reduced urine and sweat and feel that if they could sweat they could be well. The dropsy is accompanied by increased thirst. The further consequences are heart complaints caused by a waterlogged heart with arrhythmia, mitral and tricuspid value regurgitation and prolapsed. They develop a weakness from the lack of heart efficiency.
PETER CHAPPELL

SPIRITUAL PROPERTIES

I would like to thank Matthew Wood, a good friend, great herbalist, and fellow member of the American Herbalist Guild for the following insights into dogbane or werewolf root as he names it.

"The T square-like root, and the pincer like seedpods are also the symbols of Free Masonry, an analogue to the Grand Medicine Lodge in white society.

Nature is better represented by the circle, a symbol of wholeness and harmony, while mankind is represented by the square and pincers, symbols of conscious artifice. The right angle indicates the appearance of a kind of consciousness, which is at right angles to Nature. It represents the conscious mind, the ego. The pincers represent the focusing, limiting and ultimately egocentric fixation of the mind.

As a medicine, it addresses problems which arise from the juxtaposition of the ego and spirit. It is for those individuals who are losing the battle to remain a separate, conscious individual. There are times when nothing will do except total transformation.

Going further, Werewolf root is a shape-shifting medicine. It is more a matter of seeing the world in a radical, new way.

The motto of the plant is 'I will never be the same again.'"

FLOWER ESSENCES

Dogbane or Werewolf flower essence is for the emotional and spiritual issues revolving around alcoholism. It helps on several levels, the first being the awareness of addiction and attraction. It eases the pain associated with the loss or separation of "friendships" that is so necessary for the healing process to begin. Drinking buddies are only there, as long as you are one of them!

And it helps on the physical plane, by detoxifying the liver more quickly, and reducing trembling and sweating.
PRAIRIE DEVA

Dogbane essence helps us to access the courage to follow our rebellious instincts, which is an important part of growth and change.
DESERT ALCHEMY

MYTHS AND LEGENDS

Coyote's son was traveling in the sky country, when he came up to an old man, actually Spider, who was spinning Dogbane. Grandfather Spider helps the son of Coyote, by spinning coils of rope to lower him to earth. In return for this favour, Coyote's son makes Dogbane much more accessible to Spider. He plucks four hairs from his lower abdomen and throws them to the ground, which sprang into 3-4 acres of Dogbane. Spider is able to finish the rope and to lower Coyote's son back to earth.   **THOMPSON MYTHOLOGY**

In Lillooet mythology, the Transformers crossed Lillooet Lake, where they pulled hairs from their legs and threw them on the ground to create Indian Hemp plants; they then showed man and wife how to harvest, prepare it, and make dip nets for fishing with it.   **TEIT**

In more primitive and ancient thought, the dog was associated almost universally with the underworld in which it acted as both guide and guardian. Their companionship in life and their supposed knowledge of the spirit world suggested dogs as suitable guides to the afterlife. They play this role even in Central America where they carried Mayan souls across the river of death. Xoltl, the Aztec dog god, led the sun through the nocturnal underworld and was reborn with it at dawn.   **JACK TRESIDDER**

Coyote went to **SITOKTO'K** and bought a great load of **TOK** (Indian Hemp). By his magic power he was able to put it all into his carrying net and bring it all home at once…Next morning Coyote began to work with the **TOK**. He worked very fast, twisting it on the machine that he had: his thigh. Coyote twisted the **TOK** into string and made fish lines for all the important people of the village.   **TIMBROOK**

RECIPES

INFUSION- Steep one tsp of dried root in one pint of boiling water. Take one teaspoon to one-quarter ounce daily. The leaves of *A. venetum* are gathered before flowering and dried in shade. They may be steamed and dry-fried for use in infusions.

POWDER- leaf- *A. venetum*- 50 mg daily

DRY ROOT TINCTURE- 1:5 tincture at 50% alcohol. Five drops in water before meals, and up to 4-5 times daily if needed. For the fresh root, make a 1:8 at 76%.

CAUTION: According to the PDR for Herbal Medicines, serious poisoning is hardly to be expected from oral administration, due to the low resorption rate. Signs of intoxication are nausea, vomiting and a slow heartbeat.

NOTE- 0.1 grams of root possesses the potency of 2 USP digitalis units. The high content of cardenolide glycosides causes bradycardia and increased contraction of the heart. Blood pressure is lowered and a rebound vagotonic hypertension can occur. It has a lower therapeutic effect on atrial fibrillation than digitalis.

A. venetum extracts exhibit anti-platelet aggregation, suggesting caution with blood thinning medication. The coumarin isofraxidin protects leukemia cells from radiation-induced apoptosis. On the other hand, it appears effective against hepatoma cells.

POWDERED ROOT- one "O" capsule (5-10 grains) daily, or use topically. The root is collected after the plant has gone to seed. Mint tea will help any griping pain.

TWINE- Make the twine by collecting the stalks just about the time the pods are green. Cut them down and remove the branches and leaves. Flatten the stems by pulling them over a round pole. Then split open the stems from bottom to top with a knife or sharp stick and peel off the outer bark. Then twist the stems to make braids of the bark. You can then boil in hot water. This makes the fibers separate more and strengthens them. The thread is very tough.

Or when dried, the final step is to form the fibers into twine by rolling them with dampened hands on bare thigh or on a piece of buckskin over the knee. The fibre is joined for length by splitting the thick end of one piece and then thin end of another, inserting and intertwining. This splicing process can be continued indefinitely.

Finer twine is produced by splitting the stems in two; stronger ropes by plaiting two or more threads together. Stored properly, it will last for years. For garments, the twine can be spun with deer hair. Fishing lines, at least in the British Columbia Interior, were treated with lodge pole pine pitch and black bear grease, to prevent them from kinking.

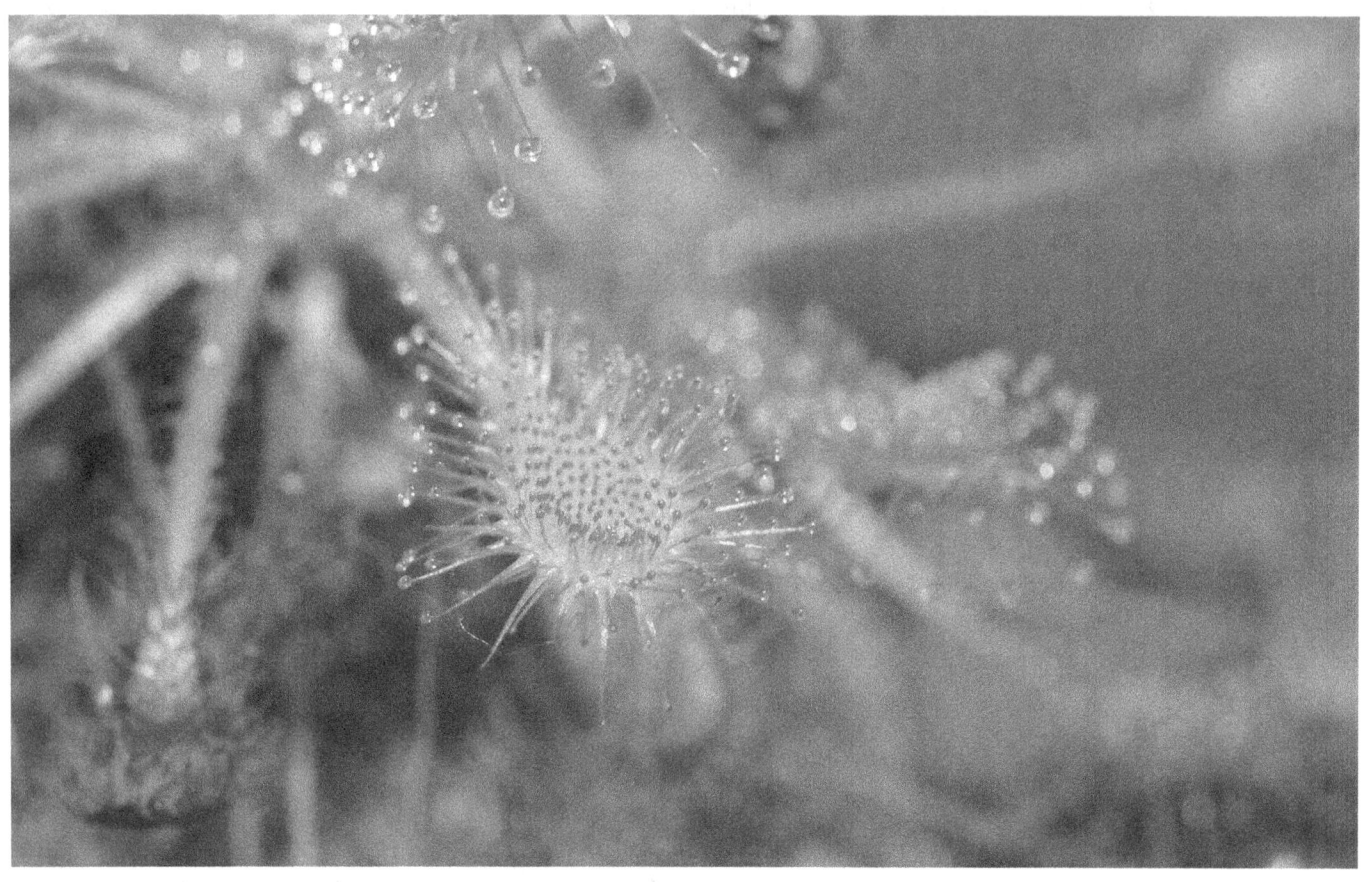

SUNDEW

DROSERA SPECIES
SUNDEW
(**Drosera rotundifolia** L.)
SLENDER LEAVED SUNDEW
(**D. linearis** Goldie)
GREAT SUNDEW
ENGLISH SUNDEW
OBLONG LEAVED SUNDEW
(**D. anglica** Huds.)
(**D. longifolia** L.) not accepted
PARTS USED- whole plant, flower

Its little feet and claws standing out as if stiff and rigid... the wicked little plant had killed it.

GARDENER'S CHRONICLE 1875

Drosera is from the Greek **DROSEROS** or dew, in reference to the sticky, shiny leaf. **ROTUNDIFOLIA** means round-leafed. The common name is thought to come from a misspelling of the Saxon **SINDEW**, "always dewy".

Anglica means England, where the plant was first described. Linearis means linear, referring to the long, slender leaves.

English Sundew symbolizes a serenade, and birth date of September 13th. This species is probably a hybrid of the other two species.

The next time you have occasion to visit a boreal bog or fen, get down low and chances are you will find Sundew. The flowers only open in full sunlight at 9-10 in morning and close by 2 pm for a single day, but the red sticky droplets on the leaves cannot be mistaken for another plant. It is small, up to the size of your thumb, but unique. In the United States, only 3-5% of the plants in original habitat have survived.

The sticky secretions are used by the plant to augment its dietary need for nitrogen, in the form of insects. Usually winged, the insects alight on the dew and become stuck, before further entrapping themselves by the enfolding leaves, as the hairs curl inward. The glandular head of sundew then excrete digestive juices that complete the meal.

The relatively slow bending of the leaf is mediated by the plant hormone auxin (indoleacetic acid).

One day, in England, a naturalist came upon a two acre meadow of sundew.

Some six million cabbage white butterflies, had tried to rest on the plants, and were in the process of being eaten.

I have a favorite spot, where I harvest sundew on an annual basis. A little goes a long way, but I find the mother tincture so much more valuable than the homeopathic preparations on the market. It is a wonderous place, with Elephant Head (Pedicularis) and other valuable herbs around a calcium-rich fen.

The Ojibwa call it **WAWIAE-NEEGAEGGUHNSH**, "round setting a-trap plant".

On the west coast, Haida peoples used this plant as a charm, and hence the name **TA7INAANG K'UUG** meaning, the heart of plenty. It was according to Nancy Turner, carried by hunters for luck.

The fresh juice has been used to remove warts, which is does, but be extremely careful as the juice is very caustic. It has also been used traditionally for curdling or clabbering milk, like nettles and cleavers.

In some Mediterranean countries, the sundew is fixed with brandy, raisins, and sugar and fermented into a cordial called **ROSSOLIS**. This is from the Latin **ROS SOLIS** meaning the dew of the sun.

In northern Russia, when the plant was somewhat plentiful, farmers used the plant in boiling water to disinfect their milk containers.

Today, in Europe, sundew *(D. rotundifolia)* is a protected species in nearly every country. The bogs of northern Finland are still used as a wild-crafted source by German homeopathic companies.

Charles Darwin was fascinated by the plant, and in 1875 published *Insectivorous Plants*. In the previous decade he observed, "At the moment I care more about Drosera than the origin of all the species of the world."

The Chinese have used sundew for headaches, dysentery and rheumatic pains, for thousands of years.

In India, the Vytans use drosera for reducing gold to powder. The fresh plants are ground to a paste, to cover a gold coin, and then enclosed in two small pieces of earthen pot cemented together with cloth and clay. When dry, the whole is place in a fire and thoroughly burnt. After cooling, the gold is found reduced to powder, and is given in grain doses as a tonic, and alterative in syphilitic conditions.

In Scotland, it was known as red rot, and Gaelic translates as very red dew or plant with shields, or sun-rose flower. The red color does not play a role in insect attraction.

The text *Regimen Sanitatis Salernitanum*, used by Gaelic herbalists in the 15th to 17th centuries recommended boiling the plant in milk for whooping cough.

In folklore, it was considered an aphrodisiac, and hence the medieval names like Youthwort or Lustwort.

Its traditional use in reproductive deficient conditions such as impotence, frigidity and amenorrhea should be more thoroughly explored.

In Traditional Chinese Medicine, these conditions are considered Kidney Yang deficient.

It has a long history of relieving morning sickness in pregnancy. However, due to the relative rarity, this plant should be protected and if used medicinally, the homeopathic form stretches a long way. Sundew is a uterine stimulant, contraindicated during pregnancy.

Work on the cultivation of sundew in Finland by Galambosi et al, showed that cultivated plants in peat beds yielded 50 times higher than in nature. The plants were fed milk powder, which increased growth by 27-113%. Up to 25 million plants a year are harvested in Finland, from the wild, for medicinal application.

At University of Craiova, Romania work on *in vitro* propagation found ferro-fluids (iron ions with oleic acid) stimulated the growth of shoots and roots, and enhanced peroxidase isoenzyme activity. Corneau et al, *Acta Hort* 1998 457.

Wowrosch et al, *Sci Pharm* 2009 77:4 found zeatin stimulated micro-propagation.

Great Sundew prefers the calcium rich, warm water fens of Alberta. At least that is where I find them in plenty. It hybridizes with *D. rotundifolia*, forming sterile plants.

MEDICINAL

CONSTITUENTS- *D. rotundifolia*- naphthaquinones (plumbagin [0.5%] and methyl-naphthazarin), hydroplumbagin, ramentaceone [7-methyl-juglone] (1.0-2.3% dry weight), various flavonoids including quercetin, isoquercetin, quercetin 3-O-galactoside (hyperoside), kaempferol, hyperoside and myricetin; quercitin-3-O-galactosylgalactoside, kaempferol 3-O-glucoside (astragalin), myricetin 3-O-galactoside, 3-chloroplumbagin, droserone (0.1%), hydroxydroserone, droserone 5-O-glucoside, droserin, hydroxydroserone-5-O-glycoside, ramenton 5-O-glycoside, ramentone, rossoliside, gossypin, gossypitrin, essential oils, anthocyanin, gossypin, carotenoids, alizarin, malic, formic, propionic, citric, gallic and butryic acids; various mineral salts including silicon, magnesium, calcium, iron, manganese, aluminum, phosphorus and sulphur; and various protelytic ferments (pepsin-like enzymes), beta-1,3-glucanase, and chitinase.
Endophytes- root- *Articulospora tetracladia, Tricoderma viride* and other fungi.
D. anglica- similar with plumbagin, and 3-chloroplumbagin; 5,8-dihydroxy-2-methyl-1,4-naphthoquinone; and 7-methyljuglone.
Glands- mucilage, digestive enzymes such as protease, esterase and acid phosphatase
Pollen- pollenkit (oil and protein)

Sundew herb is bitter, pungent, warm and sweet. It is relaxing to spasmodic coughs, and various respiratory conditions including whooping cough (specific), bronchitis, and asthma. It prevents acetylcholine or histamine-induced bronchospasms in clinical studies.

Work by Paper DH et al, *Phytother Res* 19(4): 323-6 found sundew possesses one-tenth the anti-inflammatory strength of hydrocortisone.

The herb is demulcent and expectorant, and appears to modify the vagus nerve, in some unproven manner.

It contains an antibiotic compound, plumbagin, effective against gram-positive *Streptococcus, Staphylococcus* and *Pneumococcus* species at low concentrations (1/50,000). It is also effective against gram-negative bacilli like *Salmonella*, certain pathogenic fungi and parasitic protozoa such as *Leishmania*.

Early work by Saint-Rat, Olivier and Chouteau (1946-47) found plumbagin partially inhibited *S. aureus, Streptococcus pyogenes* and *Pneumococcus* species at dilution of 1:500,000 and completely inhibited at 1:100,000.

The gram negative organisms *E. coli* and *Salmonella* typhi were inhibited at 1:10,000 while a tubercular bacillus (TB) was inhibited at 1:50,000.

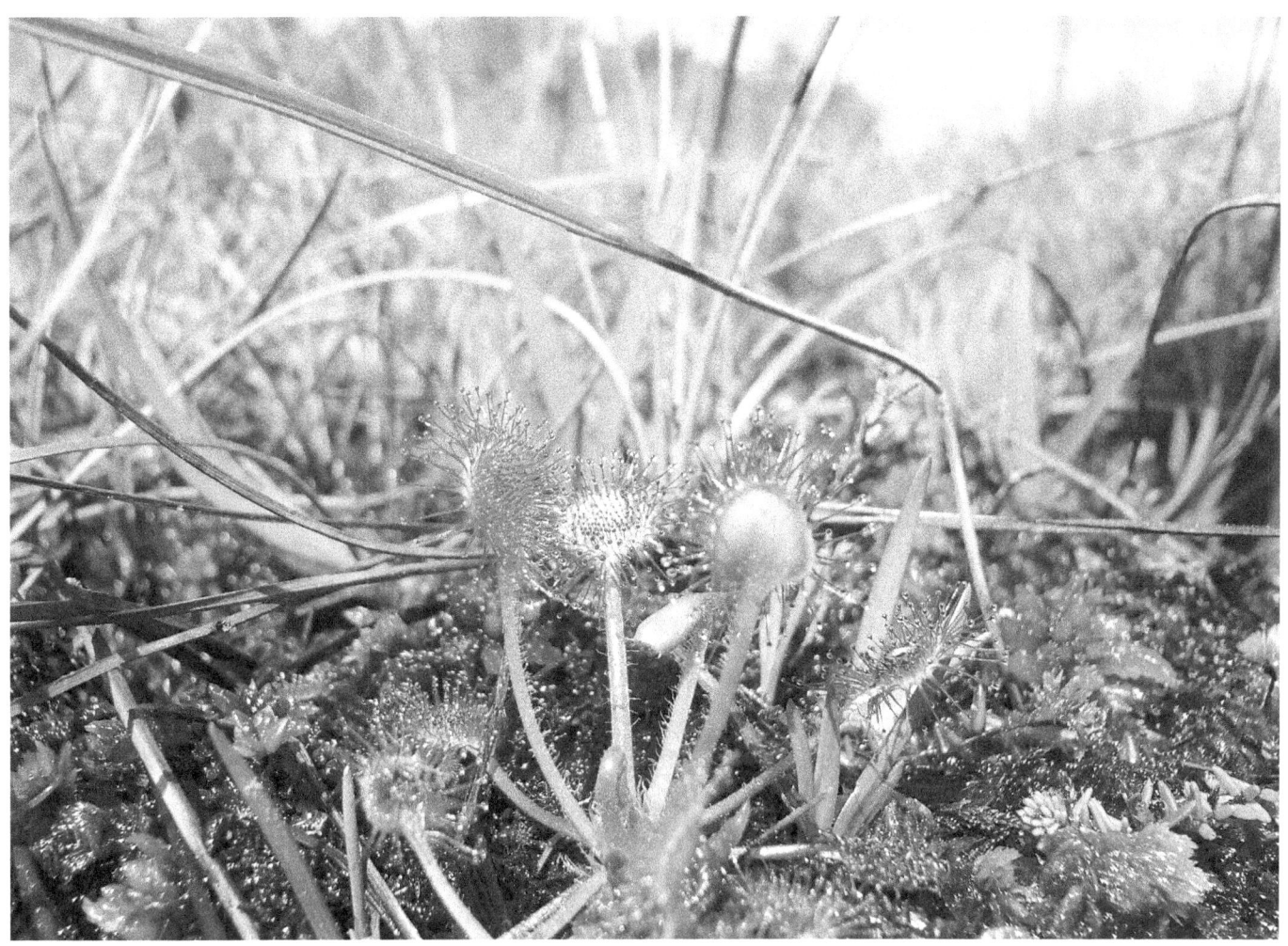

SUNDEW (*DROSERA ROTUNDIFOLIA*)

Dilutions of 1:50,000 completely inhibited *Coccidiodes immitis, Histoplasm capsulatum, Ctenomyces radicans* and *Trichophyton ferrugineum*.

Work by Towers et al, at UBC found the whole plant active against nine fungi tested.

At higher doses, of course, plumbagin is cytotoxic; one of the reasons that Venus Fly Trap, which has similar constituents, is used in treating cancer.

Devi et al, *Pharmaceutical Biology* 1999 37:3 found plumbagin is both anti-neoplastic; and in early tumor stages combines well with radiation, in both effectiveness and length of survival.

Kini et al, *Indian Journal of Exp Biol* 1997 35 related anti-tumor and anti-fertility activity to plumbagin.

Plumbagin inhibits the growth and invasion of prostate cancer. Aziz et al, *Cancer Res* 2008 68:21. It significantly reduced brain damage and neurological deficits in mice induced ischemic stroke. Son et al, *J Neurochem* 2010 112:5.

Sugie et al, *Cancer Letters* 1998 127 suggest some effect against intestinal tumors. Plumbagin may be useful in treatment of gastric cancer. Li J et al, *Altern Ther Health Med* 2017 at5382.

It prevents angiogenesis of liver carcinoma, reducing tumor growth. Wei Y et al, *Oncotarget* 2017 doi: 10. 18632/oncotarget. 14774.

Work by Kuete V et al, *BMC Pharmacol Toxicol* 2016 17(1):60 found the compound induced apoptosis in MCF-7 breast cancer cell lines.

Plumbagin inhibits thioredoxin reductase, which contributes to inducing apoptosis in HL-60 human promyelocytic leukemia cancer cells. Zhang J et al, *Arch Biochem Biophys* 2017 16L30558-6.

Plumbagin induces apoptotic and autophagic cell death in human non-small lung cancer cells, through inhibition of P13K/Akt/mTOR pathway. Li YC et al, *Cancer Lett* 2014 344(2): 239-59.

PUBMED lists over 500 studies on plumbagin. Work by Panichayupakaranant P and MI Ahmad, *Adv Exp Med Biol* 2016 929: 229-246, examines many recent studies on health benefits of plumbagin.

Naphthoquinones are not that common in nature. Pau d'arco from South America, is full of these compounds, and is used extensively in treating immune disorders, including cancer. Black walnut is rich in juglones that possess antifungal, antibacterial, antiviral and cytotoxic activity.

Sundew helps to repair genetic malfunctions, is anti-viral and enhances activity of antibiotics. A study conducted in Austria, 1994 looked at four dozen plants with vulnerary properties. Thirty-five of them showed anti-bacterial effect, while sundew, linden flower and oak bark were outstanding in their effect.

The combination of anti-spasmodic, and expectorating properties makes sundew invaluable in certain conditions, combining well with mullein, chokecherry bark, or wild licorice root. Sundew is useful for loss of voice, as both a gargle and ingested in small amounts. Sore throat, hoarseness and irritating throat tickles respond well to the herb.

It is bronchial-dilating, and also a true anti-tussive like chokecherry or wild lettuce.

Because the anti-spasmodic properties show themselves only in small doses, it seems likely that some form of catalytic or enzymatic action is involved. It has a vitamin K-like effect that assists the anti-spasmodic action in treating whooping cough.

It is likely that the naphthoquinone compounds are not responsible for anti-spasmodic activity, but perhaps the flavonoids hyperoside, quercitin and isoquercitin play a role. In one study on guinea pig ileum the antispasmodic activity is thought due to affecting an allosteric binding site of the muscarinic M3 receptors. Krenn L et al, *Arzneimittelforschung* 2004 54(7): 402-5; Kolodziej H et al, *Pharmazie* 2002 57(3): 201-3. Both 7-methyl juglone and plumbagin are moderate calcium channel blockers. Neuhaus-Carlisle K et al, *Phytomedicine* 1997 4(1): 67-71.

Gossypin inhibits mast cell-derived allergic reactions, suggesting another mode of action with sundew. Ganapaty S et al, *Ind J Biochem Biophys* 2010 47(2): 90-5.

Ramentaceone induced apoptosis in breast cancer cells, particularly for HER2-positive form. Kawiak A & E. Lojkowska, *PLoS One* 2016 11(2). It also induced apoptosis in human leukemia HL-60 cells. Kawiak A et al, *J Nat Prod* 2012 75(1):9-14.

Ramentaceone (7-methyljuglone) is anti-bacterial, anti-fungal, anti-cancer, anti-tubercular, anti-viral and anti-inflammatory. Mbaveng AT & V. Kuete, *Afr Health Sci* 2014 14(1): 201-5.

The compound is active against *Mycobacterium bovis*. McGaw LJ et al, *Biol Pharm Bull* 2008 31(7): 1429-33. In combination with isoniazid or rifampicin, the compound showed a four to six fold reduction against strains of *M. tuberculosis*. Bapela NB et al, *Phytomedicine* 2006 13(9-10): 630-5.

Gossypitrin is found in the yellow petals of Iceland Poppy, used in that country for its sedation, pain relief and insomnia.

The herb inhibits sympathetic nervous system hyperactivity, and eases vomiting, nausea and diarrhea associated with whooping cough.

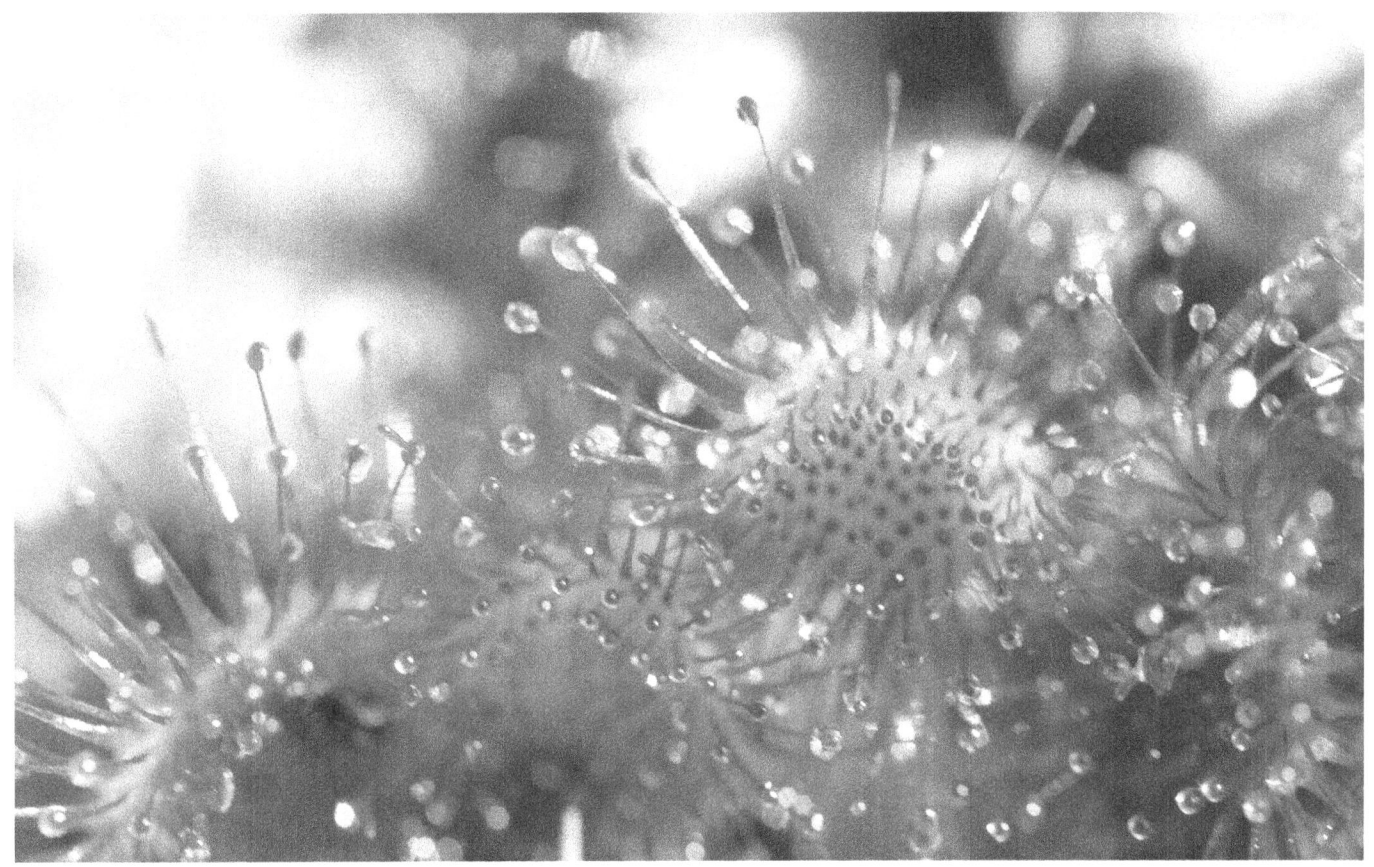

SUNDEW

Drosera rotundifolia suppresses activation of human mast cell inflammation induced by T cell membranes. Fukushima K. et al, *J Ethnopharmacology* 2009 125(1): 90-6.

It is useful juice to use externally on warts, bunions and corns, but be careful of the surrounding tissue! It is also a remedy for stomach ulcers, having a soothing effect on the gastric mucous membrane.

It combines well with gumweed and seneca root for asthma. It may be considered to possess warm, sweet energetics that remove toxins and clear heat.

Sundew combines well with cleavers or red root in the treatment of lymphadenitis, including scrofula. Although Sundew is contra-indicated, by some practitioners, in chronic tuberculosis, it can be useful in tuberculous adenitis, which is generally related to cervical lymph node involvement, and not uncommon in children.

It has tonic effect on arteriosclerosis and lowers cholesterol levels; but is contraindicated in low blood pressure.

The herbal tincture is much more effective if combined with colloidal silica (silica gel) in cases of arteriosclerosis, according to Grieve, in *A Modern Herbal*. This combination is said to reduce calcium and plaque build up on arteries, thickened with age.

It may be helpful in angina pain, helping improve arterial vascular spasms.

The plant is mildly hypoglycemic and diuretic; and will turn the urine dark- a harmless side effect not fully understood.

Pollenkit is a mixture of protein and oil that coats the pollen grains. The production of oil is expensive to plants, so it must serve an important function, possibly as an adhesive. Studies have shown the pollenkit has an individual fragrance, different from the rest of the flower.

HOMEOPATHY

This is the specific remedy for all spasmodic coughs that resemble whooping cough. The symptoms are dry and irritating and the patient can hardly breathe. The cough is deep and hoarse, and generally worse after midnight, lying down, talking, drinking, laughing or singing. There may be blood from nose or mouth.

There is often a sensation in the throat like a feather tickling, or a crumb of bread that is stuck. Some children are fine during the day, but begin to cough when their head hits the pillow at night.

Sundew also gives mild relief to gnawing, stinging pains in the hip or sciatic nerve. There may be dizziness in the open air, with a tendency to fall to the left. And the left side of the face may be cold, with a stinging pain and dry heat on the right.

Chills with hot face, cold hands, not thirst and cold feeling even covered up in bed.

Restless and anxious, full of mistrust. Imagines being deceived by spiteful, envious people; as if he enemies would not leave him quiet, envied and persecuted him.

DOSE- First to 12th potency. The mother tincture is made from the freshly extracted juice at beginning of flower; equal parts juice and alcohol. Hahnemann did first proving with five people.

PLANT OIL

A fresh plant carrier oil is extremely useful for wound healing. Like comfrey gel, it helps knit wounds, due to viscous and elastic properties, in a relatively short time.

It increases adhesion of fibroblast and smooth muscle cells, due to enhanced absorption of serum proteins.

MATERIA POETICA

Drosera, you are tubercular
With a restless energy
A cough that comes in spasms
A whoop where noses bleed
No wonder you're suspicious
Yourself, a trap for flies
They sit upon you innocent
No chance for sweet goodbyes
Persecuted in your head
A ghost could rise up from the dead
And much like Cinderella
Midnight is your foe
This time of night knows no relief
As all your problems grow
The restlessness and hoarseness
Bone pains that you so grieve
The chilliness and barking
So difficult to breathe
You'd better stop the talking
It causes wear and tear
I suggest you go out walking
You're gonna want some air.

SYLVIA CHATROUX

HYDROSOL

The distilled water thereof in wine is held fit and profitable for ...those that have a salt rheum distilling on their lungs...which water will be of a good yellow colour. The same water is held to be good for all other diseases of the lungs, as phthisicks, wheezings, shortness of breath, or cough; as also to heal the ulcers that happen in the lungs; and it comforts the heart and fainting spirits.   **CULPEPPER**

FLOWER ESSENCES

Round leafed Sundew (*D. rotundifolia*) flower essence is for relinquishing identification with the ego. It is letting go of the resistance to change to create a blending of ego and divine will.   **ALASKA**

Sundew flower essence can be used by both men and women for similar purpose.

Often times there is a turning away, or rejection of the feminine, and at the same time an aggravation of the masculine with inappropriate expressions of anger similar to symptoms of the Holly essence, developed by Dr. Bach.

It is specifically for those who find discomfort in the throat chakra due to fear they will be misunderstood or confronted on their beliefs.   **PRAIRIE DEVA**

Sundew strengthens us to focus on the task at hand. It helps us be less affected by distractions, supports us in staying calm, constant and centered. It could be helpful in some ADHD situations. It can also assist in cases of deviant behaviour, helping break the patterns of seeking attention by misbehaving.   **NETTLES AND MORE**

SPIRITUAL PROPERTIES

Sundew helps us understand how thought forms and viruses interrelate. Negative thought forms allow the entry and growth of viruses in the body.

Medically, sundew relieves both viral and negative thought form, in a manner similar to the plant working with insects.

When it captures an insect, there is gradual absorption. There is not an instantaneous or rapid motion like the Venus Fly Trap. The individual absorbs the lessons behind the negative thought form so it is understood, not simply released.

In most cases, there will be an easing of the problem, with lung difficulties symbolically related to deeper emotions.

It is these negative thought forms that affect our judgment, our misunderstanding of others, and our inability to forgive.

With Sundew, the third eye, or pineal gland, is opened. There is a sense of emotional attachment or sadness that is part of the process of dispelling negative thought form as the energy of sundew is absorbed.

Negative aspects of Pluto are released with the use of this herb.   **GURUDAS**

PERSONALITY TRAITS

Carnivorous plants have taken the unusual but not unique step of traversing the boundary between kingdoms. They live like a plant but feed like an animal. The consequence for the plant is they get both the best of both worlds and the worst of both worlds. Being hunters like animals, they are not dependent on the soil in their immediate area for nutrition and that is a plus. However, being a plant, they are stationary and must hunt from one spot, necessitating cunning.

Naturally the co-mingling of plant and animal comes through in the symptoms of these plants. Animal kingdom qualities are evident such as envy, suspicion, hatred, evil, violence, feelings of being surrounded by enemies, feeling persecuted, feeling of being maltreated, poisoned or abused by others and that one has done wrong or committed a crime. Most interesting, there are dreams of animals or insects. The person's manner of talking will also be infused with some animal energy of being animated, excited, anxious and loquacious. This can be expected to be the case since insects are an integral part of the life of these plants. **VERMEULEN**

RECIPES

INFUSION- Take one to two grams of dried herb to one pint of hot water. Steep 20 minutes. Drink one to four cups in divided doses; or thicken with honey for a useful cough syrup.

Note: The dried herb is not as useful and loses up to 60% of its activity within 30 months. Better to use fresh and immediately in below forms.

SUCCUS- Combine three parts of fresh plant juice to one part vodka. Use externally for warts and other skin blemishes.

PLANT OIL- combine one part by weight of fresh sundew (washed) with five parts of a good mono-unsaturated oil in a low temperature crock pot for four to six hours. Strain and press well. Use externally as needed.

TINCTURE- The entire fresh plant is gathered in prime and pounded to a pulp. The juice is added to an equal part of 40% alcohol and allowed to stand for one week. Strain.

Or make an extract from the fresh plant of 1:2 at 50% alcohol. Michael Moore noted that trying to wash Sundew is like trying to wash off a huge, wet Gummi Bear covered with sand.

Use 3-6 drops in water or a spoonful of honey up to six times daily. Do not use at the terminal stage of any severe lung disease or low blood pressure. A harmless side effect is a dark brown discoloration of urine after long use.

It is interesting to note that *D. rotundifolia*, *D. intermedia* and *D. anglica*, are rarely used today due to the threat of extinction in Europe. In fact, they are strictly protected in Germany. I feel fortunate to have such an abundance in my part of the boreal forest.

Drosera species from Australia, such as *D. ramentacea* and *D. peltata* are substituted, but contain only half the activity of *D. rotundifolia*.

CAUTION- Do not use during pregnancy, or with low blood pressure. Many books warn against its use in tuberculosis. I don't agree.

DUCKWEED
LESSER DUCKWEED
(***Lemna minor*** L.)
IVY LEAVED DUCKWEED
STAR DUCKWEED
(***L. trisulca*** L.)
LARGER DUCKWEED
GREATER DUCKWEED
COMMON DUCKMEAT
(***L. polyrrhiza*** [L.]) not accepted
(***Spirodela polyrrhiza*** [L.] Schleid)
PARTS USED- whole plant

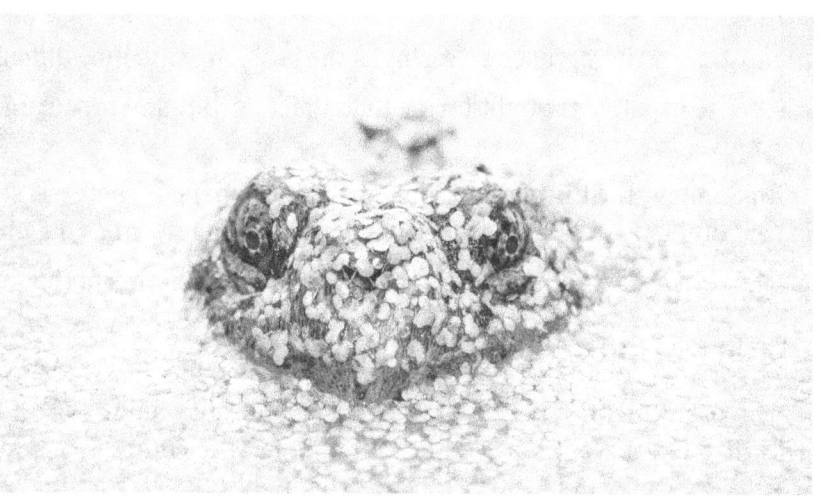

DUCKWEED AND FROG

Springtime; the pond is deep and wide.
I wait while the little boat returns.
Like a blizzard, Duckweeds close around.
A trailing Willow branch parts them again.

BUDDHIST POEM

Apparently, the pathfinder duck is a psychological archetype in certain cultures. **MICHAEL LEUNIG**

Of the more than 300,000 known flowering plants, duckweed is the smallest and simplest. The single stamen male and pinpoint female flower are difficult to find, due to their diminutive size.

Lemna is from the Greek **LIMNOS** meaning lake. Trisulca means three forked and polyrrhiza means many roots.

It floats on the surface of ponds, often mistaken for algae. In England, it was known as Ginny Greenteeth, a fairy-like inhabitant of the ponds that would drag in unwary children.

It does have distinct sexes, although it reproduces rapidly and efficiently by asexual budding. A single square foot of duckweed can completely cover five acres of water in only two months!

Like algae, it is super nutritious. The crude protein content is nearly 40%, twice that of alfalfa, and with a higher percentage of lysine and arginine.

The tea infusion is urine colored but tastes like corn silk and possesses diuretic activity.

Natives like the Iroquois mixed Ivy Duckweed with Chickweed, and applied them together for skin swellings. Various native tribes would not drink from duckweed-covered water, believing it would cause an itchy rash of the arms and hands.

In issue of *American Scientist* July/August 1978, a duckweed/dairy farm concept was proposed. In theory, one hundred cows produce 4.5 tons of manure daily. This is fermented and the methane extracted is used as a fuel. The residue is pumped to a series of lagoons totaling ten acres. The authors calculate that the total yield of duckweed is 4.8 tons, supplying 60% of the cow's protein requirements.

Harvey and Fox (1973) calculated that 4-5 hectares of duckweed would provide enough feed for up to 30,000 hens for 6-8 months.

It provides 5 to 6 times more starch than corn per acre.

Duckweed might be used to advantage in salvaging chemical waste from industry. It concentrates ten times more boron than other aquatic plants; up to 0.64mg boron/gram dry weight with no symptoms of boron toxicity.

It also concentrates aluminum. In one study conducted in California, the toxic mineral was 660,000 times higher concentration in the pond without duckweed.

Several laboratory studies have shown that duckweed can absorb up to 4000 ppm (dry weight) of zinc, 6714 ppm of copper, 1.33% cadmium and 0.47% silver.

It shows a high ability to remove uranium and thorium from tailing ponds. Sasmaz M et al, *Bull Environ Contam Toxicol* 2016 97(6):832-7.

A study at the University of Minnesota, found duckweed removed 76% of lead and 82% of nickel, suggesting use in bio-remediation of heavy metal contaminated waterways.

Work by Gallardo et al, in Florida studies, found duckweed removed 97% of lead after one week of exposure. *J Envir Sci Health* 2002 37:8. Jain et al, Bio Wastes 1989 28 found duckweed removed both copper and iron from water, with the latter mineral actually increasing copper concentration in the plants.

It can help remove nitrogen and phosphorus from water, even under certain levels of salt stress. Liu C et al, *J Environ Manage* 2017 187:497-503.

It will phyto-remediate boron. Turker OC et al, *J Hazard Mater* 2017 324(Pt B):151-9.

Government leaders in Wuhan, China, one of the hottest cities along the Yangtze River, have introduced duckweed into the lakes. It is believed the plant will be able to decrease the relative humidity. The dried herb is then burned to help drive off mosquitoes.

In parts of China, duckweed is released into ponds to kill off algae blooms, before releasing carp.

Gerald Leather has used the small plant to detect the herbicidal action of allelopathic chemicals in minute amounts.

Using a test, Leather can trace the impact of a natural herbicide on duckweed in amounts as small as a few parts per billion.

Many years later, his duckweed assays are used in industrial and academic labs throughout the world.

One plant patent for *S. polyrrhiza* was issued in China in 1989, for a shampoo to promote hair growth. This may be due to the plant signature of rootlets hanging down in tangled masses, or may actually work by some obscure biological activity.

MEDICINAL

CONSTITUENTS- *L. minor-* 40% protein, including high levels of arginine and lysine; manganese, iron, titanium, copper, radium, and cobalt. Ash yields bromine and iodine. Other unusual components are lycopersene, luteolin-7-beta-D-gluco-pyranoside, digitoxose, apiose (apiogalacturonan); 1, 3-phyadiene, 4R-hydroxy-iso-phytol, and 10R-hydroxyhexadeca and hexadeca-7Z, 10Z,13Z-trienoic acids.
The plant contains a variety of flavonoids including C-glucosyl-flavonone, orientin, isoorientin, isoscorparin, vitexin, isovitexin, lutonarin, vicenin-1, and apigenin-7-0-glucoside; cardenolides (cardiac steroids), lemnan, cyclopentane fatty acids resembling prostaglandin, and apio-galacturonans. Two percent of the whole fresh plant is extractable into solvents.
S. polyrrhiza- 18-25% protein, various C27 and C29 hydrocarbons, feruloyl and sinapoyl glucose, malonyl cyanidin 3-0-glucoside, coumaroyl and caffeoylquinic acids; lycopersene, stigmasterol, daucosterol, squalene, norspermine, norspermidine, homo-spermine, caldopentamine, potassium acetate, potassium chloride, iodine, bromine, flavones including orientin, isoorientin, luteolin-7-mono-glucoside, vitexin, isovitexin, apigenin-7-monoglucoside, malonylcyanidin-7-mon-glucoside, rutin; various organic acids including linolenic, palmitic and linoleic acids, beta carotene, lutein, epoxyluteine, violaxanthin, neoxanthin, albumins, glutelins.

Energetically, duckweed is a cold and decongesting plant. It affects the lungs and is useful in all external heat conditions, including fever, skin disease and rash. It is useful for fluid swellings, and hot, superficial edema; especially of the upper body. It can be applied both externally/ internally for bee stings.

In China, it has been used medicinally for water retention, scurvy, syphilis, and externally for eye diseases. In Mandarin, Larger duckweed is known as *FU PING*; and in Cantonese the similar *FAU PING.* Lesser Duckweed is known as **QING PING.**

In their interesting book, the Wild Plant Companion, Kathryn and Andrew March suggest:

"Ping is graphically and probably entomologically derived from another Ping that means 'level, calm or peace', and is well suited to poetry. Chinese poets have been fascinated by its rootlessness, the springtime equivalent of autumn's leaf in the wind and its prime image of what life sometimes seems: beautiful but helpless, adrift down the seasons and years in a Buddhist insubstantiality."

Jeanne Rose suggests that duckweed is a specific for the nose, and can eaten to improve the sense of taste and smell.

Hildegard of Bingen prepared a duckweed elixir that contained tormentil, field mustard (*Sinapsis arvensis*), cleavers (*Galium aparine*), duckweed and other herbs in a honey wine extract.

This was taken before breakfast and bedtime for three months as a pre-cancer therapy; or for post-operative treatment to prevent recurrence of breast tumours.

Isoorientin and isoscoparin flavonoids inhibit adipogenesis and may be useful therapeutic agents for prevention and treatment of obesity. Poudel B et al, *Mol Med Rep* 2015 12(2):3139-45.

Lutonarin, isoorientin, orientin and isovitexin exhibit neuraminidase inhibition. This compound is one of the key enzymes responsible for bacterial infection and pathogenesis. Their addition as food and additives may be useful for human health. Park MJ et al, *Nat Prod Commun* 2014 9(10):1469-72.

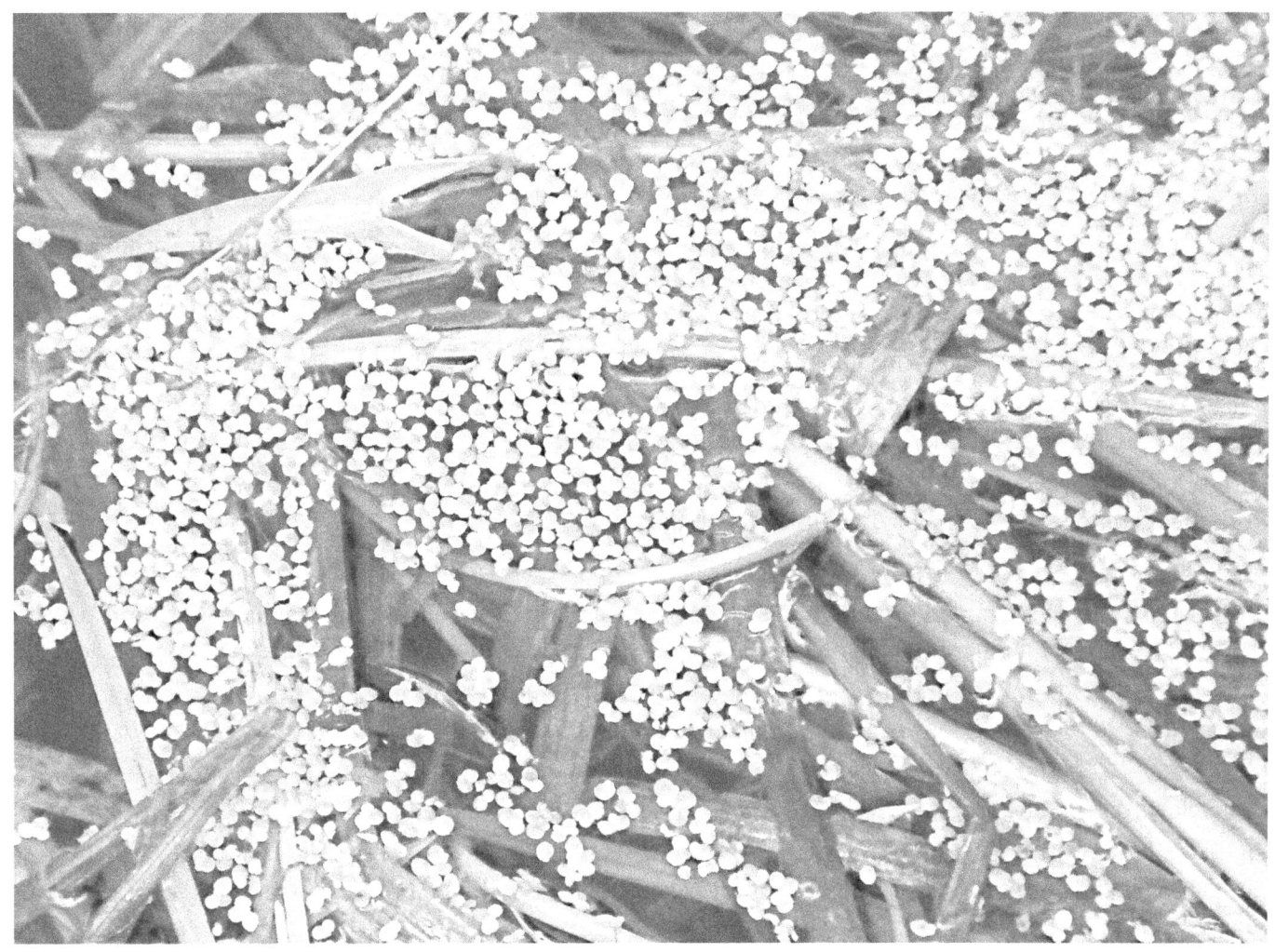

DUCKWEED

Isoorientin, vitexin, isovitexin and vicenin-2 show anti-inflammatory, anti-diarrheal and spasmolytic activity. Anzoise ML et al, *J Ethnopharm* 2016 194:137-45. This suggests benefit in colitis, or inflammatory bowel disease. Passion flower leaves contain similar flavonoids. Vicenin-2 appears to exhibit anti-spasmodic effect on gut health only when spasms are present. Verspohl EJ et al, *Phytomedicine* 2013 20(5): 427-31.

Vicenin-2 may help accelerate healing of diabetic foot ulcers. Muhammad AA et al, *Drug Des Devel Ther* 2016 10:1715-30. It also appears to be useful for reducing vascular inflammation and progression of atherosclerosis in diabetic patients. Ku SK & Bae JS, *Can J Physio Pharmacol* 2016 94(3):287-95.

It is a novel anti-coagulant, and possesses anti-thrombotic activity. Lee W & Bae JS, *Blood Coagul Fibrinolysis* 2015 26(6):628-34.

Orientin and vicenin, also present in holy basil, protects normal tissue against radiation injury. Baliga MS et al, *J Cancer Res Ther* 2016 12(1):20-7.

Vicenin-2 is synergistic with docetaxel in androgen independent prostate cancer. Nagaprashantha LD et al, *Biochem Pharmacol* 82(9):1100-9.

In Italy, the whole plant is roasted and applied to burns. I simply apply the fresh plant poultice, or previously frozen juice.

Lonicerus used duckweed to relieve symptoms of St. Anthony's fire, caused by ergoty rye.

Larger Duckweed (*S. polyrrhiza*) has cold, acrid properties useful for promoting perspiration and stimulating measles or chicken pox rash to come to surface, combining well with wild Mint and Burdock seed. It can be used in arthralgia due to damp wind, as well as erysipelas, macula and edema, helping to promote water metabolism and remove toxins. It possesses mild cardiotonic, diuretic and anti-pyretic effects. *Zhong Yao Xue* 1998 108:109. Water extracts possess a cardiotonic effect in lab studies. At high dosage, it eliminates cardiac diastole, and constricts blood vessels that raise blood pressure.

Hildegard de Bingen wrote over 800 years ago that duckweed would "reduce the useless fluids within a man." Li Shi Zhen suggests it is aligned with the yin meridian of the lungs as related to acupuncture, and associated with coughs, sore throat and pain on the front inside of arms and shoulders.

It combines well with puncture vine, forsythyia fruit and burdock seed for fever and headache from common cold.

It is used in acute cases of nephritis, hemorrhagic purpurea and urticaria in doses of 3-10 grams of dried herb in decoctions. When used in decoction combinations, add only during last five minutes to preserve potency.

Larger Duckweed contains stigmasterol and squalene that can be extracted by supercritical carbon dioxide. Both these compounds have a ready nutraceutical market.

Lycopersene exhibits anti-bacterial activity. Li JL et al, *Chin J Nat Med* 2015 13(4):307-10.

The related *L. gibba* contains a protein that is reactive in somatostatin release inhibiting factor immunoassays. Lesser Duckweed contains lemnan, composed of pectic polysaccharides with two-thirds galacturonic acid.

Lemnan exhibits immune modulation, and may be useful as an adjuvant for oral immunization. Odo et al, *Bioorg Khim* 2000 26:10; Popov et al, *Immunopharm Immunotox* 2006 28:1.

Lemnan, when combined with glycerol, helped preserve the integrity of human white blood cells at temperatures well below freezing. Khudyakov AN et al, *Biopreserv Biobank* 2015 13(4):240-6.

Duckweed (L. minor) is a fast, inexpensive and reproducible model plant system for the study of host-pathogen interactions, and large scale screening for discovery of new anti-microbial plant constituents. Zhang Y et al, *PLoS One* 2010 5(10):e13527.

HOMEOPATHY

Lemna minor (Duckweed) is a catarrhal remedy acting especially on the nostrils; where there are polyps, swellings or atrophic rhinitis. Asthma, exaggerated by nasal obstruction and made worse by wet weather may also be helped.

There may be attendant loss of smell, with a great deal of mucous discharge. There may be reflex pain from the nose to the ear; with a dry throat and mouth.

The abdomen may have disposition to noisy diarrhea.

DOSE- Third to thirtieth potency. The mother tincture is prepared from the fresh plant.

PLANT OILS

Ivy Duckweed contains 92mg/100 grams dry weight of lipids. This is composed of 31.4% neutral lipids, 42.4% glycolipids, and 26.3% phospholipids.

The phospholipids break down as follows: 36% phosphatylcholine, 20% phosphatidyl-ethanolamine, 16% phosphatidyl-glycerol, and minor amounts of phosphatidyl-serine. Fatty acid composition is 28% linolenic acid, 24% linoleic acid, and others.

Common Duckweed (*L. minor*) contains 88 mg/ 100 grams dry weight of total lipds, including 29% neutral lipids, 30% glycolipids, and 40% phospholipids.

The latter breaks down to 41% phosphatidylcholine, 3.1% phosphatidylserine, and others.

HYDROSOL

The distilled water by some is highly esteemed against all inward inflammations and pestilent fevers; as also to help the redness of the eyes, and swellings of privities, and of the breasts before they be grown to much.

CULPEPPER

FLOWER ESSENCE

Duckweed is the world's smallest flower essence, and was prepared from Lac St. Anne waters.

Duckweed is for those individuals who choose not to take time to care for themselves. The day-to-day rush pushes them further from a true sense of fulfillment and knowing. It seems that time is moving exponentially, with no way out of the "time warp" and exaggerated pace.

Duckweed flower essence instills the importance of self—particularly to those in the healing profession. It protects by allowing detached involvement; and the empowerment that brings.

PRAIRIE DEVA

PERSONALITY TRAITS

Hailed as the smallest of flowering plants, the Duckweed is a tiny aquatic dweller whose plant body may measure no more than ⅕th of an inch across.

Yet, the tiny duckweed is capable of mighty feats. A carpet of it on the surface of a lake absorbs heavy metal contaminants, and cleanses excess phosphorus and nitrogen wastes from runoff in farm areas.

Duckweed incorporates these substances into its body's biomass, thereby helping its population to expand. When the Duckweed population grows too large- threatening to steal light and nutrients from other vegetation- the tiny plants can be skimmed off.

When you're small- be it in size or stature- many avenues may seem closed to you. You may downsize your dreams, trim your expectations, or undervalue your contributions. Don't fall into that trap. You can accomplish wonders through focus and persistence. Over time, the fruits of your efforts will multiply to yield a luxuriant carpet of achievement.

G. MOHAMMED

Duckweed is a floating plant with a single round leaf, as thin as paper and no wider than a pencil eraser. It spends its winter alive at the bottom of my frozen pond, feeding on its own stored starch.

One buzzy May Day, it pops up as if arriving for an appointment, and then, to put it mildly, it multiplies.

In a matter of weeks, it has stretched a living lid of lime-green leaves across every square inch of water surface… En masse, duckweed spreads an impressive solar array- one plant, a mere quarter of an inch across, can multiply through the sheer energy of sunlight to cover an area the size of a football field in a couple of months…This spasm of photosynthesis- sunlight transformed into acres of green tissue before my eyes- is more than just my nemesis. It's a miracle.

BENYUS

Duckweed floats on the water, its body is lightweight and its qi is floating…the ancients said that its ability to induce sweating is superior to Ephedra…it is all because its body floats, so it can expel wind, because its nature is cold, so it overcomes heat, because it grows on top of water, so it is able to use water to facilitate the flow of urine.

MYTHS AND LEGENDS

In China, a pair of mandarin ducks is often kept as a symbol of faithful, committed love. In modern *Feng Shui*, ceramic mandarin ducks are set facing each other to attract love, or side by side facing the same direction to indicate a lasting relationship.

EASON

RECIPES

DRIED PLANT- 3-6 grams as needed

DECOCTION- 10-20 grams. If using the fresh herb add to decoction of other herbs at the end.

TINCTURE- 2-4 ml. A 1:2 ratio is made from the fresh plant at 70% alcohol.

CAUTION- Duckweed is contra-indicated in those individuals with spontaneous sweating or suffering blood or qi deficiency. It should be used with caution in those patients without intense or excess heat.

ELEPHANT HEAD
LITTLE RED ELEPHANT
(*Pedicularis groenlandica* Retz.)
(*Elephantella groenlandica* [Retz.] Rydb.) not accepted
WESTERN LOUSEWORT
BRACTED LOUSEWORT
(*P. bracteosa* Benth.)
COMMON LOUSEWORT
BEEFSTEAK PLANT
(*P. canadensis* Hadac.)
(*P. canadensis* L.)
CONTORTED LOUSEWORT
(*P. contorta* Benth.)
ALPINE LOUSEWORT
ARCTIC RATTLE
(*P. arctica*) not accepted
(*P. langsdorfii* **ssp.** *arctica* [R. Br.] Pennell)
HEAD SHAPED LOUSEWORT
CAPITATE LOUSEWORT
(*P. capitata* M. F. Adams)
SICKLE TOP LOUSEWORT
LEAFY LOUSEWORT
PARROT'S-BEAK
(*P. racemosa* Douglas ex Benth.)
WOOLLY LOUSEWORT
(*P. lanata* Cham & Schltdl.)
(*P. wildenowii* Vved.) not accepted
LABRADOR LOUSEWORT
(*P. labradorica* Wirsing)
(*P. euphrasioides* Stephan ex Willd.) not accepted
SWAMP LOUSEWORT
SMALL FLOWER LOUSEWORT
(*P. parviflora* Sm.)
PARTS USED- leaf, flower, root

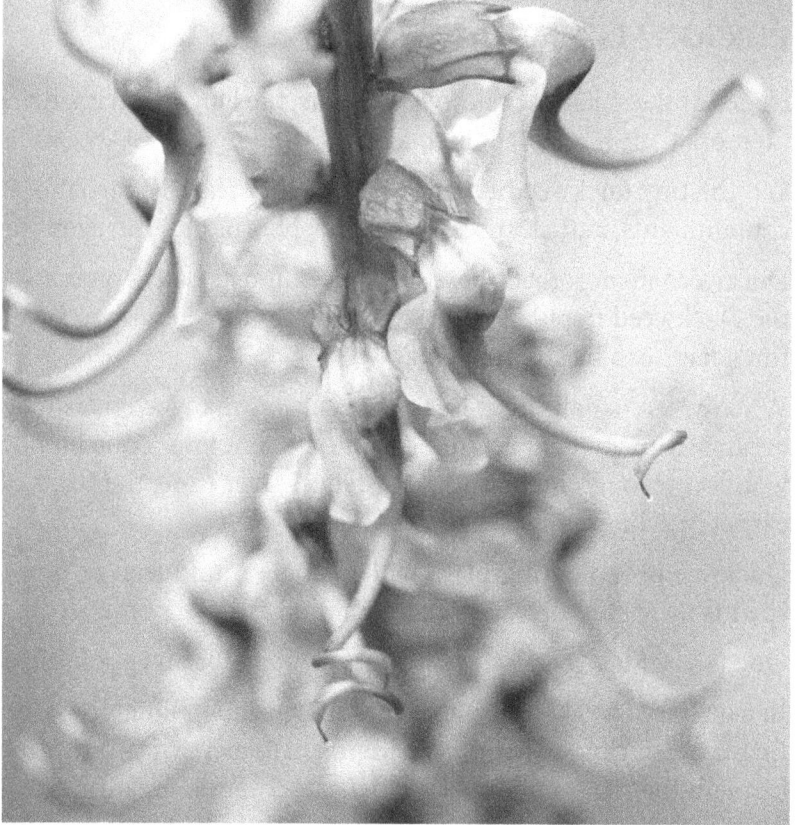

ELEPHANT HEAD CLOSE UP

Lousewort stems back to the 17th century and is related to the overgrazed fields supported weak, lice-ridden cattle. Various folk stories suggest the plants breed lice, keep them away, the seeds look like lice, the leaves look like they are filled with lice, and if livestock eat them they become infested with lice. Take your pick.

Pedicularis is Latin meaning, little louse.

Some plants, like Elephant Head, are found in alpine swamps, or generally with wet feet.

Others, like Sickle Top Lousewort, are found under spruce, or on alpine slopes, near conifers.

All the plants appear at first glance, to be dressed in thick woolly parkas.

The plants can sometimes be parasitic, and that can lend a problem to plant constituents and actions.

Sometimes Elephant Head, or Western Lousewort is parasitic on Ragwort (*Senecio* spp.), tapping into the toxic pyrrolizidine alkaloid senecionine of that plant. These should not be used.

Other times, Sickle Top Lousewort (*P. racemosa*) is parasitic on Engelmann spruce, and when dark purple, the foliage is very rich in pinidinol, a piperidine alkaloid. Or it can be parasitic at lower elevations on Silver Lupine (*Lupinus argenteus*), and accumulates toxic quinolizidine alkaloids.

Western Lousewort favors pine and spruce forests, and will pick up pinidinol from the hosts. These should also be avoided.

The rule of thumb is to see if the plants are autonomous, or if parasitic, on something rather benign. Otherwise, you can get unpredictable results, similar to that experienced by dodder.

In southern Alberta, the lousewort may tap into Golden Bean (*Thermopsis rhombifolia*) that contains anagyrine and N-methylcytisine, quinolizidine alkaloids and should be avoided.

Western Lousewort growing near *Senecio triangularis* contains senecionine, but is absent in areas outside that plant's range.

Various *Thermopsis* species are used in Russia as a natural source of cytisine.

These are active compounds responsible for the effect on uterine tissue present in Blue Cohosh. Anagyrine is present in lupine and Genista species, and is toxic, teratogenic; and yet surprisingly, a cardiac tonic.

The best advice is to use the plants free standing, and get to know your local variations.

Arctic Rattle, or Alpine Lousewort, is called **SAH TILEH** by the Slave of the boreal forest. The roots were eaten raw in times of hunger.

Head Shaped Lousewort (*P. capitata*) root was used as a trap lure for lynx and hence the name **NOTA NAYDI**, or lynx medicine. Maybe, or is the term in reference to an animal totem or medicine?

The Inuit of Baffin Island call it **KUKIUJAIT**. The long, banana-like flowers were pulled off and eaten.

Woolly Lousewort, known as **USSUSAQ** to the Inuit, is probably the second most important survival food in the alpine and arctic regions, after Alpine bistort.

The sweet, juicy, lemon-yellow roots can be boiled, baked, or stir-fried as they were by various native tribes. The stems, when small can be used as a potherb.

Inuit children suck the sweet nectar from the blossoms. In winter, the frozen, fermented greens were mixed with Sedum and served with seal oil and sugar, as a type of dessert.

The Inupiat, according to Janice Schofield, pick the flowering top and place them in a barrel, covered with water. These are fermented like sauerkraut.

Small pieces of the sun-dried root are mixed with tobacco and smoked in a pipe to relieve headaches, by the Dene and other northern groups. Other tribes dried and smoked the flowers and buds.

The fresh or dried roots are boiled to make a yellow dye for moose hides.

Elephant's Head (*P. groenlandica*) is known as Red Medicine, by the Cheyenne. For coughs, the patient drank a long brewed infusion of the pulverized leaves and stems.

Wood Betony (*P. bracteosa*) was used by the Nlaka'pamux of British Columiba as a pattern for their basket designs.

Common Lousewort (*P. canadensis*) was infused and drunk traditionally for swelling internally, stomach troubles, coughs, and bloody stools.

It was used by native tribes as a love medicine, to bring couples back together, or as an aphrodisiac by the Ojibwa. For this, the plant was chopped finely and put in the spouse's food to spark new interest. Likewise, it was used, by other indigenous tribes, as bad medicine to conjure, and cast evil spells. Gregory Tilford, a fellow member of the *American Herbalist Guild*, speculates that the aphrodisiac property may be due to mild irritation of the urinary tract by the herb. Both the Onondaga and Cayuga of the Iroquois nation called it **GWE'DIS**.

The Cherokee used Common Lousewort to de-louse dogs, or sheep.

It was an early green for soups. The chopped root was given to horses, to make them vicious to all except the owner.

As one author put it. "It's a good thing there was a natural order to these things…the only possible thing worse than a vicious girlfriend would be an amorous horse."

The Iroquois made a decoction taken to vomit for stomachaches caused by menstruation. An infusion of the root was used for heart troubles.

The Mohegan, and other tribes used leaf infusions to induce abortion.

In parts of the former USSR, the leaves are infused to make tea.

In early English herbals by Culpepper, *Pedicularis species* were boiled in wine, to cure ulcers.

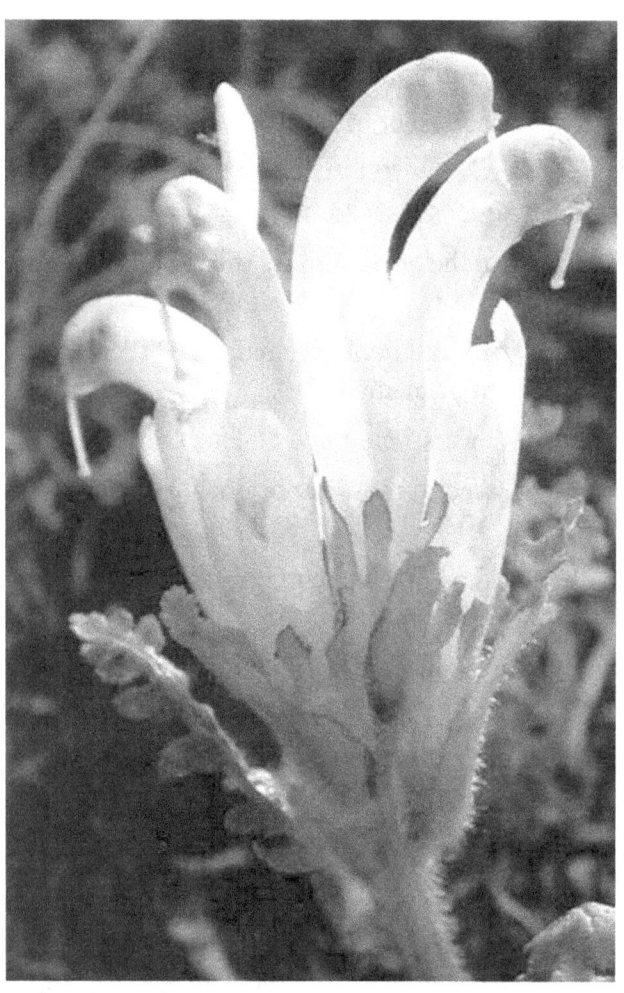

PEDICULARIS CAPITATA

The related *P. palustris*, or Red Rattle root was mixed with beef marrow or goat tallow and applied hot to areas affected by **FILLAN**. This Gaelic word describes a crippling, inflamed conditions of the knees and ankles caused by a small reddish worm that lodges under the skin of these areas. The plant contains a glycoside that is poisonous to insects and helped cure this debilitating condition that was very common on the Hebrides in the 18th century.

Labrador Lousewort is common throughout the boreal forest from northern Manitoba to Alaska, but somewhat rare in Saskatchewan. It is particularly parasitic on dwarf birch, and because of this is relatively safe to use for inflammatory conditions. The Slave name is **KOZÕ ØALLI**, perhaps derived from Kozo meaning nighthawk.

Swamp Lousewort is found in calcareous fens of the northern prairies.

The related *P. repupinata* has been used in China for fevers, rheumatism, sterility and urinary problems, as well as tinnitus, and dryness of the mouth and tongue. It is known in TCM as **MA XIAN HAO**, or **MA SHI HAO**, meaning Horse Droppings Tall Weed.

In India, the leaves of the related *P. pectinata* are used to stop spitting of blood, and as a diuretic.

The rare Furbish's Lousewort, discovered alongside a stream in Maine, prevented construction of a multi-million dollar dam. Plant Power!

MEDICINAL

CONSTITUENTS- *P. striata-* iso-verbascoside, verbascoside, cistanoside C.
P. plicata- verbascoside, martynoside.
P. groenlandica- flavonoids including luteolin; phenylpropanoids including verbascoside and echinocoside.

Much of the medicinal use of Elephant Head is derived from their various uptake constituents.

For example, the warming expectoration properties for coughs may be derived from nearby coniferous trees.

The treatment for uterine spasms, on the other hand, may come from Golden Bean alkaloids.

By itself, according to Michael Moore, it is one of the safest and most effective musculoskeletal relaxants we have in our repertory.

"It take tight, adrenalin-stressed muscles and decreases their tone and rigidity. If you have played too much tennis or moved too many boxes, drink some of the tea and relax.

Also give the tea in reduced dosage to children who can't relax after going to a scary movie, or have played so many video games that their hands, clenched around a 25 watt bulb, would light it dimly."

It is used by runners, computer addicts and a useful adjunct for massage therapists, chiropractors and rolfers who can't get into the musculature of their clients. It helps neck adjustments, TMJ or Alexander technique by lessening resistance to manipulation.

Both infused teas and tinctures work well, and alternately, the leaves and flower heads can be dried and smoked for achieving states of relaxation.

A bit of tea or tincture in evenings, helps dull some of the structured patterning of muscle hypertonicity.

Lousewort tea, for example, can be of great benefit to those suffering hemorrhoids.

Midwives have used the relaxing tea before and just after birthing, although I have no personal experience with the herb in this manner.

It helps in cases of insomnia related to fright/flight episodes, those suffering muscular jolts when falling asleep, or during first REM cycle with agitation, fear and gastritis.

A tea of the flowering tops helps ease dry, hacking coughs or calm an upset stomach.

It may lessen the nocturnal pruritis, or skin itching, associated with liver or thyroid dysfunction, combining well with fresh Marsh Scullcap tincture.

Matthew Wood writes. "Cherokee herbalist Sondra Boyd speaks highly of *Pedicularis*. She uses it for neurovascular spasm, hence in stroke and syncope, to release tension in the blood vessels caused by particles that have caught in the arteries. She also considers it to be one of the few medicines that will act on grand mal and petit mal seizures."

The roots of *P. canadensis* are used as a blood tonic, cardiac and stomachic. The tea is used in the treatment of stomachaches, ulcers, diarrhea, anemia and heart troubles.

A root poultice is applied to sore muscles, and swelling.

A leaf infusion was traditionally used internally for abortion, while fresh leaf infusions are used for a sore throat.

The leaves of this and other species is made into a tea or smoked.

Like Elephant Head, Common Lousewort can be used as a muscle relaxant and sedative.

Work by Zheng et al, 1993 indicates that *Pedicularis* species contain phenyl-propanoid glycosides, with anti-oxidant properties. Delalande et al, *SAR QSAR Environ Res* 2002 13:7-8 found cistanoside C, a phenyl propanoid glycoside from *P. spicata*, is capable of repairing DNA damaged by oxygen radicals. Pediclarioside G, isolated from this plant has been found to exhibit anti-angiogenic, anti-tumor and anti-metatastic activity. Mu et al, *Basic Clin Pharm Tox* 2008 102:1.

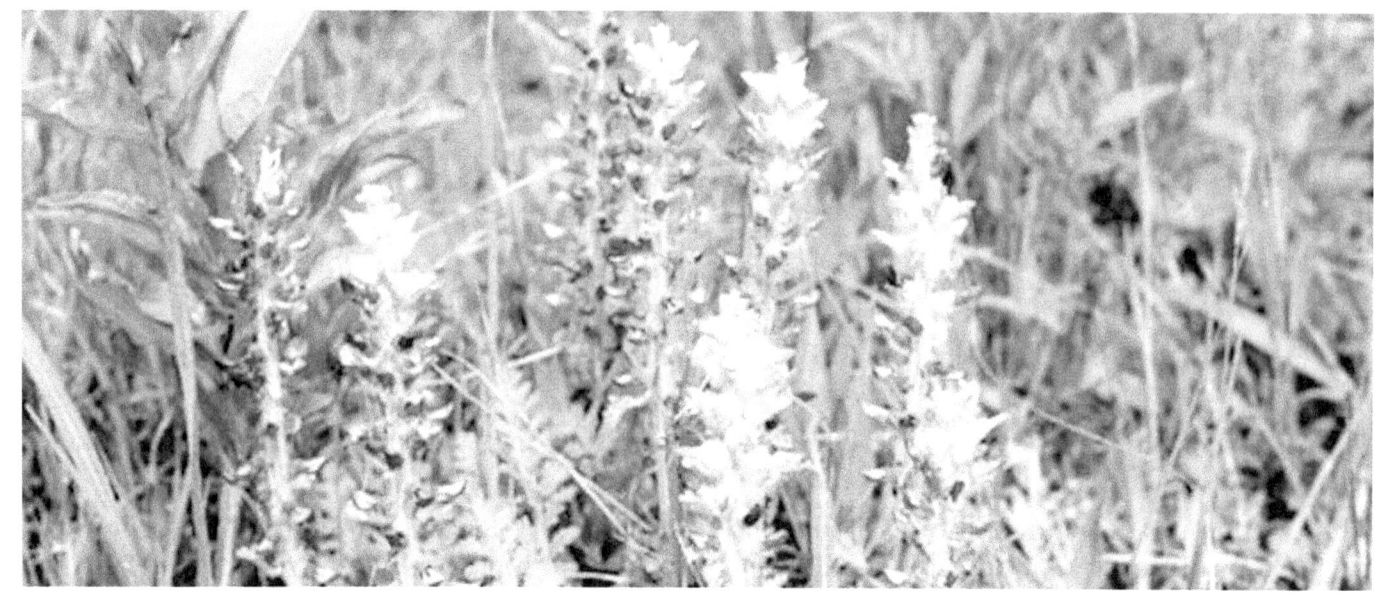

PEDICULARIS CANADENSIS

Verbascoside has been found to retard skeletal muscle fatigue. Liao et al, *Phytother Res* 1999 13:7. It also acts to alleviate fatigue due to the inhibition of exercise-induced synthesis of 5-HT (5-hydroxytryptamine) and tryptophan hydroxylase, and its increase of serotonergic type 1B inhibitory autoreceptors. Zhu M et al, *Neurosci Lett* 2016 616:75-9.

Verbascoside inhibits telomerase cell activity in tumor cells, and may be a valuable screening method for anti-tumor activity in natural products. See Mullein, under Respiratory system, for more detail on this glycoside.

Isoverbascoside possesses the activity of inducing differentiation of human hepatocellular carcinoma cell lines. *P. longiflora var. tubiformis* has been used traditionally in Nepal for the treatment of dropsy, spermatorrhea, tinnitus and carbuncles. By contrast, our species have been very poorly studied.

According to Farnsworth, acute toxicity tests conducted in mice with different lousewort species indicate lousewort is not very toxic. Orally the mean lethal dose was 8 grams/kg.

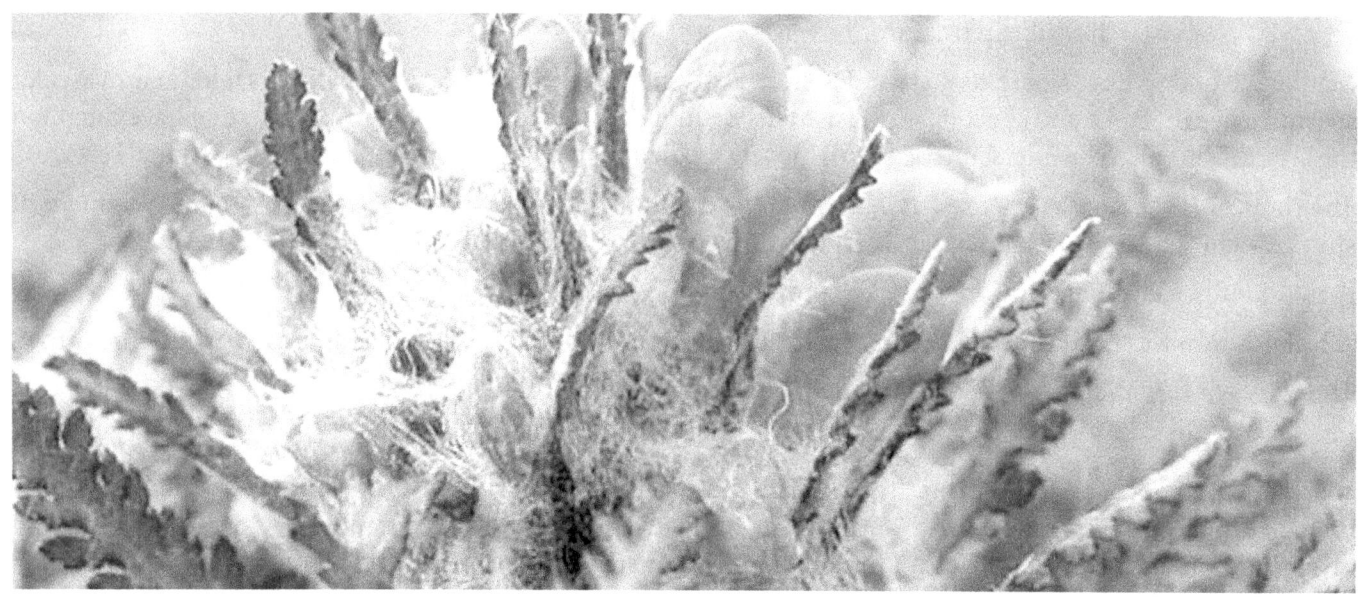

PEDICULARIS LANATUM

FLOWER ESSENCES

Elephant's Head (*P. groenlandica*) flower essence is for wisdom. It enables a deep vibrational link to the energies of the angelic kingdom that are deeply associated with humanity's own development.

The essence helps deeper attunement and awareness of angelic helpers or guides. It gives a strengthened ability to perceive and work with earth energy. **PEGASUS**

Bracted Lousewort essence helps ease blocks to getting started on a project or venture. **ROCKY MOUNTAIN**

Elephant Head essence helps one deal with issues of feeling unattractive or ugly. **ROCKY MOUNTAIN**

Pedicularis (*P. groenlandica*) is for pronounced sensitivity or hypochondria leading to seclusion or separation; fits of crying or other water imbalances; excessive emotionality which inhibits deeper understanding of one's soul pain, suffering or karma.

FLOWER ESSENCE SOCIETY

Sickletop Lousewort (*P. racemosa*) is for confidence through courage, personal stability and self-love. It enhances our ability to achieve balance in love, body self and partner. In particular, this plant enables confidence in our sexuality, in receiving or giving sexual pleasure or simply sexual energy. It could also be helpful for such imbalances as anorexia or overweight problems. **NETTLES AND MORE**

RECIPES

INFUSION- One tablespoon of dried leaf and flower; or one handful of fresh to one pint of water. Steep 20 minutes. Drink 4-6 ounces three times daily.

TINCTURE-20-40 drops as needed. The tincture can be made from the dried leaf and flower in a ratio of 1:5 with 50% alcohol. Fresh plant tincture is prepared at 1:2 and 70%.

CHEESY LOUSEWORT- Scrub and chop three cups of lousewort roots. Place in foil. Sprinkle with salt, pepper, butter and about 1/4 cup of parmesan cheese. Wrap and place on fire. **SCHOFIELD**

CAUTION- According to the late, great herbalist Michael Moore, an overdose of *Pedicularis* can cause "a befuddled lethargy and some interference with motor control, particularly in the legs.... short term discomfort of minor consequence". Also, do not use *Pedicularis* growing near groundsels or toxic legumes.

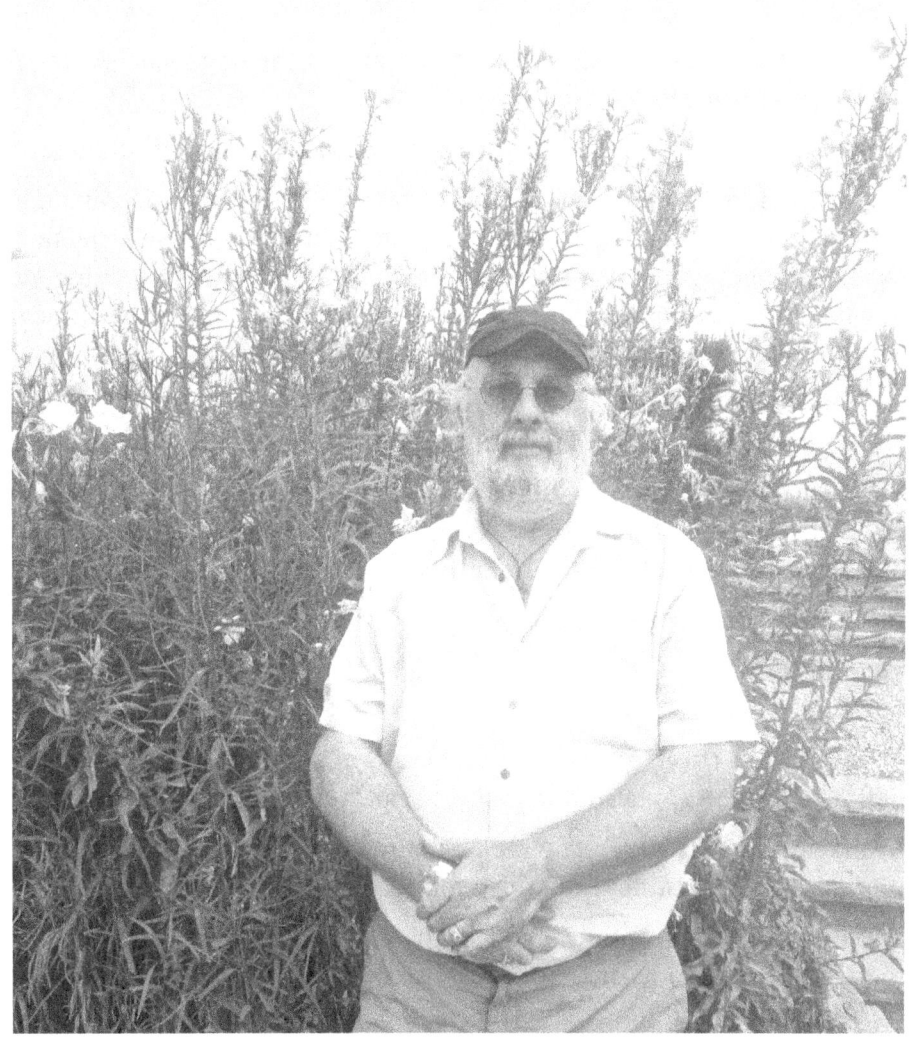

EVENING PRIMROSE AND AUTHOR

EVENING PRIMROSE
YELLOW EVENING PRIMROSE
(*Oenothera biennis* L.)
WHITE EVENING PRIMROSE
(*O. nuttallii* Sweet)
RED EVENING PRIMROSE
LARGE FLOWERED EVENING PRIMROSE
(*O. glazioviana* Micheli)
(*O. erythosepala* Borbas) not accepted
FRAGRANT EVENING PRIMROSE
BUTTE EVENING PRIMROSE
GUMBO EVENING PRIMROSE
TUFTED EVENING PRIMROSE

ALKALI LILY
(*O. caespitosa* Nutt.)
YELLOW LAVAUXIA
LONG TUBE EVENING PRIMROSE
(*O. flava* [A. Nelson] Garrett)
SHRUBBY EVENING PRIMROSE
PLAINS EVENING PRIMROSE
YELLOW SUNDROPS
(*O. serrulata* Nutt.)
PARADOXICAL EVENING PRIMROSE
(*O. paradoxa* Hudziok)
PARTS USED- leaf, root, flower, seeds

The evening primrose opes anew
Its delicate blossoms to the dew;
And, hermit-like, shunning the light,
Wastes its fair bloom upon the Night…

CLARE

And the day came when the risk to remain tight in the bud was more painful than the risk it took to blossom.

ANAIS NIN

Evening Primrose seeds itself to distraction, but the large pale-yellow flowers which open at night also add delicious perfume to the evening...

MARGERY FISH

A tuft of evening primroses o'er which the mind may hover, til it dozes.

JOHN KEATS

Oenothera is from the Greek **OINOS** for wine, and **THERA** meaning odor, pursuing or imbibing; in reference to either the dried root odor resembling wine (doubtful), or the belief that roots increased capacity for drinking wine. Another possibility is from the Greek **ONOS THERAS**, meaning "donkey catcher". The roots were infused in wine, to tame wild animals. Oenanthe was an ancient Greek perfume produced from vine leaves on Cyprus. Pliny listed it as a royal unguent for the Kings of Parthia.

Caespitosa means tufted or clumped, and refers to the low growing habit of the plant. Erythrosepala is from Greek meaning red-sepaled; biennis means biennial.

Yellow Evening Primrose is widespread in the central and southern prairies. Studies suggest many of the genera began their journey from Central America. Yellow Evening Primrose appears to be circumpolar, although many of its cousins were introduced to Europe.

As evening approaches, the yellow flowers unfurl and release a scent attractive to the night flying sphinx moth.

Well, the flowers do not so much unfurl, but if you listen carefully, the buds sound like popping soap bubbles bursting.

Even still, it has been estimated that at least half of the self-pollinated seeds die in the ovary from accumulated defects. The fruit contains hundreds of healthy seeds to ensure survival.

Its magical powers were recognized and used by indigenous people, with the plant rubbed against their bodies to ensure good hunting, and protection against snakes.

The Blackfoot dried and used the carrot-like pale pink biennial roots of yellow evening primrose for winter food. The young roots are particularly tasty, with a peppery, nutty flavor sort of like Radish. They also boiled the fresh leaves and stems as a potherb.

The seedpods are edible when young, and when dry can be pulled down along the stem to give a string fiber.

The Cherokee used the same root infusions for obesity- something just being recognized in the scientific/medical community. They used a poultice of mashed, heated root for hemorrhoids.

Natives of New Mexico use decoctions of the dried or fresh flowers for kidney trouble.

The Iroquois recognized its benefits in treating piles as well as boils and laziness. They chewed the roots and rubbed them onto athlete's muscles to improve strength.

The Potawatomi tribe used the seeds of **OWESA'WANAKUK**, or Yellow Top, medicinally in an unspecified manner.

One Cherokee name is "falling sun rose", a beautiful descriptive.

The Algonquin mashed the seeds as a poultice for skin rashes, and the women used this paste to maintain smooth, youthful skin.

The Crow simmered the flowers until water is all gone and after removing the flowers, used the oil for skin problems.

During wartime, the seeds were roasted and used as a coffee substitute.

The finely ground flowers are used in facemasks for red, irritated skin, as well as poultices for slight rheumatic pain.

While Yellow Evening-Primrose is a night blooming biennial, the other three are all day blooming perennials. Two to five yellow flowers open at dusk and wilt the following morning, to be replaced by others. The flowers have a strong lemony scent to attract moths. At regular intervals, the flowers emit small puffs of scented warm breath.

If you take the time to watch the flowers open, you will notice the petals are held together by hooks at the end of the flower cup and the segments separate first at the lower part so that the corolla can be seen for a while.

When unhooked, the corolla opens instantaneously and then halts as it takes time to spread out flat, all in about half an hour. Sometimes, you will see flowers open on a cloudy, overcast day.

Butte and White Evening-Primrose have scented flowers that open white in the morning and turn pink as the day progresses. Yellow Lavauxia starts out the day with yellow flowers that turn pink each evening. Butte or Fragrant Evening Primrose, when it opens, smells like the most exquisite perfume; a mixture of tuberose, jasmine and lemon would be one close description.

The Blackfeet used the roots of Butte Primrose, or Alkali Lily, to reduce inflammation by pounding and applying a poultice to the affected area. Their names for the plant **AP AKS IBOKN** translates roughly as "wide leaves", and **OSK PI POKU** meaning, "Sticky Root."

The Navaho used the ground plant poultices for strengthening a prolapsed uterus. A dusting powder from the flowers was used to relieve chaffing.

They used the plant in the Bead Way, Big Star Way, Red Ant Way and Blessed Way ceremonies.

Yellow Lavauxia was widely utilized by the Navaho. The ash of seedpods was smeared on burns, while a root poultice was used for large swellings, and as a "life medicine". The whole plant was used in a combination for throat troubles.

When introduced to Europe in 1612, yellow evening primrose was soon after used medicinally for calming nerves, and made into a mild sedative by infusing the flowers. The whole plant was used with spasmodic asthma and whooping cough, and was called the King's Cure-All.

In France and Germany, the first year roots are served in stews or raw in salads with flavor reminiscent of parsnips or salsify. They can be irritating to the throat when eaten alone. In France, where it is cultivated, it is known as Gardener's Ham (*Jambon du jardinier*), due to the resemblance of flavor. To the north, it is known as German Rampion.

An old legend suggested that two pounds of root would bring as much strength as 20 pounds of beef, suggesting a revitalizing effect after illness or surgery.

The red seeds can be sprinkled on baked goods or salads like poppy seed. These seeds retain their energy for up to 80 years when buried in soil, waiting for their exposure to light and a chance to germinate.

Many plants in this genus emit "phosphoresence", or luminescence from their petals at night. This is due to the storing of sunlight during the day and releasing at night. The delicately, fragrant blooms of yellow evening primrose are short-lived (often one night), and open to invite pollinating, twilight insects. Towards fall, the flowers stay open all day long.

Butte Evening Primrose (*O. caespitosa*) is a low growing, gray green plant with papery blooms on short stems. The flower buds open an hour or two before sunset and smell very similar to magnolia, or jasmine and lemon.

Red Evening Primrose is a native perennial of North America hardy to zone 3. It has red sepals and is often grown in gardens for its beauty. It is very frost and drought resistant. Both Red and Yellow Evening Primrose flowers have an unusual, not unpleasant amine-like odor, due mainly to the methyl ester mentioned below. Red Evening Primrose has a more lemon and lily-like undertone.

Red Evening Primrose symbolizes inconstancy, and birth date of March 30.

As a biennial, expect *O. biennis* seed production in the second year. The Alberta Research Council in Vegreville views it as a good native seed crop for reclamation work, and erosion control.

Large flowered evening primrose may be useful for phyto-stabilization of copper contaminated mine sites. It is not affected by high copper levels, nor hyper-accumulates the toxic metal, and will produce decent amounts of GLA. Guo P et al, *Environ Sci Pollut Res Int* 2014 21(1):631-40.

In Eastern Canada, the plants are started in greenhouses and transplanted to fields to be grown as an annual. In many respects, borage seed is a better GLA (gamma linolenic acid) oil source for the prairies commercially, but there is renewed interest in evening primrose, especially if annual varieties can be developed for the short growing season of the prairies.

The seeds are small (3.1-3.5 million per kilogram), and are planted at a rate of 150 seeds per linear meter in a row. The seeds are hardy, some have been found viable after 80 years in the soil.

Annual world production is about 4000 tonnes, with Canadians contributing less than 200 tonnes in total. Over two tonnes per hectare have been recorded in Nova Scotia, but this is on the high side, 600 lbs per acre being the average.

A Farming for the Future Project conducted in 1997 by Mike Clawson et al, looked at Evening Primrose production under irrigation in southern Alberta. Their work found that due to the longer growing season, the seed set in first year, and under proper management may happen four years out of five. Seed yields varied from 29.6 to 41.4 pounds per acre.

The left over residue from aerial parts is useful for anaerobic digestion and production of biogas. Cao Z et al, *Int J Phytoremediation* 2015 17(1-6):201-7.

The European species, *O. paradoxa* is a hybrid between *O. depressa* and either *O. parviflora* or *O. subterminalis*. It is widely grown in France, Belgium, Poland and Germany.

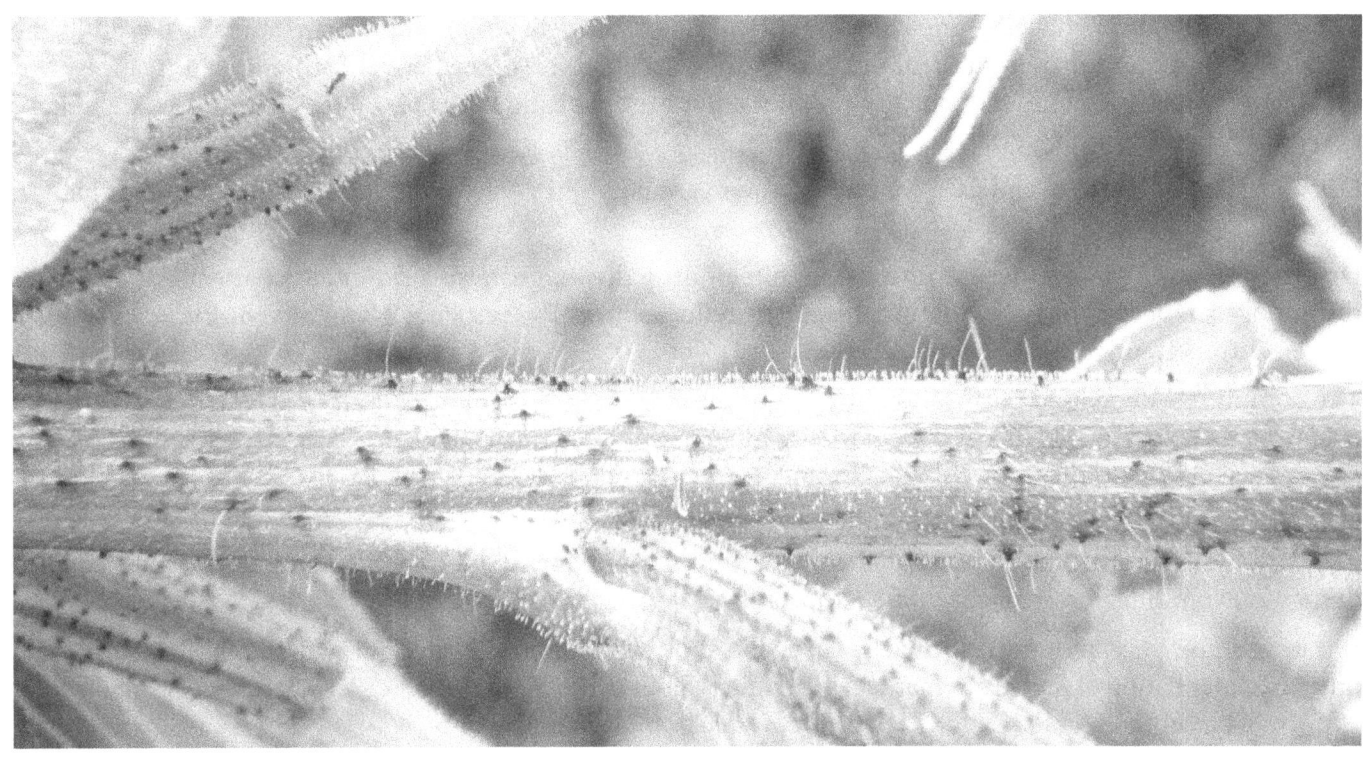

STEM OF EVENING PRIMROSE

MEDICINAL

CONSTITUENTS- *O. biennis* aerial- oenotherin, potassium nitrate, resins, and various bitter principles. The leaves contain various flavonoids, kaempferol, quercitin, and various gycosides, neochlorogenic acid, p-coumaric acid, caffeic acid derivatives, delphindin, digallic acid, ellagitannins, and gallic acid; as well as 24-methylene cycloartenol.
The leaves, stems and buds contain 24-27% protein, 4.3% fat
Roots contain mucilage, tannins, sugars, gallic acid, oenotheralanosterol A & B.
October roots contain 21% protein, the May roots only 11.5%.
seed- fatty oils (see below), as well as various amino acids, including tryptophan 1.6%, glutamic acid 2.8%, histidine 0.39%, aspartic acid 1.2%, and traces of boron.
O. caespitosa- flowers- 0.1% gallic acid
O. erythrosepala- oenothein B.
Flowers- The flowers of *Oenothera* species contain an alkaloid, Oxindole-3-acetic acid methylester.
Gallic and vanillic acids predominate in the seeds, while caffeic and ferulic acids are more common in the plants.

The fresh or dried root has soothing and anti-spasmodic action; good for coughs, asthma as well as skeletal and muscle pain in the reproductive organs.

Work by Singh R et al, *J Ethnopharm* 2012 141(1): 357-62 identified anti-inflammatory activity in roots. Oenotheralanosterol A and B, as well as gallic acid all inhibited TNF alpha and IL-6 related to inflammation.

The tops can also be used for making cough syrups, but are somewhat milder in their anti-spasmodic and sedative effect.

The dry leaves contain up to 20% of aldose reductase inhibitors, compounds that play a role in the reduction of diabetic cataracts, and support eye health. The content of polyphenols in *O. paradoxa* may be useful for inhibiting the enzymes responsible for sugar metabolism (alpha amylase and alpha glucosidase) or protein tyrosine phosphatase B, a known negative regulator in insulin signaling. This suggests possible usefulness in type two diabetes. Crampbark (*Viburnum opulus*) showed benefit in same study. Zaklos-Szyda M et al, *Curr Top Med Chem* 2015 15(23): 2431-44.

The leaves and flowers have a somewhat diuretic function that relieves kidney spasm, and sharp pain in the bladder and urethra. There is mild stimulation of the vagus nerve, somewhat validating an old treatment for underactive digestive and liver problems in seniors. Both the root and herb are mildly sedative, helping relieve nervous tension throughout the body.

Leaf tinctures are sedative and used for uterine and ovarian cramps, pelvic congestion as well as inflammation of GI tract.

Dr. Bastyr used the leaf and stem tincture, in fifteen drop doses, for nervous, irritable patients, and general respiratory support by mildly sedating the cough reflex centre. The terpene, 24-methylene cycloartenol is a proven antinociceptive.

The compound decreases postprandial hyperglycemia in mice. Okahara F et al, *Mol Nutr Food Res* 2016 60(7):1521-31. It prevents diet-induced obesity by increasing fatty acid oxidation in muscles and decreasing fatty acid synthesis in the liver. Fukuoka D et al, *J Appl Physiol* (1985). 2014 117(11):1337-48. The compound is found in dandelion leaves.

Eclectic physicians suggested leaf, root and flower tinctures for apathy, gloom and depression associated with dyspepsia, vomiting and frequent desire to urinate.

A water-soluble polysaccharide isolated by decoction showed inhibition of tumor growth in mice, and increased immune potentiating of numerous markers including lymphocytes, natural killer cells, macrophage phagocytosis and white blood cell counts. Zeng G et al, *Int J Bio Macromol* 2013 52:280-5.

The flowers can be crushed in hot water, spread on a cheesecloth, and placed on the throat and chest to ease discomfort. The leaves; either freshly bruised, or as a fomentation, can bring great relief to external skin ulcers. Or simply chew a leaf and apply as poultice to swellings, bruises, insect bites, etc.

Dr. Scudder suggested that various digestive disorders from heartburn to hepatic congestion were eased.

Glandular enlargement of the spleen, and destructive inflammation of Peyer's patches (digestive lymphatic nodes) are cleansed by the tincture.

His specific indications are sallow, dirty skin, tissues full and expressionless, face dull and apathetic, dyspepsia with vomiting of food and gastric distress, with desire to urinate frequently, choleric and dysenteric discharges, nocturnal restlessness, enervation, feeble, patient gloomy and despondent, atonic reproductive wrongs of the female, with pelvic fullness.

Dr. William Cook noted "its action is directed to the pneumongastric nerve, making it of service in asthma with gastric irritability". Many people suffer from asthma associated with esophageal reflux while trying to sleep.

William LeSassier used the whole plant collected during flower for spastic colon, crampy stools, tension in the lower pelvic area, ovarian pain, ileocecal valve pain.

HerbalGram (#44) printed a letter concerning Indian John, a Civil War herbalist. He used evening primrose leaves as a liniment for stopping goiter growth, massaged into the thyroid area. He also made an emulsion of the leaves for curing stomach cancer and other internal cancers, and leaf poultices for skin cancer sores.

The leaves are one of our richest sources of quercitin, a bioflavonoid useful in keeping healthy blood vessels, improving circulation and relieving asthma.

Dr. Winterburn wrote in *The American Homeopathist* November 1883:

'Oenothera is a useful remedy in asthma or dyspnoea associated with gastric irritability. It seems to have an especial influence on the pneumogastric, and when its function are disturbed by a morbidly sensitive gastric mucous membrane, showing itself reflexly in irritations of the laryngeal or pulmonary branches of that nerve, Oenothera is likely to prove helpful. In spasmodic asthma and whooping cough it fills a place similar to Lobelia, without its nauseant effect…I generally give ten drops of the first dilution in a half goblet of water, a teaspoonful every quarter of an hour until relieved.'

The stem bark is very mucilaginous, and astringent, and decoctions can be used for soothing skin eruptions in children.

It is worth noting that evening primrose seed bran is one of the best natural sources of tryptophan available. One kilogram of dried seeds contains up to 16,000 mg of this important sedative amino acid. The dried bran would by weight contain much more; and would be a great addition to sleep promoting foods.

Increasing the amount of serotonin, in the body, by directly stimulating dopamine D2 receptors has been shown to reduce the craving for alcohol.

The oil has long been recommended for various obsessive compulsive disorders based on the oil; but perhaps the tryptophan content is also partly responsible.

The seed extract possesses significant anti-oxidant activity at 98,563 TE/100 grams. This is nearly 30 times higher than blueberries. Borchardt et al, *J Med Plants Res* 2008 2:4.

Grind the seeds and mix with flaxseed oil to combine GLA and tryptophan with a good quality ALA oil.

GLA will certainly increase in demand. Genetic engineers are presently attempting to splice the oil capacity to canola, which would significantly change the market.

The root of evening primrose (*O. biennis*) has been found to be strongly anti-fungal (85% at 250 ppm) in studies by Shukla et al, *Journal of Ethnopharmacology*, Nov 1999. It is probably due to the gallic acid and unknown constituents.

The root can be made into syrup by chopping freshly harvested and cleaned pieces in twice the amount of honey and slowly reducing. It is great for irritating coughs or tickle that does not respond to other demulcent, relaxing expectorant herbs.

The root may possess immunosuppressive effects, and in one study blocked cytotoxic T lymphocyte mediated cytotoxicity. Hamada et al, *Biol Pharm Bull* 1997 20 1017-19.

Evening-Primrose leaves, stems, flowers, fruit and roots have been extracted with water, ethanol, ether and alkalis. Activity against gram negative, gram positive and mycobacterium have been found.

Early work by Hayes et al, Bot Gazette 1947 108 found plant extracts strongly inhibitory of *E. coli*. Recent work found plant extracts may be useful adjuncts to reduce dosage of antibiotics for the treatment of recurrent *Helicobacter pylori* infection. Kim TS et al, *Lab Anim Res* 2015 31(1):7-12.

The plant extract shows anti-viral activity, and *O. caespitosa* extracts have been patented for treatment of *Herpes simplex* lesions, *Epstein Barr and Varicella*.

Yellow Evening Primrose patents for purple pigment, and thioproline for cancer therapies have been filed.

Work by Ul'chenko et al, Chemistry of Natural Compounds 1998 34:5 compared the gamma linolenic acid content of *O. biennis*, with two other species. Both *O. lamarekiana* (6.3%), and *O. tetraptera* (5.5%) were richer in GLA than the evening primrose used commercially (5.4%). This may lead to some hybridization, or research into new strains. The oil content of *O. lamarekiana* was also impressive, at 24.7%, compared to *O. biennis* at 23.8%.

Kocourkova et al (1999) from the Czech Republic, looked at various Evening Primrose varieties for oil yield.

They found *O. ammofila* to contain 17% GLA, leading to new breeding possibilities.

Red Evening Primrose contains very interesting macrocylic hydrolyzable tannins, Oenothein B. First recognized in *Lythrum anceps* and Small flowering Willow Herb in Europe, and in Fireweed in North America, this compound has been found to effective in reducing prostate inflammation.

Earlier studies also showed it possesses both anti-viral and anti-tumor activity indicating application in both the inhibition of 5-alpha reductase responsible for benign prostatic hyperplasia as well as possible value in treating prostatic adenoma and carcinoma.

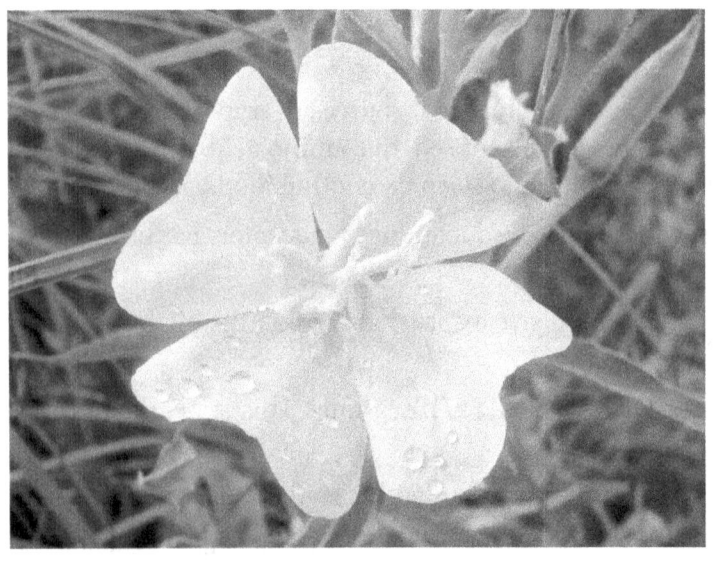

EVENING PRIMROSE FLOWER

The related *O. villosa* has been found to be active against a broad spectrum of fungal species in work by Towers et al, at University of British Columbia.

The root extract of related *O. odorata* has a positive effect on muscle atrophy. Lee YH et al, *Evid Based Complement Altern Med* 2015 :130513. An ethanol extract of seeds induces vasorelaxation of artery tissue. Kim HY et al, *J Ethnopharm* 2011 133(2)315-22.

The defatted seed of related *O. paradoxa* inhibits metallopeptidases, neutral endopeptidase and aminopeptidase. Kiss et al, *J Ag Food Chem* 2008 56:17.

The extract appears beneficial for prevention of UVA skin damage. Jaszewska E et al, *J Phytochem Phytobiol B* 2013 126:42-6.

It exhibits anti-migratory, anti-invasive and anti-metastatic potential towards prostate and breast cancer cell lines. Lewandowska U et al, *Postepy Hig Med Dosw* 2014 68:110-8. The procyanidins from defatted seeds increase apoptosis and reduce angiogenesis in MDA-MB-231 breast cancer cells. *Nutr Cancer* 2013 65(8):1219-31. Another study that year suggested the seed flavonols increased apoptosis and reduced angiogenesis of prostate cancer cells.

A polyphenol-rich extract alleviated experimental colitis, both orally and rectally, in mice. Salaga M et al, *Naunyn Schemiedebergs Arch Pharmacol* 2014 387(11):1069-78.

It induced apoptosis in human colon cancer Caco-2 cell lines. Gorlach S et al, *J Agric Food Chem* 2011 59(13):6985-97.

The seed extract increased melanoma cancer cells susceptibility to the action of vincristine. Jaszewska E et al, *J Physiol Pharmacol* 2010 61(5):637-43.

A water extract of *O. paradoxa* significantly reduced neutral endopeptidase (NEP) in patients after acute myocardial infarction. NEP inactivates protective natriuretic peptides. Kiss AK et al, *Phytotherapy Research* 2012 26(4):482-7.

Seed extracts of *O. biennis* contain polyphenols that inhibit *Streptococcus mutans* and induced dental caries, in rats. Matsumoto-Nakano M et al, *Caries Res* 2011 45(1):56-63.

A phenolic fraction from de-fatted seeds promoted selective apoptosis of colon carcinoma CaCo2 cell lines. Pellegrina CD et al, *Cancer Lett* 2005 226(1):17-25.

A decent review of Oenothera use in medicine by Singh S et al, was published in *Zhong Xi Yi Jie He Xue Bao* 2012 10(7):717-25.

HOMEOPATHY

Oenothera biennis is the remedy for effortless diarrhea with nervous exhaustion. Summer diarrhea in children, or chronic diarrhea in thin, emaciated subjects.

It is useful in whooping cough and spasmodic asthma. It has been shown to be useful in severe water retention in the brain (hydrocephalus).

Vertigo, swimming sensation in had and loss of muscular power. Numbness and pricking pain in body, accompanied by severe chills and cramping in muscles of abdomen and extremities.

DOSE- First potency. The mother tincture is prepared from the whole fresh plant in flower. First observation based on effects in forty-year old woman with first a teaspoon and then 30 drops of fluid extract in 1870s. Clinical observations by Boericke and Blackwood round out the symptoms.

SEED OIL

CONSTITUENTS- cis-linoleic acid (72%), GLA (9%), palmitic, oleic and stearic acids. The protein is rich in sulphur-bearing amino acids and tryptophan. Also contains long chain fatty alcohols such as hexacosanol, tetracosanol, docosanol, and octocosanol, and various sterols including beta sitosterol and campesterol.

A GLA, or gamma linolenic acid rich oil, with an aromatic flavour similar to poppy seed oil is produced from the ripe seeds. Over two hundred and fifty papers have been written on its medical wonders.

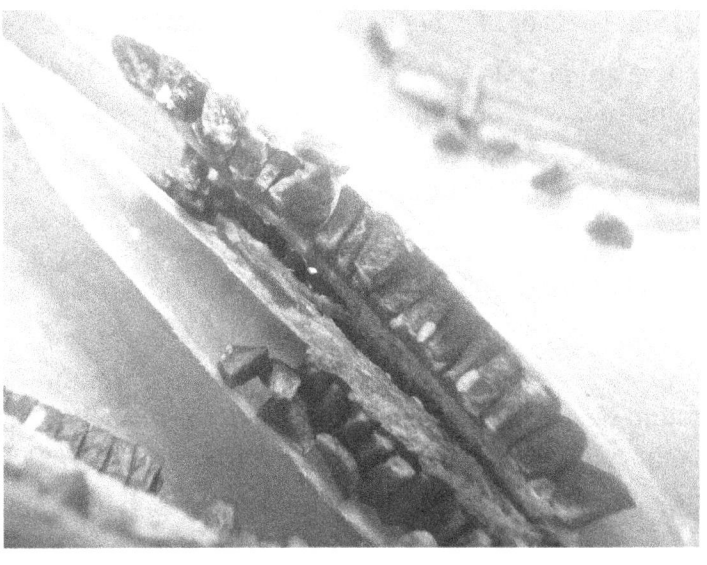

EVENING PRIMROSE SEEDS IN POD

From auto-immune disease like rheumatoid arthritis, lupus, and multiple sclerosis; to skin problems like eczema and psoriasis; to relieving PMS, diabetes, Alzheimer's, endometriosis, and heart disease.

Despite numerous warnings regarding the cardiovascular risk of Celebrex, numerous patients take this COX-2 inhibitor for osteoarthritis and joint pain. One study suggests evening primrose oil decreased blood pressure in rats given the drug, suggesting one possible way to mitigate blood pressure and stroke. Zaitone SA et al, *J Cardiovasc Pharmacol* 2011 58(1):72-9.

Evening primrose oil (EPO) is especially beneficial to patients with low delta-6-desaturase levels. Gammma linolenic acid is not normally obtained directly from dietary sources and the body relies on metabolic conversion from dietary linolenic acid. This may be affected by various concerns including ageing, diabetes, cardiovascular and cholesterol, high alcohol intake, viral infections, cancer, nutritional defects, atopic eczema and premenstrual syndrome.

Patients suffering diabetic neuropathy, in one clinical trial involving 22 males and females, showed positive benefit in a parallel double blind study.

Eleven type 1 diabetic children were given EPO for four months, in a study at Juntendo University, in Tokyo. Metabolism of prostaglandin and fat metabolism both improved and stabilized.

Two studies in England involving over 400 patients with diabetes showed nerve damage, or neuropathy was significantly reduced.

Dr. Boulton, of the Royal Hospital in Manchester found similar improvement in 146 diabetics over a one year study.

Sardine oil, vitamin E and EPO were given to diabetics in a study at the Metropolitan Geriatric Hospital in Tokyo. Lower blood lipid levels and prevention of vascular occlusions were noted, in some cases after only one month.

A human, double blind, placebo controlled clinical trial by Jamal et al, *Lancet* 1986 1098 on patients with diabetic neuropathy demonstrated reversal of symptoms with evening primrose oil.

A randomized, double blind, crossover study of fifteen healthy females by Tahvonen et al, *J Nutr Biochem* 2005 16:6 compared fish oil and black currant seed oil for two four week periods. Results showed the seed oil increased the proportion of 18:3n6 in triacylglycerols (TAG) and cholesteryl esters, and that of dihomo-gamma-linolenic (20:3n6) in TAGs, CEs and glycerophospholipids.

Serum levels of LDL cholesterol were lower after black currant seed oil compared to fish oil.

There are mixed reviews on the effectiveness of EPO in treating PMS. In some studies, remission of severe symptoms was found in up to 61% of patients.

Recent reviews of seven, placebo-controlled clinical trials (5 randomized), reported improvements in PMS. Two of the better control studies, failed to show any benefit.

In all the studies, no changes are found in plasma levels of 6-keto-prostaglandin f, FSH, LH, prolactin, progesterone, estradiol or testosterone, suggesting some other mechanism at work.

One placebo-controlled, double-blind study on 35 women suffering menopausal flushing, showed no significant difference from control. However a six-week randomized clinical trial of 56 menopausal women aged 45-59 found decreased intensity of hot flashes and ameliorated HFRDIS scores in those taking 500 mg twice daily compared to placebo. Farzaneh F et al, *Arch Gynecol Obstet* 2013 288(5): 1075-9.

The oil has been found to work synergistically with tamoxifen in a study of 38 patients by Kenny et al, *Int J Cancer* 2000 85.

Hypersensitivity to prolactin during PMS is believed due to low levels of PGE_1.

Twenty-eight women with menopausal symptoms were given EPO for six months, in a study at the Hospital for Obstetrics and Gynecology at Keele University.

Evaluation of their diaries indicated significant reduction in night-time hot flashes.

Studies from Scotland show that evening primrose oil encouraged the regeneration of liver cell damage caused by alcohol. It is also thought to stop alcohol from damaging brain cells by bolstering them with unsaturated fats.

Evening Primrose oil has been found to reduce tremors, a side effect from lithium use by manic-depressive patients.

Studies from a New York hospital found it helped reduce weight in obese people. Other studies have shown improvement in over two-thirds of hyperactive children.

Although two large trials have found no benefit in atopic eczema, other trials have found positive results in children, 1-12 years old and 320-480 mg in adults for three months. McHenry et al, *British Medical Journal* 1995 310.

Women with non-cyclic breast pain and inflammation found that taking three grams daily of EPO has equal effect to bromocriptine, or danazol but with fewer side effects (4% vs. 30-35%).

One study of 566 women with benign breast disease at Western General Hospital in Edinburgh, Scotland over seven years, found EPO and B6 of significant benefit. Another study at University Clinic in Manchester found 75% of women with breast pain were treated successfully with EPO.

A study at King's College hospital in London involving 276 physicians revealed 30% reported good results in treating mastopathy, or painful breasts. Work by Horobin, *Rev Contemp Pharmacother* 1990 1 found GLA helpful in cyclical mastalgia. Combined with EPA, the oil was found to reduce symptoms of endometriosis in 90% of women; whereas 90% of placebo group found no relief. This work also found beneficial effect in ulcerative colitis, and Sjogren's syndrome, with relief of lethargy and modest improvement in tear flow.

Midwives have found that new mothers, who would normally have 12 hours of active labor, have only 4-6 hours when taking up to four grams of evening primrose oil daily throughout pregnancy. Perineal lacerations/episiotomies and stretch marks are significantly reduced.

The oil can also be rubbed directly on the cervix to encourage softening and opening. Apply oil to fingers and rub slowly around and into the os, holding it open through 2-3 contractions.

Evening Primrose Oil appears to help prevent pre-eclampsia, a serious complication of pregnancy involving sudden rise in blood pressure and edema. A controlled, double-blind study at Tulane University in New Orleans found a combination of EPO, fish oil and magnesium oxide resulted in not one case; while the placebo group had three complications.

Animal and human cancer cell studies in South Africa and India found GLA reduced cancer growth by 70%, probably by binding to certain proteins that stimulate formation and growth of these cells.

GLA is found in breast milk. Sometimes infants switched to artificial milk formulas are deficient in delta-6-desaturase, with resultant atopic eczema. A baby's digestive system is not fully developed until at least five months of age. Massaging the oil directly into skin allows quick absorption into the body.

In England, topical creams are registered for medicinal use for this very condition.

The oil makes a superior carrier oil for use in skin care and aroma therapeutics.

Neurodermatitis is a chronic skin condition related to allergic response, causing burning and itching, especially at night. One study at the University of Turku, Finland on 14 sufferers for 12 weeks found significant reduction of infections.

A year-long multi-centre study of 609 patients found significant symptom relief after three months. In over half of patients the symptoms improved to degree that no further medication was needed.

Dr. Lepore has found that evening primrose oil appears to antidote wheat and corn allergies. The oil helps prevent formation of leukotrienes that contribute to asthma attacks. Prostaglandin E1 produced from GLA also prevents release of arachidonic acid, helping prevent inflammation.

In studies on patients with tremors from Parkinson's disease, two teaspoons of evening primrose oil daily for several months resulted in a 55% improvement.

Evening Primrose oil also helps abnormal tear production (excess or deficient), soft, brittle finger nails, and alleviates the effects of alcohol.

The oil may help patients suffering Raynaud's disease, characterized by cold hands and feet. Belch et al, *Thromb Haemost* 1985 54:2.

Synergism with colchicine in multiple sclerosis showed improvement in disability score in a human study. Co-supplementation with hemp seed and evening primrose oil showed beneficial effect in improving clinical symptoms of multiple sclerosis patients. Rezapour-Firouzi S et al, *Compl Ther Med* 2015 23(5):652-7. Earlier work, in a double-blind randomized trial of 100 MS patients, the group taking the two oils showed improved activity of liver enzymes and reduction of low grade inflammation.

And the oil reduced cyclosporine-induced kidney damage, albeit in a rat study.

Another study found EPO improved kidney function in a study where one kidney was removed from rats with chronic renal failure. Bi ZQ et al, *Zhonghua Nei Ke Za Zhi* 1992 31(1):7-10.

EPO increased the number of osteoclasts, in one study, accelerating orthodontic tooth movement. Taweechaisupapong S et al, *Angle Orthod* 2005 75(3):356-61.

In one study with a psychiatric control group and a normal control group, EPO supplementation did not produce improvement in abnormal movement measurements, but there was significant improvement in mental state, schizophrenic symptoms and memory in patients receiving essential fatty acids. In the open phase at end of trial, the supplementation of zinc, niacin, B6 and vitamin C showed more marked and significant clinical improvement.

One isolated study at Bootham Park Hospital in York, England showed marked improvement in symptoms of schizophrenia when EPO was used in combination with penicillin. No one knows why.

Another study found patients diagnosed as schizophrenic and treated with phenothiazines were later re-diagnosed with epilepsy.

A study at Tufts University in Boston in 2000 found 4.5 grams of seed oil promoted cell mediated immune function.

Numerous studies, including some above and others, suggest the efficacy of EPO in various autoimmune disease, childhood hyperactivity, chronic inflammation, ethanol toxicity and acute alcohol withdrawal syndrome, *icthyosis vulgaris*, scleroderma, Sjogren's syndrome, brittle nails, mastalgia, various psychiatric syndromes, tardive dyskinesia, ulcerative colitis, and migraine headaches.

Various patents have been filed; from vegetable derived petroleum jelly replacement to treatment of ulcerative colitis to immunosuppressive agents.

The oil may inhibit conversion of testosterone to dihydrotestosterone.

Isolated cases of EPO and B12 helping chronic fatigue syndrome have been reported from the University of Miami and New Zealand.

In one animal study, evening primrose outshone both borage and black currant oils at reversing diabetic neuropathy. This may or may not relate to humans, but each oil does have unique properties. Trials have found the oil helps reverse muscle weakness, arm tendon reflex and numbness.

In another study by Munoz et al, Nutrition 1999 15 evening primrose oil was found to enhance the body's ability to fight cancer tumors. Work by Horrobin in 1994 found high doses of GLA prolonged life, without side effects, in patients suffering from liver, breast, brain and esophageal cancers.

Faster response to tamoxifen was found in patients with estrogen sensitive breast cancer.

Evening primrose meal has great potential as a source of natural antioxidants. Schwarz et al, *Eur Food Res Technol* 2001 212.

The seed husk contains tryptophan, with some in the oil. It has been found that tryptophan boosts the effectiveness of L-dopa (found in faba beans).

Phenolics, with significant anti-oxidant potential have been found in the seed meal by Wettasinghe et al, *J. Ag. Food Chem* 2002 50. They consist of over 10.5% (+)-catechin and (-)-epicatechin.

Peschel et al, *Ind Crops and Prod* 2007 25:1 also found the seedcake to possess high anti-oxidant potential. Due to anti-oxidant and anti-inflammatory activity, the seed cake has potential application in anti-aging, moisturizing, mitigating and protective cosmetics. Ratz-Lyko A et al, *J Cosmet Laser Ther* 2015 17(2):109-15.

At the present time the growing season on the prairies is better suited to borage than evening primrose for commercial production.

Supercritical, or CO_2 extraction is a preferred process to solvents like hexane. At 122° F and 10,000 psi, more than 95% of evening primrose oil is obtained in 10 minutes.

At -25MPa, and a temperature of 25-35° C, and a CO_2 flow of 38-40 kg/h, extraction time is about three hours, to obtain the same 95%.

Solvent extraction includes the cost of solvent waste disposal, exposure of personnel to hazardous chemicals, as well as more time and less product recovery. Not to mention, a less healthy product for consumers.

Note that the wild evening primrose seed can vary greatly in oil content. Commercial suppliers and plant breeders have developed cultivar varieties with the yields noted above.

CAUTION- It is reported that some individuals suffering schizophrenia, while taking epileptogenic drugs (phenothiazines) and evening primrose oil may be subject to increased risk of temporal lobe epilepsy, or difficulty in breathing. This has been repeated numerous times, and yet, the only reference is an anonymous entry in the Date Sheet Compendium, 1994-5, with no details available.

No seizures or epileptic events were observed in a crossover study of 48 patients (mostly schizophrenic) taking phenothiazines when given EPO for four months. Vaddadi KS et al, *Psychiatry Res* 1989 27 313-23.

Phenothiazines decrease seizure threshold on their own, so any interaction report would have to be very well documented to be credible.

Borage oil may be a suitable substitute, for those concerned.

ESSENTIAL OIL

Essential oil, steam distilled from the leaves and root of evening primrose (*O. biennis*), showed 79 constituents. The main component is furfural.

The related *O. odorata* from China is made into a concrete; with linalool and indole the main constituents of 24 compounds identified so far.

LEAF AND FLOWER OIL

An oil infusion can be made of the leaves and stems of evening primrose by gently simmering in olive or canola oil. A double boiler or crockpot works best.

Use equal parts by weight and volume for superior product, for 30 minutes and then removing from heat and let sit for two more hours.

To make an ointment for treating cradle cap, eczema and other skin affections of children, simply add a small amount of pure beeswax until desired consistency.

FLOWER ESSENCES

Evening primrose (*O. biennis*) flower essence is needed often because of the over concern of parents; leading to over sensitivity of the child to ideas and influences regarding themselves.

Sometimes the caring, smothering type of concern can manifest later as a hatred of the mother.

It may never be expressed while mother is essential for life sustenance, but festers away in the personality to cause problems later in life. This can lead to feeling unsafe, or feeling uncomfortable with tears.

NEW ZEALAND

Evening primrose (*O. hookeri*) is for feelings of rejection, avoidance of commitment in relationships, or fear of parenthood. The soul is most open while in utero or in very early infancy. At this time the soul is more like a moon-being than a sun-being; it receives and reflects the soul light of the parents, but especially the mother.

FLOWER ESSENCE SOCIETY

NOTE- this essence is prepared under lunar influence.

Evening Primrose (*O. caespitosa*) flower essence is for those who lack inner strength and are overly sensitive; or prone to depression, nervousness, anxiety, rejection or sexual suppression.

They may have unhealed childhood issues related specifically to the mother, such as feeling rejected or not bonded. Or they may suffer from identity crises. **LIVING FLOWER**

Missouri Primrose (*O. missouriensis*) works on the self-esteem by helping a person learn to accept and receive love, friendship, goodness, pleasure and other forms of self-nurturing. An individual develops a sense of self-worth based on general conditions of love, respect and nurturing obtained from childhood. **DALTON**

Evening Primrose (*O. lamarckiana*) strengthens the creative forces of the moon. It helps you to rediscover and connect with the source of your self-confidence, beauty and the inner feminine. Gives insight into the old, unknown areas of darkness, such as incest, abuse and problems with sexuality. **BLOESEM**

SPIRITUAL PROPERTIES

The generous, warm message of the Evening Primrose flower spirit is one of love. It is time for you to discard all your resistance to loving and being loved and allow it to happen, naturally, with no conditions.   **ECLARE**

PERSONALITY TRAITS

The leaves of Evening primrose have a beneficial effect on the vagus nerve.

Traditionally, this nerve was thought of as a physical sensor related to digestion.

However, recent research conducted by psychologist, Robert A. Jensen, at the Southern Illinois University in Carbondale, has reported evidence the vagus nerve helps store memory, in humans.

Researchers have found stimulating the vagus nerve improves memory, and may play an important role in helping victims of stroke or head traumas recover faster.

The work by Jensen and colleagues, reported in the journal, *Nature Neuroscience*, may help explain why people remember emotionally charged events better than ordinary happenings.

The vagus nerve is a kind of two way street. It relays commands from the brain to regulate heartbeat, and keeps the brain informed about the stomach.

Studies suggest arousal hormones use the vagus nerve to tell the brain to hang onto particular memories.

Researchers looked at 10 people involved in a medical study to see if stimulating the vagus nerve could suppress epileptic seizures.

In word memory studies, an improvement of 36% better word recognition occurred in those receiving nerve stimulation. It showed that the nerve helps the brain store the memory of something that just happened, rather than alerting the brain to pay attention to what's coming up.   **PRAIRIE DEVA**

For me, Evening Primrose's primary medicine (at least, for right now), is a luminous kind of calm I feel when I taste it, and what I can only describe as a clear and quiet mind and heart—very much a gift to me.   **JANE VALENCIA**

DOCTRINE OF SIGNATURES

The flower emerges from a tuft of leaves that grown directly from the root crown, and the significance of the white flower demonstrates a magnetic healing flow of energy from the root crown to the crown at the top of the head. The flower wilts to a gentle pink colour, corresponding with the power, compassion and love of the heart or fourth chakra.

The soft yet strong velvety, hairy leaves symbolize gentle strength.

The flower appears delicate, yet its stronger than it seems; its nectar is deep and sweet, yet it can grow from dry, rocky ground. This is symbolic of having a strong foundation or connection to earth, taking in earth's nectar and giving it back to Spirit. The physical vitality of the flower lasts only one night, giving the flower a full appreciation of valuing a short life. The flowers bloom towards evening, all evening long, and in the early morning before being hit by the sun. This is a significant signature of its relationship to the moon, the feminine and the mother.   **PALLAS DOWNEY**

MYTHS AND LEGENDS

When the Old Ones of the Ani-Tsalagi tell the story of the beginning of the world, they speak of the two brothers who were made by the Father. These two brothers knew that people lived in the depths of the underground world in darkness and filth. The two descended into the earth and led the people up. The sun was so bright it made them cry, and the tears which fell grew into flowers of the sun, (and) became the evening primrose and the sunflower.

HEATHERLEY

BOTANICA POETICA

Evening Primrose
(*Oenothera biennis*)

Pretty flowers wild and plain
With special oils in its seed
Fatty acids they contain
Helps prevent deficiency
Use the plant as a poultice too
Decoct the root for hemorrhoid grief
Soothe sore throats and heal a wound
Bring a tummy ache relief
The use of the oil is fairly new
It can help with PMS
Asthma and inflammation too
Helps relieve painful breasts
For eczema, it's a great friend
Put the dryness to an end
Allergies to keep at bay
Drink the tea for obesity
A Yin tonic you might like
Seems quite safe so take it freely
Inflammation take a hike!

SYLVIA CHATROUX MD

RECIPES

TINCTURE- 30-60 drops 3X daily. The fresh aerial plant tincture is made 1:2 at 98% alcohol, or 1:5 dry tincture at 40%.

FLUID EXTRACT- five to thirty drops.

INFUSION- Prepare 1:20 with boiled water. Up to four cups daily of leaf and flower tea.

DECOCTION- Two to four ounces three times daily of simmered root.

SYRUP- Chop dried or fresh root and simmer slowly in twice the volume of honey. One tablespoon every 3-4 hours.

SEED OIL- 250 to 500 mg capsules several times daily.

FABA BEAN
FAVA BEAN
WINDSOR BEAN
HORSEBEAN
BROADBEAN
MOJO BEAN
(*Vicia faba* L.)
TICKBEAN
(*V. faba*)
CRIMSON FLOWERING FAVA
(*V. faba*)
ALPINE MILK VETCH
WILD VETCH
(*V. americana* Muhl. ex Willd.)
TUFTED VETCH
(*V. cracca* L.)
WOOLLY VETCH
HAIRY VETCH
(*V. villosa* Roth.)
PARTS USED- seed, flower

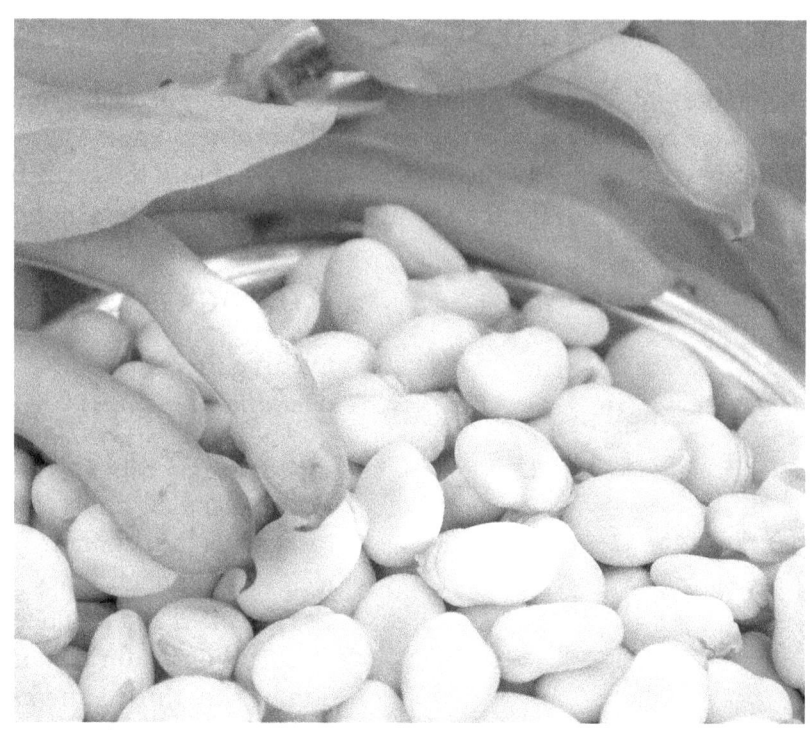

FRESH GREEN FAVA BEANS

Beans are the substance which contains…that animated matter of which our souls are particles.
DIOSGENES

First he ate some lettuce and some broad beans, then some radishes, and then, feeling rather sick, he went to look for some parsley.   **BEATRIX POTTER, THE TALE OF PETER RABBIT**

There was once a nest in a hollow,
Down in the mosses and knot grass pressed.
Soft and warm, and full to the brim,
Vetches hung over it purple and dim,
With buttercup buds to follow.   **ANON**

Vicia is from the Latin **VINCIO**, to bind. Vetch is thought to be corruption derived from the same root. Villosa means soft hairs, referring to the covered pods. Fava is an English corruption of Latin faba, meaning bean.

Faba beans were cultivated for over 6000 years, before *Phaseolus* beans reached the Old World. They reached China several thousand years late, and then moved to Japan and India. Recent work suggests it was first domesticated, by Neolithic farmers over ten thousand years ago. Wild relative seeds, fourteen thousand years old, have been found at the site el-Wad, near Mount Carmel, Israel. Caracuta V et al, *Sci Rep* 2016 6:37399.

The Israelites were familiar with faba and called them **POL** (Samuel II 17:18); which the Greeks called **POLTOS**, and the Romans **PULS**, and hence pulses.

Both the Greeks and Romans had mixed feelings about the plant.

Greek seers and oracles refused to eat them, fearing it would interfere with their prophetic visions. Pythagoras, the famed Greek philosopher, was killed by enraged folks of Crotonia when he could not cross a bean field, in order to escape. Many of his disciples were killed shortly afterwards by soldiers of Dionysus, who ambushed them in a bean field.

Pythagoras probably instituted the ban on faba because he observed the consequences of favism. To himself and his disciples, eating beans implied devouring one's own parents, causing serious disruption in the cycle of reincarnation.

The Roman Pliny believed the souls of the dead were contained in the beans. Ceres, the Roman Goddess of Grain, is said to have refused to include them as gifts to man because they beclouded the second sight of her priest. Our out of control tabby cat is named in her honor.

Ovid said that witches put beans in their mouth when calling up spirits.

The Roman scholar, Diogenes Laertius wrote: "One should abstain from eating beans because they are full of the material which contains the largest portion of that animated matter of which our souls are made."

The Greek word for soul is **ANEMOS**, which also means wind. When eaten and processed in the human intestine, soul winds are released, and eager to resume their ascension to heaven, headed straight for the nearest opening, exiting with a cry of joy. This is a most metaphoric way to look at a fart.

The Romans ate broad beans at funerals.

If all of this sounds strange, keep in mind that only recently has modern medical immunology recognized that genetically prone individuals of Mediterranean ancestry react to a substance in the beans that causes fatal dissolution of red blood cells, or favism.

When the Romans were Christianized, beans were thrown at ghosts on All Saint's Eve, our Halloween, and women who abstain from eating them for fear of being impregnated by the ghosts of frustrated men.

Some individuals are so sensitive and allergic that they faint at the light scent of the flower blossoms. Symptoms of favism can occur, after simply inhaling the pollen, in some sensitive individuals.

The scent is persistent and widespread, reminiscent of honey and auratum lily. In Suffolk, England, the scent was believed helpful to children suffering whooping cough.

In some areas of England, the scent was considered a powerful aphrodisiac. Ancient Celts applied the name beano to a funeral bean feast.

Miners in Suffolk thought more mine accidents occurred during flowering.

Two conjugates of jasmonic acid with tyrosine, dopa, and dopamine links may explain, in part, the observed benefits.

Hildegard de Bingen, the 12th century abbess, suggested "there is not much harm if sick people eat Faba beans, since they do not produce as much mucous as peas."

The Brothers Grimm tale of Jack and the Beanstalk is undoubtedly a broad bean vine.

When I lived on the shores of Lesser Slave Lake,I grew Windsor Beans as a source of winter food. The pods were huge, up to a foot long, with furry insides protecting the large, flat, kidney shaped bean.

The seeds are edible while green (like fresh peas), as well as the brown dried, after prolonged cooking (see below). The plants are nitrogen fixers, as are all legumes, and can be used as green manure.

Dr. King, the noted Eclectic physician, noted the stalks and husks when calcined and digested in white wine, are a good diuretic. The flowers, as an infusion, are reputed effective in gout and gravel. The bean flour has long been used in Europe as a remedy for diarrhea.

Fava beans are a staple in some Middle Eastern countries. They are dried and ground into flour, but more often cooked in a sauce. They were quite popular in colonial America, with fourteen varieties available from a Philadelphia seed man in 1803.

When introduced to northern Alberta, the Cree named it **MISTATIMOPEN-SAK**, or **KISTIKANIS**, meaning Horse Bean.

In the American Southwest the beans are browned in the oven, decocted with a little salt and taken as a soup to prevent pneumonia or cold lungs. If pneumonia is already present, a paste is prepared from the ground dry beans with hot water, and applied three times daily to the chest and back.

The flour is often combined with rye or spelt flour to make flat breads. In France today, faba flour is added at 2% or less to give baguettes their distinct aroma, add flavor to the bread, boost the rising process and whiten the crumb of breads made with less refined flours.

In Asia, they are fermented into a shoyu-like (soy) sauce or sprouted as a green edible. In India, the seeds are roasted and eaten like peanuts, while in China the re-hydrated beans are steamed and served cold in sesame oil dressing.

They are sometimes sprouted and cooked as a stir fry or added to soups.

Wheat pasta enriched with 35% faba flour has high protein digestibility and better amino acid profile than when enriched with 6% gluten or 5% egg. Laleg K et al, *Food Funct* 2016 7(2): 1196-207.

The shoots are boiled in oil and salt and used to rouse drunkards from their stupor in parts of China.

They have also been used as meat extenders or substitutes, as well as a skim milk substitute. A tofu-like product has been developed from faba beans by Zee et al at Laval University in Quebec.

A decantation process was used with details available in *Canadian Institutional Food Science Technology* 1987 20:4.

In certain people, an inherited form of anemia can take place when the beans are eaten in large quantities over extended time, especially raw. They are toxic only to those lacking a digestive enzyme, which normally destroys the hemolytic aspect of the seed. The substances responsible are vicine and convicine, with their oxidized forms reacting with glutathione. Young boys, especially of the eastern Mediterranean and parts of China and southeast Asia, have this congenital G6PD (glucose phosphate dehydrogenase) deficiency. This is commonly known as favaism.

The leaves are edible when cooked, or lightly steamed.

Broad bean flowers were traditionally used in the treatment of coughs, as well as uro-genital complaints, including difficulty with urination. Externally, the flowers were poulticed for skin inflammation, warts and burns, while the dry powdered bean helped heal mouth sores.

In ancient Egypt, faba beans were used as an ingredient in mouth rinses, for dressings, and in applications to "soften" stiff limbs. The bean meal was made into a paste with oil and honey, and applied to prolapsed rectums.

A modern Italian slang word for female genitals is **FAVA**, meaning bean.

In Scotland, the witches did not fly on conventional broomsticks, but used faba bean stalks instead. The pod fluff was used traditionally to remove warts, soothe chapped lips and remove the sting of nettles.

Fava Bean is now grown in North America. In 1998, just over 247 tonnes of faba beans were produced commercially in Alberta. By 2014, this had risen to nearly eighty thousand acres.

They should be planted early as they require about 115 frost free days to mature, and can take a spring frost much better than one in the fall.

St. Denis Seed Farms near St. Albert, has been growing faba for a number of years, including a white variety "Snowbird" with zero tannins. Lack of these compounds may help promote more use in livestock feed including hogs. Up to 35% faba can be added to pig rations; and would give prairie producers a replacement for soy meal at very competitive prices. Laying hens thrive when micronized-dehulled fava beans are used as substitute for soybean meal. Laudadio V et al, *Poult Sci* 2010 89(10):2299-303.

They produce an acceptable nut butter that is on the market.

Another interesting form is the Tick Bean, in reference to the tan coloured, small seed, with a distinct nutty flavor. In French, it is known as **FEVE À COUPER**, meaning "snipping" fava, in reference to the large floppy leaf buds used as a potherb. The flowers are sweet and fragrant, and the pod production higher than most other fava.

The pods contain up to 53% dietary fiber, and protein content. Up to 15% bean pod flour can be added to baked goods. Belghith-Fendri L et al, *J Food Sci* 2016 81(10).

When the top buds are picked as salad greens, the plant sets pods more quickly.

Another favorite of mine is Crimson Flowering Fava, with edible green beans, flowers and leaves. The flowers of this two foot tall Fava are intensely magenta.

The straw of broad beans burned to ash can be mixed into top soil, and quickens the germination of parsley seeds.

Intercropping faba beans with Coriander gives a good yield advantage. Biennial caraway is another good option.

Various species of *Polygonum* including Bistort, Knotweed, Water Smartweed and Lady's Thumb produce water extracts effective at controlling *Aphis fabae*.

Ants collect nectar from the leaf nectaries at the bracts. The plants benefit as the ants keep caterpillars away.

Faba bean tolerates petroleum pollution up to 10% crude oil/sand in work by Radwan et al, *Int J Phytoremed* 2000 2 suggesting their use on contaminated oil and gas well sites. The rhizobacteria assist in breakdown of hydrocarbons and removal of mercury. Sorkhoh NA et al, *Ecotoxicol Environ Saf* 2010 73(8):1998-2003.

American Vetch is a native vine-like legume very common to open woods, with white flowers, and small pods. The young shoots were cooked as greens by various Native tribes.

The Iroquois decocted the roots as a love medicine. The Navaho smudged the plant near horses to increase their endurance; and infusion of the plant as an eyewash.

The Squaxin tribe made an infusion of the crushed leaves as a bath for relieving soreness.

One magical use of vetch roots is for fidelity. If your love one has gone astray, rub the root of the vetch on your body and then wrap it in cloth and place it under your pillow. This will remind them that you're still around, waiting.

American Vetch is promoted by the Alberta Research Council as a native reclamation plant. The seed weight is 60-80 thousand per kilo, with a seeding rate of 100-150 seeds per meter row. You can expect a 78% germination rate in 3-7 days with scarification; 75% in 14 days without.

The forage is palatable to livestock, particularly sheep, and browsed by mule deer.

Tufted Vetch is an introduced perennial with purplish, blue flowers and a weak, sprawling stem. It was originally brought to North America as a fodder or green manure, which has escaped and flourished. The plant has come to symbolize reason, and dedicated to the birth date, November 24th.

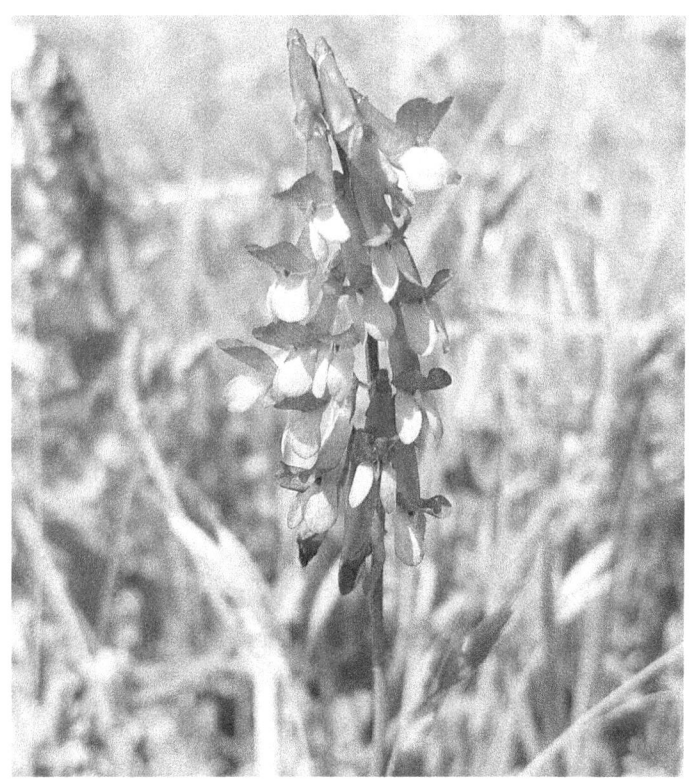

TUFTED VETCH

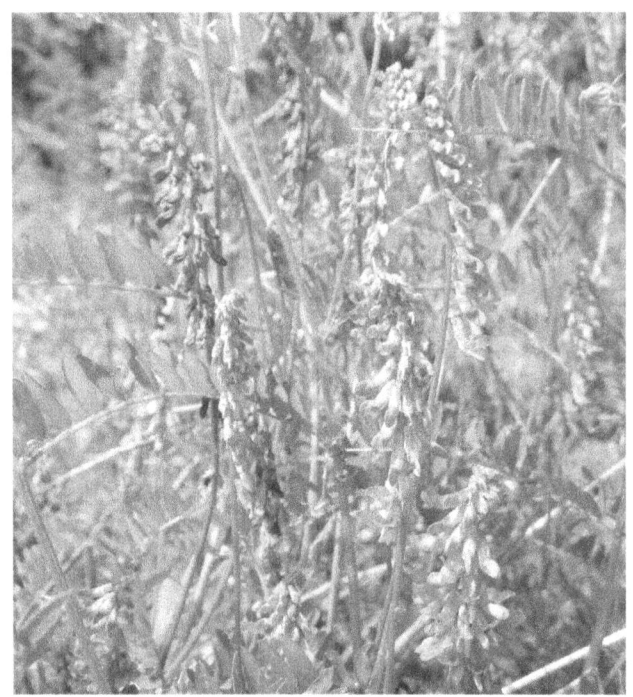

WOOLLY VETCH

The young shoots, leaves, pods and seeds are all edible after proper identification and cooking. Studies conducted in Northern Ontario and Quebec, found no increase in body weight of sheep after 3 weeks, and a loss in steers after four. The protein content and coefficient of digestibility are high, but the coefficient of cellulose is low.

The unripe seeds look like small peas, but contain traces of hydrocyanic acid, removed by cooking. The ripe seeds can be sprouted. Tufted vetch contains pyrimidin derivatives that cause photosensitivity illness.

Russell Willier, noted Cree healer, uses the roots in combinations for heart and stomach cramps. He calls the plant **PIMAHOPOKWA**, or climbing vine.

Two patents exist for *F. cracca*. One is for the lectins potential as an anti-retroviral drug; the other using affinity absorbents for isolating lectins. One-chain lectins are specific to blood type A.

The plant contains 19 phenolic compounds, nine flavonoids as well as quercetin, kaempferol, apigenin and disometin.

Woolly Vetch is an introduced annual only found in the southern part of our region. It is grown mainly to increase the nitrogen content of the soil.

As a winter annual, it is often a contaminant in fall-sown rye. Several reports indicate grazing on *V. villosa* has caused diarrhea, dermatitis, and conjunctivitis, and sexual excitement in cattle. Hair vetch poisoning can have a high mortality rate.

Beta cuamp-L-alanine, implicated in locoweed toxicity, is present in the seeds of *V. villosa*. The blue flowers contain interesting anthocyanins.

Woolly Vetch is capable of detecting the smallest intensity of light. A 25 watt lamp in clear air and complete darkness can be detected and located by the seedling tips at a distance of 19 miles; a 100 watt lamp at 44 miles. For a plant without a telescope this is truly remarkable.

Two plant physiologists in the United States have found that annual vetch works very well as an organic mulch to replace plastic sheeting in growing tomatoes; as well as other row crops like snap beans, peppers, eggplants and cantaloupe.

The annual vetch is seeded in newly plowed and disked fields about two months before winter freeze up.

They become dormant but in spring they begin to grow again vigorously. The day before planting your tomatoes, mow the vetch with a high-speed flail mower and leave the residue on beds. Transplant the young tomato plants right through the mulch, into the soil. The killed vetch forms an organic blanket that feeds nitrogen and other nutrients into the soil.

When hairy vetch and turnips are planted together, the turnip greens are aphid free, due to the vetch providing shelter for ladybugs that love to eat aphids.

Work by Fujihara et al, showed hairy vetch mulch resulted in a 60-80% reduction of weed biomass. Even more effective was to cover the row with the aerial parts of living hairy vetch; especially for root crops.

In parts of France, the seeds of *V. sativa* were traditionally used in soup and as a flour for bread. Work by Han et al, *Biotech Lett* 28(23) identified a means of producing R-cyanohydins from the seeds.

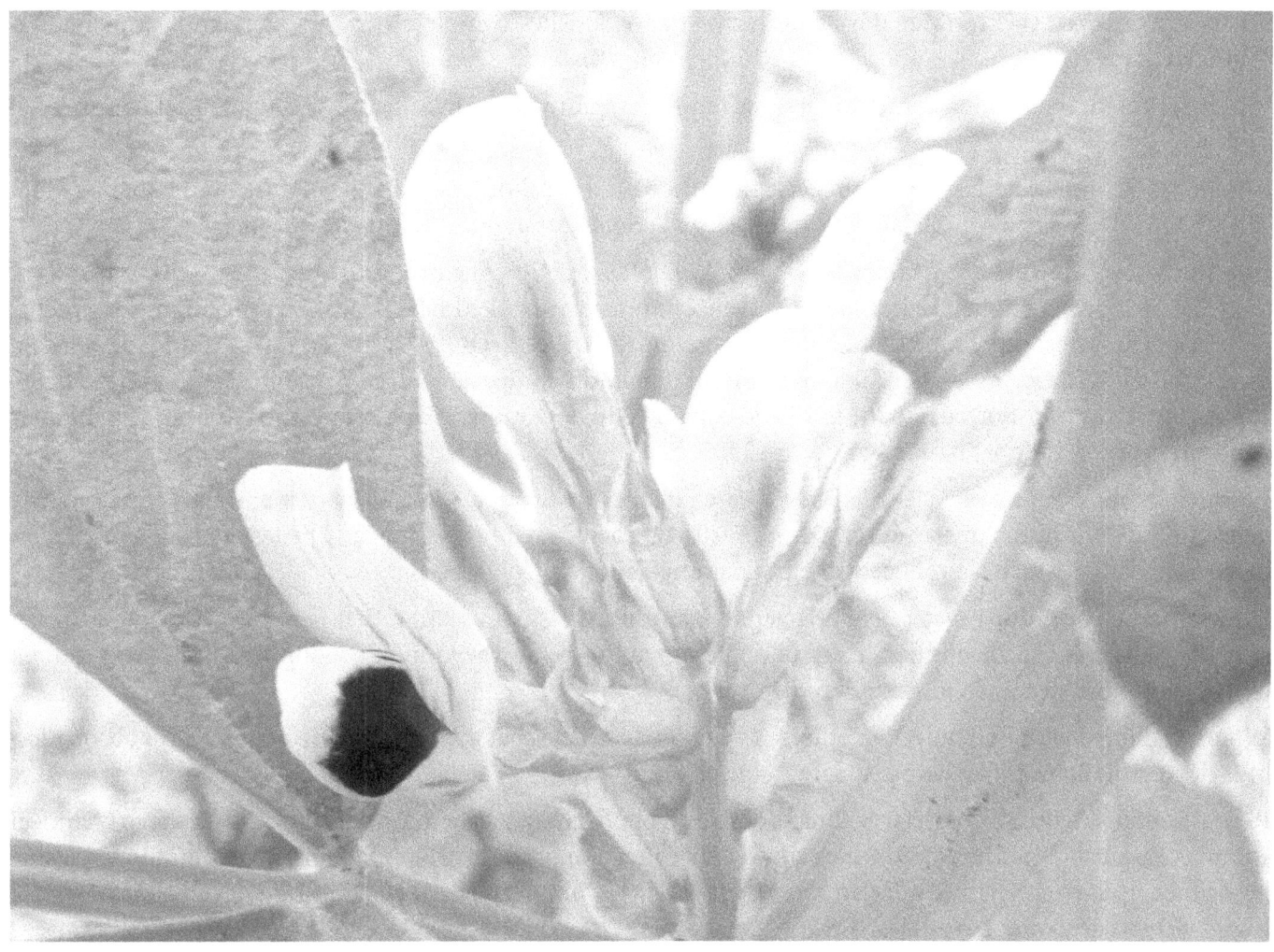

FABA BEAN FLOWERS

MEDICINAL

CONSTITUENTS - *V. cracca* -leaves- kaempferol-3-0-rhamnoside, proanthocyanidins, one chain lectins. The seed lectin of *F. cracca* is specific for human blood type A.

V. villosa- flowers- contain the 3-O-alpha-rhamnopyranoside-5-O-beta glucopyranosides of petunidin (71%), delphinidin (12%), and malvidin (9%)

Aerial parts- cyanamide

V. faba pods- five flavonoid aglycons and 8 flavonol glycosides. As the colour of the pod changes from green to reddish and finally dark brown, the flavonoids increase; and then decrease at full maturity.

seeds- 11.4 mcg/kg of estradiol monobenzoate from green seeds, including genistein, daidzein and formomonetin; wyerone, medicarpin, and epoxide (phytoalexins) ; vicine (vicioside 0.4-0.8%), convicine (0.1-0.6%), isolectins-favine-L-3.4-dihydroxyphenylalanine (L-dopa, up to 8%), tannins, starch.

sprouted seed- amylase and vitamin C activity maximum on third day, diamine oxidase.

Protein- green seeds 5.2%; dry 25%. Plant also contains convicine, wyerone epoxide, medicarpin, and gibberillin A-53, as well as jasmonic and isojasmonic acids.

stem- genistein and daidzein

Faba beans contain natural L-dopa that penetrates the intestinal epithelial cells and is transported through the blood stream to the brain capillaries where it is converted into dopamine.

The beans should be eaten, when not fully mature, but when young, with a thin skin, making them easy to digest. Up to 90% of patients afflicted with Parkinson's disease at an early age respond quickly.

It is easily oxidized two to three days after harvest and vanishes completely as the plant stops growing and begins to dry.

When sprouted, the L-dopa content increases ten times, and worth investigating as a potential commercial product.

Patient report a marked improvement each time they eat a meal of fresh faba beans. A commercial product called Dopa Bean, is now available with standardized content of natural L-dopa from faba bean.

In a study by Rabey et al, *Advanced Neurology* 1993 60 six patients with Parkinson's disease were taken off their medications, and after 12 hours were given 250 grams of cooked faba beans. Significant improvements in motor symptoms were found, compared to those on 125 mg of L-DOPA, and 12.5 mg of carbidopa. Plasma levels of L-DOPA increased after faba ingestion in a manner comparable to oral administration of the drug, suggesting it was transported into the CNS and converted to dopamine. Work in England has found the highest concentrations of L-dopa in bean variety WH 305.

Researchers at the Prince of Wales Medical Research Institute in Sydney, Australia have found a new test that may detect initial signs of Parkinson's disease from 7-20 years before symptoms appear. The test looks for antibodies to neuromelanin, which is produced when dopamine-producing nerve cells are in a degenerative state.

Large amounts of L-dopa may cause priapsim, a painful, persistent erection that is not necessarily related to sexual arousal. As Faba beans have a reputation as an aphrodisiac, they might contain that little extra L-dopa that gives a more sustained erection.

When combined with Puncture Vine, there is a synergistic effect that appears to increase the body's absorption of L-dopa. This sounds like herbal Viagra to me.

Recent work looked at a proprietary extracts derived from faba bean, called Atremorine®. This is the first clinical study on Parkinson's patients (119) which showed that after a single dose of 5 milligrams, dopamine blood plasma levels increased from 762 pg/ml to an average of 4556 pg/ml. Cacabelos R et al, *Journal of Genomic Medicine and Pharmacogenomics* 2016 1(1):1-26.

As Faba beans increase the brain's production of dopamine, this, in turn will decrease prolactin that stimulates milk production. If breastfeeding, and milk flow is deficient, do not eat the beans. Work by Koreneva, *Probl Endokrinol* 1980 26:6 found L-Dopa effective in treating women suffering amenorrhea-galactorrhea syndrome.

I used the beans for a female client that was producing breast milk, not associated with pregnancy, nor with a pituitary tumor, with success.

The medicinal uses of L-Dopa are amazingly widespread with good clinical studies on bone fracture, myocardial infarction, depression, amblyopia (lazy eye), and optic neuropathy, measles encephalitis, male sterility, peptic ulcer, restless leg syndrome, sleep disorders and various forms of dystonia. Faba may be useful in the treatment of epilepsy.

Salih et al, *Epilepsy Behav* 2008 12:1 found evidence of binding to glycine receptors and anti-convulsant properties. A synergistic pattern with diazepam was noted in the study.

As an aside, it should be noted that fresh banana peels contain 6-12 microM per gram of dopamine. Could this be the source of Mellow Yellow during the 1960s, when smoking banana peels was touted as a way to get high? The banana fruit contains (-)-salsolinol, which shows dopamine antagonism *in vivo*.

Dopamine helps alleviate cravings associated with addictions like alcohol and nicotine.

Diamine oxidase is one of the key enzymes for GABA (gamma-aminobutyric acid) formation. The compound is found in germinated fava beans.

An older study by Macarulla et al, *British Journal of Nutrition* 85:5 found both the whole bean and protein isolate from Faba was strongly anti-oxidative. Okada et al, confirmed the protein extract is water soluble. *J of Nutritional Science and Vitaminology* 2000 46:1.

Extracts induce apoptosis of HL-60 acute promyelocytic leukemia cells, and inhibit angiotensin-coverting enzyme (ACE). Proliferation of cancer cells BL 13, AGS, HepG2 and HT-29 was also noted. Siah SD et al, *British Journal Nutrition* 2012 108 Suppl 1.

A trypsin inhibitor inhibited HIV-1 reverse transcriptase activity, and showed anti-proliferative effect on HepG2 cancer cells via apoptosis. Fang EF et a, *Protein Pept Lett* 2011 18(1):64-72.

In Traditional Chinese Medicine, faba bean is used for edema, in the form of a tea. It is most commonly called **CAN COU**, meaning silkworm bean, but is also known as **HU DOU**, foreign bean, **MA CHI DOU**, horse tooth bean, and **NAN DOU**, south bean.

The fresh beans are crushed into a paste and applied externally to *tinea capitis*, while the mashed leaves help heal indolent leg ulcers.

When dry, the beans are ground into a powder. Two teaspoons are dissolved in warm water and taken three times daily for chronic diarrhea and bloody stools.

A fermented paste, doubanjiang-meju, is produced with broad beans, wheat flour and salt.

The powder is boiled with sugar to treat children with poor appetite and diarrhea; brown sugar with presence of blood from the anus. The older the powder, the stronger the effect.

One antacid product found in health food stores, contains faba bean flour for acid neutralizing effect. The beans inhibit alpha-amylase and may be useful in anti-diabetic diets. Choudhary DK & Mishra A, *Bioengineered* 2016 28 1-11.

The leaves can be juiced and 20 ml twice daily ingested for tuberculosis with coughing of blood.

The leaves, flowers, seeds and seed hull all possess anti-bacterial activity against *E. coli, Staphylococcus aureus, Shigella sp., Bacillus subtilis, Serratia marcesens,* and *Micrococcus pyogenes.* Peyvast et al, *Pak J Bio Sci* 2007 10:3.

The seed coat extracted with methanol shows activity against *S. aureus, B. subtilis, B. cereus, E. coli, Candida albicans, C. maltosa* and *Cryptococcus neoformans.* Akroum et al, *European Journal Sci Res* 2009 31:2.

Acetone extracts show inhibition of yeasts, and were most active in treating candidiasis in mice. Akroum S, *J Mycol Med* 2016 1156-5233(16)20126-3.

The aerial parts show antioxidant activity and inhibit topoisomerase I enzyme activity, suggestive of chemo-protective benefit. Spanou et al, *J Ag Food Chem* 2008 56.

Plant extracts inhibit xanthine oxidase, suggestive of benefit in gout and related rhematic conditions. Spanou C et al, *PLoS One* 2012;7(3):e32214. This is interesting as many peas and beans, due to their high content of purine, aggravate this painful condition.

The flowers combine well with corn silk in the treatment of hypertension, simmered and taken as a tea. When cooled, the flower tea helps ease the pain of kidney stones and sciatica, and stop bleeding.

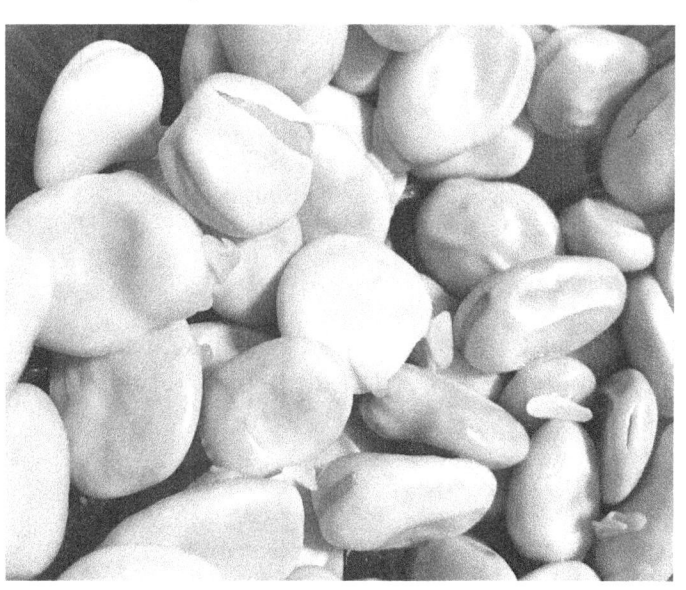

SPROUTING FABA BEANS

The shells can be simmered and the water taken for dysuria, while the stems when decocted help resolve bloody diarrhea.

Nohara et al, studied the composition and hepatoprotective properties of Faba Bean. Typical oleanene glycosides with a methyl group at C28 and having the fabatriosyl moiety showed strong hepato-protective activity. *Studies in Plant Science* 1999 6:31.

Madar and Stark, *British Journal of Nutrition* 2002 88:3, mention faba beans possess lipid lowering effects and are a source of anti-oxidative and chemopreventative factors.

Sauer, in his *Compendious Herbal*, suggests Broad Bean flour for swellings of the bosoms, and "when the member swells so that one cannot urinate, as can easily happen to those afflicted by the stone when the stone settles in the duct, then cook some broad beans in milk to a porridge consistency. Apply this thick and warm around the member".

The stems contain isoflavones at the rate of over 1 gram/kilo, and due to their prodigious growth may have some future nutraceutical application.

The biochemical composition of faba beans cooked by different extrusion temperatures and feed moisture was examined by Prakrati et al, *J of Food Science and Tech* Mysore 2000 37. Cooking them at 75 degrees Celsius increased tryptophan, methionone, and iron levels, and decreased both calcium and phosphorus.

Faba beans increase sodium excretion and diuresis through renal dopamine receptors. Vered et al, *Planta Medica* 1997 63:3.

Lectins from faba bean can alter the differentiation, adhesion and proliferation of colorectal cancer cells. Work by Jordinson et al, *Gut* 1999 44:5 found agglutinins stimulated an undifferentiated colon cancer cell line to differentiate into gland like structures, with the adhesion molecule epCAM involved. The authors suggest that dietary or therapeutic intake of faba bean lectins may slow the progression of colon cancer.

The roots are a narcotic poison. Wyeronic acid is formed when the plant is attacked by botrytis, and exhibits anti-fungal activity. Wyerone derived from faba beans has anti-fungal properties.

Tufted Vetch (*V. cracca*) leaves in water extract show activity against myco-bacteria. Two plant patents exist, one for its lectins, and their activity as an anti-retroviral drug. The lectin is blood group A specific. It accumulates cyanamide.

Woolly Vetch (*V. villosa*) seeds contain three alpha galactosides of D-pinitol. This compound, found in chickpea, lentil, and stressed pine needles, is gaining increasing importance in the maintenance of blood sugar levels.

The plant contains cyanamide, a plant growth inhibitor.

SEED OIL

CONSTITUENTS- composed mainly of oleic acid (57.5%) and linoleic acid (35%); with about 7.5% saturated fatty acids, mainly stearic acid.

ESSENTIAL OIL

Faba beans were analyzed with headspace extraction and GC mass spectrometry. Volatiles include 1-pentanol, 1-hexanol, pentanal, (E)-2-heptenal, 2-ethylfuran, 2-pentylfuran, acetone, 2-butanone, 2-heptanone and 3-octen-2-one.

HYDROSOL

The flowers and green pods are diuretic and sedative to the urinary tract. According to Culpepper, "water distilled from fresh husks drunk was effectual against the stone and to provoke urine.

Sauer also believed that "several loths (2 loths = one ounce) of water of broad bean flowers drunk in the morning before breakfast will promote urine and drive out gravel".

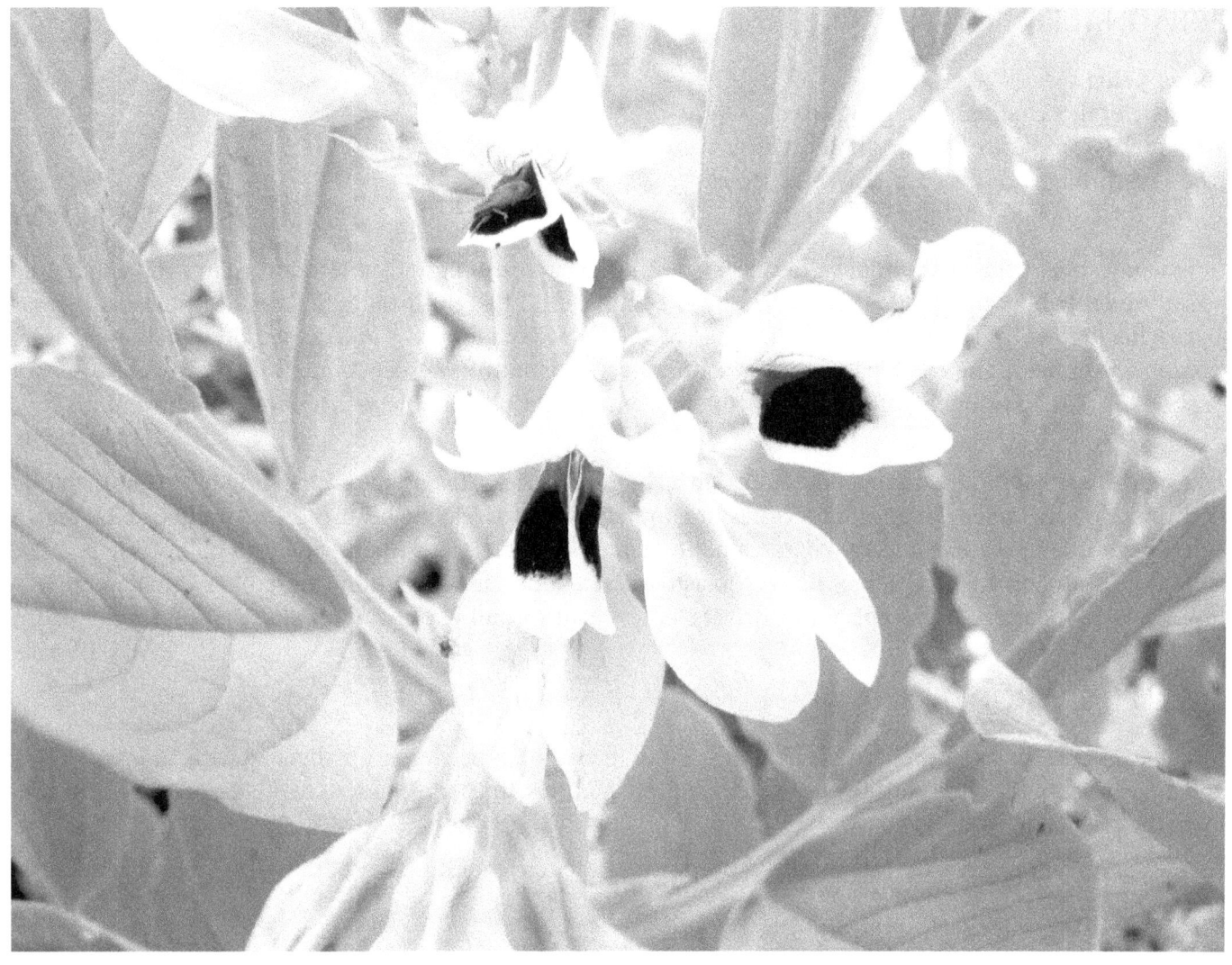

FABA BEAN FLOWERS

FLOWER ESSENCES

Tufted Vetch (*V. cracca*) flower essence is the remedy for many cases of sexual difficulty. Male or female, the difficulties are often caused by a totally incorrect " self-image". For many there is an inability to come " up-front", and accept the sexual aspect of their nature. The roots of these difficulties are nearly always in childhood, and are frequently due to heavy conditioning. There is also an inability to see the games that one plays on the sexual level, and a tendency to always blame the other sex when things do not turn out as the person would have wished. **BAILEY**

Vetch (*Vicia* sp.) flower essence helps to build healthy boundaries among members of a community, allowance for others' differences and to help teamwork and working together. **HUMMINGBIRD**

Fava (*Vicia faba*) essence facilitates all functions of brain activity, including memory, energy and sense of well-being. It is useful for balancing hormones. Strength, energy and radiant vitality come from being in balance. Good for menopause, supports a parasitic cleanse. **STAR PERUVIAN**

Tufted Vetch essence helps develop independence and self-confidence. **CHOMING**

Tufted Vetch essence strengthens self- determination and realization, helps one feel clear and free of compulsive acts and dependencies. **MARIANA**

PERSONALITY TRAITS

Tufted Vetch
I am one of those rather entangling weeds
Who makes good use of my neighbours I fear.
And I go through your garden, leaving my seeds
To make sure I come back the following year.

CAMERON

"I remember once being in the train beside the open window;I was reading and quite absorbed in a very interesting book; presently I became aware that my heart was beating and I had my 'beanfield (faba bean) feeling'\. I was just saying to myself, 'This book is as exciting as a beanfield', when I looked out of the window and saw we were passing a beanfield! The effect passed off as soon as we were out of the scent zone, which proved it was not the book. It was a most delightful sensation, and the excitement pleasurable; a sort of happy, buoyant ecstasy."

F. A. HAMPTON

Like a derelict telephone exchange, the stalks shrivel on their sticks, losing the connection between earth and sky. Their flowers, called 'letters of mourning', are now shelled pods leaving bean-money, funding an old death cult. They rattle in the bag and spill onto gambling tables to be counted. A jam jar, a roll of blotting paper, a splash of water and a soul emerges like ectoplasm—testa, root hair, cotyledon (remember the diagram?)—professors, market traders, receptionists, drivers—they're all sprouting on windowsills, waiting for Epiphany.

PAUL EVANS

SPIRITUAL PROPERTIES

Mojo beans are seen as a profound blessing from God. In Catholicism, they are associated with St. Joseph's Day and are placed on the altar. During one of Sicily's severe famines, the people prayed to St. Joseph to be delivered from the crisis.

As a result of their prayers, the Mojo beans thrived while other crops failed. They became a symbol of abundance and prosperity.

S. GREGG

OTHER PROPERTIES

Lima Beans, like their cousin Faba, have been found to be good communicators, according to new research from Japan.

Like some other plants, Lima can let its neighbors know when attacked by a pest like the spider mite. The munching releases volatile compounds that are carried through the air to neighboring plants, which then prepare chemical defenses against infestation.

This has been known for some time, but in early 2000, researchers reporting in Nature, discovered the volatile compounds that activate five defense genes in an un-infested plant.

The plants were also found to differentiate between a mite infestation and physical damage from say, stepping on the plant. These signals were ignored by the neighboring plants.

Fabaceae is the longest English word that can also be a hexadecimal numeral (consisting only of a, b, c, d, e and f). This is an old system created in the 1950s for computer ASCII code. Remember those days?

RECIPES

DOPA BEAN- One or two capsules daily of standardized faba bean extract.

A rapid reversed phase HPLC method derived by Perumal and Becker, *Food Chemistry* 2001 72:3 may prove useful in determining L-dopa percentage in beans. The variety WH305 appears to contain the highest percentage of L-dopa.

COOKED FABA BEANS- Usually broad beans require soaking overnight and cooking the hydrated beans for about two hours. A quick method involves blanching for seven minutes in boiling water, followed by hydration in a soaking medium of sodium bicarbonate, sodium carbonate and trisodium phosphate and cooking in 2.5% brine. The cooking time is reduced to fifteen, with good flavor and free from lipoxygenase, hemagglutinin and trypsin inhibitor activity.

Favism is a hemolytic anemia disease occurring in individuals suffering from a blood enzyme deficiency, glucose-6-phosphate de-hydrogenase (G6PD), that can be fatal in infants. The deficiency occurs almost exclusively in populations living around the Mediterranean, but today affects about 400 million people worldwide.

It is believed caused by the presence of faba beans, especially green pods and seeds, of two glycosidic pyrimidine derivatives, vicine and convicine, and/or their hydrolytic products (aglycones) divicine and isouramil. Some sensitive individuals react to the pollen.

It is believed a trade off for malaria resistance, as this condition produces red blood cells that starve the malaria parasite of oxygen. Or, more accurately, G6PD deficient red blood cells contain too little of a metabolite essential for the survival of the parasite.

Ironically, all known anti-malarial drugs are contraindicated for these individuals.

The gene for G6PD enzyme is carried on the X chromosome, so males are more likely to be afflicted. For a female to have the condition, genes on both of her X chromosomes would have to be affected.

Morel mushrooms should be avoided, by these same faba bean-sensitive individuals.

A recent animal study found anise essential oil decreased favism disorders, probably due to anethole content. More study is needed. Koriem KM et al, *J Diet Suppl* 2016 13(5): 505-21.

FALSE HELLEBORE
GREEN HELLEBORE
(*Veratrum eschscholtzii* A. Gray) not accepted
(*V. viride* Ait. **ssp. eschscholtzii** [R.&S.] A. Löve & D. Löve) not accepted
(*V. viride* Aiton)
PARTS USED- leaf, seeds, root

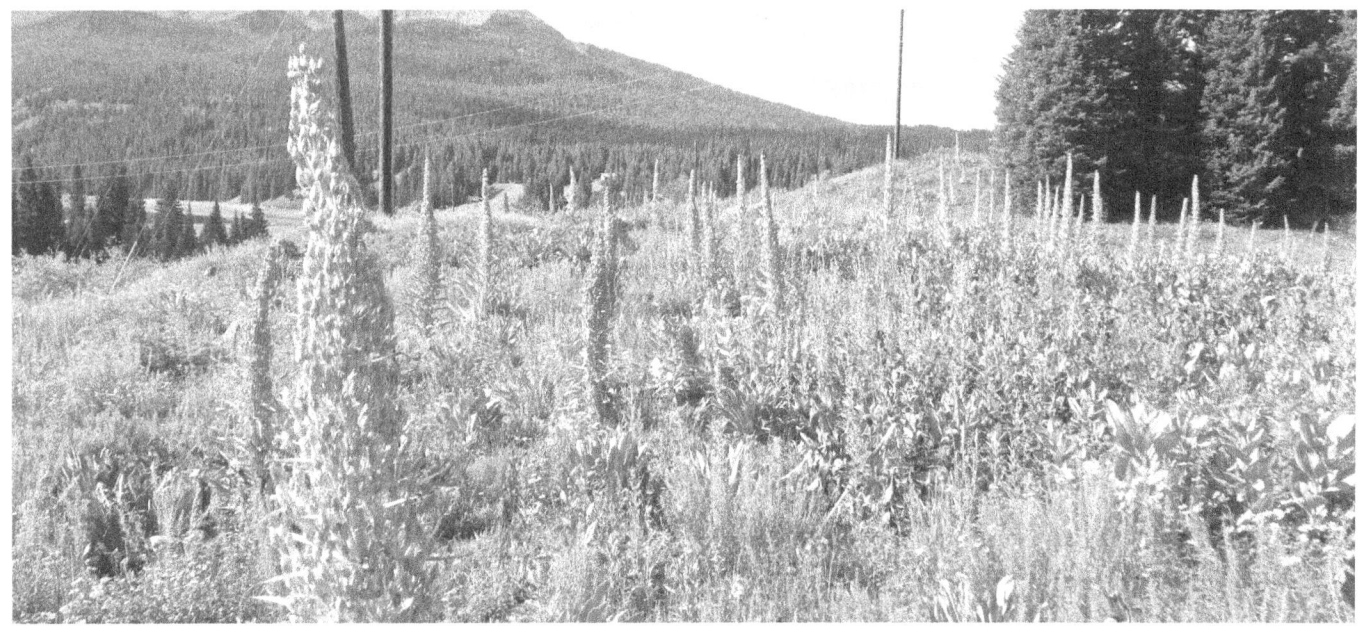

GREEN HELLEBORE

Veratrum is from **VERA** meaning true, and **ATRUM** meaning black; referring to another species of the genus. Viride means green. Eschscholtzii is named after the Russian explorer who was also honored with the species name of California poppy.

Helleborus is from a Greek name now applied to a genus of the buttercup family. Hellebore comes from the Greek **HELEIN**, meaning to injure; and **BORA**, for fodder.

Helleborus niger is Black Hellebore, an ancient poison.

White Hellebore (*Veratrum album)* with black roots, is a famous and potent herb from Europe.

False Hellebore is found in the valleys of the foothills in Alberta and throughout western North America. It is very hardy, and can survive -40° Celsius in winter with adequate snow cover.

It can grow up to ten feet tall, with massive leaves, that remind one it is a member of the lily valley. In fact, where it grows, you will likely also find False solomon seal, from the same family.

False Hellebore was used by various indigenous people, for both medicine and ritual. Josselyn (1672) reported that younger natives would elect a chief based on the ability to withstand the root poisoning the longest. It is sometimes known as Skookum Root, a Chinook jargon for strong and powerful, or Putsk, as a strong medicine.

On the plains, the Blackfoot used false hellebore root powder for headaches and itching. They call the plant **A'SIIYA'TSIS** meaning "makes you sneeze."

Further south, in corn country, the seed was soaked in a root decoction before planting. Birds who ate a few kernels would suffer from vertigo, and frighten away other birds.

Various coastal tribes would use root baths for scabies, aches and pains, and to remove human smell before hunting.

The Tlingit used it for colds, the Nisga'a for toothache.

For various indigenous tribes it was considered a cure-all; from kidney and bladder problems, to constipation, chest pains, and to abort unwanted pregnancy.

Pieces of the root were carried as good luck charms. The Lillooet tribe used the stem fibres to weave baskets and purses.

The Haida name **GWAAYK'AA** refers only to the root, as does the common name, Skookum-root. The root was mixed with urine and allowed to ferment in a woven basket, and used to conquer supernatural beings, such as under-ocean shamans or sea monsters. If this solution was sprinkled on or near them, they would lose their powers. This was a common use up and down the Northwest Coast.

It helped ward off the Land-Otter People, half man and half beast, who stole men's minds and made them pitiful creatures.

The root was believed strong enough to restore to life whole families of people whose disorganized skeletons had been recovered from the maw of a devouring monster.

The Slave call it "throw up root", or **NDAH DZEKU**. A small piece of the fresh or dried root was taken by adults to vomit and clear the stomach.

The Gitksan used the rhizome for purification and as a smudge for treating mental illness, stroke, and protection from "evil". It was also a good luck blessing for success in hunting, and for those suffering nightmares or sleep-walking.

A piece of the root was thrown into the water if rains were delayed and no salmon came to the rivers.

Recent uses involve helping cure addictions such as alcoholism and other substance abuse. Carrying a piece of root is considered a lucky amulet, and protection from evil.

The dried root was used for moxibustion in a manner similar to mugwort burning down to the skin on particular parts of the body.

The powdered root was a snuff for sinus congestion. The Dena'ina of Alaska have several names for the plant including **CH'ISHKENA** meaning "stinging root" and **NUK'ELBAQ'I** meaning "that which makes a person vomit". A small piece is used to de-worm dogs, or is placed on top of a wood stove to rid a home of germs. It is used externally for a number of ailments associated with infection, cuts, sores and inflammation.

The Wet'suwet'en of northern BC call the poisonous root **KONYE**. It was used in sweat baths and rites to ensure good hunting, but not taken internally. Men took roots from a "female" plant that has dried flowers, and women took roots from a "male" plant that lacked flowers.

The Karuk used the root for pneumonia, or strep throat, letting a one-inch length dissolve between the cheek and gums until just the wiry centre remains. Josephine Peters, an elder suggests you "don't take too much, as 'a funny feeling' on the back of your tongue can occur, akin to the paralyzing feel of a black widow bite."

Various western tribes, following the death of their chief, gave a drink of this plant to see who was least affected and therefore strongest and next chief.

Various Eclectic physicians suggested false hellebore for the treatment of hypertension (see below). In Russia, the herb is steeped in vodka (what else?) and taken internally to alleviate rheumatism and sciatica.

The powdered rhizomes are used in some commercial insecticides, cevadine and veratridine showing the greatest effect on houseflies.

There are reports (James Teit) that the Stl'atl'imx used the stem fibers to weave bags and pouches.

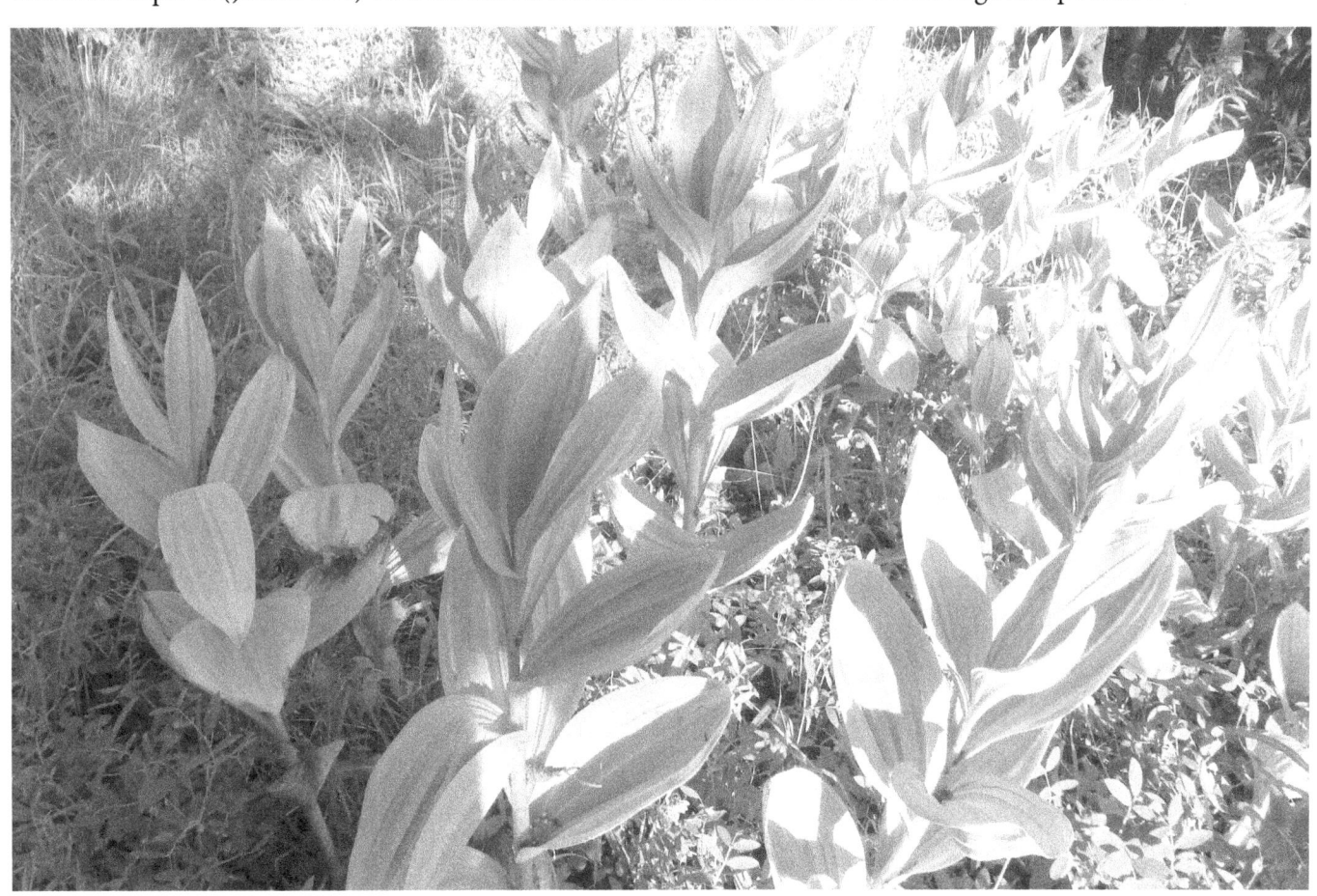

GREEN HELLEBORE

MEDICINAL

CONSTITUENTS- root- steroid alkaloids including solanidane type, isorubijervine, rubijervine, rubivirine, c-nor-D-homo-sterane-type, germine, germadine, germitrine, veramivirine, cevine, veramarine, cyclopamine, angel-oylzygadenine, zygadenine, 15-0-methylbutyroyl-germine, 1 alpha, 3 beta-dihydroxy 5 alpha-jervanin-12-en-11-one, cevadine, protoverine, veratridine, veratrosine, and protoveratrine- all alkaloids that are esters of highly hydroxylated parent alkanolamine bases. Also contains hellebrin- a glycoside, and 14-hydroxy-3-oxo-1,4,20,22-bufatrae-nolide (genin), neogermatrine and pseudo-jervine.

Veratrum alkaloids affect the brain stem, especially the medulla oblongata. Cells in the brain stem help determine the brain's general level of alertness and regulate processes such as breathing, heartbeat and blood pressure.

Veratrum root works on the afferent side of the nervous system, which it sensitizes to interpretation of blood pressure, and consequently decreases the blood pressure reactivity.

Germatrin has been found to lower blood pressure.

It is best reserved for those people who are strong and robust, and when the skin is hot and moist and pulse full and bounding.

Externally, the tincture can be painted on inflamed tonsils, or used for herpes labialis, erysipelas, boils, felons, and even inflamed acne, with care in avoiding toxicity through trans-dermal absorption.

For eczema, psoriasis and other difficult skin problems, try two parts dried root combined with three parts dried bittersweet stems in canola or olive oil in a low temperature crock pot. Add small amount of beeswax to make salve.

Active preparations cause a decrease in both systolic and diastolic blood pressure, decreased heart rate, and increased peripheral blood flow. The action is short lived, meaning that frequent small dosages must be continued for a period of time.

Eli Jones recommended false hellebore tincture for the early stages of congestive lung cancer.

Studies by Arena and Drew, 1986 indicate Veratrum alkaloids have been used in the treatment of hypertension, acute hypertensive crises, hypertensive toxemia in pregnancy, and various nephropathies.

They have been given parenterally with success in managing pulmonary edema resulting from severe acute hypertensive crises. Veratrum dissipates manic energy (excess heat and yang) due to fevers, inflammation or acute infection by slowing and sedating both mental and physical spheres.

Dr. King recommended it for cases where "the pulse is full, strong and intense, the carotids pulsate forcibly, the eyes are bloodshot, and there is a cough, headache and weight in the upper epigastrium, while the heart may beat so violently as to shake the bed, and sleep is entirely prevented."

Professor Scudder considered it preferable to aconite in asthenic diseases, high-grade fevers and pulmonary inflammations.

For pneumonia in adults, give one drop every half hour in water for 5-6 hours, according to Dr. Bastyr.

It is not appropriate for weak, asthenic individuals, and is contraindicated in those with a small weak pulse. Nausea is a sign of impending toxicity and signal to cease its use.

Jervine relaxes the myocardium, and veratroidine slows the pulse.

Isorubijervine exerts cardiac toxicity via the sodium (V) 1.5 channel.

One alkaloid, germine di-acetate, has been used experimentally to treat *myasthenia gravis*. Flacke W et al, *New England Journal of Medicine* 1966 275(22):1207-14

Veracintine, an alkaloid from the related *V. album* and its derivatives, have exhibited, *in vitro*, cytotoxic effects on leukemic cells.

Researchers from John Hopkins and Howard Hughes Medical schools have found cyclopamine blocks the growth of medulloblastomas and malignant tumors of the central nervous system.

The author Philip Beachy found it difficult to extract enough cyclopamine for more studies.

Cyclopamine comes from the reference to Cyclops, the one-eyed creature of mythology. Its tetragenic activity induces gene distortion.

Cyclopamine induces cancer signaling pathway manipulation and possible new treatment for osteosarcoma, a common bone cancer affecting young children and adults. Angulo P et al, *J Hematol Oncol* 2017 10(1):10.

Work by Houhannisyan et al, *Planta Medica* 75:13 found cyclopamine inhibits hedgehog signaling and may be useful in cancer tumors and psoriasis.

Pseudojervine is an epinephrine antagonist.

The drug, Veriloid was removed from the market, as a treatment for hypertension, due to adverse side effects in 1961.

HOMEOPATHY

Veratrum viride is indicated when the tongue is coated with a red stripe down the middle. It is useful for re-toxically treated skin diseases with consequent convulsions (impregnation phase), or in pneumonia, hypertension, cardiac asthma, and twitching and spasms of the facial muscles.

Congestion, heat and fever are prominent features.

Should be considered when high fevers in children come as they have significant development of intellect. It can also be thought of for mental pathology following fever, or a history of infections following poor recovery from fever, sunstroke, etc.

Esophagitis, with the bringing up of bloody mucous and the need to constantly swallow, are other indications.

The nose feels pointed and cold.

There may be suppurative fevers with great variation in temperature, hot in the evening and cold in the morning.

Other symptoms of note are erythema and skin itching in various parts that accompany hot sweating.

Violent electric-like shocks in the limbs, beating of pulses throughout the body, and a constant dull, aching pain in region of the heart.

In the female patient, there may be suppressed menstruation, with congestion of the head.

The patient may be thirsty, and yet the smallest amount of food or water is immediately rejected. Hiccoughs may be excessive and painful.

Frightful dreams of being on water, of persons drowning. Clearly understands former mysteries.

Clinically, it is known that diseases such as Tiegel's contracture, Thompson's Disease, athetosis, and pseudo-hypertropic muscular paralysis present symptoms quite like those produced by *V. viride* upon muscle tissue in provings.

DOSE- First to 6th potency. The mother tincture is prepared from the dried rootstock and attached rootlets.

FLOWER ESSENCES

False Hellebore essence is combined with Low Larkspur (see Delphinium) for dealing with enmeshment, playing one's part in the dysfunctional imbalance of a family or relationship. **ROCKY MTN**

[False] Hellebore essence is more about growing old gracefully. It helps you to bow down to the passing of time, whether that is getting older or accepting change over a long period of time. I think it's perfect for grumpy old men and women. **OLIVE**

False Hellebore's message is "Don't take yourself too seriously". We are not the centre of the universe. To lead fulfilling lives we need to stay calm, look, listen, not be so BUSY, caught up and self-important. Our perspective is only that, ours; we need to be reminded to approach life with respect for others' perspectives as well as our own. **NETTLES AND MORE**

PERSONALITY TRAITS

The deepest inner state here is that they have infinite knowledge and understand everything. They are a hot version of Veratrum album (which is chilly), and an overactive thyroid is common.

The Veratrum family are preachers. They know what they believe in and they tell it to you straight. They usually feel they have a direct connection to God or angels or Jesus or some profound spiritual figure, and…to the Native Americans.

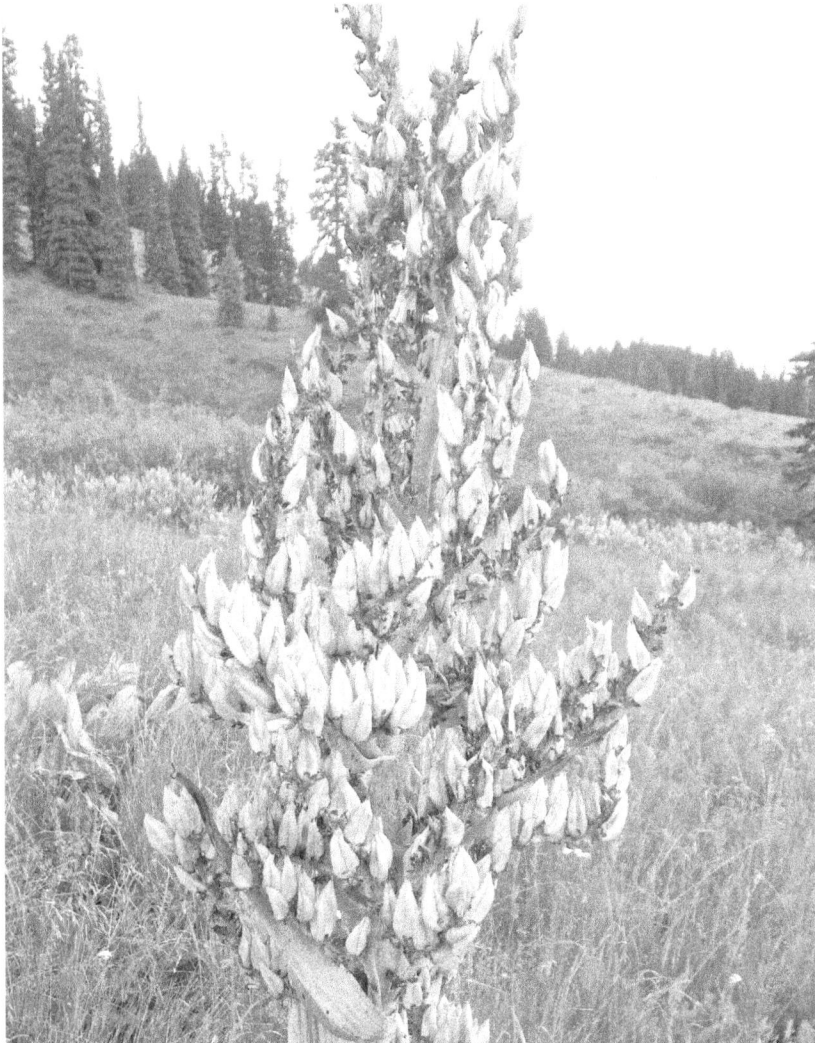

GREEN HELLEBORE

They may understand that human partners are a step on the way to divine inner union, through sex and love.

And there is the idea of wanting to be really famous, like some religious character, Mahatma Gandhi, for example. Praying can take the form of any religion, yoga, meditation, including sweat lodges. **PETER CHAPPELL**

Veratrum viride has certain "tendency, at least in the beginning, to have alternations between expressions of egotism, religiosity and expressions of despair. This despair also alternates with being critical of others…*Veratrum viride* shares with Veratrum album the rubric 'ailments from loss of social position' as well as the feeling of being unable to reach or maintain what they perceive as their lofty true potential. In this stage they can feel that their life has been ruined by others. It also shares with Veratrum album the spending addictions…May have exalted fantasies of being superior and special, yet despair of reaching this place. Tendency to get into alternative religions and to change religious affiliations frequently. **LOUIS KLEIN**

RECIPES

TINCTURE- 1-5 drops twice daily of a 1:10 tincture of the root. For congestive lung cancer, five drops in four ounces of water. Take one teaspoon per hour. It is stopped at slightest sign of nausea.

As little as one gram of the fresh root is toxic. Most potent in spring. Poisoning is seldom fatal due to rapid vomiting and poor intestinal absorption. The alkaloids act within 2 hours and effects persist for 4-6 hours, degraded in liver and excreted.

FELON- Take one part each of blue flag and veratrum root and boil for twenty minutes in half water and milk. Then soak the infected finger or toe for 20 minutes as hot as possible in mixture. Then add crushed roots to affected area for one hour.

Caution: This plant is toxic and may cause death in large doses. Poisoned individuals show cross-reaction with digoxin immunoassay, but it does not bond with DigiFab antibody fragments. Bechtel et al, *Clin Toxicol* (Phila) 2010 48:5.

It should only be used temporarily until diet and lifestyle choices help assist hypertension. As blood pressure drops, the dose of medicine can be lowered.

It is of course contraindicated in pregnancy. Three veratrum-type alkaloids, cyclopamine, jervine and cycloposine are known to cause birth defects.

VINEGAR- Soak ground rhizomes in vinegar for 7-10 days. This is a powerful insecticide, especially for controlling Colorado Potato beetle in garden plots.

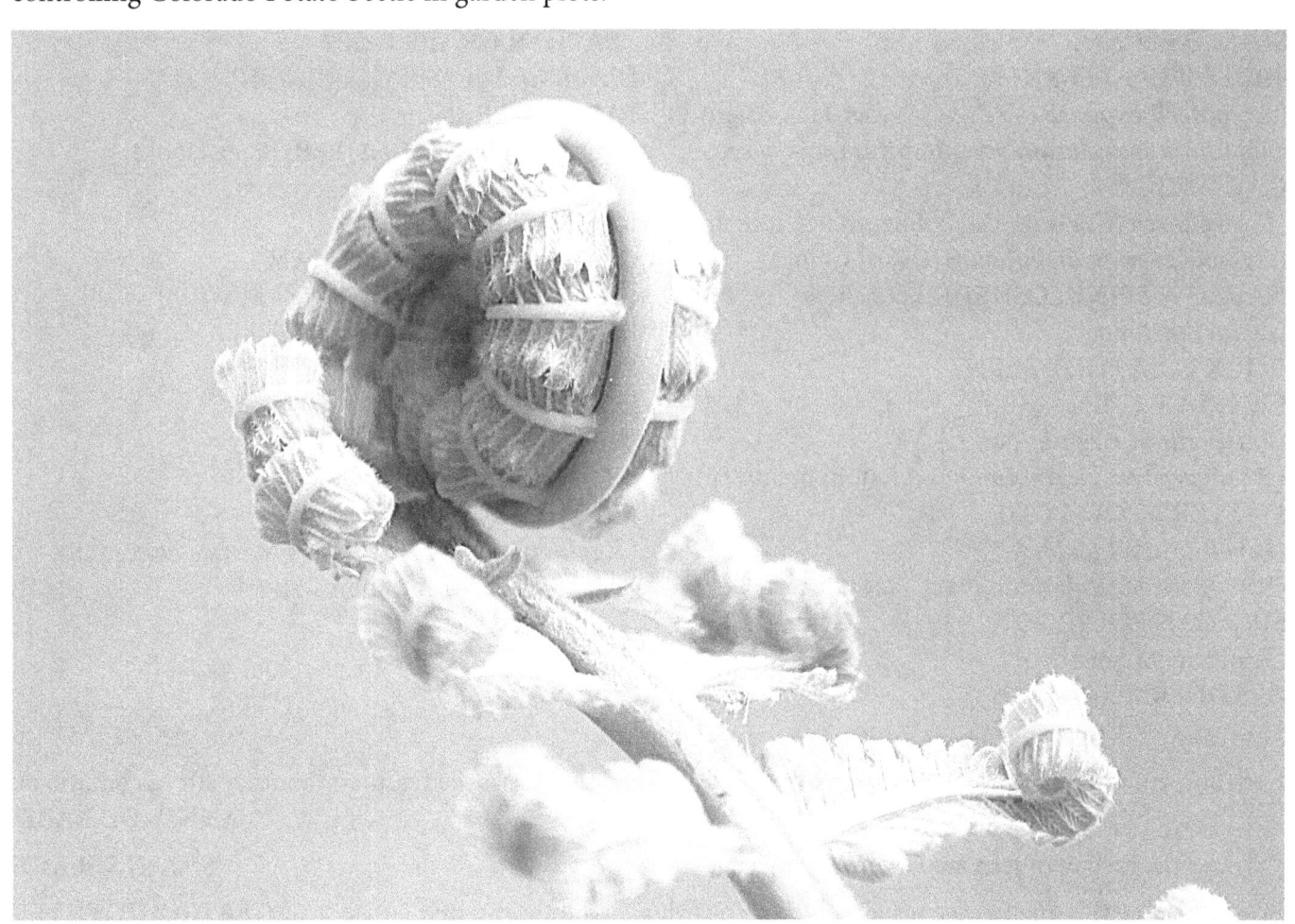

UNCURLED FERN

OSTRICH FERN
(*Matteucia struthiopteris* [L] Todaro)
(*M. struthiopteris* **var.** *pensylvanica* [Willd.] C. V. Morton)
MALE FERN
BEAR'S PAW ROOT
(*Aspidium filix-mas* [L.] Sw.) not accepted
(*Dryopteris filix-mas* [L.] Schott.)
FRAGRANT WOOD FERN
(*D. fragrans* [L.] Schott.)
NORTHERN LADY FERN
(*Athyrium filix-femina* [L.] Roth)
NORTHERN MAIDENHAIR
ALEUTIAN MAIDENHAIR
(*Adianatum pedatum* L.) not accepted
(*A. aleuticum*[Rupr.] C. A. Paris)
(*A. pedatum var. aleuticum* Rupr.) not accepted
BRACKEN FERN
EAGLE FERN
(*Pteridium aquilinum* [L.] Kuhn.)
(*Pteris aquilina* L.) not accepted
SHIELD FERN
SPINY WOOD FERN
(*Dryopteris expansa* [C. Presl.] Fraser-Jenk & Jermy)
(*Aspidium spinulosum var. dilatatum*) not accepted
OAK FERN
(*D. disjuncta* [C. Presl.] C. V. Morton) not accepted
(*Gymnocarpium disjunctum* [Rupr.] Ching)
NARROW SPINULOSE SHIELD FERN
(*D. carthusiana*)
ROCK POLYPODY FERN
LICORICE FERN
(*Polypodium virginianum* L.)
(*P. vulgare var. virginianum* [L.] Eaton) not accepted
WESTERN POLYPODY
(*P. hesperium* Maxon.)
(*P. vulgare var. columbianum* Gilb.) not accepted
SIBERIAN POLYPODY
(*P. sibiricum* Sipliv.)
BLADDER FERN

FRAGILE FERN
(*Cystopteris fragilis* [L.] Bernh.)
(*Filix fragilis* [L.] Underw.) not accepted
MOUNTAIN BLADDER FERN
(*C. montana* [Lam.] Bernh. ex Desv.)
ROCKY MOUNTAIN WOODSIA
(*Woodsia scopulina* D.C. Eaton)
WESTERN SWORD FERN
(*Polystichum munitum* [Kaulf] C. Presl.)
PURPLE CLIFF BRAKE FERN
(*Pellaea atropurpurea* [L.] Link)
SMOOTH CLIFF BRAKE
(*P. glabella* Mett ex Kuhn.)
GASTON'S CLIFF BRAKE
(*P. gastonyi* Windham)
RATTLESNAKE FERN
HEMLOCK LEAVED MOONWORT
(*Botrychium virginianum* [L.] Sw)
MOONWORT
(*B. lunaria* [L.] Sw)
(*B. onondagense* Underw.) not accepted
LEATHER GRAPE FERN
(*B. multifidum* [S G Gmel] Trevis)
PARSLEY FERN
(*Cryptogramma crispa* [L] R. Br. ex Hook)
(*Osmunda crispa* L.) not accepted
ROYAL FERN
OSMUND THE WATERMAN
(*O. regalis* L.)
(*O. regalis* **var.** *spectabilis* [Willd.] A. Gray)
SPIKEMOSS
LITTLE CLUB MOSS
(*Selaginella densa* Rydb.)
MOUNTAIN SPIKEMOSS
MARSH CLUBMOSS
(*S. selaginoides* [L.] Beauv. ex Mart. & Schrank)
PARTS USED- root, spores, shoots

Each student of ferns,I read, will have his own list of plants that for some reason or another stir his emotions.
ANNIE DILLARD

We have the receipt of fern seed- we walk invisible".
SHAKESPEARE

Bracken is like the smell of the sea as you come near it after a long absence.
GERTRUDE JEKYLL

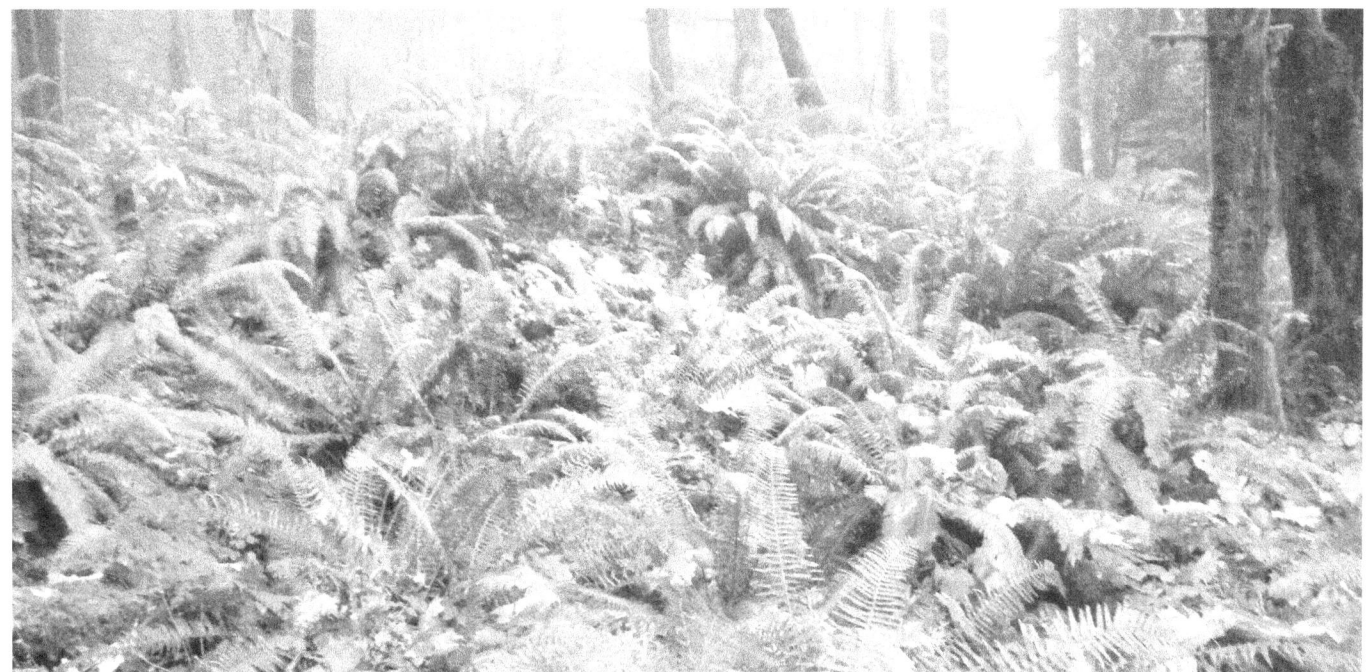

Fern is from the Anglo Saxon **FEPARN** or German **FARM** both derived from the Sanskrit **PARNA** meaning wing or feather. Fern and feather are both in reference to the pinnate leaves. Fern may derive from **FARR**, a bullock, from the use as livestock bedding.

Dryopteris is from the Greek **DRYS**, a tree or oak, and **PTERON** a wing, or feather. Aquila is Latin for eagle. Cystopteris is from the Greek **KYSTOS**, meaning bladder, and **PTERIS** fern. Fragilis means brittle. Montana is of the mountains.

Aspidium is from Greek **ASPIDION**, a little buckler. Adiantum is from the Greek meaning un-wetted or dry. Athyrium is derived from the Greek **ATHYROS**, meaning without a door, referring to the lack of protective membrane over the spore clusters.

Botrychium is from **BOTRYS** meaning a bunch of grapes. Bracken is from the Old English **BRACU**, or old German **BRACHE** meaning broken, and thought to refer to the tangle of broken stems characteristic of the fern. Aquilinum is a specific name given by Linnaeus for the appearance of a spread eagle, from the obliquely-cut lower stem. Others believe it came from the fronds spreading out like eagle wings.

Pteris is derived from **PTERON**, a feather.

Filix mas is derived from the Latin **FILIX** meaning happy, and **MAS** for man. Filices is from the Latin **FILUM**, a thread, due to their filamentary fronds. It may derive from **FILIS** for fern, and the male alludes to its asexual reproduction.

Ostrich fern is named for the plume like leaves, resembling the bird's feathers. Matteucia is named after Carlo Matteuci, an Italian physicist, and physiologist. Fiddle is from the Anglo Saxon **FITHELE**, which is in turn from the Latin **VITULA**, meaning violin. Various expressions such as fiddlesticks, fiddling around, playing second fiddle, drunk as a fiddle, and fiddle faddle, are from the English puritanical scorn of fun and belief that hard work is all that matters in life.

Fiddle-dee-dee is a corruption of the Italian **FEDIDO** meaning by the faith of God.

Osmund is from the Saxon word for domestic peace, **OS** for house and **MUND** meaning peace. The name Osmunda is said derived from the god Thor known as Osmunda.

Others believe it is from **OS**, meaning bone, and **MUNDARE** to cleanse in reference to medicinal use. A conserve of the root was used for rickets, according to Frans Vermeulen.

Ferns have long been associated with magic, fascination and sincerity. In Japan, the fern symbolizes hope, prosperity and confidence. It is a symbol of the Samurai, meaning honesty.

Male Fern was worn in the ring of Genghis Khan so that he could understand the speech of birds; and to this day represents to Mongolian people power and occultism.

Ferns originated over 380 million years ago, when the climate was warm, humid and stable.

The Maidenhead Fern was dedicated to Aphrodite and Venus, and symbolized a secret bond of love.

The Cree of Northern Alberta call all ferns by the generic **MASANAHTIK**.

As a youngster, growing up on the banks of the St. John River in New Brunswick, my entire family would take part in the spring fiddlehead (Ostrich fern) hunt. Around one million pounds per year are picked in New Brunswick. A small industry of around one ton began in northern Saskatchewan in 1993, as well as northern British Columbia.

The coiled up shoots (crosiers) looked like hairy musical treble clefs- and are so delicious! Imagine my surprise one spring day in 1974, when I found them on the south shore of Lesser Slave Lake in Northern Alberta. Fiddlehead Farms was born!

I was soon supplying a large food chain, and even wrote a cookbook on how to prepare them. The greens contain nearly 5% protein as well as alpha and beta-carotene, niacin, and riboflavin. They are high in potassium and low in sodium.

The taste is difficult to describe, but is a combination of asparagus, broccoli and artichoke, very green, sweet with a tinge of bitter.

However, it is important to cook them, as the raw fern contains thiaminase, which destroys this B vitamin. Natives of the province would dig up the underground rhizome and roast it. The outer part was peeled, and the core eaten. Other tribes ground the dried rhizomes for meal.

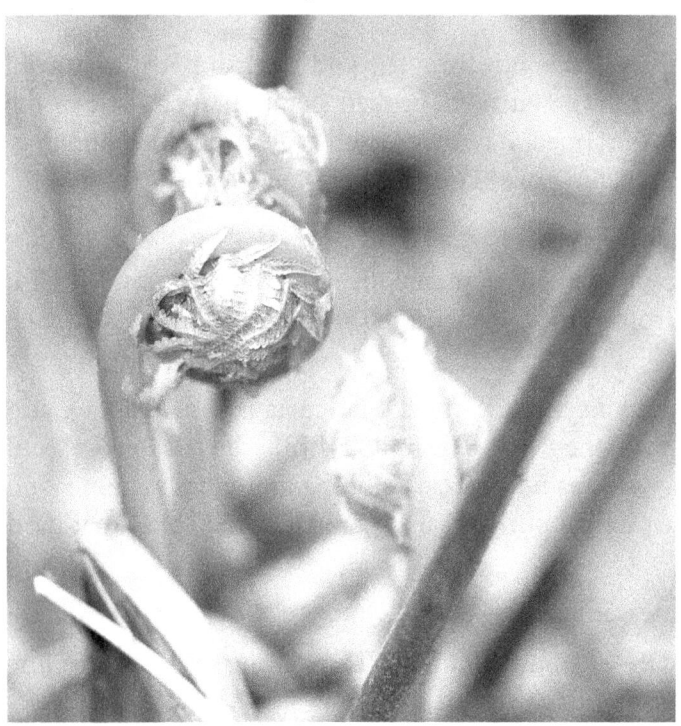

FIDDLEHEADS

The Chipewyan call it **NITELI TS' UCHOGHE**, "dry muskeg white spruce". They used the base of the stalk as a tea to treat stomach or back pain, and to remove placenta after childbirth. It was also boiled with other herbs and drunk four times daily or chewed with other plants every two hours for a racing heartbeat.

A Métis healer from the Sucker Creek region of Alberta says the stipe buds on the rhizome can be used for treating cancer and to help the patient gain weight.

Other Natives ate fiddleheads, in the belief that it would mask their scent while hunting. The Gitksan of northern BC boiled, baked or ate **DAMTX** raw with grease in early spring.

The fiddlehead is technically called a crosier, due to its resemblance to a bishop's staff.

If the urine is whitish, the root of Ostrich fern can be steeped, for a drink that assists urinary problems.

Norwegians use ostrich fern as feed for goats, and make a fern beer. Extracts from the ostrich fern root have been used in veterinary medicine for parasites.

Male Fern grows only on moist, wooded slopes, and is rare in Alberta. This is probably due to hot, dry summers and insufficient snow cover in winter; and is thus restricted to Waterton Park region of Alberta. It is common in parts of North America.

The Male fern rootstock was cut like a hand with five fingers (fronds) and carried as a good luck charm. It was called Lucky hand, Dead Man's Hand, or St. John's Hand, the latter after St. John's Eve (June 23) for extra potency.

In Finland, it was believed that only orphan children could obtain the magical, invisibility seeds, because they might be changelings. Other tales suggest Trolls guard the seeds from those hoping for promised wealth and magical powers.

It was used medicinally to relieve rheumatic pain, by sewing the fronds into clothing in the affected areas. The Greeks used it as a de-lousing potion back in 100 A.D; while the Swiss physician Peschier, introduced it into medical practice in the 18th century.

Male Fern has sori shaped like kidneys, while Lady fern is more U shaped. To be sure, cut the stalk and count the vascular bundles- seven for male fern and two for the lady.

Male Fern uncurled fronds have been boiled and eaten, and in Norway, during times of famine were mixed with flour for bread and used to brew beer.

William Cole, the English herbalist wrote, "if the Asse be oppressed with melancholy, he eats of the herbe Asplenium (Lady Fern)." You get the idea.

Male Fern can affect the optic nerve, leading to temporary or permanent blindness.

Horses and cattle poisoned by male fern have the odd tendency to stand or lie down in water, and may also go blind.

Lady fern rhizomes, known as **A'SAWAN** were cut by the Chippewa, and a handful was combined with four root lobes of nettle in decoction. This was taken internally for stoppage of urine, and as a vermifuge. Some tribes used tea from the roots to stimulate milk production in mastitis, and caked breast. The Potawatomi call it **NONAGON-A'WUSK**, meaning milkweed, in reference to above use. The WSANEC of the Saanich peninsula know it as **LEKLEKA** and they drank a tea of the shoots for tuberculosis.

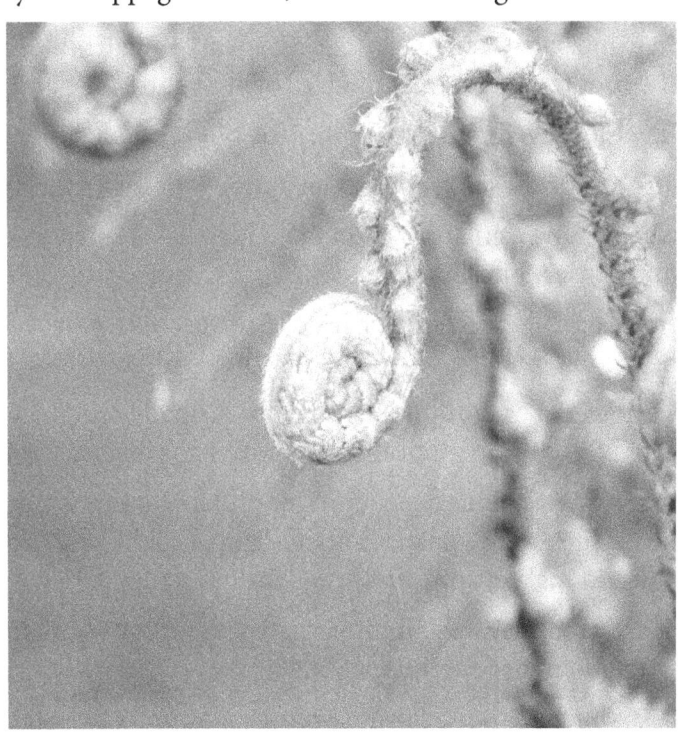

The Iroquois combined the rhizomes of **IES-KA-RON-IOKA** with New England Aster (*A. novae-angliae*) for intestinal fever, and *Rhus typhina* for frequent urination.

Tea from the stems was given to ease back pain associated with labor. Root powder was dusted on skin ulcers.

Natives of Washington State boiled the stems to halt postpartum hemorrhage, while the Thompson further north used fern infusions to stop vomiting of blood.

The Lime Village Tanaina, in Alaska, boiled lady fern for use in kidney trouble or asthma.

YOUNG LADY FERN UNFURLING

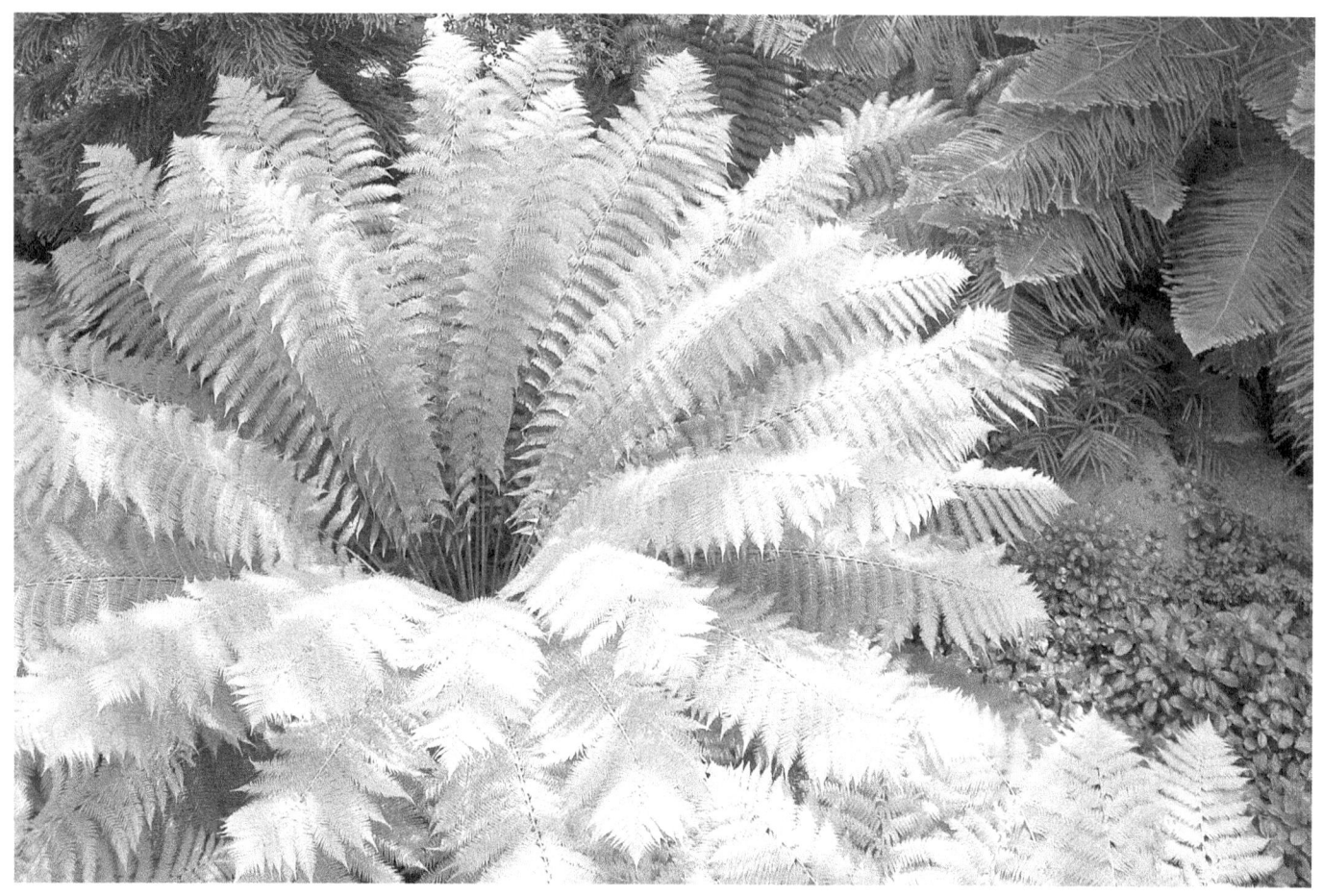

BRACKEN FERN

The Bracken Fern is often mistaken for the ostrich. It is considered one of the oldest plant species on the planet.

In some parts of England it is known as "King Charles in the Oak Tree." In West Sussex, the fern was cut above the root to predict the initial letter of a future husband or wife.

It was believed to flower only once, but of course it forms spores, but then only every seven to ten years.

The fern root was carried as an antidote to sea-sickness.

Nectar producing organs on the underside are rich in saccharine and glucose. Rub this juice on mosquito and other insect bites for quick relief.

In Ireland, it is called the Fern of God, because it was believed if the stem is cut into three sections, the first will be the letter G, the second O, and the third D.

Various tribes used the rhizome medicinally and for food. For the latter, it was dug in late fall or winter and eaten fresh, or in pit ovens to remove hairy fibers.

The Iroquois made decoctions for prolapsed uterus, and bladder control; while the Ojibwa used the root tea for headaches and female cramping. The Blackfoot ate the stems like asparagus, and the roasted roots resembled wheat dough in appearance and taste (I doubt it!).

The Cherokee used it for rheumatism, due to its signature of emerging from curled up fiddlehead and good for strengthening bent muscles and limbs.

The Montagnais used frond beds for same purpose. Steam baths or tinctures of rhizomes were used for arthritis. Decoctions were used for tuberculosis.

The fronds were used to make soft, soothing beds for elders and babies.

Today the bracken fern is used in medicine, soap making, glass, leather tanning and other industries. In Venezuela it is used for packing and wrapping heads of curing cheese. The roots have been used in place of hops in brewing herb beer.

In our area it grows to several feet but I have seen it up to fourteen feet tall in South America. It grows all over the world, including Antarctica.

In New Zealand, the rhizome known as **ARUHE** was a staple food of Maori, second only to sweet potato (kumara). It was a staple food that would not fail.

In Japan, an almond flavored starch called *WARABI* is extracted from the rootstock, and used in pastry.

The local name is **KUSASOTETSU**. The rhizomes are boiled and fried in batter as tempura or slowly cooked in soy sauce.

Raw young bracken fern contains a carcinogenic substance, ptaquiloside; as well as prunsain, thiaminase, and a radiomimetic factor, or radiation mimicking substance, that appears to be mutagenic and carcinogenic. The latter substance invades the bone marrow, causing aplastic anemia, cancers and deaths in grazing animals.

Horses become nervous, lose balance and suffer "fern staggers", while cattle lose the ability to produce leukocytes and blood platelets, bleeding to death.

Bracken fern poisoning is associated with chronic and acute enzootic hematuria in cattle (redwater disease), and causes B1, or thiamine deficiency in horses.

Work by Latorre et al, *J Immunotox* 2009 6:2 found the fern exhibits immunosuppressive effects. The carcinogen, ptaquiloside, is water soluble, but destroyed during composting.

In Japan, regular ingestion of bracken fern has been linked to esophagus and stomach cancers.

Work by Campos da Paz et al, *Mutat Res* 2008 652:2 found fern extracts cytotoxic and causing DNA damage to oral epithelial and submandibular gland cells.

On the Canary Islands, one of my favorite travel spots, the rhizome was dried and ground into flour after roasting. Without or without barley, this is called **GOFIO**, an instant food, easily digested. The freshly ground flour has a flavor similar to wild rice.

In parts of France, bracken fern root bread as a staple in times of scarcity. For emergency human food, the sprouts are soaked in water containing wood ashes for 24-36 hours to remove the free tannic acid.

It is relatively rich in nitrogen and potassium, with summer fronds composting readily due to a favorable carbon:nitrogen ratio.

Autumn harvested fronds make useful livestock bedding, with water absorbent quality, and slower degradation than cereal straw.

Bracken Fern is harvested for food in China, with annual output of 2,000 tons from Heilongijang Province alone. The related Chinese Brake Fern (*Pteris vittata*) is an efficient hyper-accumulator of arsenic. Ma et al, *Nature* 2001 409.

Bracken fern is a valuable biofuel with calorie value of 21 gigajoules per ton, and can be made into bales or briquettes. The ash left over has great potential use, containing as much as 50% potassium in June. The ash has a pH of 12, or highly alkaline. Yields of 250 kilograms of K per hectare are realized.

In pot trials, September ash increases clover yields by 150% and number of root nodules by 140%.

Less known is the production of sweet nectar from Bracken fern. Large beads of the sweet syrup, rich in saccharose and glucose flow from the fern, especially as it is unfolding as a young frond. When broken, the nectar production lasts for several days.

It also has been boiled as a solution for spraying aphids on roses. The expressed juice shows activity against Gram positive bacteria.

Many ferns, including Bracken fern, contain pterosins, or insect moulting hormones of considerable interest.

Shield Fern has been used to make infusions for dandruff. The roots were also decocted and used as foot baths in treating varicose veins. Mature fronds were stuffed in linen bags for rheumatism. The root was thrown into the fire at the summer solstice as a power charm. Some Native tribes ate the uncurled fronds before a hunt, to help mask their scent.

The Chipewyan call Shield Fern **TS'ELIDHER, NITELI TS'U CHOGHE**, or Muskeg White Spruce. The Cree know it as Raven's beak, or **KU(H)KUGUWPUK**.

Cooking was usually a slow bake over coals, or in a steaming pit. A favorite of coastal natives was to peel the rootstocks after cooking and smear with grease or fermented salmon eggs. The curled shoots of Shield Fern were taken as part of a compound decoction as an appetite stimulant.

The frond stipe bases have been traditionally decocted with other herbs for kidney pain, in other mixtures for skin washes, as cancer therapy, or smoked with other plants to treat "insanity". The roots, for food are best in spring, or fall.

Various Dryopteris roots were used for toothache, worms and other intestinal complaints. Ointment from the root healed ulcerous and cancerous tumors. This includes Spiny Wood Fern, which was used medicinally as well as for food.

The pineapple like rhizomes are dug up in fall, when they are surrounded with the scaly fingers of next year's growth. They can be picked in spring before new ferns emerge, but are harder to find.

If dark and flat inside, the rhizome is not used for food; but if light coloured and fleshy, it is steamed in pits or boiled over a fire, tasting similar to a sweet potato or yam. The Kwakwaka'wakw of British Columbia would at times cover the rhizomes with red ochre and roast them on a hemlock stick over an open fire. The finger-like spikes were then broken off, peeled like a banana, and eaten with fermented salmon roe, or grease.

The more bitter roots were used by the Nuxalk to lose weight, or to cure illness from eating shellfish infected with the red tide toxin.

The Dena'ina of Alaska call the root **UH** and gathered it widely for food, baking them in pit fires for at least 24 hours. A type of beer called **UH BIVA** was probably learned from the Russians, and involves fermenting the roots with yeast.

It was used for medicine in the form of eyewash, and internally for tuberculosis, kidney trouble, and asthma as a tea. The fiddleheads were boiled and eaten as well.

Narrow Spinulose Shield Fern (*D. carthusiana*) root, at least the middle, green part, is boiled and eaten, or the water drunk to treat worms and give people more appetite, and gain weight. Russell Willier, noted Cree Healer, calls it Fat Root, or **WIYINOHWASK**.

Oak Fern is common in the boreal forest. The Eastern Cree crushed the leaves as both an mosquito repellant and to relieve the bites already received. The Haida Gwaii know it as **HLT'AN7ANDA**.

Fragrant Wood Fern is found in the Rockies and into northeastern B.C, and throughout the Yukon and Northwest Territories. It is often found in rock crevices and is a rich dark green color, with leaves that persist for over a year. The scent is a combination of raspberry and peach, and is said to linger for years when stored as a bookmark or similar closed area.

Western Sword Fern roots are sweet and edible. The Nootka rubbed it on their hands to bring good luck while fishing. It was often used for designs in basket making, according to Steedman. Of course, the ferns were used for lining steam pits, and woven into rugs and sleeping mats. The young leaves were chewed and swallowed to ease sore throats.

Mouse Woman, in Haida tradition, lives under a clump of Western Sword Fern.

The Haida term refers to mouse mother and fern mother, in various stories. In one story, recorded by Swanton, the hero of the story helps a shrew to cross a log. The shrew [or mouse] disappears under a clump of ferns, and when the man draws the ferns aside, he finds the painted house front of the "fern-mother", with planks sewn together in the old style. The "fern-mother" calls him grandson and gives him supernatural medicine.

They were used in initiation rites and bathing rituals by **WSANEC** of Saanich peninsula on Vancouver Island. They call the fern **STXALEM**.

The Northern Maidenhair fern was often used in magic spells. The plant was immersed in water and then removed. If worn, the plant would grant you grace, beauty and love.

The water repellent, and shiny leaves were used by natives, to decorate their baskets.

The leaves were burned by the Quinault, and the ashes rubbed into the hair to make it blacker and shinier. The neighboring Lummi call it **TUNGWELTCIN**, Hair Medicine, and the Skokomish, **AIYA'O'LGAD**, meaning Hair Bigger.

The Makah chew the slightly bitter leaves for sore chest and stomach problems, or to stop internal hemorrhages associated with wounds.

The Iroquois used root decoctions to promote menstruation or abortifacient. The plant decoction was used as a wash for venereal disease and internally for children with cramps.

The Forest Potawatomi used root infusions internally to cure caked breasts in nursing mothers. The plant is known as Black Leg or **MEMAKATE'WIGA'TEUK**.

The Cherokee used the fern poultice to treat tight rheumatic muscle conditions, using the plant signature of young fronds being initially curled up and later straightening out. The name **KÂ'GA SKÛ'ⁿTAGÎ** means Crow Shin.

It was combined with hawthorn and *Aralia racemosa* as a powerful heart medicine for women with irregular beats.

A slow decoction of roots helps relieve excessive menstruation.

The plant was powdered as snuff or smoked for asthma. The Hesquiat chewed the green fronds for shortness of breath. Infusions were used by dancers in winter to keep them "light on their feet", so they could keep going for a long time.

The plant is common worldwide, and used in Egypt for hair growth. Ashes of the plant used to be mixed with olive oil and applied to bald patches on the scalp caused by ringworm. Today, it is used in commercial shampoos for hair tonics and dandruff treatment. In China, the fronds are used for impetigo and a bronchial expectorant.

The whole plant including rhizome is used for chronic catarrh and pectoral affections.

Rattlesnake fern was named for the resemblance of the yellow brown spore cases to the rattle, or simply grows in rocky woods inhabited by these reptiles. The presence of the fern is considered a sign of conditions for ginseng, bloodroot and other "sang" sign roots in Appalachia.

Gerard wrote, "of the colonies, [North America] has berries given for twenty days against poison, or administered with great success unto such as are become peevish".

Rock, Siberian and Western Polypody Fern are very similar and grow in similar habitat. Generally, Rock and Siberian are found on moist cliffs and rocks in northeastern Alberta, while Western Polypody is more likely found in the Rockies.

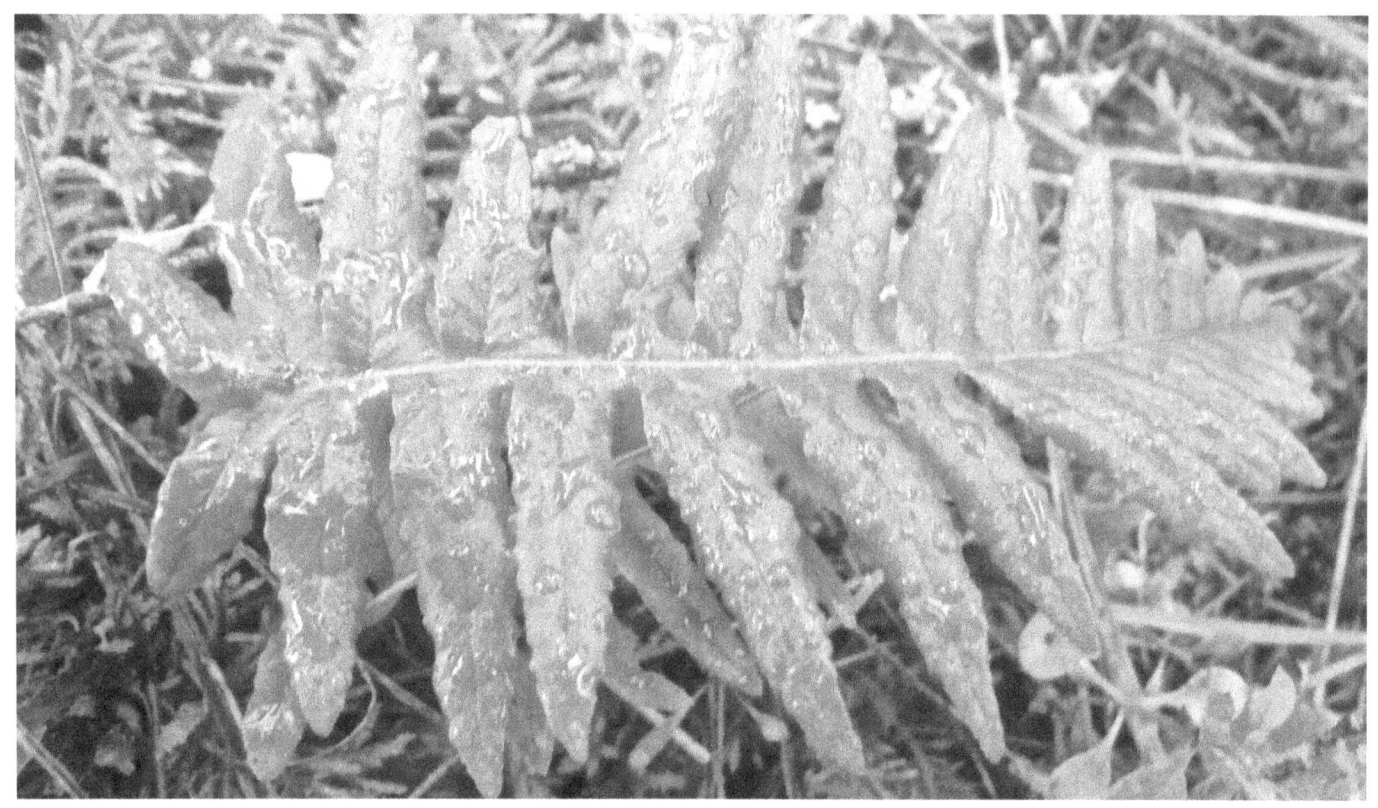

LICORICE FERN

Rock Polypody Fern is known as **KAKAKIWIKOC** by the Cree, who used leaf and rhizome decoctions, for treating tuberculosis.

Other tribes like the Bella Coola used Western Polypody in decoctions for stomach pain, or simply chewed the roots for colds and sore throats and gums.

The Cherokee used poultices of the fern for inflamed swellings and wounds, or drank infusions for hives.

The Mik'maq used the roots for pleurisy; the eastern Cree for neuralgia and kidney problems.

These roots are sweet and licorice-like, containing osladin, a steroid saponin 300 times sweeter than sucrose. In parts of France, it is sometimes called **REGLISSE**, or liquorice. Early settlers used the roots to flavor tobacco. Decoctions of the root were used to treat depression and "fearsome and troublesome" bad dreams.

It is said that chewing the root before drinking water, makes the water sweeter.

Dioscorides, in the 1st century AD, wrote polypody was used to purge mucous and an ingredient in plaster applied to dislocated fingers, or sores between the fingers.

Like other ferns, the powdered rhizomes were used to expel tapeworms.

The Polypodium ferns are of great interest to medicine. The closely related Anapsos (*P. leucotomos*) from Honduras, as an alcohol extract, has been used in the treatment of several autoimmune diseases. *Int J of Immunopharmacology* 1997 19:1. The fern provides protection against ultraviolet solar radiation. It is approved and sold in several products in Spain for treating psoriasis, and may be useful as a protective from skin cancer.

Other studies are looking at its potential for multiple sclerosis.

Bladder Fern is common to the prairies, often found in well-shaded areas on rocky slopes and shady wood. It is small, about 20-30 cm tall, with interesting constituents.

The Cherokee considered this fern to be a febrifuge, and used it as part of infusions for the chills. The Ojibwa drank a tea from the plant for stomach disorders.

The Navaho used cold compound infusions of the plant as a lotion for skin injuries.

A relative of Bladder Fern, called Bulblet Fern (*C. bulbifera*) is gathered spring or fall by the Gitksan of northern British Columbia for food. Know as **AX**, the fern has a two to six inch rhizome that has a taste and look like a woody sweet potato. The root is black when dug up, and orange when cooked, similar to a red turnip.

It is generally baked overnight in pit ovens, and then peeled. It is a good survival food.

Gaston's Cliff Brake Fern is found in the foothills and dry limestone rocks around Banff. It is an apogamous tetraploid species with purplish black stipes.

It is considered to be a hybrid of Purple and Smooth Cliff Brake. The former is considered an eastern species only, so how did it hybridize?

The Mahuna tribe infused Purple Cliff Brake to flush the kidneys, or tone and thin the blood. Infusions were also taken to prevent against sunstroke.

Moonwort, or **KANODAN** was deemed magical by the Algonquin, and used only when necessary. Gathered by moonlight, it was used in sorcerer incantations; and by alchemists who gave it credit for converting quicksilver to pure silver. The fern was gathered on the full moon for curing lunacy; and is said to wax and wane with the moon. Folklore has it that the leaves always face the moon, and that moonwort caused loss of calves in their herds.

The doctrine of signatures is the frond shaped like a crescent moon.

Assiniwi, in his excellent book on *North American Indian Medicine*, says that Moonwort is a panacea to the Algonquin, like ginseng for the Chinese, and is said to improve memory.

The Ancient Greeks made an anointing oil of rue juice and nine drops of dew from moonwort. This was sprinkled or placed upon the head of a person for protection.

In Nepal, the fronds are made into a paste and applied to boils. In Wales, the fern was boiled for dysentery.

Only the leaves were used in medicine, first boiled in red wine and drunk to "stay immoderate fluxes-vomiting-bleedings-the whites-helps blows and bruises-is good for ruptures and similar burstings-and consolidates all fractures and dislocations." The leaves in oil, ointments, and balsams were also applied to heal fresh or green wounds.

The related *B. virginiatum* roots are applied to cuts and wounds.

Leather Grape Fern (*B. multifidum*) is known as **BAYAKHRA** in Nepal. A paste of the roots is applied to the forehead for headache, as well as blemishes on the tongue. The frond juice is given for stomach troubles.

The closely related Rattlesnake Fern is said to be an indicator of ginseng habitat; to either wild craft it, or to plant it as an agro-forestry woodlot crop.

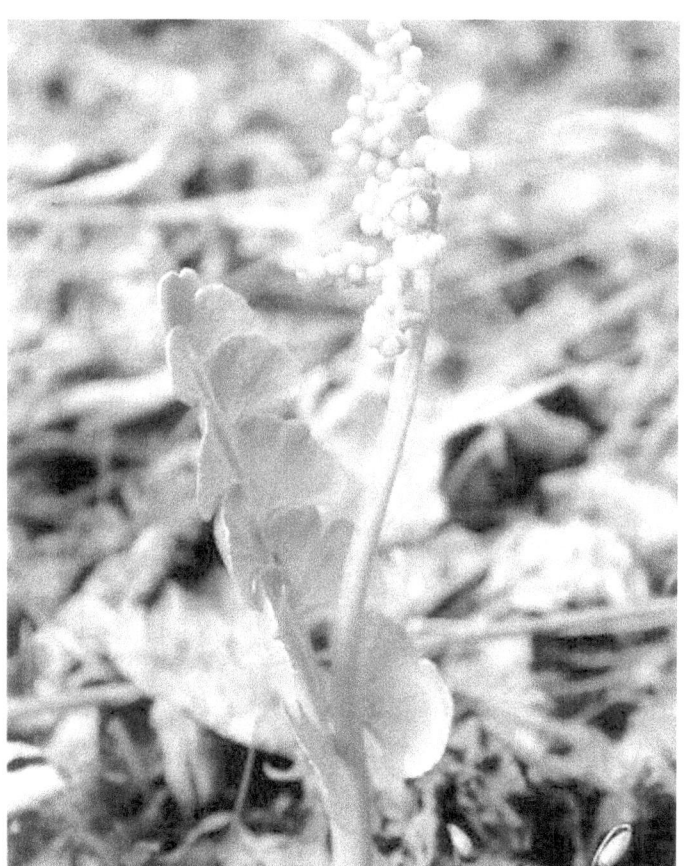

MOONWORT

99

Today, the roots of *Osmunda* species are exported from Canada to become the Osminda fiber used in the potting of orchids.

All the ferns make an acceptable stuffed mattress that fleas and bedbugs greatly dislike. For those suffering rheumatism and such a sack of the ferns will give much relief simply held on the affected region.

In Britain, the poor would mix the ashes of fern with water and form round masses called fern balls. These were heated by the fire and then made into lye for cleaning linen. In Sweden, the fern ashes were mixed with strong lye, and then formed into balls.

The ashes of fern were used in France for the manufacture of glass, due to almost pure alkali residue.

Parsley Fern is common to the Rocky Mountains and Canadian Shield of northeastern Alberta. It is small and delicate, living in rock crevices. Its common name is from the leaf shape, as it has no distinct odor.

The Thompson tribe infused and strained this fern as eyewash, and for gallstones.

Because of sporulation, it is often believed that the sex life of ferns is simple. But consider this. The mobile and independent sex cell of a fern is attracted by malic acid, and moves towards it, when it "scents" it. Only 0.000000028^{th} of a milligram is enough, a figure that even the most sophisticated scientific equipment would be hard pressed to identify.

Royal Fern is widespread throughout temperate zones and introduced to western Canada. It is hardy to zone 3 and is found in backyards and gardens in my home city of Edmonton, Alberta.

Grieve mentions its old English name is Osmund the Waterman, and the white centers of the roots have been called the Heart of Osmund. Legend has it that the wife and daughter of Osmund, a waterman of Loch Tyne, hid among Osmundas during the Danes' invasion.

The Iroquois used root decoctions for water blood and when "girls leak rotten; affected women can't raise children." They used decoctions for cold in kidneys. The fern was valued by Seminole healers, to treat chronically ill babies and steam-infused for bathing the body, in cases of insanity.

Infusions of frond have been used to treat children suffering convulsions caused by intestinal worms.

In Spain, the fern is known as **ANTOJIL** and used to set bones, and treat musculo-skeletal issues, including bone fractures, osteoporosis, rheumatic, arthritic and assorted bruises, and muscle issues. The middle part of rhizome is soaked in white wine.

Antojil wine is available commercially in northern Spain, and taken by men daily before breakfast. It is contraindicated for women of childbearing age and pregnant women, and is considered abortifacient.

To confuse things further, various Selaginella species, don't look anything like ferns, but they are taxonomically classified as such.

Little Club Moss (*Selaginella densa*) was decocted by Blackfoot "midwives" to induce labor, to expel the afterbirth and relieve pain. The flower tea was used as medicine for those spitting blood.

The powdered root was applied to the mouth of racehorses in order to make them hyperactive.

A starving man would eat the plant because it had a doping effect, making one feel unusually strong. This led to the Blackfoot name "Feels Chest". In a manner similar to Buffalo Berry (*Shepherdia canadensis*), it likely influences dopamine or serotonin levels. Research is needed.

It was given to horses to fill them with energy, suggesting some metabolic influence.

The three related species are not easily distinguished from one another, *S. densa* is more western, *S. rupestris* is found commonly in the east, and *S. sibirica* in the far north.

The whole plant of *S. wallichii* was once used as a protectant after childbirth.

Little Club Moss (*S. rupestris*) is smoked, by the southern Sotho of Africa, with Clubmoss (*L. clavatum*) for the relief of headaches. The powdered root is made into an ointment to treat venereal sores, by the Jindwe of Zimbabwe.

In Mexico, the related *S. lepidophylla* and *S. cuspidata* are called Doradilla, or the Resurrection Plant. Its name is related to its ability to curl its leaves into a ball when thirsty, and unfurl after rain. The leaves can be dried and kept in an airtight jar for years, and then resurrected by soaking in water, or exposed to a rain for as little as 15 minutes, it becomes green again.

It is a remedy for kidney stones and urinary tract irritation. It is also combined into mixtures for intestinal parasites.

Some *Selaginella* species have a deep, iridescent blue color that helps them absorb the red wavelengths of light in the deep shade of forests.

MEDICINAL

OSTRICH FERN

CONSTITUENTS- palmitic acid, astragalin, caffeic acid, various phenolic acids including chlorogenic, p-hydroxybenzoic, p-coumaric, ferulic, vanillic and protocatechuic; phytosterols including beta-sitosterol, campesterol, and stigmasterol; pinosylvin (a stilbene), ponasterone A, ecdysterone, pterosterone, filicin.
The rhizome also contains succinic acid, D-mannitol, woodwardic acid, apigenin, riboflavin, coumaric and caffeic acids, as well as ergost-6,22-diene-3beta,5alpha,8alpha-triol. One caffeic acid derivative combined with L-homoserine (L-O-caffeoylhomoserine) has been found to scavenge free radicals.
Fronds- betaine lipids, glyco- and phospholipids are high in spring "treble clefs" and reduce to zero in fully mature leaves and then increase towards fall.
82 grams of fiddleheads contain 0.7 mg iron, 13 mg. vitamin C, and small amounts of vitamins B1, B2, and B3.

Ostrich fern rhizome has been shown to possess blood sugar lowering activity, as well as activity against the polio virus.

Pinosylvin has anti-fungal and antibiotic properties (Harbourne et al, 1993).

It is used in South East Asia for the treatment of various diseases in folk medicine.

In Traditional Chinese Medicine, the root is sometimes substituted for Shield Fern (*Dropteris crassirhizoma*), root, and known as **GUAN ZHONG**.

This is considered a superior vermifuge to Male Fern (see below) as it is considerably less toxic, and yet effective for pinworms, roundworms, hookworms, tapeworms; as well as *Giardia* and *Trichomonas* species.

It is contraindicated for pregnant women, children and the feeble; as well as those with peptic ulcers.

Guan Zhong is used for its broad spectrum of anti-viral activities, and is much used in veterinary medicine, for swine ascariasis, earthworms and leeches, to bovine liver, flat and broad sucker flukes.

Ostrich Fern is known as **JIA GOU JU**, and has been used traditionally to lower blood pressure.

When young, as in fiddlehead form, the plant contains high levels of ecdysterones (Revina et al, 1985).

Anti-oxidant levels are twice that of blueberries with significant amounts of omega 3 fatty acids, according to Nova Scotia scientists.

Ostrich Fern (*M. orientalis*) contains five newly identified compounds, matteurorien, matteuorienin and matteuorienates A-C. The latter three all strongly inhibit aldose reductase. *Chemical and Pharmaceutical Bulletin* 1995 4:9.

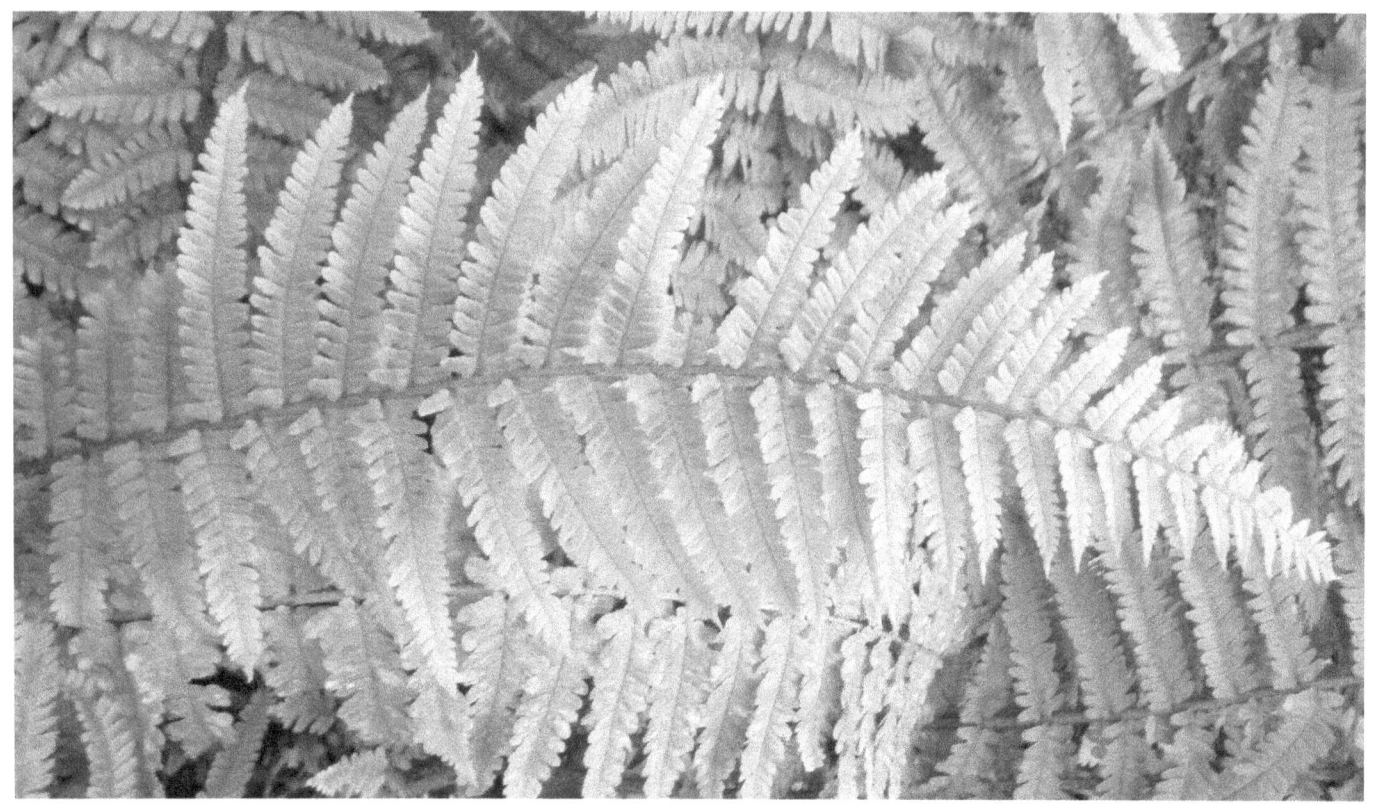

MALE FERN

MALE FERN

CONSTITUENTS- rhizomes from 6-15% oleoresins, containing up to 24% filicin, composed of filicinic acid, filicylbutanone, aspidinol. albaspidin, paraspiden and desaspidin; dryocrassin, butanon phloroglucides, filixic acid, filicinic acids, paraspidin, filmarone, aspindinole, and desaspidinol. Also includes triterpenes 9(11)-fernene, 12-hopene, 11,13(13)-hopadiene, C29 and C31 n-alkanes, resins, volatile oil.
Filicic and flavaspidic acids are inactivated in an alkaline environment.
leaf- 2.4% filicin, including flavaspidic acids, filicinic acids, paraspidin, and desaspidin.

The first recorded medicinal use of male fern in from Chinese herbal book around 200 BC. It is the only fern included in the *US Pharmacopoeia*.

The action of the root is to expel parasites like tapeworm, hookworm, roundworm and others from humans and animals. Band worms and liver flukes appear to be strongly affected, whereas roundworms and oxyuris are more resistant to treatment.

It is bitter, cold and toxic in large quantities, however.

The fresh grated root poultice is excellent for inflammation of the lymphatic glands. Decoctions are sometimes used to make baths for treating fungal disease.

The secret to making reliable male fern preparations is to make them fresh. To ensure no liver toxicity occurs, see recipes below. Studies from Russia indicate that male fern extracts, from both water and alcohol, inhibit the growth of both Gram positive and negative bacteria. Maximum potency occurs in the plants just before sporulation.

Canadian regulations forbid the internal use of male fern, due to toxicity concerns.

The reality is that male fern extracts work where other anthelmintics do not.

In one study by Alterio DL et al, *Rev Hosp Clin Fac Med Sao Paulo* 1968 23(3): 150-2 100 patients aged 5- 68 years old received 6-7 grams of male fern ethereal extract, and children 0.25-0.5 grams for every year of age. The cure rate was 97%.

This follows earlier work regarding the effectiveness of male fern by Palva et al, *Ann Med Intern Fenn* 1963 52.

In another study by Mello EB et al, *Zentralbi Bakteriol Orig A* 1978 241(3): 384-7, 29 patients aged 12-60 who had not responded to other anthelmintic therapy were given the male fern extract orally, preceded by a hypertonic magnesium sulfate solution. The cure rate was 86%.

Studies by Kapadia et al at Howard University in Washington, D.C. found aspidin and desaspidin showed significant inhibitory effect on tumour promotion. *Cancer Letters* 1996 105.

Work by Brondegaard in *Contraceptive Plant Drugs*, confirms the use of Dryopteris in modern Hungary as a contraceptive. One species of Pteris is used in TCM for the same purpose. Kong et al, *Fertility Regulating Agents*; *J Ethnopharm* 1986 15(1): 1-44.

A very interesting effect from fern was reported by Kantemir et al, *Arzneimittelforschung* 1976 26(2): 261-2. They found in male mice and rats, that one drop of a male fern extract administered orally in pure form, or suspended in sunflower oil, caused a spectacular enlargement of the penis. I did say it was interesting, not necessarily useful!

Work by Stetsenko et al 1984, showed male fern exhibiting activity against both Gram positive and negative bacteria.

The greatest activity was in plants at the height of growth at the very start of sporulation.

Work by Che et al, *Economic and Medicinal Plant Research* 1991 5, found anti-viral activity in male fern rhizome against vesicular stomatitis, herpes simplex and influenza virus type A.

The leaf is used externally for rheumatism, sciatica, muscle pain, neuralgia, and earaches as well as internally for tapeworms and flukes.

LADYFERN

CONSTITUENTS- polypodosaponin (steroid saponins), oslandin, glucocaffeic acid, methyl salicylate, triterpenes, ecdysterones (polypodine A, and 5-beta-hydroxy-ecdysterone), p-aspidin, albaspidin, margaspidin, polystichalbin, methylenebisapidinol, desapiden, various catechin tannins, including 7-L-arabino-furanoside.

Lady Fern, at the beginning of sporulation, contains its greatest anti-bacterial activity. Studies by Stetsenko et al 1984 (above) showed activity against both Gram positive and negative bacteria.

When just emerging, Lady Fern contains considerable amounts of ecdysterones.

Lady Fern rhizome is mildly expectorant, and is often used for choleric activity.

As a digestive, use 10-20 drops of the tincture are taken three times daily.

NORTHERN MAIDENHAIR

CONSTITUENTS- volatile oil, sugars, tannins, and bitter principles including naringin.

Maidenhair fern grows in the extreme southwest mountains of Alberta. It is an expectorant, stimulant, demulcent and mild astringent tonic. Decoctions are excellent for fever, coughs, hoarseness, asthma, pleurisy and streptococcus infection of the lungs.

In France and Germany, *Sirop de Capillaire* is made from a closely related fern (*A. capillus-veneris*), and used for lung problems.

Use one tablespoon of the herb in hot water, or prepare a cough syrup from the roots with two parts honey, one part water and two parts leaves (by volume) finely chopped.

It exerts similar action on the mucous membranes of the bladder and uterus, and is used for cystitis, where there is lots of mucous and burning urine.

To stimulate menstruation, take one ounce of the chopped herb, or half that of dried root to one pint of water. Simmer for twenty minutes and drink. The tea will not stimulate cramping.

Michael Moore wrote Northern Maidenhair fern "is useful for both late and lengthy periods, as it is tonic or tightening to the endometrium of the uterus. Because of its silica, unique triterpenoids, and flavonoids, it is helpful in toning the connective tissue matrix of the lungs and kidneys and can sometimes be useful as a membrane astringent in interstitial cystitis."

Dr. Cook recommended strong decoctions for irritable coughs, as well as irritated mucous membranes of the uterus and bladder; useful in scalding urine and cystic catarrh.

Naringen is very bitter, about one-fifth as strong as quinine.

Decoctions of the whole plant work well with yellow dock or Oregon grape root for jaundice and liver disorders.

Aerial parts can be infused for chronic nasal congestion or for bladder irritation associated with sand and gravel.

FRAGRANT WOOD FERN

CONSTITUENTS- aspidin PB, dryofragin, three phloroglucinol derivatives, and five terpenoids.

Studies by Vichkanova et al in 1982 looked at various Dryopteris species for anti-microbial activity. They found, in general that the fern extracts were more active against *Staphylococcus* than fungi or protozoa.

But they found Fragrant Wood Fern (*D. fragrans*) was particularly active against protozoa that cause vaginal *Trichomonas*. More study is required.

Ito et al, *Chem Pharm Bulletin* 2000 48:8 found potent inhibitory effect against Epstein-Barr virus, an indication, *in vitro*, of potential anti-tumor activity.

ROCK POLYPODY FERN
(*P. vulgare*)

CONSTITUENTS- over 30 compounds including polypodine, filicinic acid, catechol, bitters, sugars (up to 20% saccharose and glucose), resin, saponin glycosides such as osladin (500 times as sweet as sucrose), and polypodosaponin, methyl salicylate and essential oils. Three triterpenoids, dammara-17,21-diene, cyclopodmenyl acetate, and 21alpha-H-hopan-22-ol, nortriterpenoids such as 31-norcyclartenol, and various ecdysteroids (2%) have also been found. Compounds like glycyrrhizin 0.6%, catechin 3.7%, and phloroglucins 0.5% also present, as well as 15% sucrose, 6% starch and 2% fructose.

The dried root is used for stimulating bile secretions, as a laxative and for visceral obstructions and worms. It is also mildly expectorant and used for bronchial congestion, and asthma, combining well with marshmallow root. External washes are used for wounds, while poultices or sun infused liniments are used for arthritic pains in the limbs and lumbar region. It is an ingredient in plasters for dislocated fingers and applied to sores between the fingers.

The root infusions have been proven to relieve coughs in laboratory studies (Dobelis et al, 1986).

In traditional European herbal medicine, the fern has been used for treating hepatitis and jaundice, and as a remedy for indigestion and loss of appetite.

Potter's Cyclopaedia mentions, "its action is peculiar in that it occasionally produces a rash of red spots, but this disappears in a short time and causes no inconvenience"

Salmon wrote in the 1710 *English Herbal*, "it prevails against Frensies, and radically cures the most profound madness whether it be raging or otherwise."

It is considered, by many practitioners, a safe treatment for constipation in children.

Studies conducted in Kyoto, Japan in 1996 by Konoshima et al, showed that various triterpenoids isolated from various ferns, including *P. vulgare* exhibited remarkable anti-tumour effect against skin cancer. It showed inhibition of the Epstein-Barr virus, induced by the tumour promoter TPA.

Studies by Girre et al 1987, found male fern and polypody root exhibit active anti-herpetic activity, probably due to catechuic tannins.

Extracts of the plant reveal activity against Gram negative bacteria.

More research into the ecdysterone content of *P. vulgare* would be invaluable. An article by Reixach et al, *Phytochemistry* 1996 43:3, revealed an ecdysteroid composition of abutasterone, polypodine B, 20-hydroxyecdysone (ecdysterone), inokosterone, 24-hydroxyecdysterone, pterosterone, and ecdysterone. The roots contain up to 2% ecdysterones, which play a key role in insect maturity. These same sterones are used to increase the growth of farm livestock, and by athletes to increase performance and muscular development.

McCutcheon et al, *J Ethnopharmacology* 1995 49:101-110 found *P. vulgare* extracts to possess activity against bovine herpes virus type I.

Related South American *Polypodium* species have been found to exhibit anti-inflammatory activity, based mainly on their sulfono-glycolipid compounds.

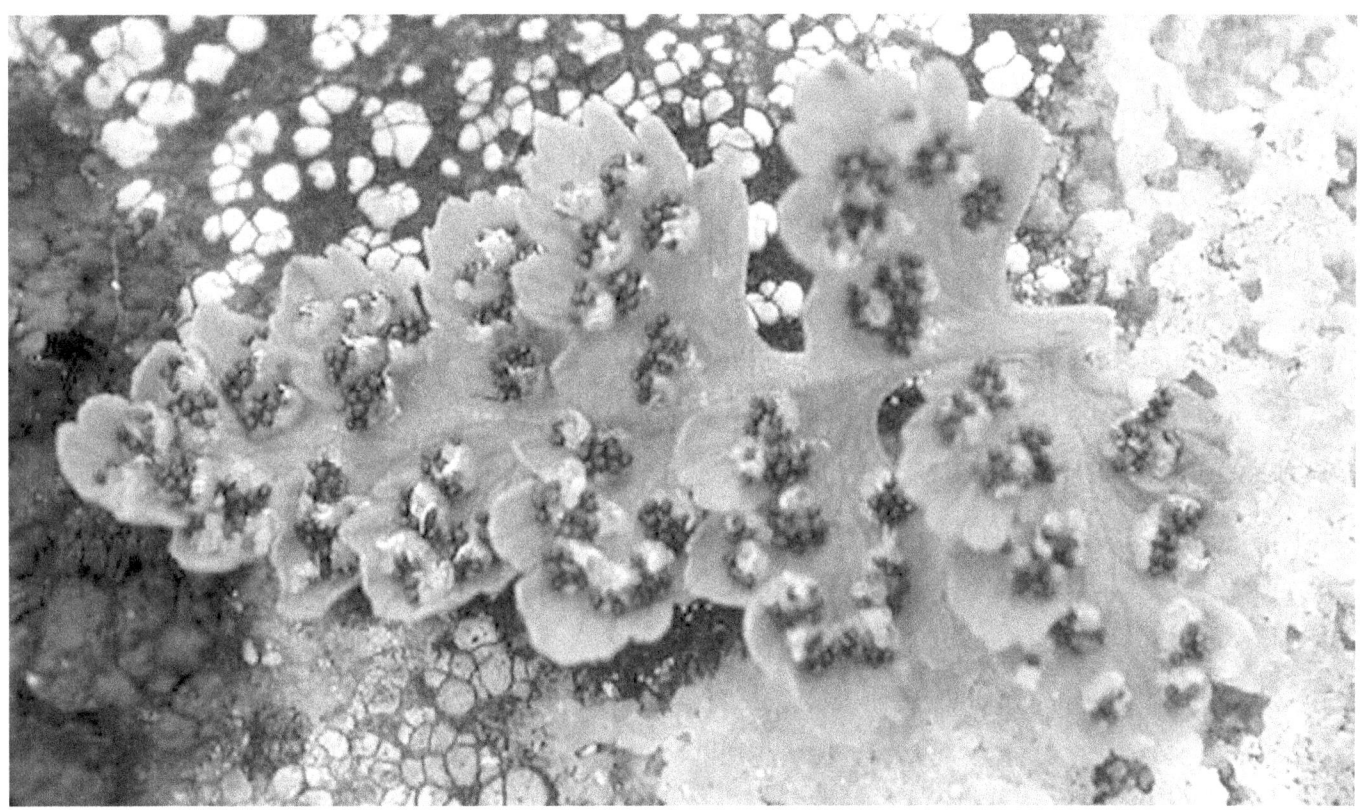

BLADDER FERN- TURNED OVER

BLADDER FERN
FRAGILE FERN
(*Cystopteris fragilis*)

CONSTITUENTS- xanthone derivatives; 1,3-dihydroxy-5, 6, 7-trimethoxy-xanthone, and 1,6-dihydro-3,5,7-trimethoxyxanthone, isomangiferin-3-methyl ether, mangiferin, isomangiferin, 1,3,6,7-tetra-hydroxyxanthone; various flavonoid compouns including astragalin, kaempferol-3,4'-O-O-bis-glucoside, kaempferol-3-O-(glucoside-3 & 6"-sulphate), caffeolyglucose 6"-sulphate, and 3"-sulphate.

Various native tribes use the fern tea to relieve stomach disorders and chills. Decoctions of the fern were used to bathe injured parts.

Bladder Fern shows activity against Gram negative and positive bacteria, according to studies by Stetsenko et al, 1984 (above). The anti-microbial activity was highest in plants at the height of their growth at the very beginning of sporulation.

SPINY WOOD FERN

This common fern has been tested for lipophilic compounds. Twenty-two lipids have been found on the glandular hairs, the most interesting being squalene.

This oil is not common from vegetative sources, and is used for the biosynthesis of triterpenoids and steroids.

Shark livers, amaranth and olives are the most well-known sources of squalene.

Spiny Wood Fern and other *Drypoteris* species contain apigenidin and luteolinidin, both antifungal agents.

WESTERN SWORD FERN

The entire fern has been expressed for juice and inhibits both gram positive bacteria and mycobacterium.

In studies conducted by McCutcheon et al, *J Ethnopharmacology* 1994 44(3): 157-69, this fern showed moderate inhibition of *Mycobacterium tuberculosis*, and *M. avium*. The rhizomes show significant activity against strains of *Pseudomonas aeruginosa* K99.

The fiddlehead, or unfurled top of this species was chewed by various First Nations as a treatment for uterine cancer. The young greens were chewed and swallowed for sore throat and tonsillitis.

RATTLESNAKE FERN

Warm infusions of the fronds induce a gentle and warm perspiration; while at the same time soothing the nervous system, and mildly diuretic. Warm decoctions of the leaves can be taken internally for poisonous animal bites.

The root was decocted by the Fox to treat tuberculosis.

ROCKY MOUNTAIN WOODSIA

Work by Towers et al, at the University of British Columbia found the whole fern active as a broad spectrum anti-fungal. See McCutcheon above.

LITTLE CLUB MOSS

CONSTITUENTS- robustaflavone, hinokiflavone, amentoflavone, apigenin.

Little Club Moss (*S. rupestris*) has been analyzed and reported to show activity on the central nervous system, smooth muscle and isolated heart tissue of frogs. Chakravarthy et al, *Planta Medica* 1981.

The leaves contain amentoflavone that increases contractability, and is an ACE inhibitor (Wagner et al, 1993).

Amentoflavone possesses potent activity against candidiasis, with arrested cell cycles during the S phase. Jung et al, *Bio Pharm Bull* 2007 30:10.

Amentoflavone induces apoptosis in *Candida albicans* by creating mitochondrial dysfunction. Hwang et al, *Mycopathologia* 2012 173(4) 207-18.

Rosbutaflavone inhibits hepatitis B virus, and xanthine oxidase associated with gout.

Little Club Moss (*S. selaginoides*) is used in Spain as an effective anthelmintic.

Related species such as *S. tamariscina, S. involvens* and *S. doederleinii* are used in Traditional Chinese Medicine. It is known as **DA YE CAI**, in Mandarin, or **SEK SONG PAAK**, in Cantonese, or commonly **CHUAN BAI**, or some variation. Grooved Spikemoss (*S. moellendorfii*) is also used, and known as **TI PO CHIH** or **DI BO ZHI**.

The fern is sweet and pungent, with calming and dissolving properties. It is used in first aid for traumatic bleeding, and coughing of blood from the lungs.

Rectal prolapse, leucorrhea, and persistent post-partum lochial discharge are also helped.

Spikemoss is used for toxicosis with boils, sore throats, coughs, and cancers involving the lungs, nasopharynx, esophagus, chorion (chorioepithelioma, choriocarcinoma) liver, and skin.

It may be useful in bronchitis, tonsillitis, chronic hepatitis with jaundice, cholecystitis, ascites, cirrhosis and acute cystitis.

Extracts from *S. doederleinii* show moderate anti-mutagenic effect. Caution should be noted, however, as there is one report of a 52 year-old female taking spike moss as an alternative cancer therapy. She developed severe bone marrow suppression after daily use for two weeks. Symptoms returned to normal after stopping the herb for one week, but it does suggest a compound that contributes to reversible bone marrow suppression.

Ginkgetin, isolated from *S. moellendoffii* shows activity against ovarian adenocarcinoma. It also exhibits activity against three human cancer cell lines and hepatitis B virus. Cao et al, Fitoterapia 81:4.

Gao et al, *Planta Med* 73:10 identified three sterols in *S. tamariscina* that inhibit leukemia cell growth.

Amentoflavone, a bioflavonoid found in both *S. tamariscina* and *Ginkgo biloba* has considerable analgesic and anti-inflammatory properties, with dual inhibition of group II phospholipase A2 and cyclooxygenase.

Work by Kang et al, *Planta Med* 2004 70 found amentoflavone relaxes vascular smooth muscle via unusual pathways.

S. articulta from South America, has been found to moderately neutralize the toxic venom of the snake, *Bothrops atrax*.

S. delicatula has been found to contain a handful of cytotoxic bioflavonoids, that significantly suppress the growth of Raji and Calu-1 tumor cell lines.

S. willdenowii from Panama contains cytotoxic bioflavonoids that show activity against a variety of human cancer cell lines.

The related *S. involvens* shows anti-acne application. *Phytother Res* 2007 22:3.

In India, the species *S. bryopteris* is known as **SANJEEVAI** meaning "one that infuses life." Work by Sah et al, *J BioSci* 2005 30:4 found it is indeed a growth promoter and protective against stress-induced cell death.

Our various species have not been examined carefully enough to determine if they share some of these properties.

DOSE- 2-5 ml of tincture, 15-30 grams in decoction. For cancer doses of up to 100 grams of spikemoss decocted for 3-4 hours are used.

HOMEOPATHY

Male fern is a specific for expelling internal worms, especially when accompanied by constipation. Tuberculosis in young patients, with no fever and limited ulcerated lesions, would be helped. Lymphatic congestion, and lymph node enlargement may be present; as well as recurrent sterility or miscarriage that has no hormonal basis.

When there is loss of sharpness of vision, not traceable to any eye disease, male fern may be tried. This includes yellow vision, retinal hemorrhage and hemianopsia.

Often the abdomen is bloated with a gnawing pain made worse by sweets. There may be diarrhea and vomiting; or the telltale signs of worms like itchy nose, pale face, and blue rings around eyes. Sometimes there is a painless hiccough.

A be-numbed sensation creeps over body.

DOSE- First to third potency. The mother tincture is made from the fresh rootstalk with the leaf bases; but separated from the roots in Autumn. First fragmentary proving by Berridge with two females and one male at 101st and 102nd dilutions in 1876.

Toxic effects from therapeutic anthelmintic use observed by Allen and Clarke. Clinical observations by Boericke.

Bracken Fern (*P. aquilinum*) is for a detached, distant feeling, a desire to hide, dis-inclined to make small talk. Patient is irritable, short-tempered, negative with thoughts of verbal and physical violence.

Lethargic, woolly, fuzzy, and inability to focus. Delusions of being a failure, haggard and old, with erratic behavior in traffic. Claustrophobia, and dreams of death of horses due to starvation, being criminal, underground activities, theft and capture, or of traveling.

Sensations of head constriction, lump in throat, eye, nose and tongue thicker and exhibiting stuck feelings. Dizziness, light headed, sensitive sense of smell. Ovarian pain on alternating sides.

DOSE- 6-30C. Proving by Lisa Griffiths with three females and one male at 30C in 1998. Another proving was conducted by Marie Geary with five females and one male at 6C, 12C and 30C in 2000.

The most striking characteristic of bracken is its capacity for rapid and invisible travel. What is particularly intriguing about the recurring theme of India in the dreams is that the spores are exceptionally good at colonizing poor and devastated land. The huge rhizome that moves outward and engulfs everything in its path is evoked in the dream of the octopus in the sea pool, which the dreamers cannot escape as it approaches with its tentacles reaching out to consume her.

Its increased vigour, aggression and suppressive abilities when exposed to higher light intensity are echoed in several incidences of uncharacteristic behavior of some provers. There are great waves or rushes of energy and outbursts of anger and aggression towards others who threaten or obstruct in some way. There is also claustrophobia, with an overwhelming desire to be out in the open air. Attempt to control bracken involved the beating, cutting, spraying and burning of the fronds, which are the 'head' of the plant body. It seems quite extraordinary therefore to find repeated head pain, and dreams of the tops of heads being cut off or blown off.

SUMMARIZED by LISA GRIFFITHS

There will be big issues around being overwhelmed and being overwhelming. The rage is overwhelming, the person is overwhelmed with rage, nausea is an overwhelming feeling, cancer is a disease that 'takes over'. Things come in waves, waves of nausea, waves of rage. Waves are overwhelming.

MARY GEARY

Selaginella is macerated in milk and used locally and internally for the bites of snakes and spiders.

OLEORESIN

An oily extract that is sweet, woody, earthy and tenacious is made from the male fern root. This is a traditional vermifuge, for expelling worms and parasites. The oleoresin is made by soaking the powdered, dry root in pure ether, filtering, and then evaporating the ether, from the tincture. The resultant product is a thick black oil.

The resin is used as a fixative in Oriental perfume, and in face powders.

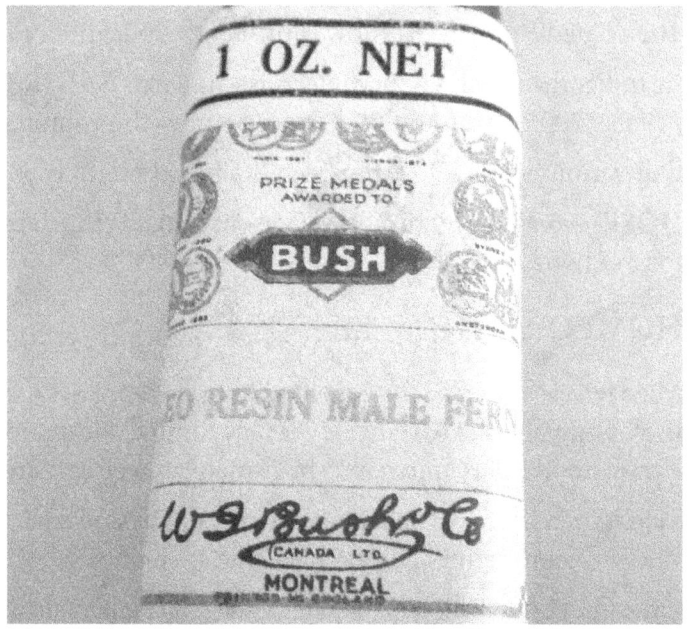

OLEORESIN OF MALE FERN ROOT
- FROM MY PRIVATE COLLECTION

ROOT OIL

CONSTITUENTS- hexyl and octyl esters, butyric acid and pelargonic acid.

Oily extracts of male fern have been used by perfumers and aromatherapists for years. Male fern oil is prepared from air-dried rhizomes collected in June.

The yield is .025% of light yellow oil with intense male fern odour, and is usually extracted with volatile solvents. It has an iodine value of 85.4.

The fern, or fougere, oils are usually fresh, green and aromatic; and combine well with the dry notes of usnea and other tree moss absolutes.

Fougere perfumes may be classified as deep-noted, sophisticated lavenders. They are appreciated by masculine taste, especially in aftershave and cologne. Coumarin notes, like sweet clover are very complementary.

Fougere oil is used as an aid in astral projection and psychic development.

Ostrich fern has been steam-distilled and contains 103 compounds, including (E)-phytol 25%, nonanal 15%, decanal 7.6% and two aldehydes with seaweed like odor. Miyazawa et al, *J Oleo Sci* 2007 56:9.

The lipids of *S. selagnoides* have been examined with the vegetative runners containing 67 mg/g and runner with spikelets containing 140 mg/gram. They consists of 60-70% neutral lipids, 13-17% glycolipids, 10-16% phospholipids, and 3-5% betaine DGTS.

In the neutral fraction, 11-12% DAG, or diacylglycerol, and 30% TAG.

HYDROSOLS

Maidenhair distilled in May, the water cleanses both liver and lungs, clarifies the blood and breaks the stone.

CULPEPPER

Brunschwig suggests a water of the whole Maidenhair fern be applied to alopecia of the head to cause the hairs to hold, as well as break stone, clear yellow jaundice, and modify colic humors of the stomach and gut.

Water from Polypody ferns is used to clean the blood, soothe irritated coughs, soften the belly and soothe the melancholic.

BRUNSCHWIG

FERN ESSENCES

Bracken fern essence is very helpful where there is fear of psychic sensitivity, and the pressure felt to accept and use these gifts. These imbalances are often caused by a left brain dominant approach to living. There is a need to search out and examine the artistic and creative side. It is useful to use this remedy with a program of artistic and creative endeavors.

BAILEY

Bracken essence with alcohol and water is for feelings of frustration and defeat. It is for people who have difficulty expressing their true selves to the world. Because of this, they often play the childlike role in life; with the frustration that goes with not accepting their own power. It is often useful in cases with cancer involved.

BAILEY

Moonwort essence is associated with childbirth and the first time mother. Often times, fears projected from the unconscious, or even well-meaning friends, can create stress in the mother to be, and anxiety over the birth process. Moonwort can assist by helping both mother and fetus trust in the natural rhythms of labour; and have faith in the timing of the birth experience. It will, on the physical level, alleviate some of the back pain associated with labour and ensure the placenta is fully expelled. This essence is prepared, of course, at full moon.

PRAIRIE DEVA

Male fern essence is made from the dark red blossoms that open for one night only around the summer solstice. It is useful to those desiring to know more about the nature of plants, and their metaphysical associations. It is taken, along with the flower essence of the plant you are requesting information, so that much clearer transmission of information can take place. Only one drop is added to the mixture; or taken under the tongue if you are sitting and meditating with a plant.   **PRAIRIE DEVA**

SPIRITUAL PROPERTIES

For millenia, the Fern was known for magical powers. Humans saw in this plant a deep metaphor, an inner image that is barely comprehended today.

It was the spiral shape that attracted people to ferns. From early Paleolithic rock art to decorative vases and wall paintings in all cultures, we find spirals wherever people have wanted to symbolically portray the path of spiritual development- moving in circles yet always ascending to higher levels.

We see this universal symbol in the huge spiral nebulas of galaxies, in the spirals of our fingertips, in the whirl shaped hair growth of our bodies, and in the whirl shaped muscles fibres of our hearts.

People imitated in spiral dances this movement to integrate themselves into the cosmic energies, especially on Solstice.

The spiral is an ancient symbol of good luck and healing, and fern fronds, especially still curled have long been incorporated into feasts and ceremonies.

In his book The Spiritual Earth, P. Cyrill von Crasinski suggests that the paper spiral noisemakers of birthday parties are really stylized fern spirals.

During the Roman festival Saturnalia, partygoers threw fern fronds at each other for good luck. They also sprinkled fern spores, today's confetti, on each other to bring love and fertility. Called the flower of lovers, these were a potent sexual charm in the Middle Ages.

Every child knew that fern seeds could make those who possessed them happy, wealthy, and able to find treasures, and understand the language of animals.   **FISCHER-RIZZI**

For the Coastal Salish, fronds of Sword fern (*P. munitum*) were seen as spiritual helpers, according to Saanich elder Elsie Claxton. In the winter initiation ceremonies for new dancers in the big house, the new dancers dance around the fronds, which are then carefully gathered and placed in a special location where no one should touch them because they have been transformed through the dance to hold special powers.   **NANCY TURNER 2005**

PERSONALITY TRAITS

The seedpods of Moonwort are broad, round and moon-shaped and are of a silver hue. The silver film makes them look like coins, and is also somewhat similar to an old French cake which was named **OUBLIE**- forgetfulness. A French count, taken prisoner in battle and left too long un-ransomed, painted a branch of Moonwort and sent it to his feudal estate to reproach his retainers for their delay in securing his freedom.   **POWELL**

Bracken is a good young man's name. It is a name for youth, inexperience, and great potential. This is a person who is very impressive, if a bit too brash and sometimes boastful. This is a lover, a drinker, and an energetic person. Bracken is the name for a passionate young drummer, or a shy fellow who wishes he were more outgoing.   **MCFARLAND**

One sweet steroid saponin of the polypody is called osladin. It is a true agent for change. It causes genetic mutation. In a planet saturated with osladins, change came as biodiversity. We see these changes today in the cones of the conifers, the display of our tropical forests, and in the ultimate coronation, the forest crown of the Boreal north.   **BERESFORD-KROEGER**

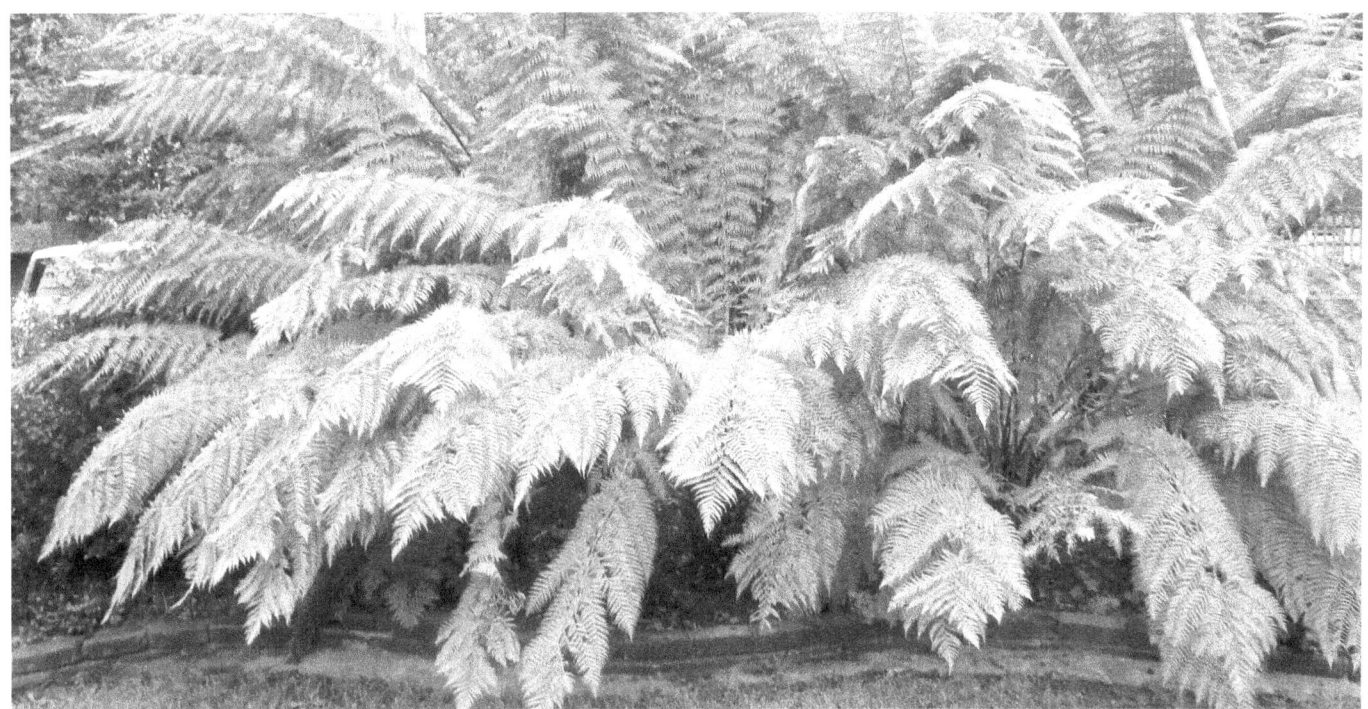

FERNS CAN BE HUGE- NOTE THE CAR ON LEFT SIDE FOR COMPARISON

Rudolf Steiner compares ferns with the stage of development of the child when it says 'I' for the first time. Grohmann concurs. 'In the fern the plant comes to itself. For the first time it forms leaves and at least superficially, stems and roots. The frond is nature's image of the 'I' feeling of the child.'

Despite their firm rooting in the earth, they have come from millions of years of being microscopic floating plants. The long held bait of being invisible and covert is hard to give up.

Even in their newly established environment, there is still a tendency to hide, be concealed, secretive and in the shadows… To advance, one must have the 'I' and eye to see through appearances into the invisible, convert meanings and hidden treasures and decide for oneself. Otherwise one might become blinded by adherence to past influences, dependencies or others' pints of view. Opening one's eyes to life, in all its variety, the joys and dangers, nourishment and toxins means to be fully alive in oneself, ready and able to imbibe the sweetness of life and live on the new terrestrial home of one's identity. **VERMEULEN**

Bracken, with its aversion to diversity, seems like a cancer on the "skin" of the planet…Bracken is a "keynote" in the diagnosis of the ailing planet…Bracken is an indicator species that things are not OK when it is growing rampantly. The world's immune system is strained. Cancer breaks out in an individual when the immune system is weakened. **MARY GEARY**

MYTHS AND LEGENDS

Polypodium Barometz
"Cradled in snow, and fanned by Arctic air,
Shines, gentle Barometz, thy golden hair;
Rooted in earth each cloven hoof descends,
And round and round her flexile neck she bends;
Crops the green coral moss, and hoary thyme,
Or laps with rosy tongue the melting rime;
Eyes with mute tenderness her distant dam,
Or seems to bleat-a vegetable Lamb. **DR. DARWIN**

Legend has it that when Adam and Eve were banished from the Garden of Eden, the Archangel Gabriel guarded the gate through which they left to earn their bread by the sweat of their brows in the wilderness. Stepping aside to let them pass, Gabriel brushed a wing against a boulder and a feather dropped to the ground. The feather took root and grew into the fiddlehead fern, which has ever since been sacred to the archangel.

HENDRICKSON

A long time after that they began to starve…Then they gathered edible fern stumps right behind them. Those they ate. They hunted outward and inward. Finally, after the hero, Big-tail, performed shamanistic rituals all night, Supernatural-Being-Looking-Landward promised to feed his people if they would "stop making the little supernatural being living along the shore cry…" He was referring to the fern spirit woman, who cried because the ferns were being eaten…"But still they all went out to look for food again up and down the inlet… That night, [Big-tail] again sang a song for himself. In the night the wind blew in from the sea. At daybreak he stopped singing. The day after that one went out very early…Now they were saved. They stopped starving."

SWANTON

In mythology, it [bracken] is said by some to originate from Tane-pukupukurangi, involved in rendering asunder Rangi, the Sky Father and Papa, the Earth Mother. It is also said to descend from Haumia Tiketike, one of their sons. Haumia at one time clung as hair to the back of Rangi, but when the two parents were separated by their children, Haumia fell down and buried himself in the Earth Mother. Only the hair of his head, now recognized as fern fronds, was visible. Despite his attempt at concealment man found and dug up the root for food. The tohunga expert made much use of the bracken fern as a medium to consult various spiritual entities…The Maori put great store on its use as a medium to contact the atua [supernatural beings].

RILEY

RECIPES

MALE FERN POWDERED ROOT- one to four drams

OLEORESIN- 2-3 grams given once

TINCTURE- 45-90 drops of root tincture on empty stomach in morning.

Chop fresh fern leaves and cover with 60% alcohol in a glass jar for 4-6 days in the sun or a warm place. This can be used as an embrocation like eucalptus oil.

EXTRACT- one half to one teaspoon. The single and daily dose of *Filicus extractum* is 6-8 grams for adults and 4-6 grams for children. If unsuccessful do not repeat until a few weeks have passed. Extracts contain approx. 25% filicin.

CAUTION- The filicin has a poisoning effect, if absorbed. The patient should prepare by taking a bland diet of complex carbohydrates to protect the liver. On the second day, take two to four milk thistle capsules and follow with 8-10 grams of male fern extract in two portions at fifteen minute intervals in the morning. A laxative tea should also be taken. Antacids inactivate the herb, and should not be taken within 1-2 hours.

Castor oil and other fats increase absorption and risk of toxicity.

Male fern root should not be administered in the presence of anemia, cardiac, liver or kidney disease or diabetes. It is not advisable for children, during pregnancy or the elderly. Overdose can lead to central nervous system disorders like spasm, paralysis, visual disorders and even blindness. Benzodiazepines and oxygen may be need in case of seizure or respiratory failure. The drug is stored over charcoaled calcium for a maximum of one year at a relative humidity below 0.05 in a sealed container in the dark. This is not recommended but simply noted for educational purposes.

OSTRICH FERN ROOT DECOCTION- 6-16 grams

TINCTURE- 10-25 drops. Prepare from dry rhizome 1:5 and 40% alcohol

POWDER IN CAPSULE- 0.5-1.0 gram.

STORAGE- Fiddleheads picked and stored at 0°C, and 100% humidity, provide 95% marketable product after 16 days and 76% after 32 days. Storage in water at same temperature for 15 days resulted in 97% marketability. Not much difference for the added cost and labor.

MAIDENHAIR FERN DECOCTION- One ounce herb, or one half oz. root to a pint of water. Use the whole amount in divided doses over twelve hours.

POLYPODY ROOT DECOCTION Boil one half ounce of chopped root in one pint of water for 30 minutes. **DOSE**- Four ounces as needed, taken cooled.

POWDERED ROOT- two grams two to four times daily.

RATTLESNAKE FERN- One ounce of fronds to one pint of water. Take two ounces of infusion or decoction every hour.

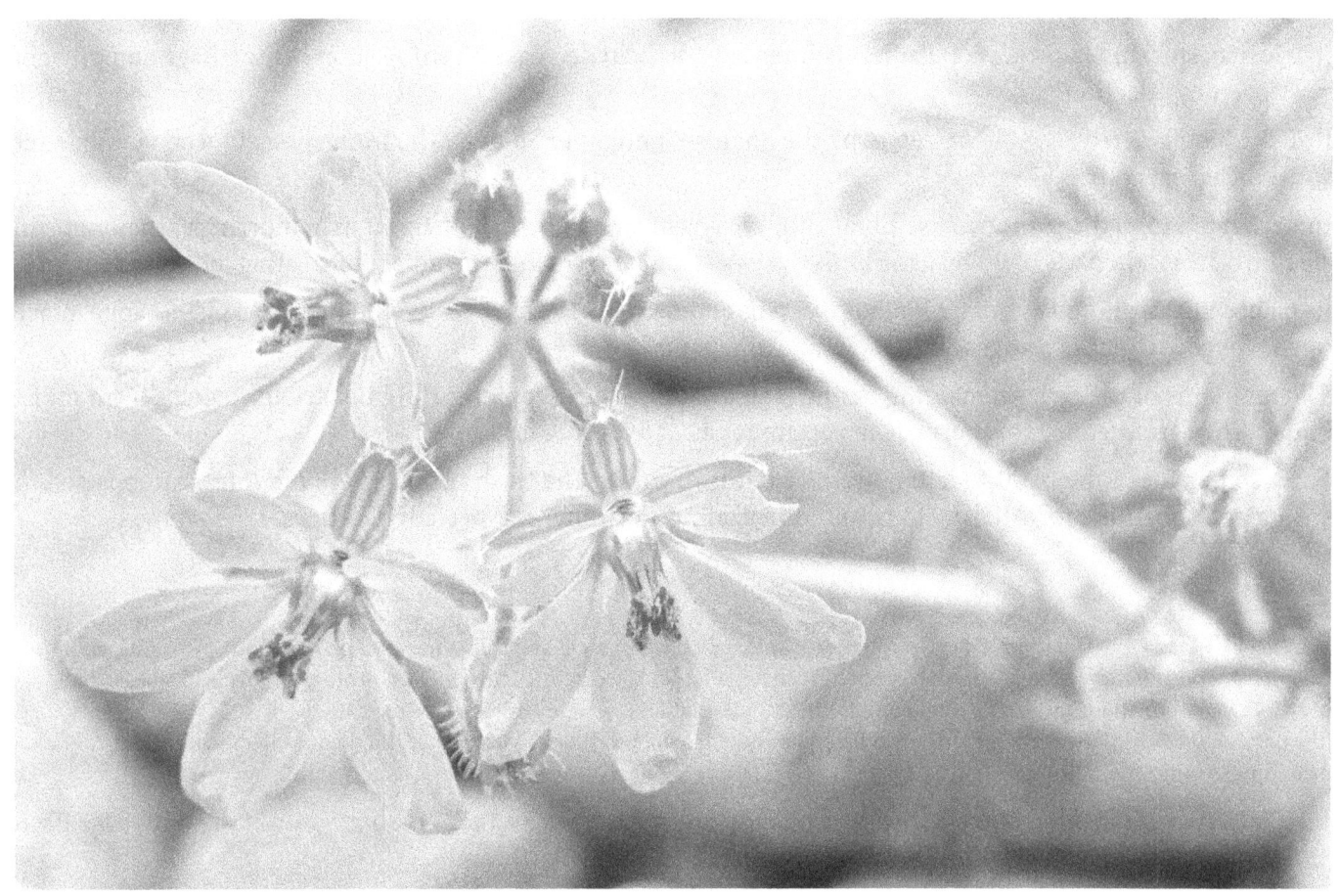

FILAREE

FILAREE
REDSTEM STORK'S BILL
(***Erodium cicutarium*** [L.] L'Hér. ex Ait.)
(***Geranium cicutarium*** L.) not accepted
PARTS USED- leaves, flowers, root

Erodium is from the Greek **HERODIOS** for "heron", a reference to the slender seed vessel resembling a bird's beak. The seed head looks somewhat like an anemic bird of paradise. Cicutarium used to mean "resembling poison hemlock leaves", which the plant certainly does, although filaree is hairy. Filaree probably comes from the Arabic **AL-FILAL**, which means "stork fingers", or from the Spanish **ALFILER** meaning, pin.

The possess a unique seed dispersal mechanism, flinging seeds up to a half meter away, and then drilling into the ground, twisting and untwisting in response to humidity.

Redstem Filaree, or Storkbill has a history of use by native people of North America, despite its late introduction by Europeans. The Costanoan used infusions of the leaves for typhoid fever. The Navaho used the plant for infections, including wildcat and mountain lion bites. Jemez mothers ate the roots to increase breast milk production. The Zuni applied the crushed root to sores, and decocted the root for stomach aches.

The Blackfeet made use of the early spring plant, eating it raw or cooked. It is tastiest before flower.

The tender leaves can be added to salads or steamed like as a potherb. They can be added to omelets, sauces or soups with good results. The flavor is mild and nut-like with a slight bitter aftertaste.

European herbalists used the plant for its astringent, diuretic, emmenagogue, hemostatic, oxytocic and sudorific properties, but mainly for water retention and excessive menstruation.

In Mexico, storkbill is a traditional afterbirth remedy; to help decrease bleeding, stop hemorrhage and prevent post-partum infection.

In Peru the plant is called *Aguja Aguja* by the Spanish, and *Sanu Sanu* by the indigenous Quechua, the latter word meaning, comb.

In herbal folklore, the plant was useful for dropsy, dysentery, gonorrhea, menstrual hemorrhage, rheumatism, sore throats, etc. In parts of Bolivia, the fresh leaves are eaten raw in salads with oil for treating kidney conditions.

Its plant signature is quite obvious, looking like pins and needles. The long beaks with a surgical phallic appearance open clogged urinary passages and relieve sticking pains.

The remnants of the styles remaining on the fruit are very hygroscopic, curling in various degrees from moist to dry. They are used for this purpose in certain types of hygrometers.

Early settlers used the plant to fatten up their herds of cattle. The fresh plant, where plentiful, can be used in spring as a substitute for Alfalfa. Dogs, and other domestic animals, especially racehorses, relish the herb.

MEDICINAL

CONSTITUENTS- Vitamin K, beta-carotene, thiamin, riboflavin, niacin and calcium; catechol, histamine, tyramine, choline, caffeine and putrescine; essential oils, polyphenols, such as gallic acid, geraniin, methyl gallate, protocatechuic acid, ellagic acid, brevifolin, and brevifolin carboxylic acid, tannins, flavonoids, quercitin, kaempferol, myricetin.
The petals contain various anthocyanins including glucosides like petunidin, malvidin, cyanidin, peonidin, malvidin; and cyanidin-3-rutinoside.

Filaree is useful for mild urinary tract and bladder infections, where there is sharp pain. It also relieves PMS and water retention associated with the discomfort.

The dried tops make a tea infusion that is green and hay-like in taste.

The whole plant, including root, can be infused and used for its astringent properties in relieving sore throat by gargling; and nausea and diarrhea by ingesting. It makes an effective wash for scratches, cuts and abrasions. It combines well with borage for cervicitis that follows vaginal inflammation.

The root is hemostatic against uterine hemorrhage; probably due to its high potassium salt content; and has been used as a substitute for goldenseal root.

The tea can also be added to a hot bath to relieve arthritic pain, or taken internally. The fresh leaves can be applied to affected areas to reduce swelling.

Filaree is a galactagogue, increasing the supply of milk in both humans and animals.

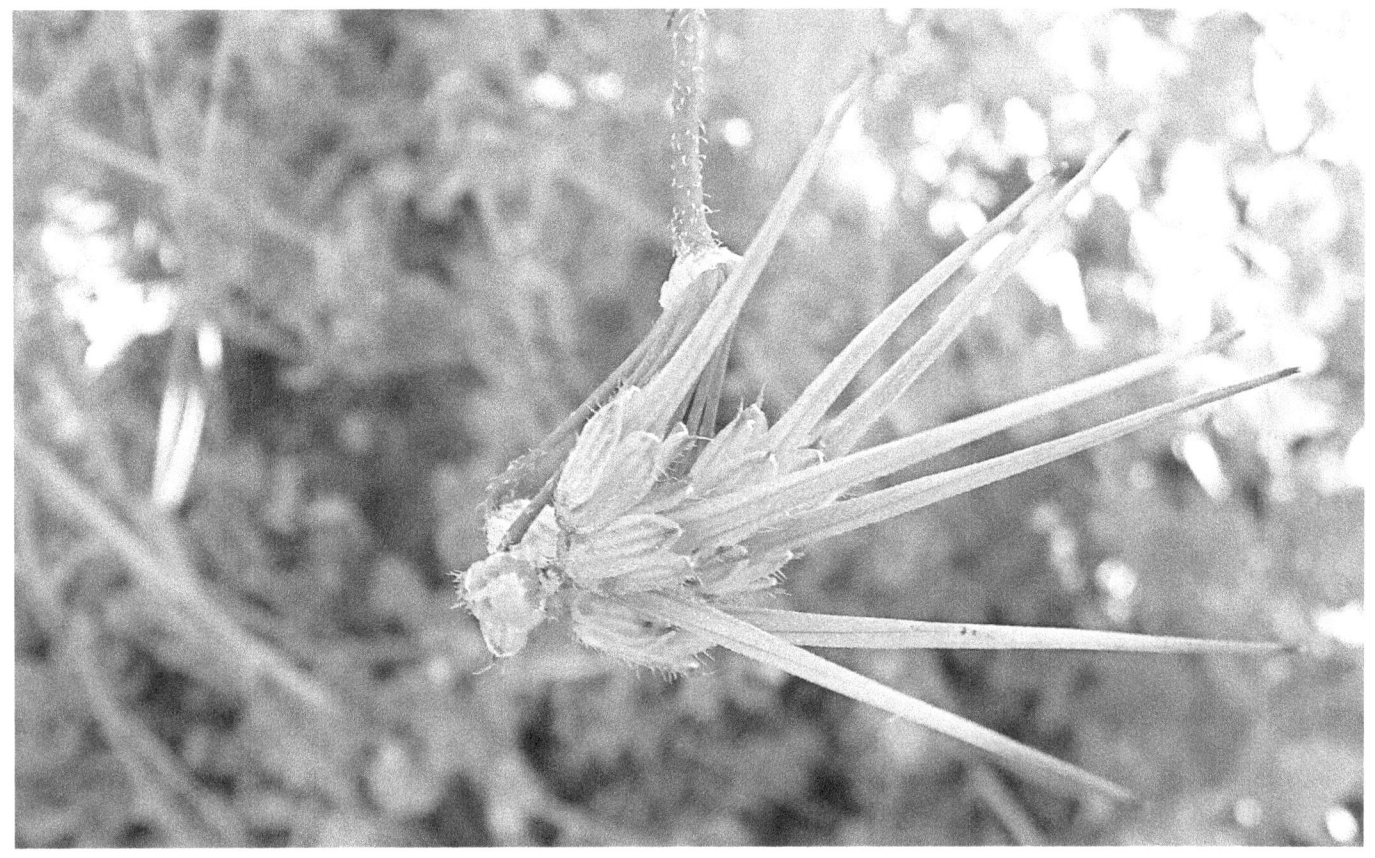

STORKBILL

Filaree has little adverse affect on the kidneys, despite its diuretic effect, and is used in China for kidney trauma, including blood in the urine. It is called **LAO GUAN CAO**, and noted for its warm nature and bitter, acrid flavor.

Jaio Shu De, a brilliant TCM practitioner, used 30 grams of filaree for rheumatoid arthritis patients who have trouble bending and stretching. He suggests that it can be steeped as an infusion, or made into a medicinal wine.

Laboratory studies have shown filaree to increase the tone and reduce the strength or inhibited contraction, of guinea pig ileum. Extracts also stimulated contractions in rat uterus, providing insight into folkloric usage.

Methanol extracts from filaree were shown to exert stimulatory effect on the synthesis of interferon inducted with Newcastle disease virus in cell cultures. Studies by Zielinska-Jenczylik et al, in Poland, found the extract was effective before, or after the virus was introduced. Influenza A was also inhibited. *Arch Immun Ther Exp* 1988 36:5.

Water-soluble extracts show activity against myxoviruses, herpes simplex 1, vesicular stomatitis and vaccinia virus. Above journal 1987 35(2):211-20.

Studies by Sroka in 1994, showed filaree extracts to have strong antioxidative properties. Follow up by Fecka et al, *Herba Polonica* 1997 43:3 found low concentrations of filaree extracts stimulated, and high concentrations inhibited, the free radical activity of human granulocytes, *in vitro*.

Balchin et al, *Acta Botanica Gallica* 1995 142:1 confirmed the anti-spasmodic activity of Filaree and other *Erodium* species.

Work by Gohar on *E. glaucophyllum* found geraniin exhibits both anti-bacterial and anti-fungal activity. *Z Naturforsch* 2003, 58:9-10.

HOMEOPATHY

Erodium, or Stork's bill is a popular hemostat used in Russia, especially for in between menstrual bleeding, or continued excessive blood loss during the period. Cervical and uterine polyps, uterine cancer.

DOSE- Tincture to third potency. Clarke.

ESSENTIAL OIL

Essential oil, steam distilled from the leaves of *Erodium cicutarium* contain isomenthone (11.2%), citronellol (15.4%), geraniol (16.7%), and methyl eugenol (10.6%).

The leaves and stems contain 22% hexadecanoic acid, whole plants 36% and 10-11% hexahydrofarnesyl acetone. Radulovic et al, *Centre Eur J Bio* 2010 4:3.

FLOWER ESSENCE

Filaree flower essence is for those with disproportionate and obsessive worry, or those unable to gain a wider perspective of daily events. It helps develop star-like vision, and a cosmic overview, which holds the events of ordinary life in perspective.   **FLOWER ESSENCE SOCIETY**

SPIRITUAL PROPERTIES

Filaree is a pretty little plant (that) has lacy fern-like leaves and magenta star-shaped flowers. The spirit of this plant offered itself to me as a kind of spiritual messenger service.

I returned to the filaree spirit and asked if it could summon the spirits of other plants I might need to help heal my patients. The spirit said it would be delighted to do this. It was hard for me to believe this would work, but I either had to take him at his word or abandon plant spirit medicine altogether. I took him at his word and found he delivers a purer, more specific medicine than the laboratory does.

Currently, I most often give drops of filaree flower essence, asking my messenger to summon a specific plant spirit.   **COWAN**

MYTHS AND LEGENDS

The Stork was a popular emblem of longevity and, in Taoism, of immortality. There are elsewhere, storks symbolize filial devotion because they were thought to feed their elderly parents. Its nursing care and association with new life as a migratory bird of spring made it sacred to the Greek goddess Hera as a protective divinity of nursing mothers – the basis of the Western fable that storks bring babies. Christian symbolism links the stork with purity, piety and resurrection.   **JACK TRESIDDER**

RECIPES

INFUSION- 3-4 oz. three times daily

TINCTURE- 10-15 drops. Fresh plant tinctures are made 1:4 ratio, and 60%.

CAUTION- Because of the oxytocin effect, the plant is best avoided during pregnancy.

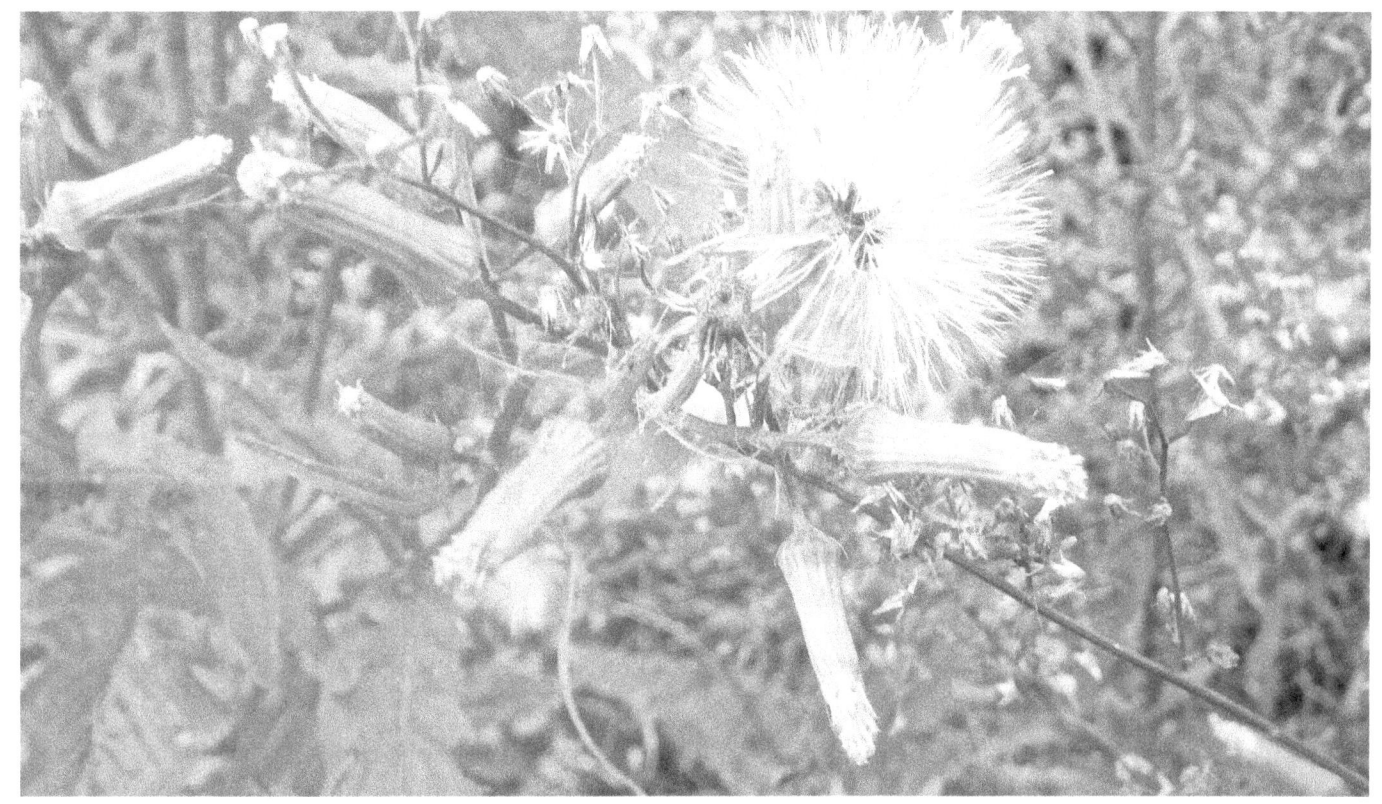

CANADA FLEABANE

CANADA FLEABANE
(***Conyza canadensis*** [L.] Cronq.)
(***Erigeron canadensis*** L.) not accepted
WHITETOP FLEABANE
ANNUAL FLEABANE
DAISY FLEABANE
(***E. annuus*** [L.] Pers.)
PRAIRIE FLEABANE
(***E. strigosus*** Muhl. Ex Willd.)
SMOOTH FLEABANE
(***E. glabellus*** Nutt.)
NORTHERN DAISY FLEABANE
BITTER FLEABANE
(***E. acris*** L.)
(***E. acris ssp. debilis*** [Gray] Piper [L.] S.F. Gray p.p.) not accepted
(***E. acris ssp. politus*** [Fries] Schinz & R. Keller) not accepted
PHILADELPHIA FLEABANE
SKEVISH
(***E. philadelphicus*** L.)
SUBALPINE DAISY
(***E. peregrinus*** [Banks ex Pursh] Greene)
(***E. peregrinus var. thompsonii*** [S. F. Blake ex J. W. Thompson]Cronquist)
(***E. peregrinus ssp. callianthemus*** [Greene] Cronq.) not accepted

TUFTED FLEABANE
WILD DAISY
(*E. caespitosus* Nutt.)
CUT LEAF FLEABANE
DWARF MOUNTAIN FLEABANE
(*E. compositus* Pursh.)
ALBERTA FLEABANE
(*E. trifidus* Hooke.)
SPREADING FLEABANE
(*E. divergens* Torrey & A Gray)
(*E. divaricatus* Michx.) not accepted
LARGE FLOWER FLEABANE
(*E. grandiflorus* Hook.)
HIRSUTE FLEABANE

LOW MEADOW FLEABANE
(*E. lonchophyllus* Hook.)
TRAILING FLEABANE
(*E. flagellaris* A. Gray)
GOLDEN FLEABANE
ALPINE YELLOW FLEABANE
(*E. aureus* Greene.)
(*Haplopappus brandegeei* A. Gray)
SHOWY FLEABANE
ASPEN FLEABANE
THREE NERVE FLEABANE
(*E. speciosus* [Lindl.] DC.)
PARTS USED- roots, flowers, leaves

Erigeron means "soon becoming old", from the Greek **ERI** meaning early or spring, and **GERON** meaning aged. The plant is often overlooked, due to its plain and unattractive nature that looks old even when a young plant. Conyza is the name used by Pliny for some kinds of fleabane, possibly from **KONOPS**, for flea. Caespitosus means, tufted.

Glabellus means smooth, although the plant is actually quite hairy. Divergens is from the Latin **DIS**, meaning apart, and **VERGER**, meaning to turn; in reference to the spreading hairs of the plant. Flagellaris is from the Latin, meaning to whip; referring to the whip-like trailing stems.

The fleabanes and asters look very similar, but the former are spring and summer flowers and have very narrow, numerous rays.

In Norse mythology, the fleabane was the flower of the god Odin; and later became associated with St. Christopher.

Its common name comes from burning it for smoke protections from gnats, and fleas; the seeds even look like fleas. The leaves, when crushed, have a distinct carrot-like odour.

The Cree and Blackfoot used both Canada and Philadelphia fleabane for chronic diarrhea; and saving young mothers from uterine hemorrhage. The roots were boiled to extract the strong volatile oils for menstrual difficulties.

The Chippewa steeped Canada Fleabane, **GABABI'KWUNA'TIG**, "Knotted Tree" for "female weakness". The roots and leaves from just two plants were decocted and drunk for stomach pain. The neighboring Iroquois infused the plant with Wild Ginger root to treat fevers and convulsions.

When picked before flowering, the plant can be poulticed for cancerous lesions on the legs.

The Navaho used the powdered, dried leaves as a snuff for acute hay fever with nasal congestion and sore, itchy eyes.

In Argentina, the leaves are also used as a snuff for relieving rhinitis, while the Zuni tribe crushed the ray flowers between fingers and into the nostril for the same purpose. They call it **HA'MO U'TEAWE**, or Leaf Ball Flowers.

The Lakota made a root and lower stalk tea to treat bowel pain and diarrhea, especially in children. It was known as a sweet smelling weed. The Mesquakie name for fleabane is **TCATCA' MOSIKANI**, meaning sneezing.

The flowers were added to smoking mixtures, with mullein, and uva ursi. It was also boiled to make steam for sweat lodges.

Jethro Kloss recommended hot (112-115° F) enemas for cholera, dysentery and summer complaints in both adults and children, when other remedies have failed. Alum root, and catnip may be added to a tea for treating bladder troubles, scalding urine and hemorrhage from the bowels or uterus.

John William Fyfe wrote (1909). "This old remedy constitutes a valuable medicament in many wrongs of life. In diseases of the kidneys and bladder, especially when a tonic and stimulant action is desired, it is used with gratifying results. In albuminaria much benefit is derived from its employment, and in diabetes insipidus it exercises a restraining influence. In painful diseases of the kidneys and bladder its action is decidedly corrective, and in chronic nephritis and chronic cystitis it is deemed a remedial agent of great value…in chronic catarrhal affections of the genitourinary organs of the female, especially when there is a profuse discharge, it is often useful.

In chronic cough with much expectoration it exercises a quieting influence, and its astringency is of marked benefit in diarrhea, and dysentery, as well as in cholera infantum."

The plant is native to North America, and believed to have been introduced in 17th century to France in bales of animal skins. Some authors suggest it was in the stuffing of a bird, but who really remembers.

It spreads quickly, and can release up to 400,000 seeds from one plant.

In medieval Europe, fleabane seeds were placed on bed sheets to promote chastity.

In Africa, the plant is used as a wash for eczema and ringworm. Tincture of fleabane is used for cystitis, gonorrhea and other genito-urinary disease.

In Cuba, fleabane infusions are used for hemorrhage, diarrhea and edema. In the Yucatan and Peru, where it is known as **HUAMANTARO**, very similar uses are observed.

Studies conducted at the *Instituto Medico Nacional* in Mexico City found fleabane is effective in relieving gastric inflammation and vomiting. The plant is known in Mexico as Simonillo. It is used for relieving hemorrhoids and colitis.

In Japan, fleabane is known as a railway weed and is used in folk medicine for treating jaundice. The leaves are also boiled, chopped and dried, and are sometimes cooked with rice for a tarragon-like flavor.

In African folk medicine, fleabane is used in the treatment of *granuloma annulare*, sore throats, and urinary tract infections. Starlings incorporate fleabane into their nests; and it has been found that young birds in these nests have far fewer parasitical mites than young birds in nests with no fleabane.

Fleabane hyper-accumulates cadmium, zinc and chromium. Krgovic R et al, *Environ Sci Pollut Res Int* 2015 22(14):10506-15. It also hyper-accumulates lead in its root.

Both Northern Daisy Fleabane and Whitetop are common throughout wooded regions of the more northern prairies. Whitetop was used by the Flambeau Ojibwa as a perfume to cure sick headaches; and by the Catawba as a root decoction for heart ailments.

Fleabane and Whitetop were brewed and used as rectal injections for chronic diarrhea by the Fox and other tribes.

The Lakota infused the whole plant to treat sore mouths in children, or adults suffering from difficult urination. They had three different names for the plant, **INIJAN PEXUTA** or **INIJANPI**, sore mouth medicine, or **ONWAHINJUN-TONPI**, meaning "tanning substance".

The latter name applies to the blossoms being mixed with buffalo brain, gall and spleen, and then rubbed into a hide as part of the tanning process.

Whitetop Fleabane seedlings release up to ten different matricaria and lachnophyllum esters to inhibit other plant growth and make room for their own family. One compound, dehydro-matricaria ester causes 50% inhibition at only 10 ppm, during its short half-life of one to two days.

Philadelphia Fleabane is a native perennial with pink to purple to white flowers, fairly common to the prairies. Barton called it a powerful diuretic and sudorific useful in gouty and gravelly complaints. The Houma tribe boiled the root for menstrual and kidney troubles.

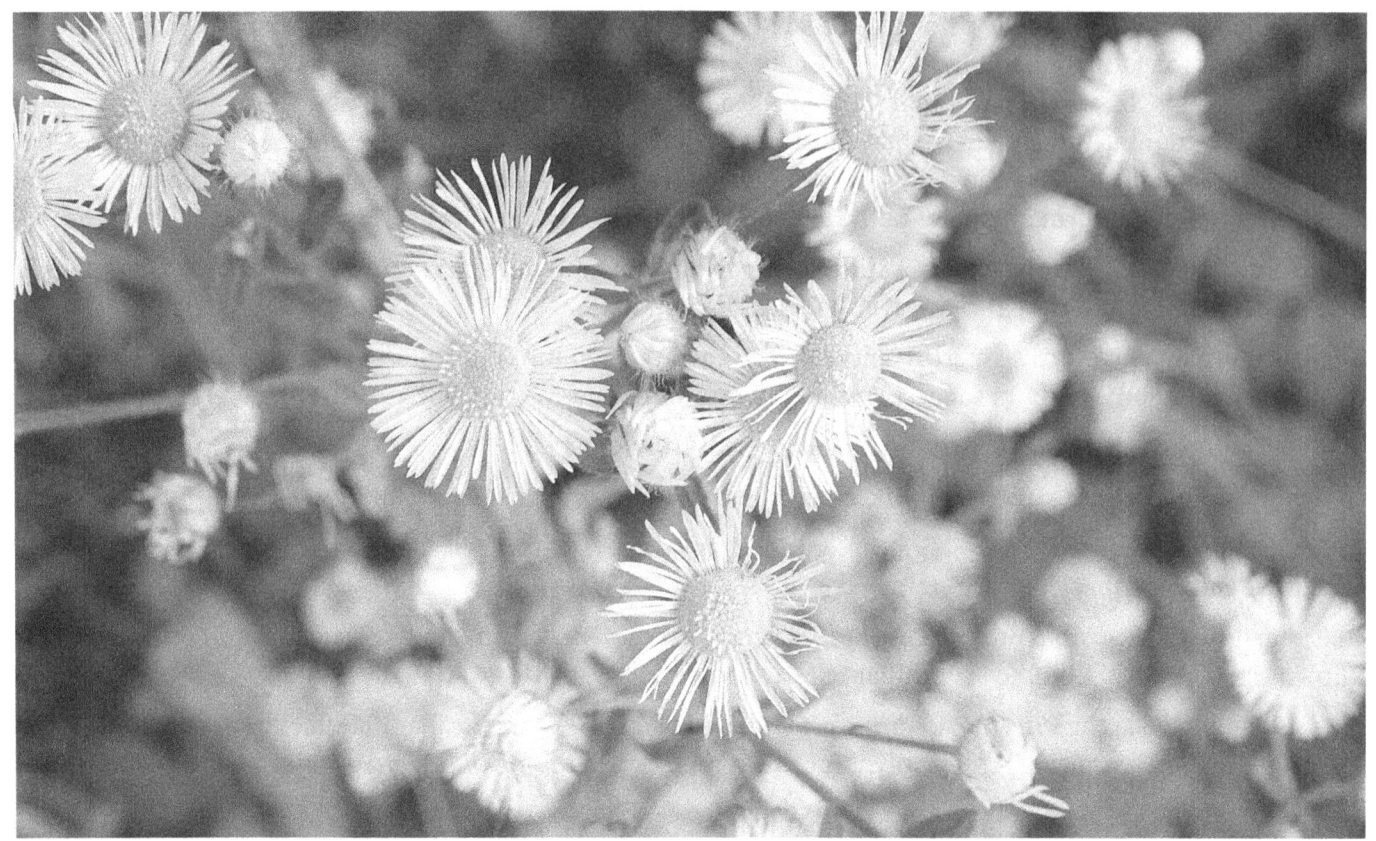

WHITE TOP FLEABANE

The Fox tribe, and others, infused the flowers to help break fevers, by inducing sweating. They call the plant **NO'SOWINI** meaning "sweat", and used it in their steam baths to keep healthy.

Other tribes used this plant for treating chronic diarrhea and hemorrhage during childbirth.

Others used the leaf tea for bloody sputum, water retention, delayed menstruation, bronchial congestion, headaches and fever.

The flowers were dried and powdered and then used as a snuff for headaches and sinus congestion, often combined with wild bergamot and stems of flowers of Golden Alexander, or Meadow Parsnip.

Northern Daisy (*E. acris*) has been introduced to Europe. In Italy, the roots are used for toothache and arthritic pain, and in Spain the aerial parts are used as digestive.

Sub-Alpine Daisy is confined to the foothills and open montane forests in Alberta. It gets smaller with increases in elevation, with beautiful pink flowers.

The Nlaka'pamux of British Columbia call it Star Flower, and use the flower head design in basketry.

The Cheyenne call it Pink Color Medicine, **MA HOM' A UTS IS SE' E AO**, or **MA?OMA?OHTSE-HESEEO?OTSE**.

They used the plant as a medicine to cure dizziness, drowsiness or backache.

Hot infusions were prepared from the dried and pulverized roots, stems and flowers. The patients was covered in a blanket and sat over a steaming infusion to induce sweating. For aches between the shoulders, the patient drank the infusion and rubbed the painful part with some of the tea.

Tufted Fleabane is widespread in the province of Alberta, from the coulees and badlands, all the way to the Peace River country.

Tufted fleabane contains volatile oils, and many Native tribes boiled the roots and leaves to extract these oils, for rheumatism, hemorrhoids and other inflammatory conditions.

The Cree boiled the plant and drank it for diarrhea, as did the Paiute. They would cool the decoction further and use it as eyewash.

Compound Fleabane is a low native perennial of the drier areas of the southwest prairies. It has pink, blue or white flowers. The Thompson tribe chewed the plant and spit it on sores.

Spreading Fleabane (*E. divergens*) was infused by Navaho women as an aid in childbirth delivery. It was also used as a snuff for headaches, and as part of a compound remedy for snakebite.

A cold infusion was used as eyewash and for "lightning infection". The root was considered a life medicine.

The Kiowas, for example, believed **A KENT EIN**, or white flower plant, an omen of good fortune, and used it to enrich their lodging.

E. flagellaris leaves were chewed by the Navaho and applied to spider bites or to stop bleeding.

The Fleabane, *E. formossissimus* was taken as part of a cold infusion and used as a lotion for good luck in hunting.

Large flowered Fleabane *(E. grandiflorus)* roots were used by the Gosiute to poison their arrows.

The Thompsons made a salve of the toasted and crushed plant and animal fat to rub on sores, cuts, wounds and painful areas; as well as swollen glands and sore throat. For the latter, the plant was also chewed.

Hirsute, or Low Meadow Fleabane is an uncommon biennial found throughout moister parts of the prairies.

Showy Fleabane root has been decocted and then cooled as eyewash, or used internally for diarrhea and/or hemorrhage associated with childbirth.

The Ojibwa call it **NOKWE' SIGUN**, and used an unspecified part of the plant, possibly the root, as a perfume to treat headache.

The related *E. glaucum* has evergreen leaves that are glaucous and clammy to touch, yielding a balsamic perfume on the fingers.

Trailing Daisy (*E. flagellaris*) is known as **ZARZILLA** to Hispanic healers, of the American Southwest. The plant is used, in the form of an infused tea, for kidney trouble.

MEDICINAL

CONSTITUENTS- *C. canadensis-* limonene, dipentene, proprionic and gallic acid, terpenol, C10 polyacetylenes, polyenes, polyines, beta himachalene, and methyl caprate derivatives, as well as caffeic acid, alpha spinosterol, apigenin, succinic acid, syringic acid, trans alpha bergamotene, vanillic acid and its benzenoid, centaur X, cumulene, 0-benzylbenzoic acid, dephenyl methane-2-carboxylic acid, 3-beta-erythrodiol.
Also contains 8 sesquiterpenes, B-santalen, B-himachalen, cuparene, alpha-curcumene, delta cadinene, and 3 unidentified as yet), as well as matricaria methyl esters. Twelve flavonoids including querctin-7-O-beta-D-galactopyranosides, quercitin, luteolin, apigenin, baicalein, rutin and others.
root- various enoic and diynoic acid methyl esters, 5-hexa 1-4-diene-2-ynylidenyl-2-(5-H)-furanone, and 5-hexa-1-en-2-ynylidenyl-2-(5-H)-furanone; conyzapyranone A and B; 4Z,8Z-matricaria-y-lactone, 4E, 8Z-matricaria-y-lactone, epifriedelaol, friedeline, taraxerol, simiarenol, spinasterol, apigenin, stigmasterol, conyzagenin A and B
E. annuus- pyromeconic acid, 5-hydroxy-alpha-pyrone (and glycoside), alpha spinasterol, catechol, germacrene, chlorogenic acid, erigeroside, cis- and trans-matricaria esters, cis-lachrophyllum esters, erigerenone B, C10 polyacetylenes, and numerous flavonoids, including apigenin-7-glucuronide, erigeroflavanone.
E. acris- pyromeconic acid, beta D glucosides, apigenin, kaempferol, luteolin, quercitin, and variety of flavonoids including luteolin-7-0-glucoside, caffeic acid, scutellarin, 6'-caffeoylerigeroside; phytosterols including campesterol, chondrillasterol, stigmasterol, stigmast-7-en-3ol (3alpha,5alpha) and spinasterol. Leaves are rich in scutellarin and chlorogenic acid. Flowers are rich in quercitin 3-O-glucoside.
E. philadelphicus- 2 matricaria lactones, erigerol (diterpenoid), erigerenones A & B, philadelphinone (diterpenoid).

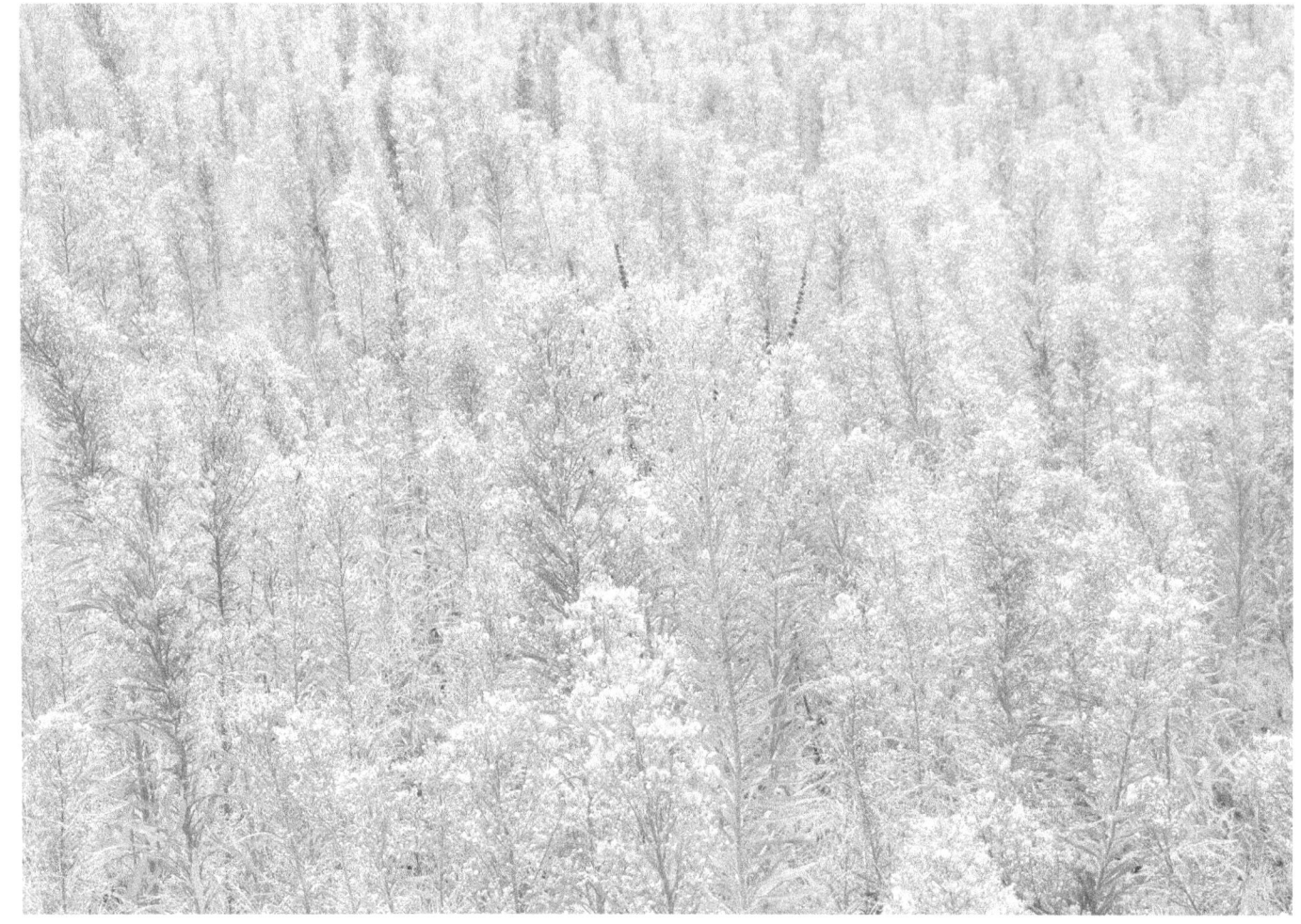

FIELD OF CANADA FLEABANE

Fleabane is an extremely useful, and gentle drying astringent. It is most helpful during heavy menstrual periods, or when breakthrough bleeding occurs. Postpartum hemorrhage, as well as stomach, bowel, or kidney and bladder bleeding, also calls for its use, and it combines well with nettles and shepherd's purse in these conditions.

It is useful for treating chronic nephrotic syndromes, glomerulonephritis and proteinuria, associated with renal weakness or failure; as well as chronic diarrhea, and metrorrhagia.

Fleabane acts as both a nerve relaxant and a stimulant for the lungs; to expel excessive phlegm. Fleabane is for congestion, but not acute inflammation. In bloody bronchitis, it combines well with mullein, and plantain, especially in the form of a honey syrup.

Summer complaints in children, especially persistent diarrhea, respond quickly to a cup or two of fleabane tea. Dr. Bastyr said that Erigeron could be used to treat infantile diarrhea caused by soy allergy. Likewise, diverticulitis, IBS and recurrent ulcerative colitis with repeated diarrhea are all relieved. Leaky gut syndrome related to allergies, malabsorption and immune response is likewise relieved.

Cool infusions of the leaf support the kidneys by constricting the renal capillaries. This action is often useful in excessive urination that accompanies diabetes. It also has a gentle action removing stones and gravel from the kidneys; and chronic bladder irritations.

Fleabane is a powerful diuretic that helps eliminate uric acid, by doubling the quantity of urine passed, as well as encouraging discharge of wastes from edema tissue. It is of value in conditions like cellulitis and gouty arthritis.

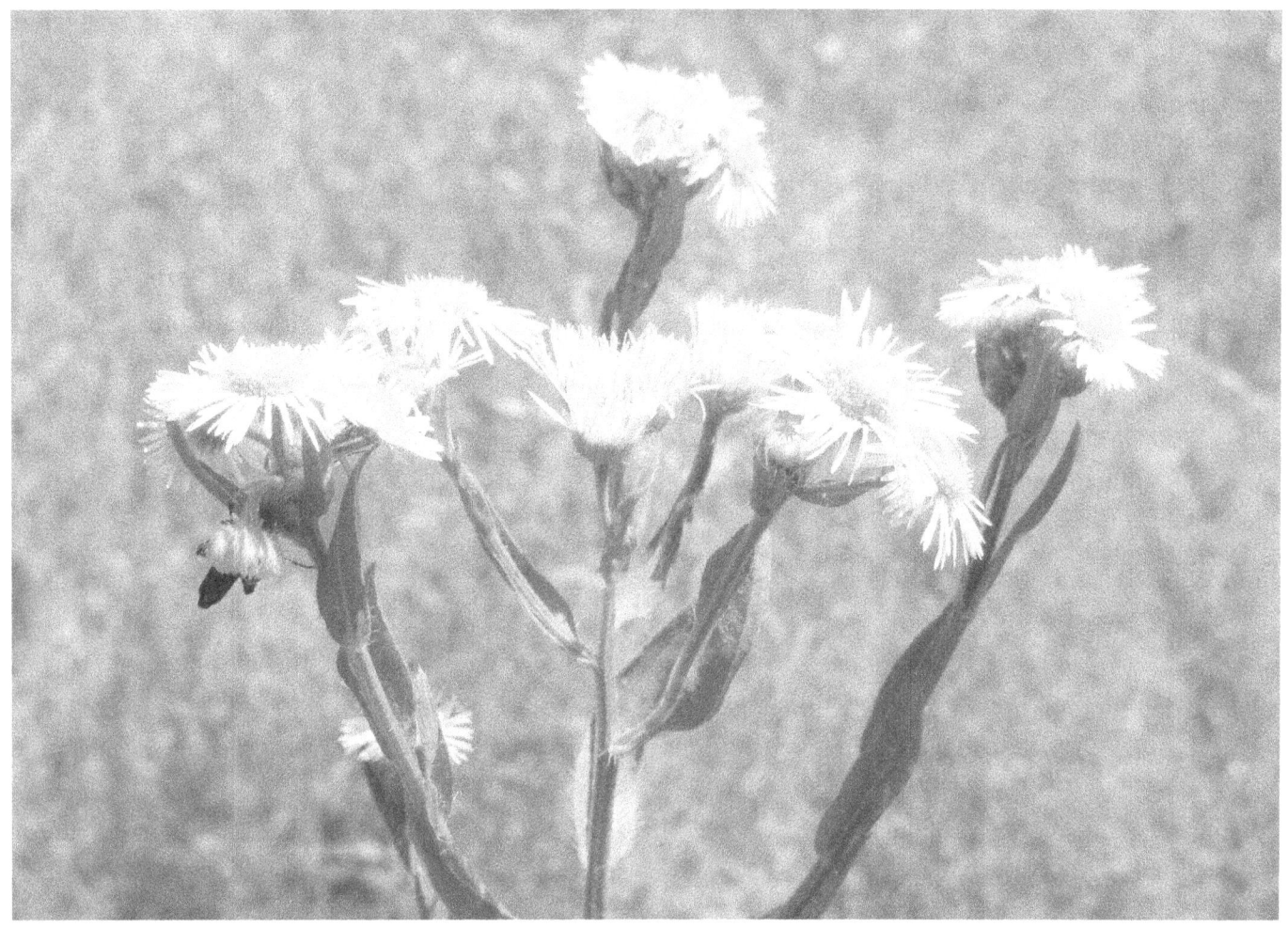

WHITETOP FLEABANE

Hemorrhoids that linger, but never bleed excessively, respond to the tea, as well as retention enemas.

The anti-inflammatory nature of the polyines, and sesquiterpenes helps in some cases of osteoarthritis.

The leaf and flower have shown activity against both gram positive and negative bacteria; as well as activity against tuberculin mycobacterium, and anti-fungal activity against *Helminthosporium turciccin*. Use external washes for ringworm, eczema and other skin conditions, as well as a hair rinse for lice.

In vitro screening shows alcohol extracts active against liver flukes. Shafiq A et al, *Trop Biomed* 2015 32(3):407-12.

Beta-himachalene, one constituent of the leaves and flowers has been demonstrated to have anti-inflammatory activity in laboratory tests.

Work by Lenfeld and Motl, in the former Czechoslovakia confirmed various sesquiterpenes may be responsible for the plant's anti-inflammatory effect.

It appears that a number of mechanisms are responsible for the anti-inflammatory nature of the herb. Sohn et al, *Ann Nutr Metab* 2009 54:3; Sung J et al, *Nutr Res Pract* 2014 8(4):352-9.

The herb contains anti-coagulant and anti-platelet activity. Pawlaczyk I et al, *Thromb Res* 2011 127(4):328-40.

Fleabane extracts modulate plasma protein oxidation induced by peroxynitrate, at least in vitro, suggesting anti-oxidant properties. Saluk-Juszczak et al, *Centr Eur J Biol* 5:6.

Water-soluble compounds, isolated from flowers, show potential to protect lymphocytes from gamma radiation-induced damage. Szejk M et al, *Int J Biol Macromol* 2017 94 (ptA):585-93.

The herb contains a derivation of octulosonic acid that inhibits catecholamine secretion induced by acetylcholine. Ding et al, *J Nat Prod* 2010 73:2.

Extracts of the plant show activity against neuroblastoma SH-SY5 Y cells, suggesting of playing a role in treatment of Alzheimer's disease. Huang et al, *Zhong guo Zhong Yao Za Zhi* 2010 35:8.

Fleabane leaf infusions possess anti-hypertensive activity. Lasserre et al, *Naturwissen* 1983 70.

The plant is being investigated for treating peri-menopausal symptoms with some positive results.

Fleabane shows potent activity against MCF-7 breast cancer cell lines. Abu-Dahab et al, *Sci Pharm* 2007 75.

The root contains compounds active against human cervix adenocarcinoma, skin carcinoma and breast (MCF-7) cancer cell lines. Csupor-Loffler B et al, *Planta Medica* 77:11 1183-88.

Both Fleabane and Whitetop show activity against skin, breast, and cervical human cancer cell lines. Rethy et al, *Phyto Res* 21:12; Loffler et al, *Planta Med* 77:1.

The compound 3-beta-erythrodiol induces early and late apoptosis and cell cycle arrest in human gastric cancer. Liu K et al, *Oncol Rep* 2016 35(4):2328-38.

Both Whitetop and Philadephia Fleabane are more diuretic and less astringent than *E. canadensis*, but can be substituted when needed.

The dried leaves and stems of *E. annuus* have compounds with hypotensive action. This may be due in part to apigenin compounds that also exhibit estrogen receptor and benzodiazepine receptor activity.

The leaf contains caffeic acid that exhibits anti-oxidant and neuroprotective activity against neuronal cells. Jeong CH et al, *Chin Med* 2011 6:25.

Patents in Japan have been obtained for the use of 5- hydroxy-a-pyrone and its glucoside as an aging inhibitor for plants and glycosidase.

Pyromeconic acid, isolated from *E. annuus,* was granted a patent in Japan in 1952. A similar claim for *E. acris* was made in the former USSR in 1982.

Whitetop Fleabane (*E. annus*) contains pyromeconic acid. Studies conducted by Hashidoko in Japan in 1995, found pyromeconic acid has an affinity for siderophilic activity, meaning it has an affinity for iron.

Cantrell et al, looked at some 230 plant extracts for activity against mycobacterium. Whitetop Fleabane showed 100% inhibition of both *M. tuberculosis* and *M. avium. Phytomedicine* 1998 5:2.

Even more exciting is recent work on the anti-oxidative and protein glycation inhibition of Whitetop Fleabane. Glycation, in brief, is the process of normal aging and age-related diseases.

Glycated hemoglobin, is a measure of low term elevated blood sugar levels.

Kim et al, *J Agric Food Chem* 2003 51 the whole plant showed significant bioactivity in both areas, leading to potential treatment in age prevention and diabetic complications. Work by Jang DS et al, *Biol Pharm Bull* 2010 33(2):329-33 found a caffeoylquinic compound in leaf and stem that inhibit protein glycation, aldose reductase and prevention of cataracts.

The flowers contain erigeroflavanone, found to inhibit advanced glycation and aldose lens reductase associated with diabetic complications. Yoo et al, *J Nat Prod* 2008 71:4.

Erigeroflavanone may be useful in the treatment of renal complications associated with diabetes. Kim OS et al, Chem Biol Interact 2009 180(3): 414-20.

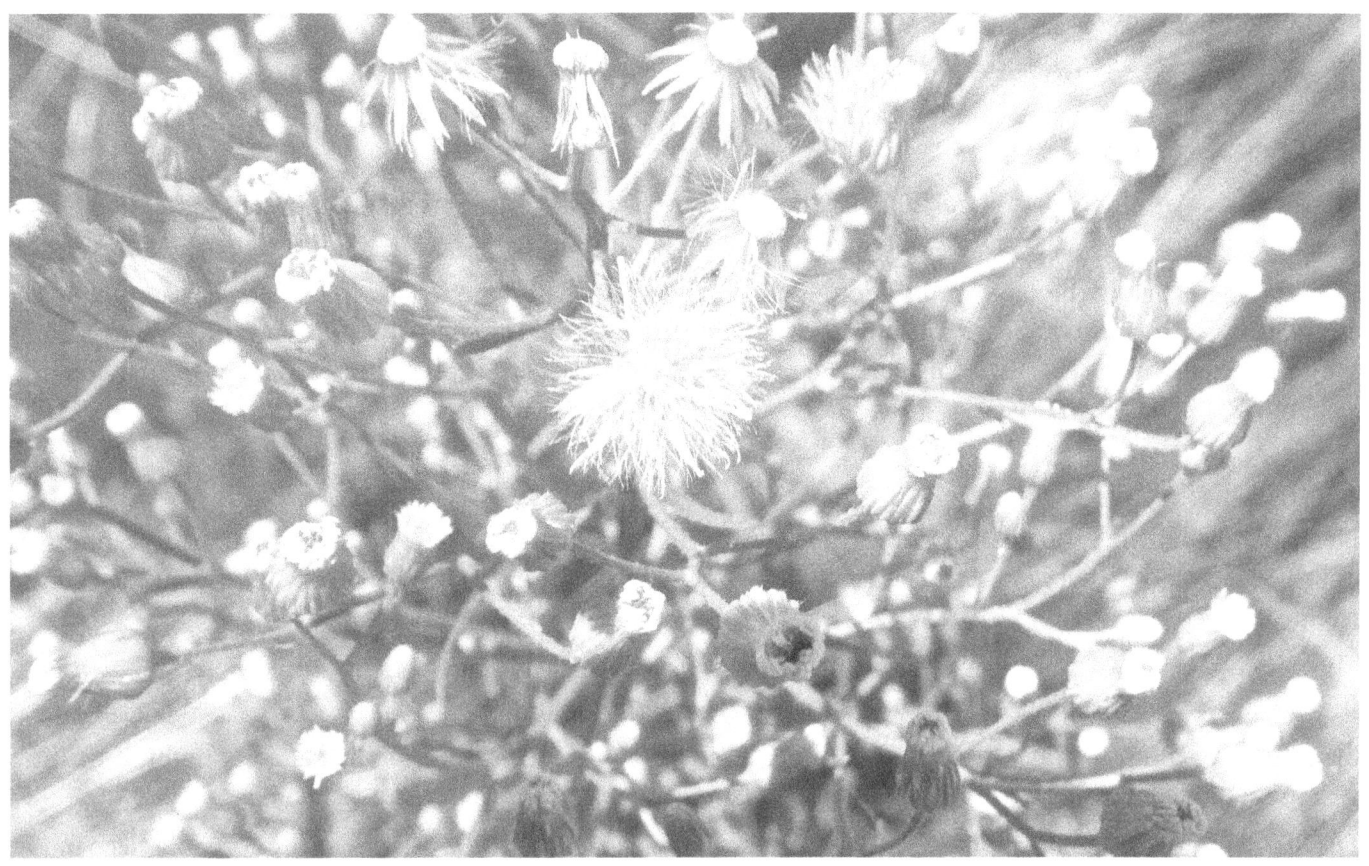

CANADA FLEABANE

Jang et al, *Arch Pharm Res* 2008 31:7; and *Bio Pharm Bull* 2010 33:2, identified 3,5-di-0-caffeoyl epi-quinic acid as most active flower compound against advanced glycation. Caffeic acid, 3,6-di-0-ferulolysucrose and above compound were most active at inhibiting aldose reductase. Clinical applications for diabetic complications are possible.

The flowers contain ergosterol peroxide, an anti-atherosclerosis agent. Kim DH et al, *Arch Pharm Res* 2005 28(5): 541-5.

Whitetop contains gamma pyranone, a compound that exhibits anti-tumor activity against human hepatoma, liver and leukemia cell lines. Li X et al, *Pharmazie* 2006 61(5):474-7.

The roots ameliorate acute inflammation through inhibition of NFalphaB activation. Jo MJ et al, *Evid Based Complement Alternat Med* 2013 Feb 24.

Philadelphia fleabane was researched by Deutsch and colleagues. They found water extracts of plant effective in lowering the intraocular eye pressure, similar to *Cannabis sativa*. *Current Eye Research* 1987 6:7.

The flowers can be used for fever, especially if chills are present as a hot infusion. Dysmenorrhea with back pain responds well.

Acetone extracts of the plant exhibit activity against both gram positive and gram negative bacteria.

Two matricaria lactones isolated from *E. philadelphicus* have been found active against *Mycobacterium tuberculosis* and *M. avium*, with MICs of 12.5 ug/ml and 50 ug/ml respectively. TianSheng et al, *Planta Medica* 1998 64:7.

The expressed juice of the whole plant of *E. divergens* has been studied, and shown to exhibit activity against both gram positive and mycobacterium.

Smooth Fleabane water extracts show no activity but 80% acetone extracts possess moderate activity against *S. aureus*. Osborn et al, *Br J Exp Path* 1943 24.

The related *E. breviscapus* is standardized to 98% breviscapine, and used in China for ischemic heart disease and to alleviate after effects of stroke.

Work by Wang et al, *Zhong Yao Cai* 2003 26:9 found anti-coagulation effect is result of inhibiting platelet factor III, and prothrombin V; as well as enhancing the activity of fibrimolysis.

Work by Liao et al, in the same publication, issue 28:2, found the herb beneficial in re-establishment of blood circulation in the ischemic brain, and improvement of neuronal metabolism and survival. Other work has found the constituent scutellarin, also present in Scullcap species, helps protect neuronal damage after cerebral ischemia/reperfusion.

HOMEOPATHY

Fleabane is used wherever there is hemorrhage of the bladder; or where the uterus is expelling large amounts of bright red blood. There may be an accompanied pain in the left hip or ovary area; or noise or buzzing in the right ear.

The pain is usually worse with every movement, or after a restless night, the patient is tired, weak and irritated. In between period bleeding, or nosebleeds in place of a period, call for fleabane.

Symptoms of mind include great depression, excessive languor, delusion of being called at night, intruding sexual thoughts, mistakes in writing, leaving out words and letters, as well as masochism.

DOSE- Tincture to the third potency. The mother tincture is made from the whole fresh Canada fleabane in flower. First proving based on work of Burt with tincture, third trituration of oil and decoction of dried plant about 1866. A proving with tincture and 3x was conducted by Mezger with five females and 11 males in 1950.

ESSENTIAL OIL

CONSTITUENTS- *E. canadensis*-aerial cumin aldehyde, limonene (up to 78%), methyl octanoates, beta pinenes, sesquiterpenes, polyacetyl esters, matricaria esters (up to 30%), lachnophylum ester, d-limonene, d'pentene, delta-l-terpineol, p-cymene, camphene, mycrene, germacrene, alpha-cis-bergamots, beta-trans-farnesene, and cuminaldehydes. Over 47 volatile components have been identified, of which 91% are terpenoids.
The root contains the above, as well as a 2Z,8Z matricaria ester (C11H8O2).
European research found 18 compounds with 76% limonene, 5.8% cis santalene, 3.8% delta three carene, and 3.62% beta mycrene.
E. philadelphicus- The yield is about 0.15% of dried plant material. It contains up to 80% cis-2, cis-8-matricaria ester, with smaller amounts of trans-2, cis-8-matricaria ester (17.4%), 3Z-hexenol (11.4%), delta cadiene (9.4%), germacrene D (7.5%), cis-2-lachrophyllum ester (5.3%), trans-2-lachrophyllum ester (4.2%), beta eudesmol (4.9%), para-cresol (4.4%) and other terpenes. It also contains 0.73% by weight of C10 polyacetylenes.
E. acris- limonene, beta pinene, (E)-beta-ocimene, alphamuurolen, germacrene D, (E)-beta farnasene.
Roots- 1.0% yield containing 49% (Z, Z)-matricaria ester, and 37% lachnophyllum ester, as well as elemenes and tricyclic sesquiterpene hydrocarbons.
E. annuus- flower- germacrene D 47%, (Z) lachnophyllum esters 20%. The root contains 59.9% matricaria esters, and 34.9% lachnophyllum esters.
Roots- 0.05% yield containing 46% (Z, Z)-matricaria ester, and 27% (Z)-lachnophyllum ester, beta sesquiphellandrene and beta bisabolene.
E. speciosus- methyl 2Z,8Z-deca-2,8-diene-4,6-diynoate and its 2E,8E isomer.

The steam-distilled oil from the entire flowering Canada Fleabane is herbaceous and ethereal, with a sweet cumin amber-like undertone. On dilution, the oil resembles neroli.

It varies from a pale yellow green to dark yellow, and produces 0.33-0.66% from the fresh leaf; and 0.2-1.7% from the dried. Specific gravity is 0.8464.

It is one of the most diffusive stimulants in the plant kingdom. It is used in the perfumery industry to modify the top note of fern and cypress type blends and for adding unusual nuances.

In the food and flavor industry it is used for candy, ice cream and soft drinks in 0.2-5 ppm.

The oil will arrest most uterine hemorrhage with two or three drops on a sugar cube. In emergency, this can be repeated 3-4 times every fifteen minutes.

The oil is excellent for prolapse of the intestine, with resultant gas and bloating. Old herbals recommended one dram of the oil mixed with egg yolk and milk for various intestinal complaints.

The oil is highly prized in France, where medical aromatherapists use the oil for pancreatic and hepatic stimulation. It is also a powerful anti-spasmodic, anti-rheumatic and coronary dilator.

It has been used in the stimulation of retarded puberty in young women. The essential oil contains human growth hormones, one of the very few plants containing this unique compound.

The oil has been used in gonorrhea, bladder complaints, lung infections, intestinal parasites, and even neat on cystic pimples. It clears excessive protein from the urine, and reduces kidney inflammation.

Diluted with carrier oil such as coconut oil and made into suppositories, it reduces inflamed hemorrhoids.

Eclectic practitioners dissolved one dram of oil to an ounce of pure alcohol. They employed this as an application to inflamed and enlarged tonsils, or other inflammations of the throat.

Topical application may be useful for middle ear infections. Do not put in ear canal, but massage neat into adjacent areas.

The essential oil was official in the *US Pharmacopoeia* from 1863-1916, and used to accelerate uterine contractions immediately before childbirth, suggestive of oxytocic activity.

In China, the essential oil is given to prevent allergic diarrhea in children due to ingesting cow milk.

The oil is being researched for treating hypertension in veterinary medicine. It inhibits the growth of mold.

Moderate anti-fungal activity against *Cryptococcus neoformans* and *Trichophyton interdigitalis* was noted. Veres K et al, *Scientific World Journal* 2012:489646.

Steamed-distilled aerial parts of Showy Fleabane, possess activity against a number of fungi that attack strawberry plants, including *Botrytis cinerea, Colletotrichum acutatum, C. fragariae,* and *C. gloeosporioides*. Meepagala et al, *Pest Manag Sci* 2002 58 (10):1043-7.

Bitter Fleabane (*E. acris*) essential oil from the root shows high anti-proliferative activity against human breast MCF-7 cancer cell lines. The aerial essential oil showed activity against all five Candida species tested.

Whitetop essential oil tested active against the same lines, but not as powerfully. Nazaruk J et al, *Z Naturforsch C* 2010 65(11-12):642-6.

PLANT OILS

Whitetop *(E. annuus)* collects unsaturated fatty acids in the stems and leaves. This is somewhat unusual, and presents the possibility of hypocholesterolemic action from a dry plant material. The specifics are linoleic 46.7%, and linolenic acids 26.6%, with stearic, palmitic, oleic, and palmitoleic acids also present.

HYDROSOL

Fleabane hydrosol is weedy and unpleasant to both smell and taste. The pH is 3.9, indicating good shelf stability.

Suzanne Catty has trialed it for blackflies and mosquitoes with some success.

She suggests the hydrosol is anti-bacterial, digestive and diuretic for kidney infections.

FLOWER ESSENCES

Fleabane is for the "beautiful people". That is, many people with considerable external beauty find it difficult to forge deep and lasting relationships. Fleabane flower essence works in two ways.

It helps to ward off those "parasitic encounters" that stem from other's need to be near them.

It also helps the individual discover their own needs, with less reliance on the flattery of others.

PRAIRIE DEVA

Canadian Fleabane is for those feeling empty, that laughter has gone out of one's life. It is a grief essence, for bereavement some time ago. It helps a person move back into the world when they have experienced a loss.

NEW MILLENIUM

Fleabane essence is for those experiencing menopause, helping temper hot flashes, ease passage and rebalance male female energies.

CHOMING

Golden Fleabane essence is for dealing with being a black sheep in a family.

ROCKY MTN

Annual Fleabane flower essence is for when one feels hindered by others, or feels the need to be freed from feelings and influence of others.

MIRIANA

Fleabane is a major help when experiencing menopause; helps to temper those hot flashes and many of irritants of menopause including that crawly feeling on your skin; helps rebalance masculine and feminine energies that are out of balance.

RAVENWORKS

RECIPES

INFUSION- One-quarter ounce of Fleabane to one pint of boiling water. Steep twenty minutes. Drink 2-4 ounces three times daily. Warm for lungs and uterine problems. Cool for problems of bladder and kidney.

TINCTURE- 10-20 drops 3X daily. Fresh aerial parts are prepared at 1:4 and 50% alcohol. Fleabane is contraindicated during pregnancy.

FLUID EXTRACT- 4-8 ml daily

POWDERED CAPSULE- 1-2 capsules three times daily of a 1:10 dry extract containing 50-200 mg per capsule

ESSENTIAL OIL- 5-10 drops every two hours as needed for hemorrhage. Inhalation of fleabane essential oil stimulates hypothalamus and in turn pituitary.

FRESH JUICE- 50 grams daily.

FULLER'S TEASEL
COMMON TEASEL
WILD TEASEL
VENUS' BASIN
(***Dipsacus sylvestris*** Huds.) not accepted
(***D. fullonum*** L.)
CULTIVATED TEASEL
(***D. sativus*** [L.] Honck.)
(***D. fullonum*** ssp. ***sativus*** [L.] Thell.)
CUTLEAF TEASEL
(***D. lanciniatus*** L.)

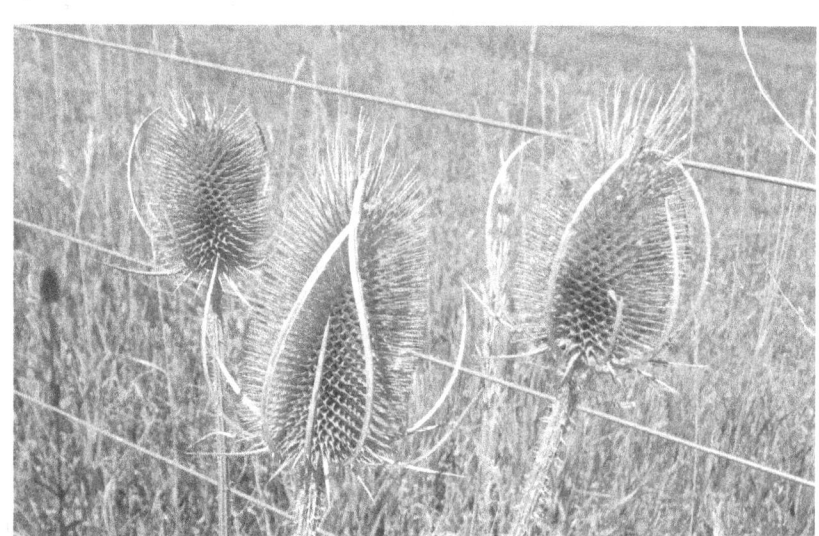

TEASEL ALONG FENCE LINE IN COLORADO

ASIAN TEASEL
SICHUAN TEASEL
(*D. asper* Wallich ex Candolle)
(*D. asperoides* C. Y Cheng & Ai)
JAPANESE TEASEL
(*D. japonica* Miquel.)
CHINESE TEASEL
(*D. chinensis* Batalin)
PARTS USED- root, stem, leaf, flower

Teasel is from the English Teazle, and in turn from the Anglo-Saxon *Taesen*.

Sylvestris means found in dense woods, and thus makes no sense for a plant that loves full sun. Dipsacus is a transliteration into botanical Latin of a Greek word coined by Galen. Dipsa means thirst, but dipsacus has a different meaning. Galen used the word to suggest the raving thirst experienced by diabetics.

The idea the axil of the leaf holds a drop of water, to help quench the plant's thirst is absurd. Water does collect there, and may prevent sap-sucking aphids from climbing the stem.

Insects collect in the water and this addition of dead insect protein, causes a 30% increase in seed set and the seed mass:biomass ratio. Shaw PJ & Shackleton K, *PLoS One* 2011 6(3):e17935.

Teasel heads were traditionally used to card wool, full the cloth and comb certain clothes. Cashmere still calls for its use. Today, they are used on the green baize used on billiard tables, to raise the nap. The name Fuller refers to an ancestor who teased up the nap with teasel. He put sizing in cloth and used a fine clay called Fuller's Earth. Now you know.

The European species, *D. fullonum* meaning teasel of the fullers, was often found planted near woolen factories. It is identifiable in the early 6th century Vienna Dioscorides, an illuminated manuscript of *De Materia Medica*.

I have come upon it in British Columbia, Idaho and Montana, but it has not introduced itself to Alberta as of yet. It will not be long.

Cutleaf Teasel is both an introduced and invasive perennial. It was first known in New York and Michigan since before 1900. It is now in Oregon and throughout the mid-west from Ontario down to Colorado and across to Virginia.

Each seed head may contain up to 1500 flowers, that each last just twenty four hours. It has white flowers and deep cut leaves, whereas common teasel has purple flowers and toothed leaves. One plant can produce over three thousand seeds.

Cutleaf Teasel is more aggressive, but Common Teasel is more widespread.

Biological control of this invasive herb with the mite, *Leipothrix dipsacivagus*, has been moderately successful.

Asian Teasel is widely used for medicine in that continent. It is known as **CHUAN XU DUAN**, Liu Han (Mandarin), Chyun Dyun (Cantonese), Ru Duan (reconnect that which is severed), Jie Gu (bone-mending) and Shan Lo Bo. In Japan it is known as **ZOKUDAN** meaning, Solder Fracture. Chinese teasel is also known as **DA TOU XU DUAN**. The Chinese name for *D. japonica* means "restore what is broken".

The wild plant is widely over-harvested and endangered by urbanization.

The root is bitter, pungent, warm, dry and slightly sweet. It is astringent, restorative, stabilizing, stimulating and decongesting. In TCM terms, it is yang tonifying.

Asian teasel and Japanese teasel look similar, but the former is perennial and has a white or yellow corolla, and the latter is biennial with pink corolla.

MEDICINAL

CONSTITUENTS- *D. fullonum*- theine, tannin, gallotannins, bobeic acid, theophylline.
D. asper- asperosaponin A-C, various triterpene saponins, phenolic acids including caffeic acid, 2,6-dihydroxycinnamic acid, ursolic acid, oleanolic acid, vanillic acid, 2'-O-caffeoyl-D-glucopyranoside ester, caffeoylquinic acid, iridoid glucosides, triterpenoids, oleanic acid and akebia saponin D (asperosaponin VI), lamine, phytosterols, iridoid glycosides including loganin, loganin acid, cantleyoside, tripolostoside A and sweroside derivatives, dipsalignan A-D, beta sitosterol, vogeloside, epi-vogeloside, cauloside A, deoxyloganic acid.

A tincture of the fresh flowering head can be useful for relief of headaches.

Cold infusions of the leaves relieve redness and inflammation of eyes. Strain well and use an eyecup. Traditionally, water was gathered from cup formed by sessile leaves as eye wash and to clear skin blemishes.

Warm infusions are taken internally for improving digestion and soothing the intestinal tract. John Hill (1740), the English herbalist noted. "The root is used: it is bitter, and given in infusion, strengthens the stomach and creates an appetite. It is also good against obstructions of the liver and jaundice. People have an opinion of the water that stands in the hollow of the leaves, being good to take away freckles."

A mild flower infusion helps promote liver and gall bladder health, including jaundice.

The root oil is considered excellent for warts, boils and abscesses.

The root is stimulating to the nervous system and helps result in feelings of comfort and exhilaration, similar to drinking too much coffee. Use the tea for mental alertness when needed. The compound theine is also known as caffeine.

Bobeic acid is also found in tea leaves. Theophylline is also similar in structure to caffeine and a well-known bronchial smooth muscle relaxant. It is also found in cocoa beans.

Common teasel is used in Peru for liver and digestive concerns.

Matthew Wood writes. "The late William LeSassier introduced *D. sylvestris* into practice in North America as a substitute for the Eastern species [*D. japonica*] and I learned from him to use it for catastrophic injuries of the joints and tendons. Later, when I was searching for a remedy for Lyme disease I remembered that teasel was said to act on the kidney jing. Syphilis is viewed as an attack on the kidney essence in traditional medicine (East or West), and since Lyme disease is due to a syphilitic spirochete, I surmised that teasel would be a possible remedy for this dreadful disease. Besides which, it acts on the connective tissue, joints, bones, tendons, and muscles, very much like Lyme. This has been verified in my practice and that of many others and in fact there is now medical research on the subject." He continues in his book The Earthwise Herbal (Old World): "Teasel is an important remedy for conditions where the muscles are torn, badly injured or inflamed. Especially where the large joints (shoulders, hips) are torn and damaged...In addition, it is specific for Lyme disease; unfortunately, it only works in some cases."

The physio-medicalist, Christopher Menzies-Trull adds ocular inflammation, excessive wrinkles on the face, eczema, psoriasis, acne and impetigo, lack of appetite, and parasites in intestine, as symptoms of teasel use. Many of these are from the homeopathic provings noted below.

Matthew also notes it is good for large, bulky people who throw their joints out with special force, and chronic inflammation of the muscles, with limitations of movement and great pain. "If you have ever suffered from the experience of having something 'broken' in your life, so that a major piece, a part of your path, does not come into play, cannot become manifest, then you know how important it is that there is a medicine to 'Restore What is Broken'." He shares several case studies of interest in my all time favorite herbal, *The Book of Herbal Wisdom* pages 237-40.

Fresh first year roots were extracted with ethanol and ethyl acetate; and the latter was found active against *Borrelia burgforferi*, associated with Lyme disease. Liebold T et al, *Pharmazie* 2011 66(8):628-30. A 70% ethanol extract showed no growth inhibition.

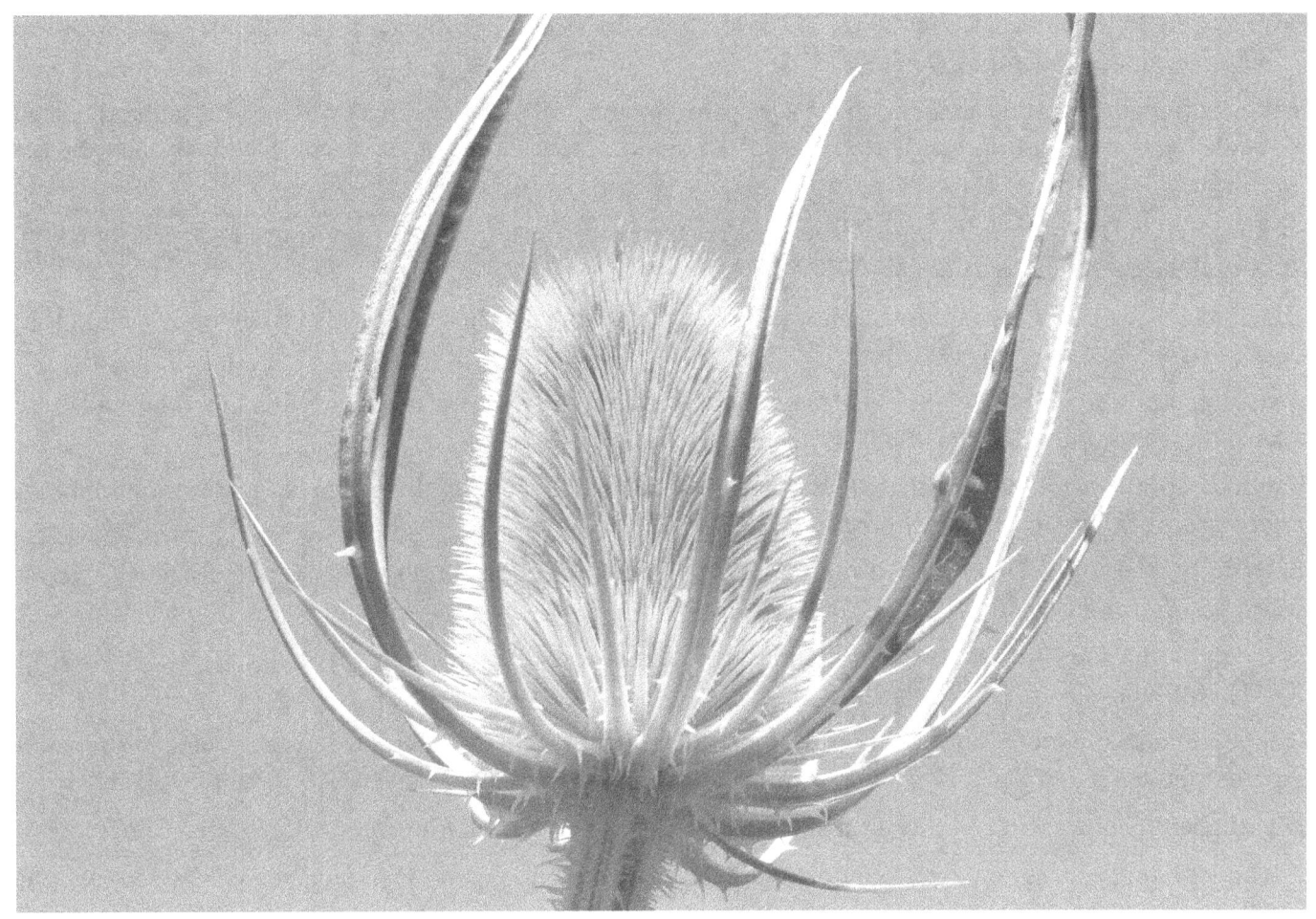

COMMON TEASEL

Asian Teasel root is useful for bone, ligament and muscle weakness, especially of the lumbar, knees and legs. It relieves pain of the lower back and arthritis associated with knees. It can be used in traumatic injuries with swelling, ruptured tendons, and fractures.

It is a uterine stimulant and is contraindicated in pregnancy, except when there is fetal unrest and threatened miscarriage.

Progesterone is an important hormone in first trimester miscarriage. A study by Gao J et al, *Fitoterapia* 2016 113:58-63 found alcohol extractions of dipsacus root and asperosaponin VI significantly increased effect on the progesterone receptor. In another study, the root of *D. asperoides* exhibited progesteronic activity. Ahmed HM et al, *J Biosci* 2014 39(3):453-61. The activity of 100 (mu)g/ml was equivalent to 31.45 ng/ml progesterone.

It is useful for damp cold conditions of the urogenital system including white leucorrhea, seminal incontinence, metrorrhagia and heavy or painful menses.

In TCM, the kidney dominates the bone and generates the marrow. That is, when the bone is strong and powerful, so is the kidney essence and qi.

A polysaccharide from root of *D. asperoides* prevented kidney damage after renal ischemia-reperfusion injury. Cong G et al, *Int J Biol Macromol* 2013 56:14-9.

It may be useful in helping protect brain tissue and preventing or treating amyloid plaquing associated with senile dementia and Alzheimer's disease.

Qian YH et al, *Anatomical Sci Int* 2002 77(3):196-200; Kim SS et al, *Phytotherapy Res* 2005 19(3):243-5; and Zhou YQ et al, *Cell Biol Int* 2009 33(10):1102-1110.

Saponins from the root appear to improve the learning and memory in Alzheimer's disease rats, perhaps related to regulating acetylcholinesterase metabolism of the hippocampus. Wan QY, *Zhongguo Ying Yong Sheng Li Xue Za Zhi* 2015 31(1):82-4.

Abekia saponin D appears to suppress Alzheimer's related neuro-inflammation and memory system dysfunction. Yu X et al, *Behav Brain Res* 2012 235(2):200-9.

Loganic acid ethyl ester, loganin and cantleyoside show moderate neuroprotective effects against toxin induced cell death in PC 12 cells. Ji D et al, *Molecules* 2012 17(2):1419-24.

Asperosaponins A-C protect PC12 cells against induced cytotoxicity. This suggests benefit in neuronal and brain related disorders. Ji D et al, *Fitoterapia* 2012 83(5):843-8.

The root of *D. asperoides* contains polysaccharides that may be potentially effective in preventing human osteosarcoma. Chen J et al, *Carbohydr Polym* 2013 95(2):780-4.

Both decoctions and wine processed *D. asper* appear beneficial in prevention of osteoporosis, albeit in a rat study. Tao Y et al, *J Ethnopharm* 2017 January 27.

The polysaccharides increase osteoblast and decrease osteoclast activity. Niu YB et al, *Osteoporos Int* 2012 23(11):2649-60.

It appears that wine processing enhances the bioavailability of 4-caffeoylquinic acid, loganic acid, loganin and asperosaponin VI. Tao Y et al, *J Chromatogr B Analyt Technol Biomed Life Sci* 2016 15:1036-1037:33-41.

Dipsalignan A shows weak activity against HIV-1 integrase. Sun X et al, *Molecules* 2015 20(2):2165-75.

Akebiasaponin induces apoptosis in human gastric cancer cell lines. Xu MY et al, *Food Chem Toxicol* 2013 59:703-8.

Dipsacus saponin C may have prothrombotic risks, at least in a rat *in vivo* study. Song JS et al, *J Thromb Haemostat* 2012 10(5):895-906. Human relevance to whole root extracts is unknown.

HOMEOPATHY

The teasel (*D. sylvestris*) mind is dejected and depressed in morning upon awakening and better in afternoon.

There is nostalgia about past friendships and older things and buildings.

Dreams are of fire, hotels and holidays, journeys that are laborious, strenuous and colourful, in pink and purple range.

Delusions include eye, closed eyes, animal eyes, being looked at and looking away.

There are night sweats, eyes are swollen, noise in ears as if from water and thistly prickles in throat.

Involuntary loss of urine in early morning in bed.

DOSE- lower potencies to 200c. Proving by Benedikt Pawlita with eight females and three males at 12c, 30c, and 200c in 2005. In same year Pawlita proved six others with C1-C4 trituration.

ESSENTIAL OIL

The aerial parts of D. japonicus in flower were steam distilled and found to yield 46 compounds by GC-MS. The main compounds are linalool (11.78%), trans-geraniol (8.58%), 1,8-cineole (7.91%)), beta-caryophyllene (5.58%), alpha terpineol (5.32%), beta selinene (5.15%), and spathulenol (5.04%).

The oil exhibits pronounced fumigant toxicity against the grain pests *Sitophilus zeamais* and *Tribolium castaneum*. Liu ZL et al, *Z Naturforsch C* 2013 68(1-2):13-18.

FLOWER ESSENCES

Teasel flower essence is for those who are tired, weak, depleted, emotionally exhausted, confused, lost and dissatisfied; are in a toxic relationship, are codependent, abused and taken advantage of. **DALTON**

Teasel (*D. fullonum*) is for imbalances in giving and receiving; heals energy "leaks" in chakras; for holding and maintaining energy within the system; and for treating emotional pain which causes energy depletion. **DARCY WILLIAMSON**

PERSONALITY TRAITS

When I first looked at Teasel I was impressed with the potential of the plant as a medicine. The large, hard, tall stalks, which remain dead but still strong through the winter, seemed to indicate an affinity for bones. At intervals along the stem the opposite leaves merge together to form a cup which holds water after a rain. Surely,I thought, this must be a remedy for the joints and the kidney essence. **MATTHEW WOOD**

RECIPES

ROOT TINCTURE- Use fall roots of first year. 1-3 drops up to three times daily for six weeks in cases of Lyme disease. Larger doses for inflamed joints and muscle. Matthew notes that chronic cases of Lyme will aggravate after two or three weeks.

If you mix antibiotics and teasel root, you may create a Herxheimer reaction that can be very unpleasant.

DECOCTION- 8-14 grams 1:20 ratio. One to two cups daily.

CAUTION- Do not take during pregnancy, except in cases of threatened miscarriage.

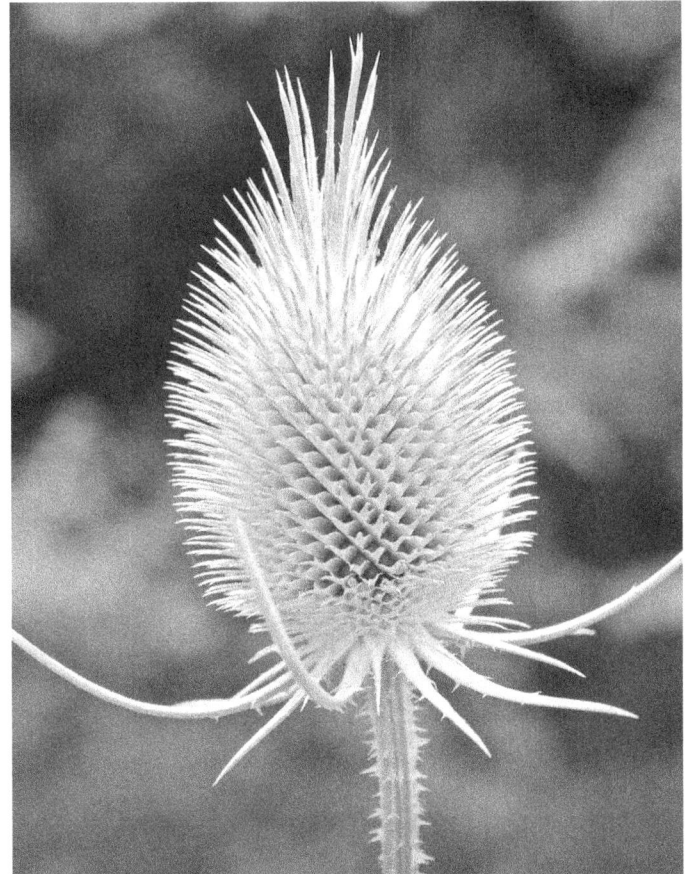

FULLER'S TEASEL

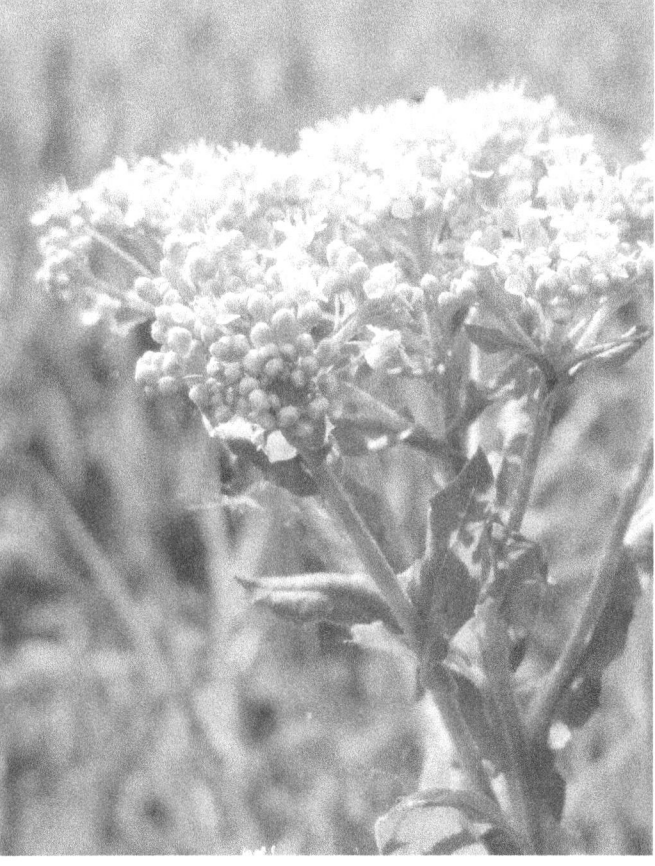

LEPIDIUM DRABA

GARDEN CRESS
GARDEN PEPPERWORT
(*Lepidium sativum* L.)
RISHAD CRESS
(*L. sativum*)
PERENNIAL PEPPERCRESS
TALL WHITETOP
DITTANDER
(*L. latifolium* L.)
(*Cardaria latifolia* [L.] Spach) not accepted
PEPPERWORT
FIELD PEPPERWEED
FIELD PEPPERGRASS
(*L. campestre* [L.] W. T. Aiton)
(*Neolepia campestris*
        [L.] W. A. Weber) not accepted
(*Thlaspi campestre* L.) not accepted
COMMON PEPPERGRASS
MINER'S PEPPERWEED
(*L. densiflorum* Schrad.)
(*L. neglectum* Thell.) not accepted
(*L. elongatum* Rydb.) not accepted
PEPPERGRASS
(*L. apetalum* Willd.)
PENNYCRESS
STINKWEED
FANWEED
BOOR'S MUSTARD
(*Thlaspi arvense* L.)
MOUNTAIN CANDYTUFT
ALPINE PENNYCRESS
(*T. montanum*) not accepted
(*Noccaea fendleri* ssp. *glauca*
        [A. Nelson] Al-Shehbaz & M. Koch)
BITTER CRESS
LADY'S SMOCK
CUCKOO FLOWER
MEADOWFOAM CABBAGE
(*Cardamine pratensis* L.)
QUAKER BITTER CRESS
(*C. pennsylvanica* Muhl. ex Willd.)
SIBERIAN BITTER CRESS
(*C. umbellata* Greene)
(*C. oligosperma* ssp. *kamtschatica*
        [Regel] Cody) not accepted
BREWER'S BITTERCRESS
(*C. brewerii* S. Watson)

TOWER MUSTARD
(*Arabis glabra* [L.] Bernh.) not accepted
(*Turritis glabra* L.)
REFLEXED ROCKCRESS
(*A. retrofracta* Graham) not accepted
(*Boechera retrofracta* [Graham] A. Love & D. Love)
(*A. holboelli* Hornem.) not accepted
HAIRY ROCKCRESS
(*A. hirsuta* [L.] Scop)
LYALL'S ROCKCRESS
(*A. lyallii*) not accepted
(*B. lyallii* [S. Watson] Dom.)
LYRE-LEAVED ROCKCRESS
(*A. lyrata*) not accepted
(*Arabidopsis lyrata* ssp. *lyrata*
        [L.] O'Kane & Al-Shezbah)
ROCK CRESS
(*A. drummondii* A. Gray) not accepted
(*B. stricta* [Graham] Al-Shezbah)
EARLY WINTER CRESS
UPLAND CRESS
(*Barbarea verna* [Mill.] Asch.)
(*B. praecox* [Sm.] R. Br.) not accepted
YELLOW ROCKET
WINTER CRESS
(*B. vulgaris* W. T. Aiton)
ERECT POD WINTER CRESS
(*B. orthoceras* Ledeb.)
(*B. americana* Rydb.) not accepted
HEART-PODDED HOARY CRESS
(*Cardaria draba* [L.] Desv.) not accepted
(*Lepidium draba* L.)
SIBERIAN MUSTARD
(*C. pubescens* [C. A. Meyer] Jarm.) not accepted
(*L. appelianum* Al-Shehbaz)
LENS PODDED HOARYCRESS
(*C. chlapensis* [L.] Hand.-Maz.) not accepted
(*L. chalepensis* L.)
MARSH YELLOW CRESS
(*Rorripa palustris* [L.] Besser)
NORTHERN YELLOW CRESS
(*R. islandica* [Oeder] Borbás)
SPREADING YELLOW CRESS
(*R. sinuata* [Nutt.] Hitch)
CREEPING YELLOW CRESS
(*R. sylvestris* [L.] Besser)

MOUNTAIN CRESS
(*R. indica* [L.] Hiern)
SLENDER CRESS
(*R. tenerrima* Greene)
COMMON WATERCRESS
(*R. nasturtium-aquaticum* [L.] Hayek) not accepted
(*Nasturtium officinale* W. T. Aiton)
SMALL LEAVED WATERCRESS
(*N. microphyllum* Boenn. ex Rchb.)
PART USED- leaves and seeds

Eat Cresses and get wit.   **GREEK PROVERB**

I linger round my shingly bars,
I loiter round my cresses.   **TENNYSON**

Steep for Danewulf leaves of Lady Smock,
For they keep strong the heart.   **UNKNOWN**

When daisies pied and violets blue
And lady-smocks all silver white
And cuckoo-buds of yellow hue
Do paint the meadows with delight.   **LOVE'S LOST LABOUR**

Watery cress, Queen of the stream,
in salads, fine you have no peer;
poor man's bread, rich man's cream,
all men's delight for half the year.   **BELSINGER**

I regard the Watercress seller as one of the saviours.   **DOCTOR KING CHAMBERS**

Lepidium is from the Greek **LEPIS** meaning "scale", and the diminutive **IUM**, for little; referring to the small scale covering of the seed pods. Lepisma is derived from Greek meaning, scale or rind. Campestre is Latin meaning, of the fields.

Cress may derive from the Latin, **CRESCERE** to grow fast, or the Greek **GRASTIS**, meaning, "green fodder".

Related English words are crescent, increase, decrease, recruit, and accrue. The early Germanic **KRESSE**, from the Old High German verb **KRESON**, means to creep or to crawl. It may also derive from the Indo-European "to nibble", or "to eat".

The name Stinkweed originated from the disagreeable odor that is released from the whole plant when crushed. Pennycress is from the resemblance of the round, flat pods to old silver three penny coins.

Today, in Germany, the plant is called **FELD PFENNIGKRAUT**, or Field Pennywort, after **PFENNING**, a copper coin. In France, it is known as **MONNOYERE**, from the Old French **MONNOIE**, for money.

Thlaspi was a name given to this plant by Dioscorides in 1st century AD, as the "cress of corruption and ruination".

It comes from the Greek *THLAO* meaning "to crush or compress", probably in reference to the flat fruit, and *ASPIS* for shield. Arvensis means, "of the field".

Cardamine is said to derive from the Greek **KARDAMON**, a name Dioscorides used for a member of the mustard family.

Other authors including myself, feel it comes from the Greek **KARDIA**, meaning heart, and **DAMAO**, to overpower, or to calm; hence heart subdue, or strengthen.

Brewerii is named after Professor William Brewer, of Yale University, in honor of his Californian botanical field trips of the 19th century.

Ladies' Smock was named in honor of the Virgin Mary, as it flowers around Lady Day.

Smock is a lady's undergarment that in the 18th century became shift and then replace by chemise. Smock became smick and then smicker, which means, "to have amorous looks and purpose."

Arabis may stem from Arabo, a complex and elaborate design of intertwined flowers and geometrical patterns of the Moors, or simply in reference to the country. Arabesque would be a related form, meaning fantastic and elaborate. Hirsuta means hairy.

Barbarea originates from the old name *Herba Sanctae Barbarae*, or Herb of Saint Barbara. She is the patron saint of artillerymen and miners; and protectress of lightning, tornadoes and thunderstorms. The Saint's special Feast day is December 4th. She was beheaded, by her own father in 225 AD because she converted to Christianity, and refused to marry the man of his choice.

In 1969, the Roman Catholic Church declared her to be a non-historical person and took her feast day off the church calendar.

A German interpretation of the name derives from winter cress eaten by "barbel", a type of fresh water carp. In France, the plant is known as **BARBARÉE**.

Another possibility, put forward by Leonhart Fuchs in the early 16th century, is that Barbarea and the German common name Barbarakraut derive from the Latin, *Carpentarium herba*, used for wounds to joiners, wagoneers and carpenters.

Draba is from the Greek **DRABE**, meaning bitter or acrid. Cardaria refers to the heart.

Rorripa is from the Saxon name **RORIPPEN**, and in turn from the Latin **RORO** to be moist and **RIPA** for riverbank. It may be from **RORIDUS**, meaning covered with dew.

The Latin vulgar phrase, **ROSE RIPAE**, meaning "dew of the riverbank", also makes sense.

Water Nasturium is from the Greek **MNASTORGION**, or "one that longs for wet soil".

Nasturium may also derive from the Latin **NASUS**, meaning nose and **TORTUS** turned away; referring to the volatile pungency of the bruised plant. For this reason it is called **NASITROD** in France.

Common garden cress has been introduced and now naturalized itself in Alberta. It frequents roadsides and waste areas near civilization.

Originally from Persia, or perhaps Southwest Asia, it was first mentioned by Xenophon in about 400 BC, as a food to eat, even before bread was known. It is consumed as a vegetable in Maori communities of New Zealand.

Ibn al-Awwam refers to its anti-histamine action, since it was used against insect bites and insect repellent. Other early authors, like El Farcy, wrote that garden cress incites coitus and stimulates the appetite. In the Talmud, the herb is known as **SHIHLAYIM**.

Ibn Massa reported the herb dissipates colic and gets rid of tapeworms and other intestinal worms.

Early German settlers to North America would put the ground seeds in plantain water as a vermifuge treatment.

The root was used traditionally in Mexico for diarrhea and dysentery.

Today, in Morocco and Iran, the seeds are still used as an aphrodisiac.

Garden Cress used to be known as Passerage, believed to drive away madness.

The plant symbolizes stability and is associated with birth date of January 11.

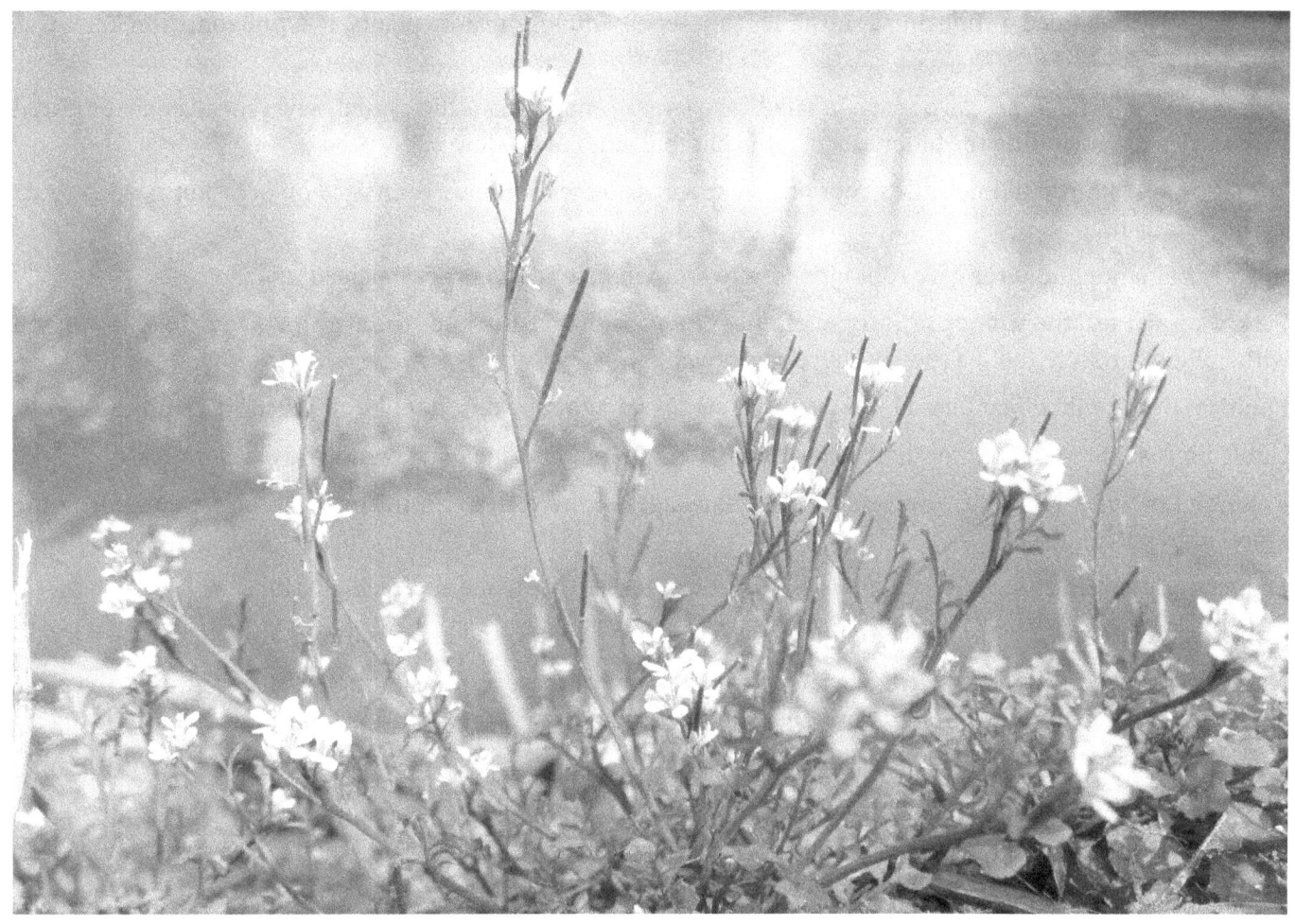

BITTER CRESS

Oxygala, a type of curd cheese with herbs, is made with either fresh or dried garden cress.

Dioscorides wrote, "lepidium is a little herb well known, preserved in brine with milk. The facultie of the leaves is sharp, exulcerating, wherefore it is a most singular plaster for the Sciatica, being beaten small with the root of Elycampane, and laid on for a quarter of an hour."

One unusual form from Iraq is Rishad Cress, with leaves that resemble the fern-like leaves of carrot. It is still very popular today on donairs, made from fresh clay oven-baked flatbread, and filled with grilled meat, yogurt and the spicy, hot Rishad Cress. Mmmmm.

In Ireland, the plant is known as tongue grass; and the young shoots, leaves and unripe seedpods are eaten as a potherb.

The seeds germinate in a few days, and by sowing onto your compost pile, you can determine if the soil is mature.

Seed powder, up to 0.75% of total rations, resulted in better health status and performance in chicken broilers up to age of six weeks. Shawle et al, *Springerplus* 2016 5(1):1441. The need to remove antibiotics from feed is crucial, given the higher levels of antibiotic resistance in the human population related to ingesting commercial livestock protein.

The plant is able to hyper-accumulate mercury from contaminated soil. Smolinska B, Szczodrowska A, *N Biotechnol* 2016 6784(16):32314-7.

Tall Whitetop, or peppergrass, was introduced to North America in a bag of sugar beet seed from Europe near the turn of the last century.

It is an aggressive weed, producing a substance that repels and kills nearby plants, in a phenomenon known as allelopathy.

Peppergrass (*L. latifolium*) can be used in salads; the Greeks and Romans did as well. Several sauces are prepared with the leaves, including the bitter sauce of the paschal lamb of the Jews.

The seeds were known in England as Poor man's pepper. And the roots have been used on occasion as a substitute for horseradish.

In early England, midwives gave root infusions to women in labor, in order to speed up labor.

Parkinson wrote, "the women of Bury in Suffolk doe usually give the juice thereof in ale to drinke to women with child to procure them a speedy delivery in travail."

Poultices of the wilted plant have been used on sciatica and gouty pains, but like all mustards, with caution.

Cooled infusions were used for diarrhea and summer complaint, usually taken during or after meals.

Preserved in wine, Dittander was said to open blockages of the spleen, rid the body of scurvy and purify the blood of hypochondriacs.

Pepperwort, also introduced to the prairies, has edible leaves that make an excellent sauce for fish.

Common peppergrass is the most common species on the prairies, and an introduced annual.

Native tribes like the Mahuna were quick to take advantage of these European imports. They infused the plant and drank the tea for weight reduction. The Navaho-Kayenta used the plant for the effects of swallowing an ant, headaches, sunburn and kidney complaints.

They also rubbed the plant on a baby's face to help put them to sleep.

Peppergrass is often called Sciatica Cress in the southern United States. Fresh plant poultices are applied externally to affected areas, working in a similar manner to mustard plasters.

All the seeds can be sprouted for commercial markets.

Common Pepper Cress seed is used in Traditional Chinese Medicine, and known as bitter **BEI TING LI ZI**. Another mustard relative *Descurainia sophia* is **TING LI ZI** and used interchangeably. The latter is milder in potency, and used to sedate the lung and relieve wheezing.

The raw seed is used to drain fluid from the chest and lungs; edema associated with oliguria and dysuria, and ascites due to accumulation of fluids in the abdomen. It has been used to treat pleurisy and water retention in thoracic cavity.

The seed is stir-fried until scorched, for lung abscesses, asthma, and phlegm.

The seeds are combined with a demulcent, sweet herb to avoid damage to the stomach lining.

It combines well with astragalus root and prepared aconite root for congestive heart failure or cardiac disease with reduced urination, edema of the face and wheezing.

An ancient saying is, "acute sensations of fullness in the chest due to water qi within the Lung cannot be eliminated without this herb." It is therefore useful for phlegm and thin mucus obstructing Lung Qi, made worse when the patient lies flat, with edema in chest and abdomen, but not to be used in cases of deficiency.

Garden Cress can bio-accumulate arsenic, and could be useful in bioremediation.

In India and Pakistan, the plant is used for bronchitis, and rheumatic conditions, the seed for bleeding piles and the root for secondary syphilis.

The related *L. nitidum* leaves were boiled and used to wash hair and prevent baldness by Cahuilla of California.

Perennial Peppergrass (*L. latifolium*) is a widely used leafy green in parts of India.

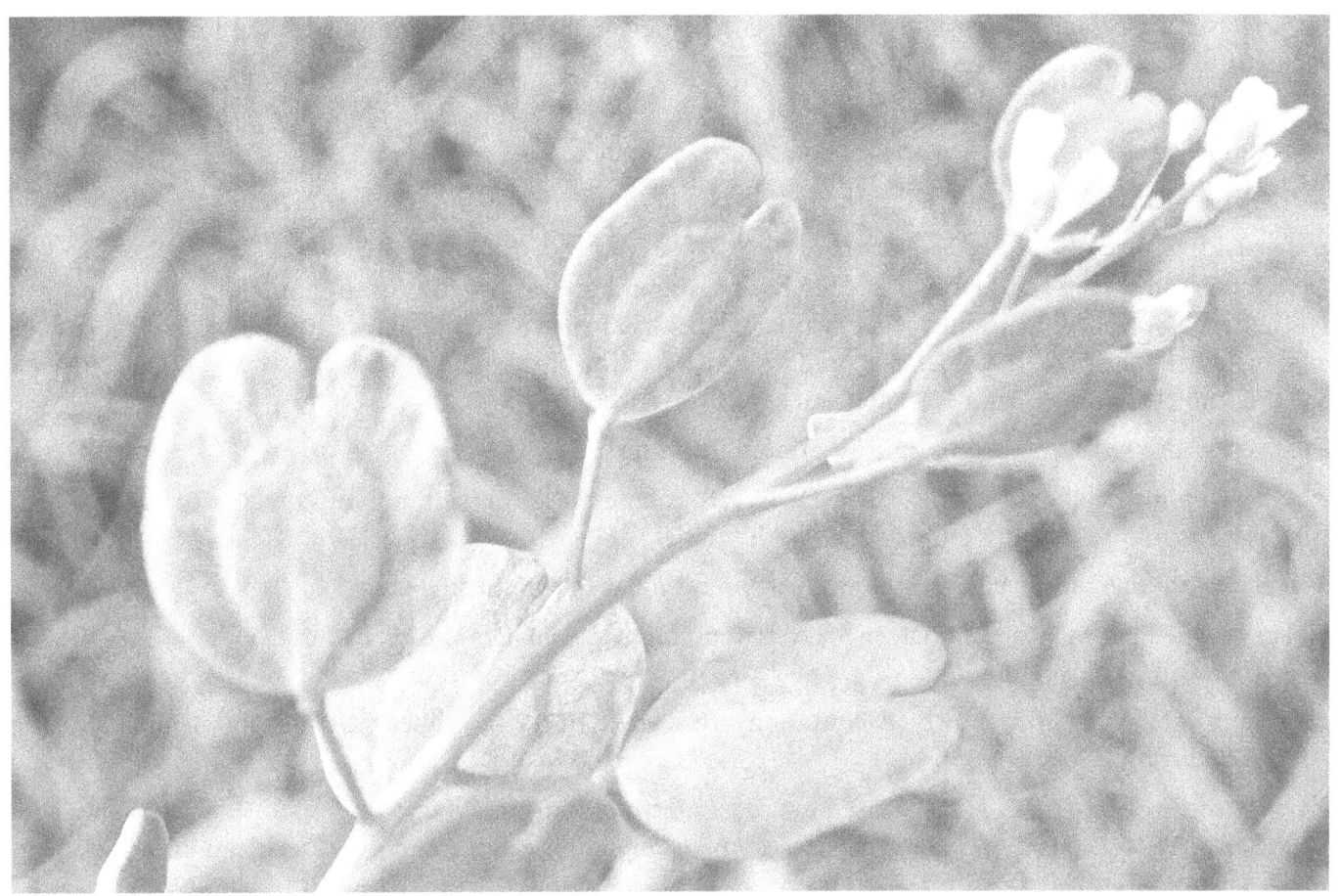

PENNYCRESS- NOTE COIN SHAPED PODS

Pennycress leaves, picked before flowering, have a mustard-like flavor, that make an acceptable potherb, or raw in salads. The small, black seeds can be ground and used for seasoning, giving a spicy, cayenne like flavor to wild game.

It is high in vitamin C and contains large amounts of organic sulphur. In Eurasia, the plant has been used for their astringent, stimulating and diuretic effects.

Externally, poultices of the plant have been used to treat lumbago, but be careful of burning the skin tissue.

The flowers, leaves and seeds in water extracts, show activity against mycobacterium.

Milk from cows that have eaten stinkweed is unpleasant and unpalatable. The flavor and odor does not disappear until 7-8 hours after the weed is eaten.

It spreads readily, producing up to 15,000 seeds per plant. One Canadian study showed a 16% infestation, reduced wheat production by 36% over five years.

Ironically, a study by Stefureac et al in Romania (1979), found pennycress seed stimulates the germination and early growth of red and white clover, birds foot trefoil, and perennial rye (*Lolium perenne*).

An interesting study conducted by Hartmann and Nezadal in Germany 1990, discovered weeds including pennycress, cleavers and field bindweed could be reduced from 80%, to less than 2% by night time tillage.

Ironically, horsetail, couch grass, and ryegrass increased, using this nocturnal approach.

More research on photo-control of weeds is needed.

The roots contain anti-fungal compounds.

Pennycress, and some of its relatives are being used experimentally to reclaim soils contaminated with heavy metals, in a process called green remediation.

Rufus Chaney, an agronomist in Maryland, has experimented with various *Thlaspi* species, including Pennycress, and Alpine Pennycress (*T. caerulescens*), from southern France.

In 1865, pennycress was identified as the first hyper-accumulating plant, when incinerated ash from plants growing on zinc and cadmium rich soil near the Belgian-German border was found to contain over 17% zinc.

Pennycress can take in zinc at the rate of 125 kilograms per hectare, as well as cadmium at 2 kg/ha. Pennycress is especially good at taking in zinc, accumulating up to 30,000 parts per million, whereas most plants experience zinc toxicity by the time they reach 500 ppm. Up to 16% of the burnt plant ash can constitute zinc, making it a suitable choice for organic mineral supplements.

Pennycress also pulls lead, arsenic and aluminum from the soil.

About 1.5 billion people suffer zinc deficiency, and 30% of the world's agricultural soil contains low levels. Crops that use zinc more efficiently could address both problems.

The plants can then be burned and the ash recovered similar to commercial ore.

Chaney says, "Plants that accumulate high levels of uranium and cobalt have been found, but no work has been done to maximize this removal."

Cadmium is taken up efficiently by Alpine Pennycress, absorbing 15-20 times other genera members. Chang et al, *Z Naturforsch* 2005 60c 3-4.

Phytoextraction Associates LLC is licensed to use this technology. At remedial costs of $250 to $1000 per acre per year this is still considerably less than the estimated one million dollars in the older clean up, remove and replace procedures.

In one Boston suburb, alpine pennycress was used to take up lead, zinc and cadmium from a contaminated backyard.

A New York Sculptor, Mel Chin, read about hyper-accumulator plants, and was struck by the poetic nature of the process.

He designed a circular field with pennycress planting following Chaney's advice. Two main walkways, on a site contaminated with cadmium, lead and zinc near St. Paul, Minnesota, divided the field like the crosshairs of a riflescope, symbolizing a targeting of the earth for cleanup.

Revival Field, as Chin calls it, relates "to my interest in alchemy and my understanding of transformative processes and the mutable nature of materials."

The Métis of Alberta know the plant as **LARB A PALET** or **KÂ-WIHCÎKI-MACIPAKWAHK**. Further east, the Anishinaabemowin name is **ZHAABOOMIN**.

Pennycress seeds, and shoots are used in medicine by the Chinese. The plant is known as **NAN BAI JIANG**, or Southern Bai Jiang. It is used as a substitute for *Patrinia villosa* and *P. scabiosifolia*, especially in Hong Kong and Taiwan.

The seeds are used to enhance the acuity of vision, and indicated for conjunctive congestion with swelling, pain and tears.

In Spain, the plant is considered astringent and the seeds stimulating. When studying in Barcelona, I learned the Catalonian name for the plant is Traspic.

The seeds are a principal constituent of wheat, and could be used as a source of oil.

The residual meal, after oil extraction, is comparable in protein content to cottonseed meal, and quite adequate as livestock feed.

It has the disadvantage in dairy cows of imparting an unpleasant flavor to milk.

In test plantings in Montana, irrigated land produced 1500 pounds of seed per acre. Autumn grown plants produced yields of 1500 kg/hectare in North Dakota studies.

Fan weed has potential as an industrial oil crop, with seeds containing up to 26% oil by weight.

Mountain Candytuft is a native species of the western prairies and one of our first spring flowers. Only about four inches tall with small white flowers, it has an incredible sweet perfume.

Siberian Bitter Cress is a northern perennial that grows in moist montane and subalpine sites. In spring, the young leaves often have a purplish hue.

All bitter cress can add a hot and peppery taste to wilderness dishes. They can be eaten raw, or cooked in soups, stews for better effect. The small rosettes are best. The spring leaves are oily and quite unpleasant, on their own.

Bitter Cress is one of the prettiest flowers of spring. In Britain it is called Cuckoo Flower, either because it blooms when the cuckoo arrives for the summer; or because the basal and stem leaves are so different, making the plant look Cuckoo. A more likely explanation is Cuckoo Spit, for the foamy deposit that often covers the plant. This is not from Cuckoos however, but the nymph of an insect called the Frog Hopper or spittlebug (*Philaenus spumarius*).

Cuckoo-bud was invented by Shakespeare as an allusion to cuckold, a term for a man whose wife has committed adultery.

In Austria, it was believed that picking the plant would lead to being bitten by a snake.

Galen believed the plant had the same virtues as watercress, being gently stimulating and diuretic.

Cardamine pratensis was the favorite beauty herb of Mumtaz Mahal, the wife of Shah Jehan, in India. She ate some every day and always remained so beautiful and loving, that when she died in 1631 during the birth of their 14th child, the broken hearted Shah forced 22000 men to work for 22 years on her $230 million white marble tomb at Agar- the famous Taj Mahal.

In some parts of Europe, the plant is used in the treatment of nervous affections. In the Cornwall region of England, the flowering tops were used for curing epilepsy, spasmodic asthma and nervous hysteria.

Dr. King, the Eclectic physician noted the plant loses its characteristic benefits upon drying. The fresh plant, or tincture "has been used in chorea, asthma, dropsy, bronchitis, intermittent fever, laryngitis, and scaly skin affections, and locally to cancer and other sores."

The herb is infused and taken to improve the health of both arteries and veins.

It encourages digestion and flow of bile.

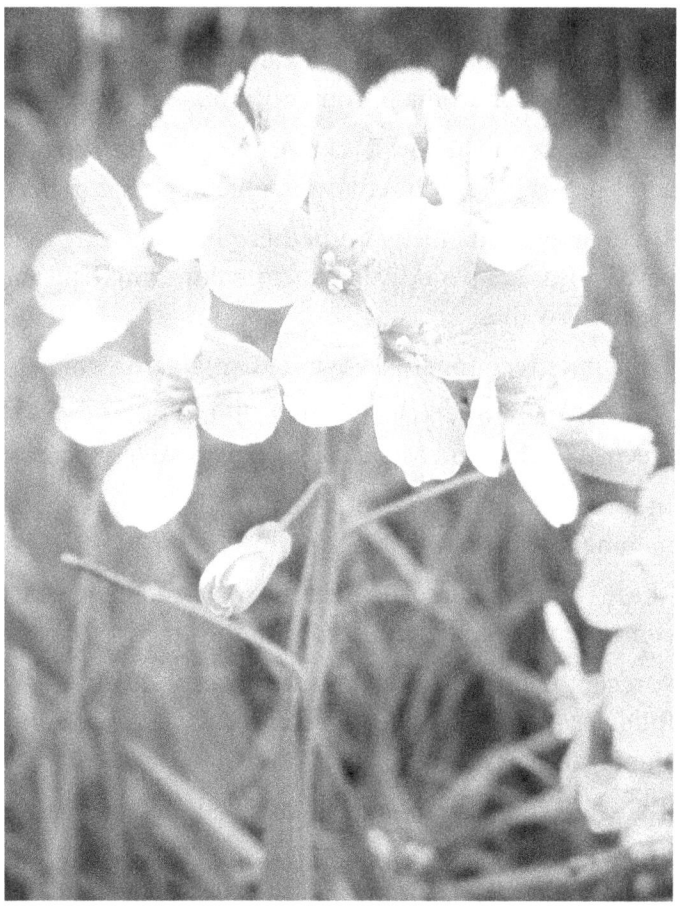

CUCKOO FLOWER

141

The seeds contain myronic acid. Cuckoo flower is unusual for mustards, in that the basal leaves root at the tip. The plant has an efficient seed dispersal system that can fling seeds, from the siliques, up to two meters, when ripe.

Both goats and sheep enjoy eating the plant, but horses and cattle will ignore it. Veterinarians often give a tea to animals suffering nervous disorders.

The related *C. angulata*, an introduced plant, exhibits activity against herpes virus type 1.

The related *C. cordifolia*, with heart shaped leaves, was used traditionally for heart problems, following the doctrine of signatures.

The seeds are often eaten after meals in India, to stimulate digestion, relieve flatulence and act as a soothing carminative.

Tower Mustard is used by the Cheyenne as a medicine. It is known as "Yellow Medicine", or **HEOVE-HESEEO?OTSE.**

A tea was infused and taken as a beverage for colds, as a general preventative and to treat sick children.

All Rock cresses are sub-alpine in nature, growing on gravel sites at higher altitudes.

They are all edible, with a sharp flavor typical of the mustard family.

The leaves and flowers have a horseradish type flavor that goes well with sandwiches, and salads.

Rock Cress aerial parts were decocted by the Okanagan and Thompson, for pains in the lumbar, kidney and bladder regions. They applied fresh poultices to skin sores.

Both the Thompson and Salishan decocted the plant to treat gonorrhea; and used a stronger decoction for diarrhea.

Many of the *Arabis* species have snow-white flowers that have a delicate heliotrope odor. I don't know if it can be captured for aroma purposes or not.

Wintercress and Yellow Rocket are very similar in appearance and usage, the former considered native and the latter naturalized. Wintercress is a biennial that prefers the moisture of boreal forests and mountains.

The young plants are good potherb like so many members of the mustard family. The tender young leaves have a pleasant, peppery taste before flowering. The young flower buds add flavor to salads, soups, quiches and vegetable dishes.

Culpepper recommended Winter Cress "to provoke urine, to help strangury, and expel gravel and stone."

A variegated form was introduced into France in 1827, and is still a popular edible ornamental spring salad green. Mesclun and Misticanza salads have led to a resurgence of popularity.

In Sweden, during the 18th Century, Wintercress was eaten in spring and fall salads, and boiled like other members of the family.

The leaves remain green under the snow and hence their name. A breeding program in Sweden to produce seed condiments was abandoned due to the longevity of seeds in the soil.

A recent hybrid between yellow rocket and Chinese cabbage has been developed in Russia as a protein-rich fodder. When feed to cattle vs. control it showed an average body weight gain of 11.2%; with feed costs were significantly reduced.

The seeds can be sprouted; or edible oil pressed from them.

The Cherokee ate the boiled "creasy" greens, according to Duke, to purify the blood. The Mohegans and Shinnecock used leaf infusions, drunk every half hour for coughs.

Like plantain, the plant can be poulticed and applied to bee stings and other skin inflammations.

The tea is used to stimulate appetite, as a source of Vitamin C in the winter, and a diuretic. Vitamin C content is over 60 mg per 100 grams.

Yellow Rocket has been found to effectively germinate in oil-saturated soil, making it another option for land reclamation from damaged, deserted oil and gas sites.

Yellow Rocket causes the third greatest reductions in crop yields, of seven major weeds in spring wheat in Russia.

A triterpenoid saponin from Yellow Rocket has been found to be a feeding deterrent against the diamondback moth.

A variegated cultivar, *variegatum*, is sometimes grown as an ornamental edible landscape plant.

In Spain, Yellow Rocket leaves are vulnerary, while in La Reunion the plant is considered a stimulant and anti-scorbutic.

Hoary cress is an introduced, noxious weed, common to the southern prairies. It would be difficult to convince farmers that this perennial pest plant has any redeeming qualities. It grows where many other plants would have a difficult time, preferring a very acidic soil pH of 3.6-4.3.The heart-shaped seedpods lack hairs, hence their name and identification.

The plant seed can be dried, ground and used as a pepper-like spice.

If picked and eaten early in spring, the young flower heads are an excellent edible.

Rorripa nasturtium-aquaticum is a rare, introduced member of the mustard family found in ditches and creeks in shallow water of Alberta. Watercress is an aquatic plant, or hydrophyte, that has spread across North America. Early botanists believed it was introduced from Europe, but this may not be correct.

One day, on a mushroom walk near Drayton Valley,I found it growing for a long distance in two running sloughs caused by tire tracks through a swamp. The same thing happened on another mushroom foray near Pincher Creek, with abundant growth.

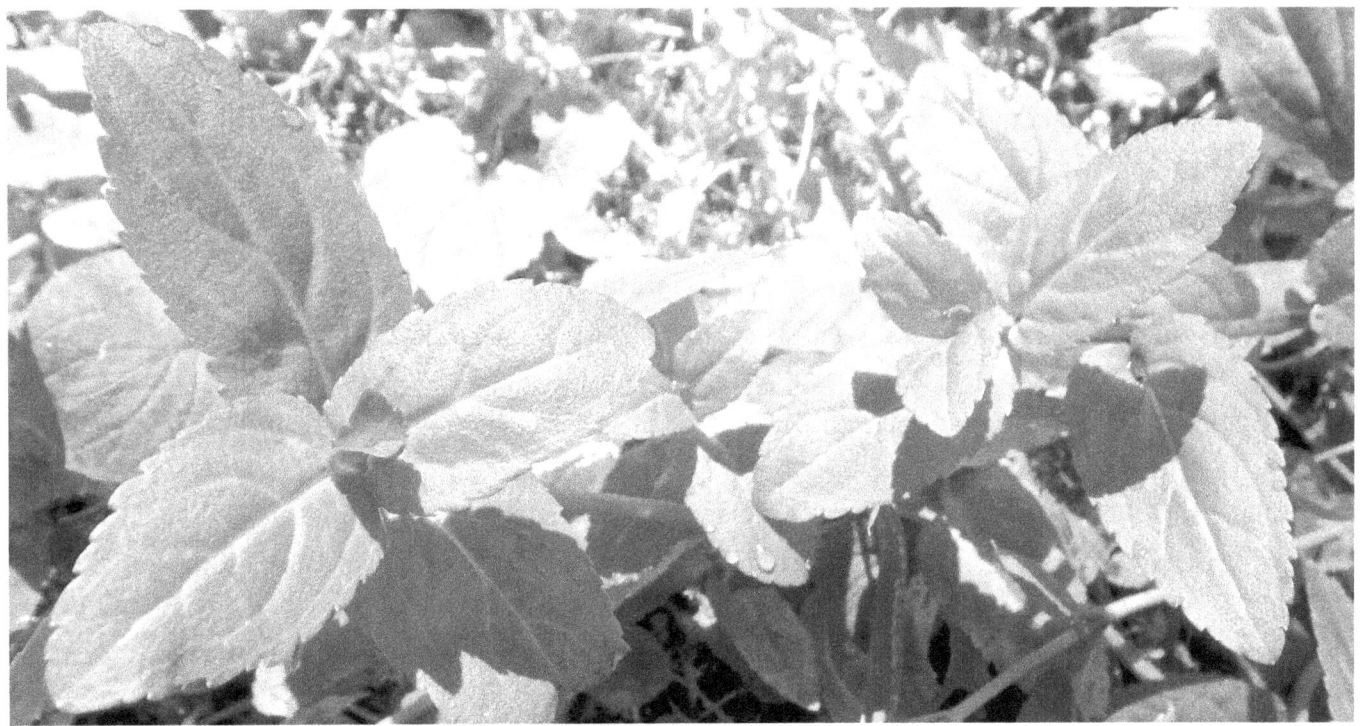

WATERCRESS

It is highly prized for salads, extremely nourishing and rich in minerals, and widely available in supermarkets. Ducks and muskrats also enjoy a nibble.

The Romans used a mixture of watercress and vinegar to treat mental illness. The proverb "Eat Cress and learn more wit", came from this practice. Years before, the Persians ate watercress raw, when subjected to heavy physical labour.

Watercress had various ancient names including **KARDAMON**, meaning head-subduer from the Greek, as well as Sisymbrium, Rorippa and Nasturium from the Latin.

Watercress was THE herb that cured stupidity or idiocy. In The Clouds, a 4th century Greek writer, Aristophanes wrote, "The earth would draw their essence to herself; the same too is the case with Watercress. Thought draws the essence into Watercress."

Hippocrates said it was stimulant and expectorant, while Dioscorides believed it an aphrodisiac. It is said that the former "father of medicine" set his first healing centre near a watercress stream.

Spartan athletes, in the 7th century BC, relaxed nude after exercising in public gymnasiums (from the Greek **GYMNOS**, meaning nude). Their coaches gave them heavily buttered, open face sandwiches (?) with yogurt and watercress for optimum conditioning. I thought the Earl of Sandwich invented the two slices of bread meal.

Zenophon advised Persians to feed their children on Watercress so they might grow in stature and have active minds.

Well Grass, an ancient name, says a lot about the herb's medicinal repute. Paracelsus said that watercress draws all toxins to itself and transforms it, in the human body as well as in nature.

The ancient Egyptian pharaohs had freshly squeezed watercress juice served to their slaves each morning and afternoon to increase their productivity.

The Salernitan School of Medicine recommended rubbing the juice into the scalp to strengthen and thicken hair.

Langham, the English herbalist, said Watercress seed "provoketh venery and lust". Mrs. Leyel, the British herbal writer explained, "both it and its cousin, spinach, contain *radioactive calcium* that has a decided influence on rhythmatic heartbeat. It encouraged good circulation to build strong arteries and veins."

Old German herbals suggest that the seeds of watercress and garden cress be taken together to dissolve blood clots.

Gerard talks about the green sickness, a mysterious illness that affected young women until the beginning of the century. Also known as Disease of Virgins, it was found to be chlorosis, a form of iron deficiency anemia. His use of watercress was appropriate as it is full of organic iron, and copper.

In Victorian England, it was known as "poor man's bread" by the working class.

In Twelfth Night, Viola told of the young woman who..."let concealment like a worm i' the bud, Feed on her damask cheek: she pin'd in thought; And with a green and yellow melancholy, She sat like patience on a monument smiling at grief."

In Ireland, the plant was known as St. Patrick's Cabbage. Early Anglo-Saxons named it **STUNE** or **STIME**.

Evelyne Winter, in Mexico's Ancient and Native Remedies, suggests "for weak lungs or tuberculosis, crush the raw plant and add three parts water; add sugar to taste. Let stand a few hours; strain; drink only that when thirsty".

In parts of Africa, the herb is used for treating anthrax, in parts of Venezuela the fresh plant juice is given for tuberculosis.

The Cayuga of the Iroquois First Nation call it **DIUSAI"DAWIT**, translating roughly as tastes like pepper.

The Chumash of California call it **SPE'EI HE'SO'O** meaning "flower of the water". It was eaten raw for liver ailments. Recent information from the Santa Ynez Reservation reports using it for illness caused by drinking too much alcohol.

The Cahuilla ate the leaves and reportedly used the plant for liver ailments and low blood pressure. A good book by Bean and Saubel is, *Temalpakh: Cahuilla Indian Knowledge and Uses of Plants,* Malki Museum Press, 1972.

Use is widespread throughout the southwestern United States for heart and kidney ailments, tuberculosis and influenza. Karen Ford, *Las Yerbas de la Gente*, U Michigan Museum Anthro Papers No. 60, 1975.

Watercress has been rubbed on the scalp to strengthen and thicken hair. An old French saying is loosely translated "a bald man has no watercress on his head".

It has been combined with honey for bleaching freckles and clearing the complexion. It is found in Jumping Curls, a personal care item for hair.

Plant extracts induce the expression of aquaporin 3, a protein essential for skin hydration. Sugiyama et al, *Fragrance Journal* 2006 34.

Extracts of watercress may be useful American foulbrood, a serious disease in bees. Piana M et al, *An Acad Bras Cienc* 2015 87(2): 1041-7. No toxicity to bees was noted.

The Chinese extracted the pure juice of **TING LI**, and stored it in cool basements and caves. The Turks said the seeds of **SU TERESI** could be kept for up to five years.

The mesmerization of seeds, and observation of the effect on growth was recorded in Raoul Montadon's, *Les radiations humaines* 1927. Work on radish seed, watercress and other seed sprouts showed significant effect on size, color and flavor.

Watercress is a bright green in shade, but becomes purple brown in full sunlight due to its iron content, according to Dr. Fernie.

Watercress concentrations of gluco-nasturtiin are significantly increased, by growing the plants at lower temperatures, during longer days, and increased exposure to red light. Engelen-Eigles et al, *J Ag Food Chem* 2006 54. Sulphur, as an additive, increases constituent content by up to 40%. Watercress is fed to horses to increase their red blood cell count, due in large part to high content of iron and folates.

Oral adminstration of 1% watercress extract, added to food pellets, improved rainbow trout immune systems. Asadi MS et al, *Open Vet Journal* 2012 2(1):32-9.

In parts of New Zealand, it is considered a riverweed. We should be so lucky!

Rorippa contains a variety of alkaloids. The related Marsh Yellow Grass *(R. islandica)*, a native annual, contains hirsutin.

The Navaho-Ramah used the plant as ceremonial eyewash.

Spreading Yellow Grass is a native perennial mostly found in the aspen parklands and further south. It was traditionally used by Zuni healers as an infused wash, while the blossom smoke was used for inflamed eyes.

Creeping Yellow Cress, an introduced species, was decocted and given to mothers nursing a baby with fever.

The roots release hirsutin, a degradation product of gluco-hirsutin as well as arabin, camelinin and other compounds that are phytotoxic.

Mountain Cress Seed *(R. montana)* is used in Traditional Chinese Medicine, and called **HAN CAI**. Other names are **YE YOU CAI**, meaning wild oil vegetable, **JIANG JIAN DAO CAO**, river scissors grass, **TANG GE CAI**, pond kudzu vine vegetable, and **GAN YOU CAI**, dry oil vegetable.

Small-leaved Nasturtium with longer, more slender fruits, is found in Saskatchewan.

MEDICINAL

CONSTITUENTS-*L. sativum* herbage- quercitin, kaempferol, sepharose (lectin), merulidial, glucotro-paeolin, a glucoside, which yields benzyl cyanide when fresh plant is bruised; cucurbitacins, and cardiac steroids (cardenolides). Phytosterol content is quite high with ergost-5-en-3-ol, gamma sitosterol, stigmasta-5, 24-dien-3(3beta)-ol, and unusual 9,19-cyclolanost-24-en-3-ol,(3beta).

seeds- essential oils including benzyl and allyl isothisocyanate; allyl disulfide;linoleic/linolenic/erucic/palmitic/stearic acid, lepidines A-F (alkaloid), sitosterol, helveticoside, vitamins B and C, 18% mucilage; mainly cellulose and polysaccharides; acylated flavonol glycosides.

L. latifolium seed- myrosin

T. arvense- seed- sinigrin, myrosin, lecithin, sucrose, fixed oils, indole, eicosanoic-(11)-acid, protein.

Leaf- 54% protein, vitamin C 1900mg/g.

L. apetalum- aerial parts- evomonoside

Seed- helveticoside, apetalumosides A, B1-B12, and C

Barbarea verna seed- gluconasturtiin.

B. orthoceras- barbarin

B. vulgaris- Vitamin C (60 mg/100g), sinigrin, glucobarbarin.

C. draba- 4-methyl-sulfinylbutyl glucosinolate, glucoraphanin, isothiocyanate, thiophene-A, erysolin, sulphoraphen, phenylhepatriyne

flowerhead- L-prolinium 4-(methylsulfinyl)butyl glucosinolate.

Arabis hirsuta- contains sulfuraphene, 8-methylsulfinyul-octylglucosinolate, & 5-(4-methoxyphenyl)-2-oxazolidinethione.

*N. officinale-*raphanolide, raphanol, diastase, gluconasturin, bitters, tryptophan, essential oils including phenyl ethyl mustard oil, flavonols, megastigmane glucosides, vitamins A (4700 IU) C (43 mg/100g),D, E (34 mg/100g), and niacin (B3); as well as calcium, iron, chlorine, chromium, iodine, fluorine, phosphorus, sulphur, manganese silica, arsenic, zinc, copper, and germanium. Leaves contain 14 phenolic compounds including coumaric acid and its derivatives caftaric acid and quercitin derivatives.

When bruised the destruction of cells releases phenyl ethyl isothiocyanate, and benzyl isothiocyanate.

seeds- defatted- 5.32 grams of gluconasturtiin per 100 grams.

Root- 20 compounds including coumaric acid, sinapic acid, caftaric acid and quercitin derivatives.

R. indica- rorippin, rorifone, rorifamide, and two cardiotonics helveticoside and evomonoside; as well as gluconasturtin and alpha-phenylethyl-isothiocyanate, among 33 glucosinolates, 40 flavonol glycosides and 18 phenolics and organic compounds.

R. sylvestris- salicylic, p-hydroxybenzoic, vanillic and syringic acid, hirsutin, 4-methoxyindole-3-acetonitrile, pyrocatechol.

Garden cress is widely used in various traditional medicine systems throughout the world, including anti-inflammatory, anti-pyretic, anti-hypertensive, anti-asthmatic, anti-cancer and anti-oxidant properties.

Garden Cress is mainly used for asthma, with a moist cough; bleeding hemorrhoids, or enlarged lymph glands.

One recipe from Ethiopia combines garden cress, Indian mustard seed, and *Nigella sativa* seed with garlic and butter for pneumonia.

The leaves are a stimulating diuretic. The seeds are the most important medicine and are tonic, aperient and alterative- all meaning they restore balance and health to a weakened body. Infusions or decoctions of the seeds are useful in diarrhea, or in skin disease due to impure blood related to spleen enlargement like mononucleosis. Emulsions of the seed, made by crushing them, soothe the intestinal mucous membranes. Soaked in water, they become mucilaginous, and valuable for diarrhea, dysentery and such; and externally as a liniment for dressing the sores of horses and other farm animals.

The whole herb, and especially the seed, contains anti-fungal and anti-bacterial activity. Cooked as a soup, it is effective for treating bronchitis and coughs.

The seeds mediate bronchial dilation via anticholinergic activity and inhibition of Ca^{++} channels and phospohodiesrase enzymes. Khan AU & Gilani AH, *Phytotherapy Research* 2015 June 10.

The infused seeds are boiled with milk and given to children suffering measles.

The taste is similar to nasturtium, and contains the same glucoside, glucotropaeolin.

This breaks down by hydrolysis into glucose and substances with antibiotic effect (benzyl isothiocyanate) under the activity of an enzyme such as tropaeolase or myronsinase.

This ferment is not activated, however, if the temperature is too low or high, in which case toxic benzyl cyanate is formed. Chewing it well with saliva for a few minutes will produce desired results.

Benzyl isothiocyanate inhibits prostate cancer development, in a mice study, via induction of cell cycle G1 arrest. Cho HJ et al, *Int J Mol Sci* 17(2):264.

It also shows potential as a preventative agent for metastatic breast cancer. Kim EJ et al, *Breast Cancer Res Treat* 2011 130(1):61-71.

The compound inhibits migration and invasion of human gastric cancer cells. Ho CC et al, *Human Exp Toxicol* 2011 30(4): 296-306.

Porridge of the seeds has been given, traditionally, to a nursing mother to help increase breast milk production.

The seeds are ingested for impotence, and mild aphrodisiac quality. The crushed seeds are eaten with bread for asthenia, in Africa.

The seeds show hypotensive and anti-spasmodic activity. Work by Maghrani et al, *J Ethnopharm* 2005 100:1-2 193-7 found water extracts exhibit significant systolic-lowering activity in cases of high blood pressure.

Poultices of the seeds relieve rheumatism and acute inflammatory pain; but use a vegetable carrier oil to ensure the skin is not burned. A hot infusion or poultice with fresh leaves will relieve poison ivy.

Studies suggest the herb has strong inhibitory effect on the proliferation of fibroblasts and exhibits modulation of connective tissue, confirming traditional use for inflammatory conditions, such as arthritis. Raval ND et al, *Ayu* 2013 34(3):302-4.

Studies in Saudi Arabia indicate that the traditional use of the seeds of *Lepidium sativum* for fracture healing have a basis in fact. Extracts of the plant were tested for their effect on collagen deposition and tensile strength in the tibia of rats. The extract significantly increased collagen deposition and tensile strength.

Work by Juma et al, *Med Gen Med* 2007 9:2 on rabbit fractures found a significant increase in healing of fractures at six and twelve weeks compared to control.

The seeds may be beneficial in reducing the effect of glucocorticoids induced osteoporosis. It may be synergistic with alendronate (biphosphonates). Elshal MF et al, *Afr J Tradit Complement Altern Med* 2013 10(5): 267-73.

Pharmacological studies conducted by Vohora and Khan (1977) suggest the presence of a cardio-active substance, that is unstable in solution. They concluded it probably exerts its action through adrenergic mechanisms.

In 1995, a study conducted by Eskander et al, at the *National Research Centre* in Cairo looked at garden cress *(L. sativum)* in an experiment with alloxan-induced diabetic rats. Ten days of an herbal decoction that included garden cress, normalized blood glucose levels. It also increased serum insulin levels, and restored SGOT and other levels to normal range.

Another study, by Patole et al, *The Journal of Medicinal and Aromatic Plant Sciences* 1998 20(4) followed the 21 treatment of diabetics with 15 grams daily of garden cress seeds. Nine out of 11 subjects showed reduction in the levels of blood glucose from 10.2 to 8.3 mM; proving their use as a hypoglycemic herb.

Further work by Eddouks et al, *J Ethnopharm* 97:1, and *Phytother Res* 2008 22:1 appears to confirm the plant's hypoglycemic activity.

A recent study found a garden cress seed extract significantly decreased fasting blood sugar and other diabetic parameters in a rat model. Qusti S et al, *Evid Based Complement Alternat Med* 2016:5614564.

The herb exhibits anti-viral effect against the encephalitis virus Columbia SH in mice studies.

Kalaycioglu and Oner, found garden cress extracts exhibit anti-mutagen effect. *Turkish Journal of Botany* 1994 18:3.

Sepharose, a lectin, isolated from *Lepidium sativum* extracts, has been shown to react with human erythrocytes.

Navarro E et al, *Journal of Ethnopharmacology* 1994 41(1-2): 65-9 showed water extracts given orally and intra-peritoneal to rats, considerably increased urinary excretion.

More recent work by Wright in the same journal 2007 114(1):1-31 found *L. sativa and L. latifolium* exhibit diuretic activity.

Work by Harjit et al, published in the *Indian Journal of Animal Nutrition* 1998 15:3 looked at the total phyto-estrogenic content of different herbs used in galactagogue products. Garden Cress content measured 161, while Fenugreek seed only measured 130 by the same standards.

Work by Kassie et al, found garden cress juice to be highly protective towards benzopyrene induced DNA damage, but that the effect cannot be explained by isothiocyanate content. *Chem Biol Interact* 2003 142:3. Earlier work by the same author in *Carcinogenesis* 2002 23:7 suggested that the chemoprotective mechanism of Garden Cress may be related to increased activity of hepatic UDP glucuronosyltransferase. The amount of juice to produce protective mechanism is about the same as the level of glucosinolates found in a regular salad.

Pretreatment with ethanol extracts of the seeds protected live health in a manner similar to silymarin derived from Milk Thistle seeds. The animal model suggests it down regulates the caspase 3 and up-regulates the BCL_2 protein expression. Raish M et al, *BMC Complement Altern Med* 2016 16(1): 501.

Work by Al-Sheddi ES et al, *Pharm Biol* 2016 54(2):314-21 found cytoprotective benefit from seed extracts against hydrogen induced toxicity in human liver cells.

The seeds may protect the kidneys from toxicity during cisplatin treatment for cancer. Yadav et al, *Int J Phytomed* 2010 2:3.

Rehman et al, *Phytother Res* 26:1 found the seeds possess anti-spasmodic and anti-diarrheal properties, possibly via muscarinic and calcium channels.

The root exhibits anti-protozoa activity. Calzada et al, *Phytother Res* 17:6.

Work by Adam at King Saud University found that rats fed diets where this plant comprised 50% of their weight for six weeks proved lethal. Pet owners raising rats, you have been warned!

The related Pepper Grass *L. latifolium* (perennial) has been introduced and found occasionally in southern Alberta around Lethbridge. It is used in the Canary Islands as a medicinal stomach tonic and diuretic. Human studies conducted on Tenerife in 1994 confirmed the diuretic and possibly hypotensive action of this plant. It is known as rompepiedra, or break stone, due to its use for kidney stones.

Both *L. latifolium* and *L. sativum* aerial parts possess diuretic effect. Wright CI et al, *Journal of Ethnopharmacology* 2007 114(1):1-31.

Caballero et al, *Fitoterapia* 2004 75(2):187-91 found the herb fed orally to rats decreased prostatic hypertrophy.

L. capitatum, a related member of the genus, has been found to be an effective post-coital contraceptive. Animal studies confirm the estrogenicity of plant extracts. Singh MM et al, *Planta Medica* 1984 50(2):154-7.

Ethanol extracts showed a 60-70% anti-implantation in female albino rats.

Field Peppergrass (*L. campestre*) has been studied for biological activity.

Saline and water extracts of the flowers, leaves, root and stem (entire plant) indicate activity against gram negative and mycobacterium.

Dr. Bernhard Juurlink is looking at Field Peppergrass as a source of glucoraphinin for creating dietary phase two enzyme inducers. All members of the Cabbage family contain glucoraphinin, with broccoli sprouts being especially rich.

Field Peppergrass is an aggressive plant that is rich in this, as well as the anti-nuritive compound, glucosinalbin.

He has worked with colleagues, in hopes to develop a glucoraphanin extraction technology, and to develop a domesticated cultivar high in the desired compound and low in glycosinolates.

Hoary Cress (*Cardaria draba*) is also rich in glucoraphanin.

The oilseed residue contains significant phenolic content, with 44.7 mg/gram of total content, and a direct correlation with anti-oxidant activity sinapine content was negligible.

Common Peppergrass (*L. densiflorum*) has also been studied with acetone and ether extracts showing activity against gram-positive bacteria. Bishop and MacDonald, *Can J Botany* 1956 29.

Water extracts of Common Peppergrass (*L. apetalum*) increase left ventricular myocardial contractility, function of pump blood and coronary flow, in a manner similar to isoperaline. The herb did not obviously change heart rate, but increased coronary flow instead of enhancing oxygen consumption of cardiac muscle. Wu X et al, *Zhong Yao Cai* 1998 21(5):243-5.

Both water and methanol extracts of the plant exhibit activity against Hep 3B and Hep G2 carcinoma cell lines. Park et al, *Pharm Bio* 40:3.

It is used for cough with copious sputum, stuffy chest and asthma due to excessive phlegm. For acute asthma it brings immediate and excellent action, removing excess mucus and reducing inflammation, in hot irritated conditions.

In fact, the ripe seed is reserved for excess conditions due to its acrid, bitter, cold and draining properties.

It works well for congestive heart failure with dyspnea and edema, combining well with tonic herbs to prevent side effects.

The seeds are known as **TINGLIZI** in China, and **JUNGRYUKZA** in Korea. Traditionally, the seed is called **BEITINGLIZI**, to distinguish it from the ripe seed of *Descurainia sophia*. In TCM, the seed is used to purge lung fire, relieve dyspnea when lying down, reduce edema through diuresis and indicated mainly for phlegm accumulation, coughs with excessive sputum and general swelling. A thorough review is available in Chinese. Zhou XD et al, *Zhongguo Zhong Yao Za Zhi* 3014 39(24):4699-708.

An ethanol extract of seeds induce positive inotropic atrial activity as least in part, due to the digitalis-like activity of helveticoside, rather than increase in cAMP efflux. Kim SJ et al, *Evid Based Complement Alternat Med* 2013:404713.

It is a potential compound for chronic obstructive pulmonary disease, due to its interaction with gene expression. Bao H et al, *Lung* 2014 192(1):87-93.

Helveticoside also induces reciprocal gene regulation and signaling processes in A459 human lung cancer cells. Kim BY et al, *BMC Genomics* 2015 16:713.

The seeds contain flavonoid glycosides that inhibit triglyceride accumulation in liver cells. Shi P et al, *Fitoterapia* 2015 103:197-205.

Thirty children with cough and dyspnea from bronchitis were treated with seed decoctions with a 96.7% success rate. *Zhong Yi Za Zhi* 1961 4:27.

Extracts of the plant inhibit hyper-pigmentation via 1L-6 mediated down-regulation of Mitf, rather than direct inhibition of tyrosinase activity. Choi H et al, *Pigment Cell Research* 2005 18(6):439-46.

The plant contains the cardiac glycoside, evomonoside, which inhibits cancer cell proliferation and induces apoptosis in osteosarcoma cell line 143B. Delebinski CI et al, *Cell Prolif* 2015 48(5):600-10. It shows moderate activity against herpes simplex types 1 and 2. Wangteeraprasert R et al, *Phytother Res* 2012 26(10): 1496-9.

The related *L. virginicum* root is used for treating excessive mucus of the respiratory tract. The seeds possess a very high anti-oxidant activity, 25948 TE/100 grams. Keep in mind that blueberries are only 3300 TE/100 grams.

Pennycress herb is used in Traditional Chinese Medicine for its bitter pungent flavour, and cold properties. It is known as **SU BAI JIANG**, which translates roughly as "spoiled bean paste from Su". It is also known as **BAI JIANG CAO.**

The plant acts mainly on the stomach, large intestine, and liver meridians, helping to remove toxic heat, eliminate furuncles, erysipelas, hyperemia, and pinkish leucorrhea mixed with whitish discharge. It is used for pelvic inflammatory disease (PID) and inflammation of the uterus.

The herb cools and relieves ulcerations, pus, inflammation, bronchitis and colitis.

The herb is used in cases of stagnant blood, abdominal pain, including appendicitis, combining well with dandelion root, and barley malt for indigestion accompanied with abdominal pain. The direction is lifting and disperses stagnation and relieves pain. Mumps and mastitis are two other lymphatic indications of use.

Pennycress has significant anti-fungal and anti-microbial activity against *Candida albicans*, and *Staphylococcus and Streptococcus* bacterium.

The leaf tea is used externally for poison ivy.

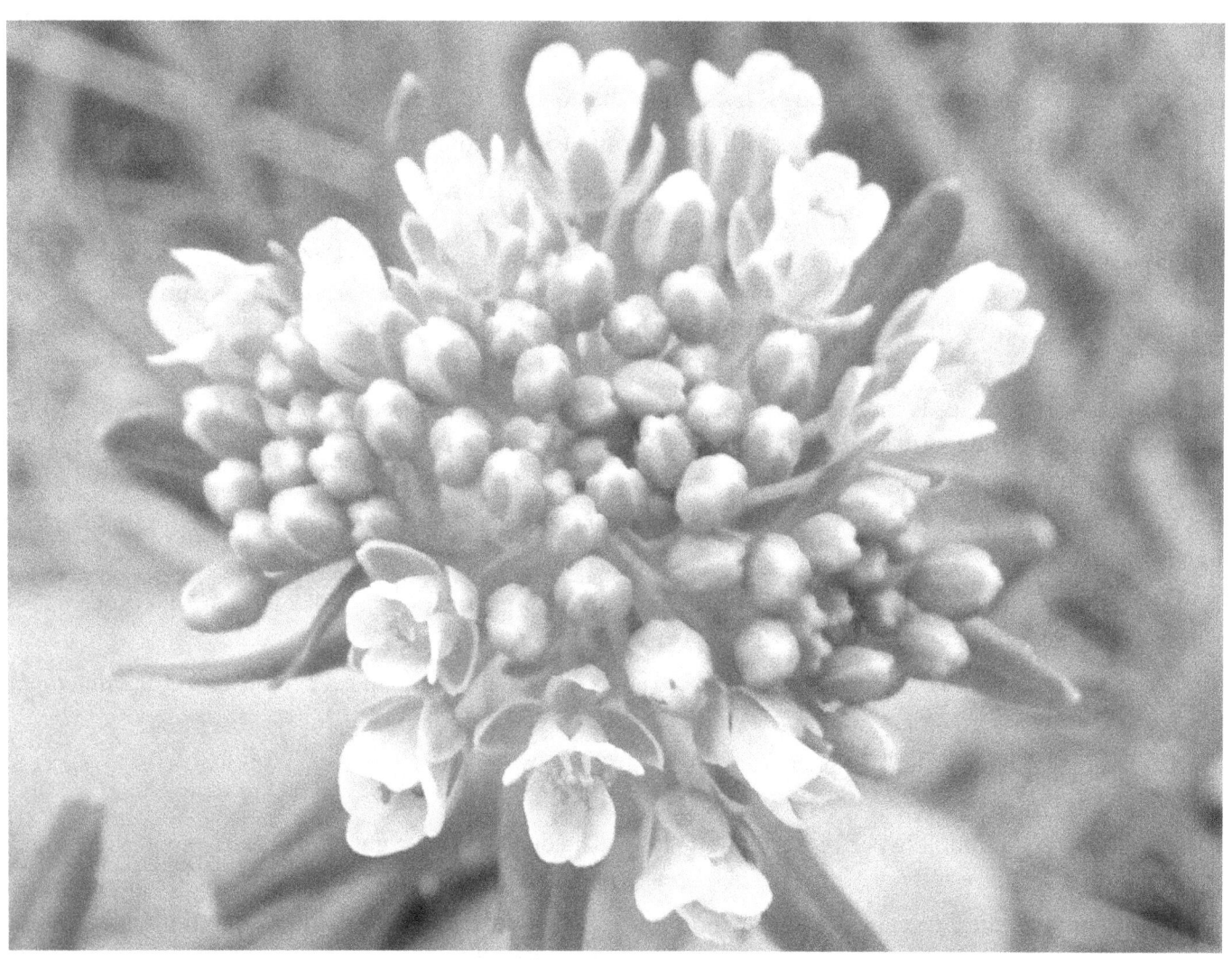

PENNY CRESS FLOWERS

It combines well with Job's Tears for purulent discharge due to damp heat, and with red peony root for postpartum fevers, blood stasis and abdominal pain.

A combination of pennycress, *Panax ginseng*, *Agrimonia pilosa* and arginine was given to a 75 year old female, diagnosed with pancreatic cancer, and multiple metastases in the liver and lymph nodes. She survived eleven months without the side-effects of a severity greater than grade one. Li Y et al, *Oncol Lett* 2015 10(1):263-7.

The seed is known as **XI MING ZI**, and is considered acrid, and slightly warm. They are used to brighten the eyes, treat eye pain and tearing, and balance the five viscera. When taken over time, the seeds are said to make the body light and prevent senility.

The seedpods kill intestinal parasites.

Other names include **MA XIN**, Horse Acrid, and **BI XIN**, meaning Grate Firewood.

Yellow Rocket (*B. vulgaris*) has been studied for anti-bacterial activity. The leaves, stems and flowers all exhibit mycobacterium activity in both water and ethanol extracts. Seven flavonoid glycosides have been recently identified by Senatore et al, *Journal of Agricultural and Food Chemistry* 2000 48.

Early Winter Cress (*B. verna*) seed is a rich source of 2-phenethyl glucosinolate; a break down product of glucosinolates with well-known anti-cancer activity, analogous to the sulphoraphane in broccoli sprouts. It is present in watercress, and has shown significant ability to neutralize the carcinogenic effects of tobacco smoke, nitrosamines, or acetaminophen toxicity.

Other benefits of the derived phenethyl isothiocyanate supplementation include both phase I, and phase II liver detoxification.

Work by Barillari et al, *Fitoterapia* 2001 72:7 looked at isolating this compound from the seed, as they contain only this gluconasturtiin. This could be a valuable precursor of the cancer preventative.

It may be an important dietary supplement for the treatment of neuro-degenerative diseases such as Alzhemier's and Parkinson's by preventing apoptosis of nerve cells.

Research by David Ribnicky et al at Rutgers University has discovered a method for maximizing the release of this compound. These include temperatures at 22° C, and pH 7.2 for twenty minutes.

Upland Cress seeds, under optimal conditions release 186 micrograms of active compound, PEITC, compared to Watercress at 75 mcg, and horseradish at 28 mcg.

Entire study is available in *The Journal of Nutraceuticals, Functional and Medical Foods* 2001 3:3 by Ribnicky et al.

The seeds, rich in PEITC possess anti-inflammatory properties. Dey et al, *J Pharm Exp Ther* 2006 317.

PEITC has been found to be effective in IBS or irritable and inflammatory bowel syndromes. Dey et al, *BMC Chemical Bio* 2010 10:1.

The phenolics present in oilseed residue possess anti-oxidant properties, with one study showing water extracts yielding 25.2 mg/gram of extractable compounds.

Barbarin is a tyrosinase inhibitor isolated from Winter Cress. It exhibits significant inhibitory effect against mushroom and murine tyrosinases. In the study, conducted by Seo-BoRam et al, *Planta Medica* 1999 65:8, using various concentrations of L-DOPA as the substrate, barbarin was identified as an uncompetitive inhibitor.

Early German settlers to North America used the seed of Hoary Cress medicinally. This seed is probably the source of its successful escape.

Hoary Cress seeds were used to purify the blood, to loosen internal blockages of the lungs, spleen, liver and mesenteric tissue. The seeds were taken to cleanse the kidneys and as a de-wormer.

Extracts of the plant have been found to exhibit anti-microbial activity. Research carried out at Kerman University in Iran by Sabahi et al in 1987 showed the plant had marked inhibitory action against bacteria.

Various constituents show activity against meningo-virus and Newcastle disease virus.

Research by Dornberger K & Lich H, *Pharmazie* 1982 37(3):215-21 screened 700 plant species for new chemical substances that may halt or delay the growth of cancer cells.

Material from aerial parts of this plant was amongst the three highest in cytotoxic activity and the greatest, to produce interference with nucleic acid metabolism.

Erysolin, isolated from Hoary Cress seed, inhibited ATR (ataxia telangiectasia and RAD3 related) selective phosphorylation and sensitized p53-deficient cancer cells to chemo agents both in vitro and in vivo. Kawasumi M et al, *Cancer Research* 2014 74(24):7534-45. It induces apoptosis in human colon cancer cell lines, inducing caspase-8 activation. Kim MJ et al, *Anticancer Res* 2010 30(9):3611-9.

Erysolin, erucin and sulforaphane are found in various cruciferous vegetables such as cabbage, broccoli, cauliflower, etc; as well as many of the cresses.

Glucuraphanins are common to the cabbage family and especially rich in broccoli sprouts. They help decrease both cancer formation and oxidative stress that leads to atherosclerosis.

Hoary Cress is rich in this precious compound, and scientists will be working to develop a glucoraphanin extraction technology.

At the same time, other research will be working at domesticating hybrids that are low in the anti-nutritive glycosinolates. *Canadian Journal of Physiology and Pharmacology*, 2001 79.

Watercress is one of our super foods with a strong cleansing and nourishing function.

Growing in cold, running waters, it absorbs a plethora of trace minerals vital to health. It is vitamin rich with four times the vitamin C of lettuce and more calcium than whole milk, as well as large amounts of vitamin A.

Taken daily, watercress increases plasma lutein levels by 100% and beta-carotene levels by 33%.

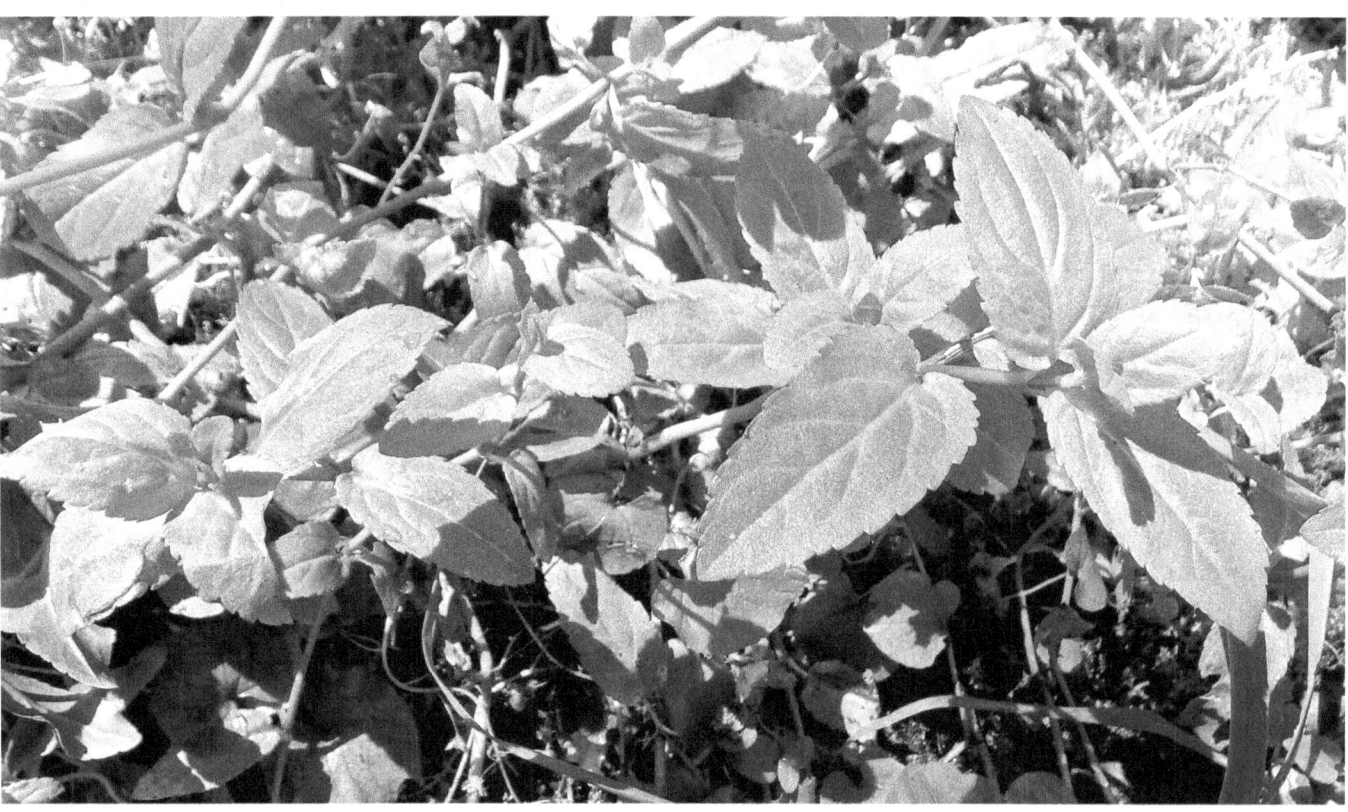

WATERCRESS

And although it contains only small amounts of iodine, its many trace minerals make it very useful for balancing the thyroid, whether under or overactive.

Because of this, it is considered by herbalists to be a blood builder. It restores, according to Peter Holmes "every aspect of the blood, both in a structural and a functional sense: as a bearer of oxygen, as a fluid tissue, as an immune vehicle. This is mostly due to its amazing range of minerals and trace elements. In this connection, Watercress should prove excellent for balancing and regulating calcium metabolism and blood levels.

Closely connected are diuretic activities which not only cleanse fluids, blood and tissues, but also exert a global regulating effect on these."

The nature of watercress is warming and drying, and in TCM is used for liver Qi stagnation and in Ayurvedic medicine for kapha and vata tendencies.

Work by Chen et al, *Clin Pharm & Therapeutics* 1996 60 suggests watercress exerts influence on liver and kidney protection from, and detoxification of acetaminophen.

This makes watercress an excellent addition to lymphatic and digestive cleansing. Its organic sulphur content, in part, aids in proper functioning of the pancreas. Daily consumption helps to reduce lymphocyte DNA damage.

Associated conditions such as prostate irritation, vaginal pruritis, and chronic skin irritations can be relieved with the addition of watercress.

Watercress tea should be chilled in the fridge, and then used for dermatitis, rashes, and eczema, applied several times daily as a wash, or fomentation. It is reputed excellent as a hair tonic.

Watercress helps heal mouth sores, gingivitis, as well as freshen the breath of those suffering halitosis.

The respiratory system is stimulated, helping expel thin, white mucous and clearing head colds and congestion with a hot tea.

Watercress contains flavonols and megastigmanes that inhibit histamine release. Goda et al, *Bio & Pharm Bulletin* 1999 22:12.

It promotes biliary insufficiency, including the breaking up and removal of urinary and bile stones. Rheumatism associated with liver and gall bladder congestion is also relieved.

Daily regimes have been shown to decrease plasma triglyceride levels by about ten percent. Recent work suggests the leaves may be beneficial in lowering blood sugar and lipid levels associated with diabetes. Hadjzadeh MA et al, *Indian J Physiol Pharmacol* 2015 59(2):223-30.

Pituitary and thyroid deficiencies and the associated weakness, fatigue, depression and exhaustion are helped enormously by watercress, due in part to the rich source of manganese. The fresh juice helps relieve menopausal hot flashes when taken cold.

Watercress is the richest green source of tryptophan, which helps boost brain levels of serotonin.

Insufficient breast milk, and anemia are both improved with watercress in the diet, the latter due to its rich organic source of iron, copper and manganese.

Watercress is known in China as West Foreign Vegetable or **XI YANG CAI**, or simply Segment Vegetable, BAN CAI. The cooked soup is used in TCM for tuberculosis, coughing and burning of lungs; as well as pruritus and cloudy, painful urination.

Rebecca Wood has done an enormous amount of research in her book *The New Whole Foods Encyclopedia*.

She suggests raw watercress is not recommended for the young, the elderly, or anyone with compromised health, a propensity for yeast infections, or with a history of internal parasites.

With all issues except the parasites,I take exception. In fact, watercress is excellent for rebuilding poor health, and does not affect young and old in any negative way. It may affect those with a cold, empty feeling and lacking strength if taken in large amounts, and may be cooked, in this case.

Parasites are a problem, especially in wild watercress, due to giardia and other water borne concerns. Wash it well, and be aware of where you harvest.

The nutritional value of watercress was first revealed in a 1920s study on school age children. Watercress was found to duplicate the benefits in growing children as milk. Sherman's *Essentials of Nutrition* from the 1930s found that when watercress juice was added to children's diet, their growth and development was enhanced.

Watercress contains rich stores of gluconasturtiin, a precursor of PEITC, or phenethyl isothiocyanate. This substance has been found to prevent the development of lung cancer in both mice and humans, and remains an exciting development. Research continues on initial work by Hecht, *Advances in Experimental Medicine and Biology* 1996 401. Since this first study, hundreds of research publications have shown PEITC to slow or kill various cancer cell lines.

Recent work by Casanova et al, 2011 25:12 found it an antioxidant that is a "powerful tool for improving health and quality of life."

A dose of 2 ounces of fresh watercress juice three times daily was used in human clinical trials. Fortunately commercially prepared organic juice is available for those wanting to protect themselves, or do periodic cleansing.

Dr. Graham Packham of Southhampton General Hospital found the compound to block the function of a protein called hypoxia-inducible factor, which plays a key role in cancer development. HIF turns on blood vessel promoting factors, and watercress blocks supply of blood vessels to tumors. PEITC also turns off the HIF signal by changing the function of a second protein called 4EBP1. In a study with female breast cancer survivors, PEITC was found in the blood following a watercress meal showing a down regulation of the pathway leading to development of breast cancer.

Watercress juice is a useful morning tonic for those who have over-indulged in alcohol the previous evening.

The three key stages of carcinogenesis (initiation, proliferation and metastasis) were blocked in a study of watercress extract and colon cancer cells.

It appears that watercress modulates anti-cancer pathways via 4E binding protein 1 phosphorylation. Work by Syed et al, *Br J Nutr* 2010 104:9 drew blood on former breast cancer patients taking watercress juice.

Work by Palaniswamy et al, *J Agric Food Chem* 2003 51 found PEITC and ascorbic acid levels highest in leaves harvested at 40 days. This suggests greenhouse propagation for health benefits is very feasible.

Watercress ingestion may protect against exercise-induced DNA damage and lipid peroxidation. A randomized, controlled study of ten healthy, young males for eight weeks, showed prevention of damage in both acute and chronic ingestion. Fogarty MC et al, *British Journal of Nutrition* 2013 109(2): 293-301.

Watercress juice has been found active against tubercular mycobacterium. The freshly made juice is significantly anti-inflammatory and useful externally on burns.

In Brazil, researchers found that extracts possess anti-tumour properties in experiments with mice. In one study, mice supplemented with PEITC and grafted with human prostate tumors, found a 50% reduction in tumor weight.

The plant exhibits significant anti-oxidant activity. Ozen et al, *Acta Pol Pharm* 2009 66:2.

Further work by Hofmann et al, *Eur J Nutrition* 2009 48:8 found the herb modulates enzymes SOD and GPX both *in vitro* and *in vivo*.

The plant has potent anti-inflammatory activity. Sadeghi H et al, *Pharm Biol* 2014 52(2).

Watercress may be useful against *Escherichia coli* infections. Freitas E et al, *Lett Appl Microbiol* 2013 57(4):266-73. In fact, it shows synergistic effect with standard antibiotics.

The plant appears to prevent gentamicin-induced kidney toxicity. Shahani S et al, *Toxicol Mech Methods* 2016 23:1-8.

It also appears, in small amounts, to prevent renal stone formation. Mehrabi S et al, *Journal Nephropathol* 2016 5(4):123-7.

NOTE-I am fully aware watercress is a member of cabbage or mustard family. Most members, especially ingested raw, are potential goitergens. Watercress is NOT!

Rorippa indica, formerly *R. montana*, is known as **HAN CAI** in Traditional Chinese Medicine. It consists mainly of rorifone and rotifamide, and is used chiefly as an anti-tussive, in the treatment of chronic bronchitis, and asthma.

Han Cai is an anti-tussive, expectorant, diuretic and detoxicant, but is combined with one-half part plantain leaf in treating painful, frequent urination.

The plant juice is used in China to relieve dermatitis caused by paint spills.

It is often used interchangeably with garden cress (*L. viriginicum*), and other mustard family like *Draba nemorosa* and *Descurainia sophia*.

Like Common Peppergrass, it contains helveticoside and evomonoside. See above for medicinal properties.

Mountain Cress (*N. montanum*) glucosinolates have been shown to rapidly increase by the addition of tryptophan to their growing environment. *Fitoterapia* 75:2.

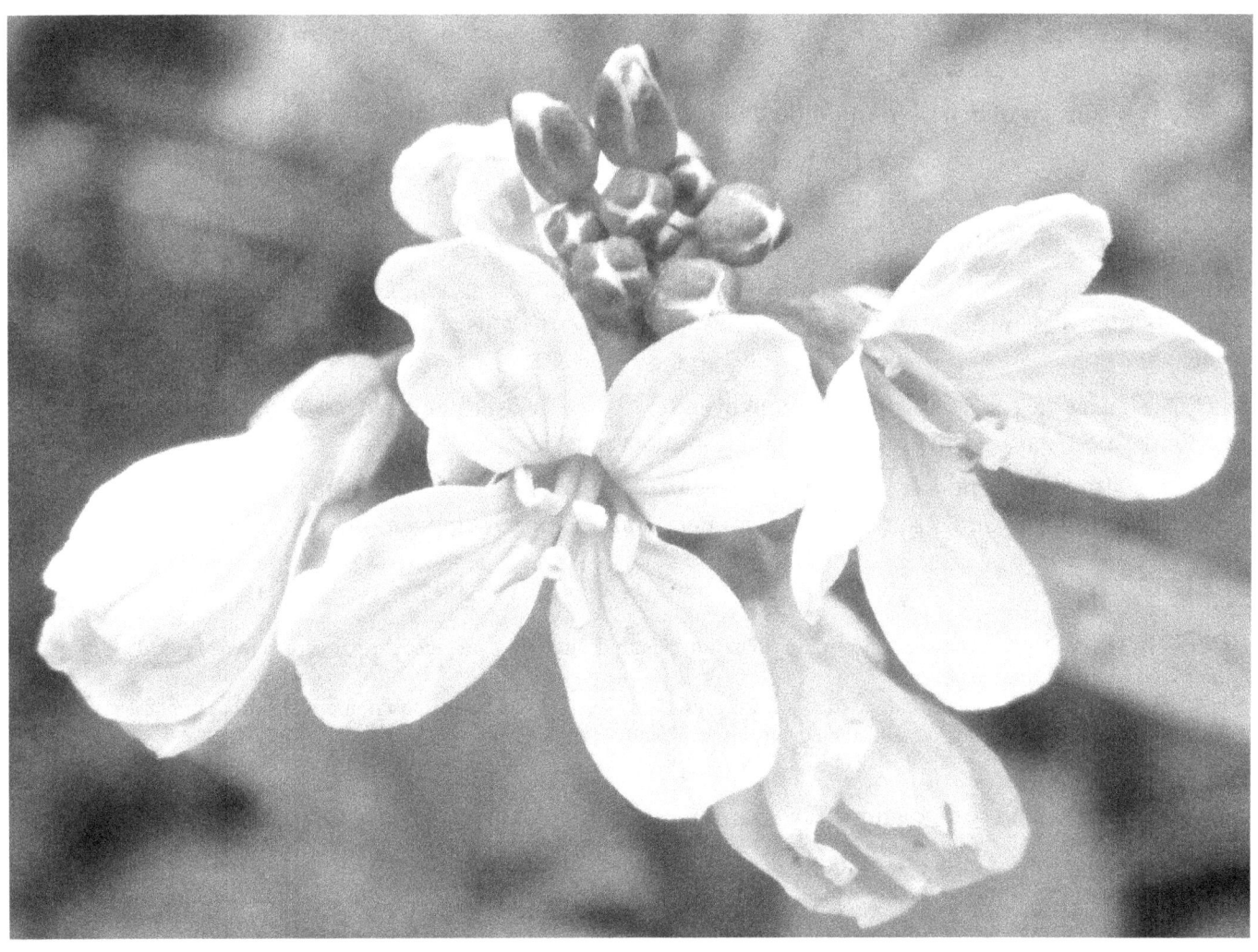

BITTER CRESS FLOWERS

HOMEOPATHY

The mother tincture of Bitter Cress, prepared from the dried herb, is used for diabetes.

Nasturium aquaticum- Watercress is useful in scorbutic affections and constipation, related to strictures of urinary apparatus. It is supposed to be aphrodisiacal in its action. It antidotes tobacco narcosis and is sedative to neurotic affections, neurasthenia, hysteria and the like. It is also indicated in cirrhosis of the liver and dropsy.

DOSE- Tincture- Eight drops as needed. Use 1X potency to stimulate gall bladder function, as well as for diuretic and detoxification.

The mother tincture is prepared from the fresh plant in flower of *N. officinale*.

ESSENTIAL OILS

Essential oils have been produced from the seeds of *Lepidium sativum*. *Journal of Essential Oil Research* 1993 5:5 465-479.

Major constituents of the leaf oil, known as Cress oil, are 53% phenylacetonitrile and 26% aromatic benzyl isothiocyanates. The leaf and seed oil both sink in water. The roots contain 65% of the latter compound.

The essential oil shows moderate larvicial activity agains the mosquito carrying West Nile virus. Kimbaris AC et al, *Parasitol Research* 2012 111(6):2403-10.

Upon distillation, the fresh herb of *L. latifolium* yields a sulphur containing oil that also sinks in water, composed mainly of allyl isothiocyanates.

The seed oil consists of benzyl mustard oil that owes its formation to a glucoside called glucotropaelin.

The volatile oil has been shown to inhibit the growth of *Bacillus subtilis and Staphylococcus aureus*. The active ingredients, the benzyl isothiocyanates, are excreted within an hour of ingestion.

Copper stills should be avoided when dealing with sulphur containing oils, as copper sulphide can form too easily.

Early winter Cress (*B. praecox*) contains the glucoside gluconasturtiin, also found in Nasturium. Upon distillation, both plants yield identical oils, consisting mainly of phenyl ethyl mustard oil. The melting point of thiourea is 135°C.

The flowering aerial parts of *C. draba* contain over 80% 3-butenyl isothiocyanate, the seeds and roots over 72% and 30% respectively of 4-methylsulfinyl butyl isothiocyanate.

Watercress absolute is produced from the fresh plant, using alcohol as a solvent. Although it is produced mainly for the flavor industry, it has some use in perfumery and fragrance compositions.

SEED OILS

CONSTITUENTS- *T. arvense*- allyl isothio-cyanate, allyl sulphide and other oil glucocides. It also contains over 30% of unsaturated fatty acid from C18:1 to C24:1.
A breakdown reveals 20% linoleic acid, up to 23% linolenic acid, 13.8% oleic acid, 9% eicosenoioc acid, and nearly 38% erucic acid. The seed contains 16-24% crude protein, and 20 fatty acids. Yield is 26-31%.

The seed oil composition of *L. campestre* is about 35% linolenic acid and 23% erucic acid, with about 20% content. The thousand seed weight is 1.99 grams, large enough to use in oil crop production.

Other species of the genus contain up to 47% linolenic, and yield more than 30%.

Garden Cress (*L. sativum*) seeds have been trialed in Poland as an alternative source of oil. The plant produces in excess of one tonne/hectare of seed. More information is found in Musnicki, *Rosliny-Oleiste* 1997 18:2.

Yield is around 26%, comprised of 42% polyunsaturated and 40% monounsaturated oils. Tocopherols are quite high and phytosterols are 14.4 mg/g. Moser et al, *Indust Crops Prod* 2009 30:2.

Other studies found the content of alpha linolenic acid from seeds was 33.6%. It may be useful when blended with other seed oils, such as sesame or sunflower, to increase ALA, and decrease the omega 6 to omega 3 ratio. Umesha SS, *Food Chem* 2012 135(4):2845-51.

A combination of rice bran and garden cress seed oil appears to attenuate ulcerative colitis. Reddy KV et al, *Int J Colorectal Disease* 2014 29(2):267-9.

The fast growing annual may have potential to supplement biodiesel production.

Pennycress oil is a potential substitute for rapeseed oil as an additive for special lubricants. This is especially true of blown lubricants, due to the marked ability to adhere to metal surfaces under heavy loads. It also resists flushing by water.

The use of the oil in coating compositions has been partially investigated in past years.

Pouring boiling water over feed containing stinkweed inactivates the enzymes that release the mustard-like oils.

If the herb or seeds are covered with cold water, and allowed to stand before distilling, a colour-less oil with a peculiar, penetrating odor that reminds one of both mustard and garlic. The taste is leek-like.

The oil has potential as an industrial crop, but probably not for human consumption. It yields from 30-48%. In 1949, Lips and Grace, *Can Journal of Research* discussed the edible properties of stinkweed oil and shortening made from it. The oil is 33% erucic acid and 22% linoleic acid.

It was traditionally used as a lamp oil.

Stan Peacock, a High Prairie farmer trialed the plant on his marginal land, and obtained a good yield of oil suitable for biofuel. Pennycress biofuel performs to -28° C compared to -7° C for canola biofuel. The environmental footprint is also significant, with one unit of biodiesel yielding 4.5 units for canola and even higher for pennycress. Ethanol, by comparison, yields 1.1 units of energy for each unit, barely saving anything.

Dr. Ampong-Nyarko, from CDC North, looked at seeding times and potential for leftover meal. It has potential as a natural herbicide, among other uses.

Research in Europe is looking at biotech manipulation (GMO) to increase high quality biodiesel production. Claver A et al, *J Plant Physiol* 2017 208:7-16.

The seeds of the perennial Yellow Rocket *(B. vulgaris)* contain about 30% erucic acid, and 22% each of oleic and linoleic acids. The thousand seed weight (TSW) is 0.53 grams.

Early Winter Cress *(B. verna)* is well over 50% erucic acid. TSW is 0.86 grams.

HYDROSOLS

The distilled water of garden cress will open a blocked liver, spleen, and urinary vessels; drive grit and sand from the kidneys and bladder; cleanse the chest of phlegm; kill and expel worms, and is good for consumption. If drawn up into the nose, it will cleanse the head and cause vigorous sneezing. If it is held in the mouth, it will draw down phlegm from the head. When washed with it, all manner of corruptions of the skin, black moles, itch, pox, and abscesses will be heated.

If a small piece of cloth is dipped into the water of garden cress and laid over these corruptions, it will cleanse the same. If a few loths of this same water are drunk, it will prove especially good for blood spitting. **SAUER**

Pennycress is distilled in June. The water comforts the heart and body, relieves yellow jaundice and rids the belly of all worms.

BRUNSCHWIG

Watercress water cleanses the blood, and provokes urine exceedingly, kills worms, outwardly mixed with honey, it clears the skin of morphew and sun-burning.   **CULPEPPER**

Watercress water is good for worms, gravel, preventing loss of hair, ill tongue. Do not drink too much as it might do great harm to stomach. It is combined with strawberry water for blood on ankles, or fresh chilblains. It helps draw red spots away. It relieves teeth pain and swellings.   **BRUNSCHWIG**

FLOWER ESSENCES

Lady's Smock essence is used for a better understanding of family history and the part it has to play in your own development as an individual.   **OLIVE**

Cuckoo Flower essence helps to release anger directed at others. It helps attune to love at the unconditional level.   **BRYNAHERB**

Meadowfoam Cabbage essence helps bring old knowledge back to surface. It opens up access to won feelings and basic fundamentals of life.   **MIRIANA**

Yellow Rocket essence helps provide comfort in personal crisis such as divorce, bankruptcy, and helps promote concentrated work.   **MIRIANA**

PERSONALITY TRAITS

Soil is a kind of language, and the plants that grow in it are a particularly engrossing story for the gardener. Clover's tale is all about nitrogen deficiency...Horsetail is a run-on sentence about acidic or low-lime soil.

Wild Carrot and Stinkweed natter on about high-lime conditions, while Field Bindweed and Sheep Sorrel talk sand. Plantain, Canada Thistle and Dandelions won't shut up about heavy clay, common Mullein about low fertility. Plants, especially weeds, tell us all kinds of things about soil, if we're willing to listen.   **L. JOHNSON**

Within a few weeks now Draba, the smallest flower that blows, will sprinkle every sandy place with small blooms.

He who hopes for spring with upturned eye never sees so small a thing as Draba. He who despairs of spring with downcast eye steps on it, unknowing. He who searches for spring with his knees in the mud finds it, in abundance.

Draba asks and gets, but scant allowance of warmth and comfort; it subsists on the leavings of unwanted time and space. Botany books give it two or three lines, but never a plate or portrait. Sand too poor and sun too weak for bigger, better blooms are good enough for Draba. After all, it is no spring flower, but only a postscript to a hope.

Draba plucks no heartstrings. Its perfume, if there is any, is lost in the gusty winds. Its color is plain white. Its leaves wear a sensible woolly coat. Nothing eats it; it is too small. No poets sing of it. Some botanist once gave it a Latin name, and then forgot it. Altogether it is of no importance- just a small creature that does a small job quickly and well.   **ALDO LEOPOLD**

SPIRITUAL PROPERTIES

Winter cress has the ability to cure or relieve a number of minor illnesses and complaints pertaining to the reproductive system.

A tea made by steeping the fresh flowers and leaves for ten minutes in hot water can greatly relieve menstrual cramps if taken three times a day starting one week before the onset of the menses. The root can be chopped, stewed and eaten to reduce pressure on the fallopian tubes during pregnancy. The stem may be chopped and soaked in olive oil to yield an oily rub for genitals when inflamed due to chafing, etc.   **HILARION**

MYTHS AND LEGENDS

According to legend, the beautiful Saint Barbara was locked in a tower by her pagan father, to keep her from her many suitors. However, she managed to admit a Christian priest disguised as a doctor, and was converted. On discovering her new faith, her faith, her father handed her over to the authorities, who ordered him to cut off her head, but he was struck dead by lightning before he could behead her. It became the custom to invoke Barbara against sudden death.

TRESIDDER

St. Barbara was the legendary Barbara of Nicomedia, said to have been martyred in 306. According to legend, Barbara lived in Asia Minor, in Turkey. Her father, the pagan emperor Dioscorus, persecuted Christians, and when she became a Christian he ordered that she be tortured and beheaded. While in her cell, Barbara found a dried up cherry branch, which blossomed profusely before her execution.

Immediately following her execution, Dioscorus was struck dead by lightning, explaining why St. Barbara is often called on for protection during thunderstorms. Saint Barbara is also the patron saint of artillerymen and miners. Traditionally in German-speaking countries, particularly in Austria and Catholic regions of Germany, a small cherry branch is cut off and placed in water on Dec. 4th, a custom known as Barbarazweig or Barbara Branch. If the branch blooms precisely on Dec. 25th, it is regarded as a particularly good sign for the future.

SMALL

Watercress is one of the ingredients of the sacred elixir used in the initiation ceremony of the Santeria religion. The species are claimed by the Yoruba deities, Yemaya and Oshun, who are generally reputed, to have dominion over stomach irritations. Yemaya corresponds with Our Lady of Regla, and Oshun related to La Caridad del Cobre.

Yemay is universally equated with Yesod, the plane of love and mercy of the Qabalistic Tree of Life, corresponding with Artemis, the Greek goddess and coming under the rulership of the Moon. Oshun, on the other hand, corresponds with Netzach, the emotional sensitivity plane of the Tree of Life, equating with the Greek goddess of love, Aphrodite, and having Venus as her ruling planet.

ANDOH

RECIPES

TINCTURE- 6-20 drops. A fresh plant tincture is prepared at 1:4 and 40% alcohol.

POWDER- 0.3-1 gram

DECOCTION- 1-3 grams. Crush seeds first. Use 1:20 ratio.

INFUSION- pennycress aerial parts- 1:20 ratio. 60-100 ml twice daily.

Hoary Cress- 30-40 grains as needed.

TINCTURE-watercress 30-40 drops as needed. Prepare 1:4 fresh at 45%.

FRESH JUICE- 10 mls diluted in water, three times daily. Take a 3 day break every eight days to avoid an irritation of the bladder. Use with care in pregnancy, peptic ulcers, and kidney inflammation. It freezes well as ice cubes.

R. montana- 3-6 grams.

CAUTION: Do not take pennycress in excess internally, as it may decrease levels of white blood cells, and cause nausea and dizziness. The seedpods can irritate the mucous membranes of the throat and stomach.

Best dried in isolation due to the strong odor it releases after picking.

Studies on beagles found garden cress may interfere with theophylline, cyclosporine, carbamazepine, phenytoin and sildenafil pharmacokinetics. Caution is advised.

Watercress may inhibit the oxidative metabolism of acetaminophen, and should not be combined. It may be used as a chaser, to ensure liver and kidney toxicity is minimized.

It is a mild uterine stimulant and should not be used during pregnancy; and may irritate gastric or duodenal ulcers, and those suffering acute kidney inflammation.

SLENDER GILIA
PINK TWINK
(*Gilia gracilis* Hook) not accepted
(*Microsteris gracilis* **var.** *gracilis* [Hook.] Greene)
(*Phlox gracilis*) not accepted
SCARLET GILIA
DESERT TRUMPET
SKY ROCKETS
(*G. aggregata* [Pursh] Spreng.) not accepted
(*Ipomopsis aggregata* **ssp.** *aggregata* [Pursh] V. E. Grant)
(*Cantua aggregata*) not accepted
CLUSTERED GILIA
(*G. congesta* Hook) not accepted
(*I. congesta* **ssp.** *congesta* [Hook.] V. E. Grant)
MOSS PHLOX
HOOD'S PHLOX
SPINY PHLOX
(*P. hoodii* Richardson)
DOWNY PILOSA
(*P. pilosa* L.)
BLUE PHLOX
ALYSSUM LEAF PHLOX
(*P. alyssifolia* Greene)

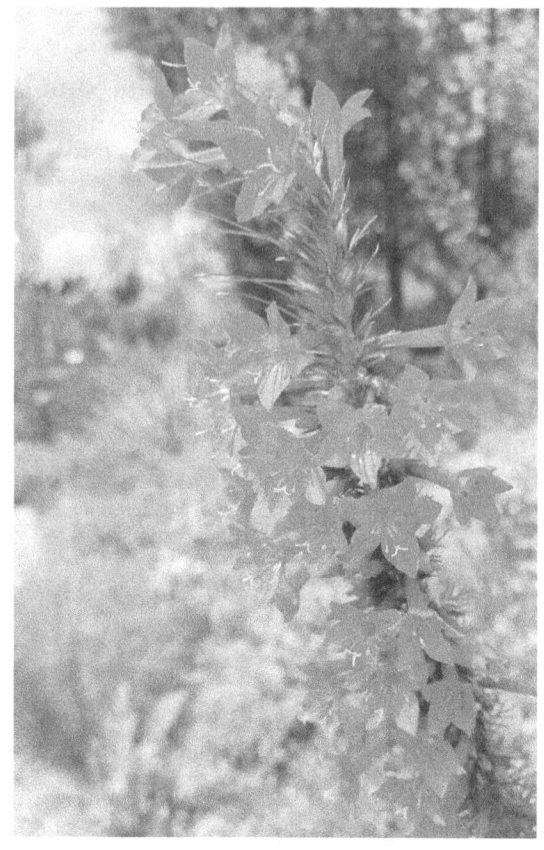

IPOMOPSIS RUBRA

Gilia is named after Filipo Luigi Gili, a famous scientist, astronomer and botanist, who lived in 18ᵗʰ century Rome. He was originally from Spain, where his name was Felipe S. Gil. Some authors believe they were two different people. Who knows!

Gracilis is from the Latin meaning scanty, slender or graceful. Ipomopsis means worm-like, aggregata means clustered, referring to close carpels. Congesta is from the Latin, **CONGESTUS**, from **COM** meaning "together", and **GERERE**, to carry.

Microsteris is from the Greek **MIKROS**, meaning small, and **STEIRA**, meaning sterile or barren.

Phlox is also from the Greek meaning a plant with flame colored petals. Robert Hood was a midshipman on one of Sir John Franklin's expeditions.

Moss Phlox was infused as a tea by the Blackfoot as a mild laxative for children and chest pain.

A dye was made from the plant, in the manner of lichens, by both the Blackfoot and Blood tribes. The white to violet flowers give a yellow dye.

Blue Phlox is less common, and confined in Alberta to south of the Old Man river. The name is confusing, as the fresh flowers are white to pink, only turning blue after they dry.

Slender Gilia is an annual, restricted to the southwest montane region of Alberta, and introduced into the Yukon.

The Gosiute poulticed the whole plant on wounds and bruises, a use shared with the Navaho-Ramah.

The latter people made cold infusions as a mouthwash for sores of the gums and mouth.

Scarlet Gilia is found in the south-central prairies, while the white flowered Clustered Gilia is not common, but sometimes found in the southwest region. Both are native perennials. The former has a skunky scent.

Scarlet Gilia was traditionally used by the Navaho as an emetic, a wash for spider bites, and for general stomach problems. A cold infusion was used as a hunting medicine, and applied to both the hunter and his weapon of choice.

The Paiute decocted the roots for treating colds, or combined it with other plants as a physic or ceremonial emetic.

The Shoshone poulticed the whole plant for rheumatism, and a decoction for washing the skin, especially for itch or venereal ulcers. It was also drunk as a blood tonic, or as part of decoctions to treat gonorrhea or syphilis.

The plant tea was considered a blood tonic, or postpartum rejuvenator.

The Okanagan used the leaves tea as a tonic, steeping it in hot water until a bright green, and taken in small doses.

Clustered Gilia was decocted by the Paiute to treat colds, diarrhea, indigestion and other stomach troubles.

The Shoshone favored it as eyewash, pimples or wounds, or internally to treat kidney or liver problems. A poultice of the mashed plant was applied to erysipelas.

The Washoe infused the crushed plant and applied it as a poultice to cases of dropsy. And the Zuni used warm infusions for headache, as a diuretic or laxative, and even rubbed onto the body for fevers, as well as the neck for swollen throats.

Downy Phlox (*P. pilosa*) was used as a leaf infusion by the Fox tribe as a wash for eczema, and swallowed to cure and purify the blood.

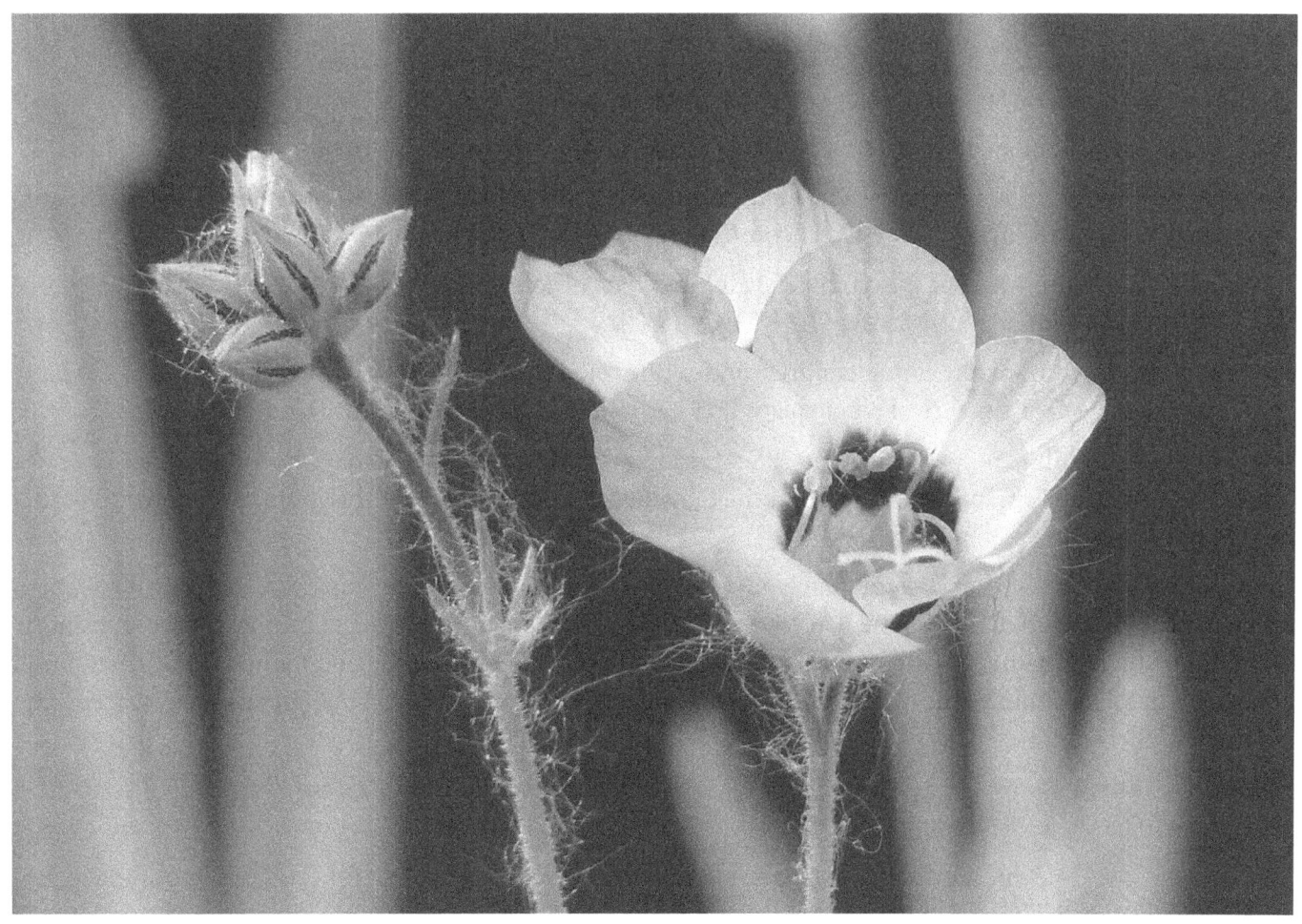

GILIA TRICOLOR

The root was part of a compound mixture, used as a love medicine.

It is surprising that no ethnobotanical record of use for snakebites is recorded in the literature. The compound patuletin inhibits phospholipase activity and shows potential against snake venom in work by Fernandes JM et al, *PLoS One* 2016 11(12): e0168658.

Several Phlox species were used by Native tribes of the West, including Long leaf Phlox (*P. longifolia*), Desert Phlox (*P. austromontana*) and *P. stansburyi*.

The latter plant was used by the Navaho to regulate the menstrual cycle; while Desert Phlox root was given to babies for stomachaches, or rubbed onto the body for muscle aches and colds.

Long leaf Phlox root treat was used for similar purposes, including diarrhea, venereal disease, anemia, and to ease the pain of childbirth.

P. multiflora leaves and flowers were infused by the Cheyenne of Montana as a stimulant. According to Grinnell, "the fluid was rubbed over the body of the patient, and some of it was drunk, reputedly restoring a light and natural feeling."

It has long been assumed that plants associated with mycorrhizal fungi, have a higher tolerance for herbivore grazing. One study suggests that fungi on scarlet gilia appear to be parasitic, after aerial parts are eaten by ungulates. Allsup CM & Paige KN, *Oecologia* 2016 180(2): 463-74.

MEDICINAL

CONSTITUENTS- *P. pilosa-* various flavonoids including apigenin and luteolin.
I. aggregata- eupalitin, eupatolitin and patuletin glycosides, schottenol glucoside, liliacoumarin.

Various Ipomopsis species have shown anti-viral activity, and cytotoxicity against various cancer cell lines.

Work at UBC found aerial parts and roots of Scarlet Gilia active against all nine fungal species tested, in some cases equal to activity of nystatin. McCutcheon AR et al, *J Ethnopharm* 1994 44(3): 157-69.

An extract of the plant was found to completely inhibit cytopathology induced by para-influenza virus type 3. McCutcheon et al, *J Ethnopharm* 1995 49 101-110.

Bronchitis and pneumonia in young children under one one year old, is often associated with this endemic infection. Use the tea or tincture of whole plant that has removed alcohol with hot water evaporation.

The root extract inhibits herpes virus type 3. Six tumor-inhibiting compounds have been identified. Arisawa et al, *J Pharm Sci* 1985 73. Ipomopsin was identified by the same author as a new biscoumarin in *J Nat Products* 1984 47.

Large doses of the plant are toxic, so caution is advised. However, a tincture of the whole flowering plant including root can be given in small doses (one half teaspoon) three times daily. Watch for vomiting, diarrhea, clammy skin). If no side effects increase to one teaspoon three times daily and use for one month. Take a two-week break with dandelion and burdock root tea. Repeat as necessary for viral-related malignant cancers, according to Darcy Williamson, noted herbalist.

Eupalitin induces apoptosis in prostate carcinoma cells via caspase-3 pathway. Kaleem S et al, *Cell Biol Int* 2016 40(2): 196-203.

Eupalitin appears to exhibit cytotoxicity against drug-sensitive T-lymphoblastoid cell lines and multi-drug-resistant leukemia cell lines. Tacchini M et al, *Nat Prod Res* 2015 29(22): 2071-9.

It also induces activation of caspases 3/7 in human colorectal tumor cells. Ghallib RM et al, *Journal of Medicinal Plants Research* 2013 7(20): 1401-5.

Another coumarin identified as liliacoumarin was found active against *Staphylococcus aureus, E. coli, Pseudomonas aeruginosa, Bacillus subtilis,* and *Candida albicans.*

Patuletin is found in Scarlet Gilia, as well as the flower heads of various Arnica species. It is anti-microbial, anti-inflammatory and anti-oxidant. Abdel-Wahhab et al, *Pharm Bio* 2005 43:6.

Patuletin protects brain neurons from glutamate induced oxidative stress. Kim SR et al, *Free Radic Biol Med* 2002 32(7): 596-604.

It is a lens aldose reductase inhibitor, which means it may have benefit in preventing eye disease, associated with diabetes; and may be useful against rheumatoid arthritis. Li et al, *Yan Ke Xue Bao* 1991 7:1.

Patuletin shows significant anti-inflammatory and anti-arthritic activity in rodent models, particularly for rheumatoid arthritis. Jabeen A et al, *Int Immunopharmacol* 2016 36: 232-40. The compound is both cytotoxic and inhibits growth of HeLa human cancer cell line. Kashif M et al, *Pharm Biol* 2015 53(5): 672-81. Patuletin is also found in French marigold flowers (*Tagetes patula*), German Chamomile, spinach and Nettles (*U. urens*).

Scarlet Gilia can be used in anti-fungal ointments. The dried plant is infused for discomforts associated with colds, or taken in capsules for constipation.

The eastern *P. subuta* leaf contains higher phenols and vitamin C than green tea and is a potent anti-oxidant. Nagai et al, *J Food Ag Envir* 5:1.

ESSENTIAL OIL

Scarlet Gilia buds contain large amounts of alpha pinene, and lesser amounts of beta pinene. The corollas contain alpha pinene, beta carophyllene, four terpenoids, three esters and one ketone. Irwin et al, *J Chem Ecol* 2002 28:3.

SPIRITUAL PROPERTIES

The Klamath Indian name of the plant, (Scarlet Gilia) derived from ÕHLS, meaning dove, **AM**, meaning plant, and **BON-WÄS**, for drink, commemorates the legend, current among the Indian children, who pluck the flowers and suck the nectar, that in the old days when the beasts and birds lived together and understood each other's language the wild dove's drink was the nectar of this flower and nothing else.　　　　**COLVILLE**

PERSONALITY TRAITS

The tundra is an inhospitable environment. Yet the Alpine Phlox does just fine there. Forming an inconspicuous mound of tiny leaves and small white flowers, a 150 year-old alpine phlox may grow no larger than a baseball. It is a conservative plant-slow growing and energy efficient- yet, amazingly, its compactness allows it to maintain a temperature inside the mound about 20 degrees warmer than its cold environment. Now that's a plant with fire in its belly!

Of course, we also are apt to get ourselves all heated up. But sometimes that heat builds and builds until it gets the better of us, and we explode in a fiery tantrum. Rather than using our energy for warmth and growth, we waste it- and usually do harm in the process. How much healthier to stay quiet, controlled and totally energized.　　　　**G. MOHAMMED**

GLASSWORT
RED SAMPHIRE
FALSE SAMPHIRE
RED SWAMPFIRE
(*Salicornia rubra* A. Nelson)
(*S. europaea* **ssp.** *rubra*
                [A. Nelson] Breitung) not accepted
(*S. borealis* S. L. Wolff & Jefferies) not accepted
SLENDER GLASSWORT
(*S. maritima* S. L. Wolff & Jefferies)
(*S. europaea* auct. non L.)
(*S. herbacea* auct. non [L.] L.)
(*S. prostrata* auct. non Pall.) not accepted
(*S. ramosissima* auct. non J. Woods) not accepted
DWARF SALTWORT
(*S. bigelovii* Torr.)
AMERICAN GLASSWORT
PICKLEWEED
(*S. virginica* L.) not accepted
(*S. depressa* Standl.)
PACIFIC SALICORNIA
(*Sarcocornia pacifica* [Standl.] A. J. Scott)
PERENNIAL GLASSWORT
(*S. perennis* Mill.) not accepted
(*Sarcocornia perrennis* [Mill.] A. J. Scott)
(*S. ambigua* Michx.) not accepted
PARTS USED- succulent tips

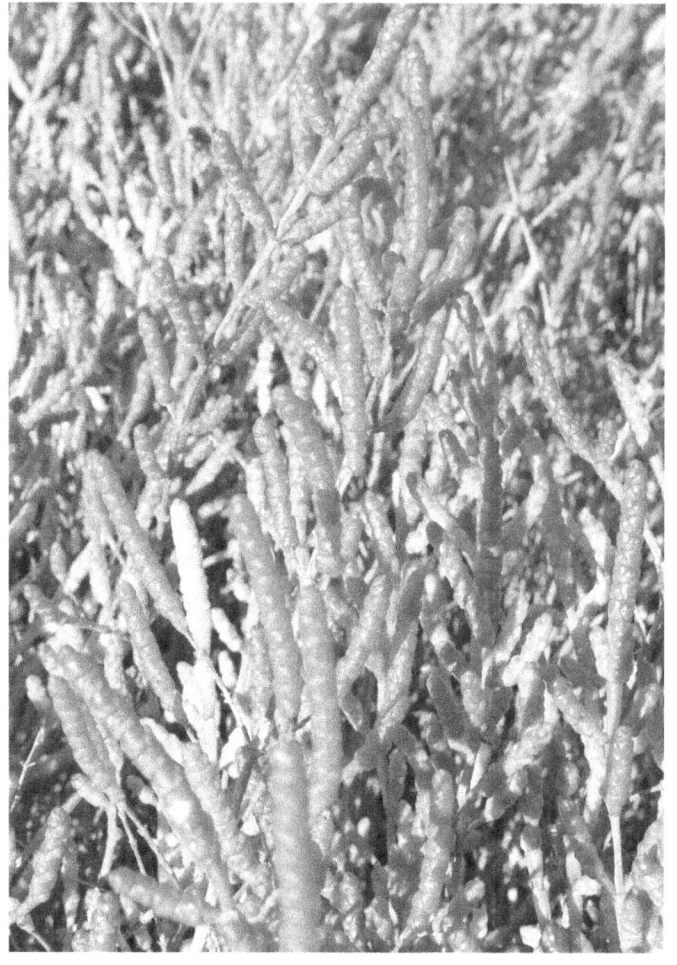

GLASSWORT

Half way down Hangs one that gathers samphire, dreadful trade! Methinks he seems no bigger than his head.
SHAKESPEARE

Salicornia is from the Italian **SAL**, for salt; and **CORNU**, meaning horn; hence Salt horn. Europaea means from Europe. Rubra is red. Samphire comes from the French, l'herbe de Saint-Pierre, and then Sampierre, sampere, and finally samphire.

Some authors believe samphire derived from the French name *Herbe de Saint-Pierre*.

Glasswort may derive from its use to make glass, or because it is so brittle, and the sound of walking across it makes a crackling sound.

The genus is a taxonomic nightmare. Kadereit G et al, *Taxon* 2007 56:1143-70. It is considered the most complicated group of vascular plants, and that is saying something.

Red Samphire is a fascinating example of a plant's ability to adapt. This succulent, annual, salt loving glasswort grows on alkaline mud flats throughout the prairies. It begins as green in spring, and as the glycoside betanin (as in beets) is formed, the plant turns crimson. It is found from Alaska to New Mexico and east to Nova Scotia.

The beautiful shades of red, often contrasted on white, saline soil, sometimes cover several acres. It occupies saline and alkaline soils, and is often found ringing a small, alkaline pond, or where farmers have extensively irrigated and created a soil that will not grow anything else. The plant pumps the salts into cells at the end of stem, and when they cannot hold any more salt, they die and drop off. This is repeated.

The minerals salts were extracted by the Cree of Saskatchewan and elsewhere, to season food and supply needed nutrients. The plants were washed and boiled and the decoction evaporated for dry salt. Mudie PJ et al, *Can J Botany* 2005 83:111-123.

In fact, the Cree name **SIWITAKAN**, means "Salt".

The red samphire stems were boiled, strained, and then the water evaporated away to concentrate the various minerals, including valuable trace minerals. As Robin Marles notes in his excellent book, *Aboriginal Plant Use in Canada's Northwest Boreal Forest*, "consumption of small amounts of chromium, manganese, and magnesium salts has been shown to be beneficial in the treatment of non-insulin dependent diabetes".

The Gosiute of Utah and Nevada ground the seed heads into flour.

Long Ago Person Found (Kwädäy Dän Ts'ìnchí) died on a British Columbia glacier over 560 years ago. Like Oetze, the Iceman of the Swiss Alps, the contents of his stomach revealed early indigenous dietary habits.

One of the pollens found in his stomach was from the succulent perennial glasswort (*S. perennis*).

His robe was made from skins of arctic ground squirrels, his hat from the roots of Sitka spruce.

Glassworts contain a lot of soda, and since Biblical times have been used for making glass and soap.

Early glassmakers in England imported the glasswort ashes from the Mediterranean where they were called Barilla. This was mixed with fine sand and made into beautiful glass.

Travelers to North America in the 1700s, found glasswort growing abundantly in salt marshes and sloughs, and found the Spanish had already found and named the plant here Barilla.

Soap, made from the ashes of glasswort, was spread on a piece of thick brown paper cut to the shape of shoe sole, and bound to the soles of the feet. This was a common remedy for persons casually taken speechless or struck dumb, according to Parkinson.

Coles, another English botanist, suggested glasswort as a purge, for dropsy, to provoke urine, to expel the dead birth, to open obstructions of the liver and spleen, to consume proud flesh, to clear the skin of spots and freckles and to squirt into a horse's eye "to take away the skin that beginneth to grow there and dimm the sight...to dry up running sores and scabs, tetters and ring-worms...and to help the itch."

William Turner named the jointed salt marsh plant "saltwurt" due to its salty taste. He reported the seeds were eaten by larks in East Friesland, but mentions no medicinal use.

In Norfolk, the plant is gathered as a spring tonic, and made into an ointment for cracked hands and skin conditions.

The ashes of Glasswort were mixed with special sand and boiled in furnaces to make glass. Different metals added at the last minute would give different colored glass, greatly prized in those days. Unfortunately, the combination of toxic metals and intense brightness, led to early blindness and death for the glassmaker. There are references in the Bible to the use of Glasswort for soap and glass.

The ashes were leached with limewater to make a solution of caustic soda.

The soap was made after the manner of the Castilians, who were said to have invented the special recipes. Today, Castille soap is a prized, non-clogging pore vegetable soap.

The caustic soda was combined with animal fats, for a cruder, but still effective cleanser. Another approach was to combine the alkali ash from *Salicornia* species with the abietic acids in the resin of coniferous trees such as pine or spruce.

Red Samphire is edible, and a great hiking snack, if not a little salty.

Chewed in mid summer, they taste like lettuce hearts with a bit of salt. They can be added raw to salads, or quickly simmer for no more than 2-3 minutes, drained and cooled.

They can also be pickled in vinegar for later use. In France, *S. herbacea* is gathered commercially for pickling or to eat raw with fish. The Acadians of Nova Scotia nicknamed the plant **TETINES DE SOURIS**, or mouse nipples, after the small clusters on the stem.

The crunchy tips are sold as Sea Asparagus to trendy European restaurants for salad or fish dishes. Also known as Crow's Foot Greens, in Nova Scotia, the aerial parts of *S. europaea*, from the saltwater marshes, are a delicious and exported snack.

In Korea, it is known as Hamcho, or Tungtungmadi. It is used for constipation, obesity, diabetes and cancer, indigestion, hepatitis, nephropathy, asthma and arthritis.

It was combined at 0.5-1% with probiotics and found as effective as antibiotics in raising commercial chicken. Sarker et al, *J Med Plants Res* 2010 4:5.

Glasswort, along with dandelion, ginger root, licorice root and a few other herbs, is a Korean Traditional Health Drink (*Taemyeongcheong*).

The drink appears to prevent liver damage associated with acetominophen. Yi RK et al, *Prev Nutr Food Sci* 2015 20(1):52-9.

Glasswort vinegar, in lab studies, appears to alleviate fatigue, and increased running endurance. Cho HD et al, *J Sci Food Agric* 2016 96(4):1085-92.

The herb is used in the process of making NURUK and to add nutrition to MAKEGEOLLI. Bo Young Jeon et al, *Food Sci Biotech* 19:4.

Plants that can tolerate saline or salt spills are of interest in reclamation work; especially oil well drilling.

A recent listing of 517 salt tolerant plant species in China, all with economic benefit, can be found in the *Journal of Nanjing Forestry University* 1999 23:4.

Work at the U. of California, in the lab of Norman Terry, has found Annual Pickleweed (*S. bigelovii*) removes selenium from contaminated drainage water more efficiently than any plant tested.

The plant absorbs and then releases selenium into the atmosphere as a gas.

MEDICINAL

CONSTITUENTS- various betanin derivatives, including betalains, betanidin-5-0-(2-0-glucuronyl) glycoside; various flavanones and chromone derivatives; isorhamnetin-3-0-glucoside, isorhamnetin 3-O-beta-D-glucopyranoside, quercitin-3-0-(6"-malonyl)glucoside; rutoside, quercetin, quercitin-3-0-glucoside; 6,7-dimeth-oxychromone; 6,7-methylenedioxy-chromone, four dicaffeoylquinic acid derivatives, salbige A & B (noroleanane-type triterpene saponins, echinocystic acid, gypsogenin, pheophorbide A, various polysaccharides, icariside B2, longifloroside B.

Salicornia herbacea has been found to possess immune modulating activity due to polysaccharides soluble in hot water. Sun-A Im et al, *J Ethnopharm* 111:2.

It also is a potent tyrosinase inhibitor, suggesting anti-oxidant and skin rejuvenation possibilities. Sung et al, *Biosci Biotech Biochem* 2009 73:3.

Polysaccharides from *Salicornia* genus have been found to stimulate macrophages to express iNOS generation through activation of NF-kappaB. Lee et al, *J Ethnopharm* 103:3.

Work by Kim MS et al, found an ethanol extract and a methylene chloride fraction show strong protective effect glutamate-induced cell death of hippocampal HT22 cells.

A potential neuroprotective salt substitute or dietary supplement may be developed. *Journal Med Foods* 2017 20(2):140-151.

A vegetable salt, Saloni, has been developed and is marketed in India.

Although the salt contains 55% sodium chloride, it also contain 5-(hydroxymethyl) furfural, p-coumaric acid and trans-ferulic acid, the latter responsible for vascular protection. In rats fed high salt diets, both systolic and diastolic pressures increased, as did arterial pressure, whereas the salicornia extract did not effect either. Panth N et al, *Int J Mol Sci* 2016 17(7).

Its potential as a functional food for glucose metabolism, was studied in STZ-induced diabetic rats. Lee SS et al, *J Exercise Nutrition Biochem* 2015 19(3):235-45.

Mice studies suggest glasswort is a potential natural anti-obesity agent that can take the place of regular salt. Pichiah PB et al, *J Sci Food Agric* 2015 95(15):3150-9.

The compound isorhamnetin 3-O-beta-D-glucopyranoside exhibits anti-adipogenic activity, and alleviates lipid accumulation associated with obesity. Kong CS & Seo Y, *Immunopharmacol Immunotoxicol* 2012 34(6):907-11.

The flavanones and chromone derivatives appear to alleviate serious septicemia, in lab studies. Tuan NQ et al, *J Agric Food Chem* 2015 63(46):10121-30.

The seeds show potent anti-oxidant activity and ethyl ether extracts show cytotoxicity against human colon cancer cell lines. Kang et al, *J Ethnopharmacology*.

Betalains reduce COX-2, suggestive of anti-inflammatory activity. Farabegoli F et al, *Food Chem* 2017 218:356-64.

Salbige A and B exhibit potent anti-proliferative activity to A549 cancer cells, and pheophorbide A shows inhibition of A549 and HepG2 cancer cell lines. Zhao Y et al, *Food Chem* 2014 151:101-9.

Polysaccharides from S. herbacea exhibit activity against human colon cancer cells. Ryu DS et al, *J Microbiol Biotechnol* 2009 19(11):1482-9.

Perennial Glasswort may be useful in protecting against lead-induced toxicity in kidney cells. Gargouri M et al, *Ecotoxicol Environ Saf* 2013 95:44-51.

Glasswort extracts (*S. freitagii*) exhibit high anti-proliferative activity against HT-29 and Caco-2 cancer cell lines. Altay A et al, *Chem Biodivers* 2016 October 4.

PERSONALITY TRAITS

Since Glasswort droops over the water by which it grows, it has been compared to a woman with some pretension to beauty spending her time admiring her reflected image.   **POWELL**

Leaf and flower seem at first sight to have disappeared, both being reduced to an extreme degree. The dried herb has a high content of common salt, and may be considered vegetabilised salt…The reader who has gain perceptive awareness of form-giving forces will have realized how the plant archetype takes on different shapes, and indeed become excessively active within it. To balance this, he might consider plant families, which link themselves to extreme degree to the opposite pole, to animal nature.

In the one type of plant, the root element hypertrophies; in the other, the flowering element gains the upper hand, the root process wastes away and they have to become parasitic flowers.

The root-stressed plant on the other hand lose their flowering nature. One might mentally compare the glasswort and, say, a tropical orchid (one which is parasitic on trees), with its bemusing scent, its animal-like flower, its colouring which speaks of astral spheres, being almost an aura. With such images, such forms created by the magic of life, it is possible to enhance one's ability to penetrate, through contemplation of form, to the forces which give form.   **WILHELM PELIKAN**

RECIPES

SAMPHIRE PICKLE- Wash and drain two cups of fresh samphire. Pack loosely in a jar with a pinch of horseradish, some nasturtium or mustard seeds and peppercorns. Some people use onions and lemon slices.

Boil together one cup of vinegar, and one cup of cider (or two cups apple cider vinegar), a pinch of salt and pour over samphire. Place in a warm oven for one hour. Cover and cool. Store in fridge.

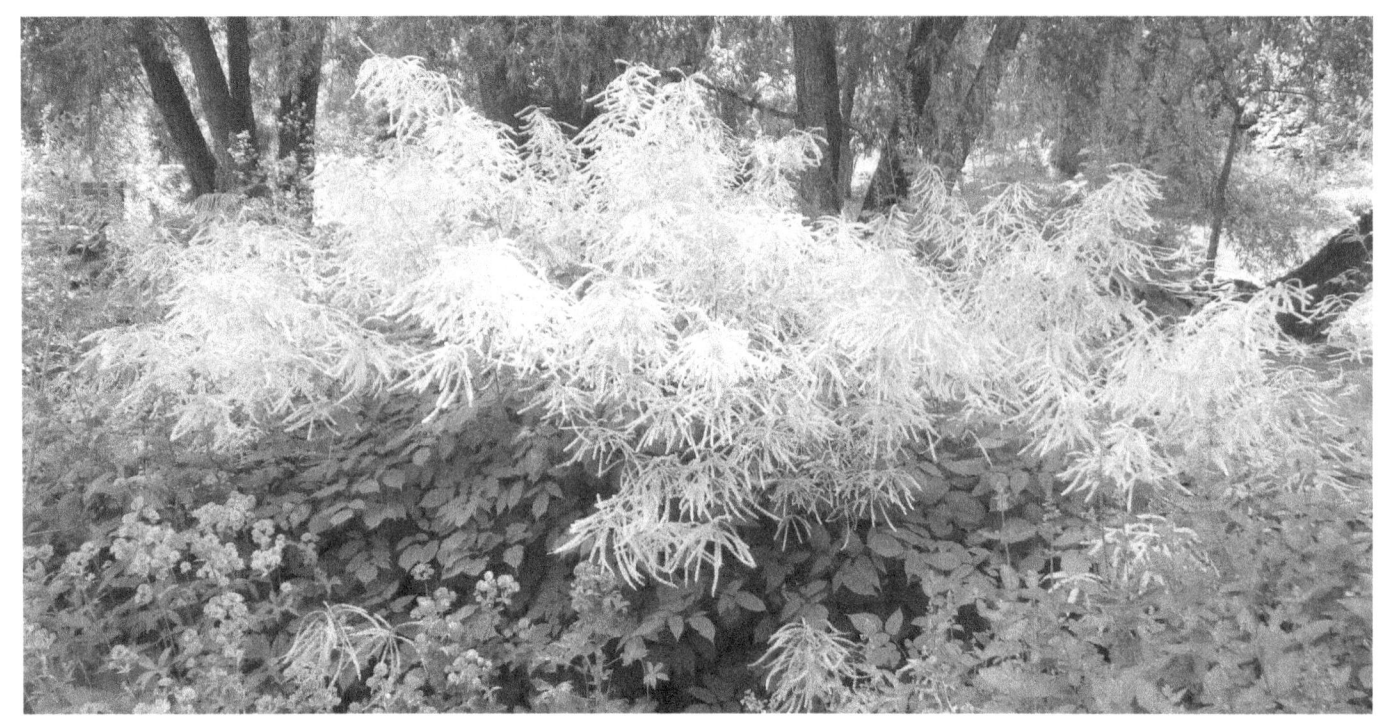

GOAT'S BEARD

GOAT'S BEARD
SYLVAN GOAT'S BEARD
SPAGHETTI FLOWER
(**Aruncus dioicus** [Walter] Fern)
BRIDE'S FEATHERS
(**A. sylvester** Kostel. ex Maxim.) not accepted
(**A. dioicus var vulgaris** [Maxim.] H. Hara)
(**A. acuminatus** Rydb.) not accepted
PARTS USED- root, stems

Aruncus may be from the Latin **ARUNDO** means reed-like, or more likely from the Greek **ARYNGOS** meaning, Goat's beard.

Goat's Beard, or Spaghetti Flower is a tall perennial (1-2 metres) of the moist forests, and found alongside roads and clearings. It is dioecious, meaning it has male and female flowers on separate plants.

It shares a common name with *Trogopogon dubius*, a low growing yellow flower, with a seed head resembling a large dandelion fluff. That is the only similarity.

This Goat's Beard, named for its large, fluffy white flower clusters, is a member of the rose family.

In northern Italy, the young shoots are gathered and eaten as a vegetable.

The plant was used in various ways by First Nations peoples of British Columbia. The Tlingit decocted the root for blood problems, while the Nuxalk and Bella Coola used the tea for stomach trouble, gonorrhea and as a diuretic. The Makah decocted the root tea for kidney trouble and gonorrhea. They call the plant **XA'XA'TSBUKKUK**, or flowers that look like herring eggs.

The leaves were chewed as a remedy for spitting up blood from the lungs, and tuberculosis.

The roots were simmered in mountain goat fat for application to the deadly smallpox, while the Lummi tried the leaves, chewing them up and applying them to the skin vesicles.

168

The Kwakwaka'wakw made a cough medicine from the root, which was dried and then soaked, scraped and held in the mouth.

The Skagit burned the twigs and mixed the ashes with bear grease to make a salve for swellings, particularly for the throat region.

In fact, they call the plant **PESDE'DA'TS** meaning, "swollen part goes down".

The Klallam used root salve for indolent sores and ulcers that would not heal.

The Sagkit made a root infusion that was taken for colds and sore throats; while the Comox steeped the roots and drank it for swellings in the body.

Squamish women took an infusion of the roots just before childbirth, in order to "help heal the insides". Small sips were often given to pregnant women to prevent excessive hemorrhage following labor.

The Thompson tribe made a salve of the stalk ashes and grease to relieve paralysis, and a decoction of the roots for colds, flu, and internal ailments, including swellings, indigestion, and general stomach upset. Teit made note that the Uta'mkt used it during the "Spanish Influenza" of 1918 and to relieve paralysis.

The Cherokee, further southeast, made a poultice of the root for bee stings on the face or eye. An infusion of the root was used to prevent excessive bleeding at childbirth; to bath swollen feet; or to stop excessive urination.

Folk healers of the Appalachians call it Ghost Breath. You made a tea of the root if you suffered a bad dream.

The leaves and stems contain hydrocyanic glycoside, and the seeds contain saponins.

It is used in central Europe for digestive complaints and reducing fevers. The variety *kamtschaticus* is eaten as a wild vegetable in Korea. It is also used for skin care, detoxification and tonsillitis. It is sometimes referred to as Mountain Asparagus.

Research by Kim DH et al, suggests plant extracts may be used to reduce UV-B induced skin aging and as a potential cosmoceutical material. *J Nat Med* 2012 66(4):631-6.

Today, it is a common nursery plant, used at the back of gardens as a border. Be careful, as it will take over a small garden. The cultivar *Kneiffii* is shorter with more finely divided foliage.

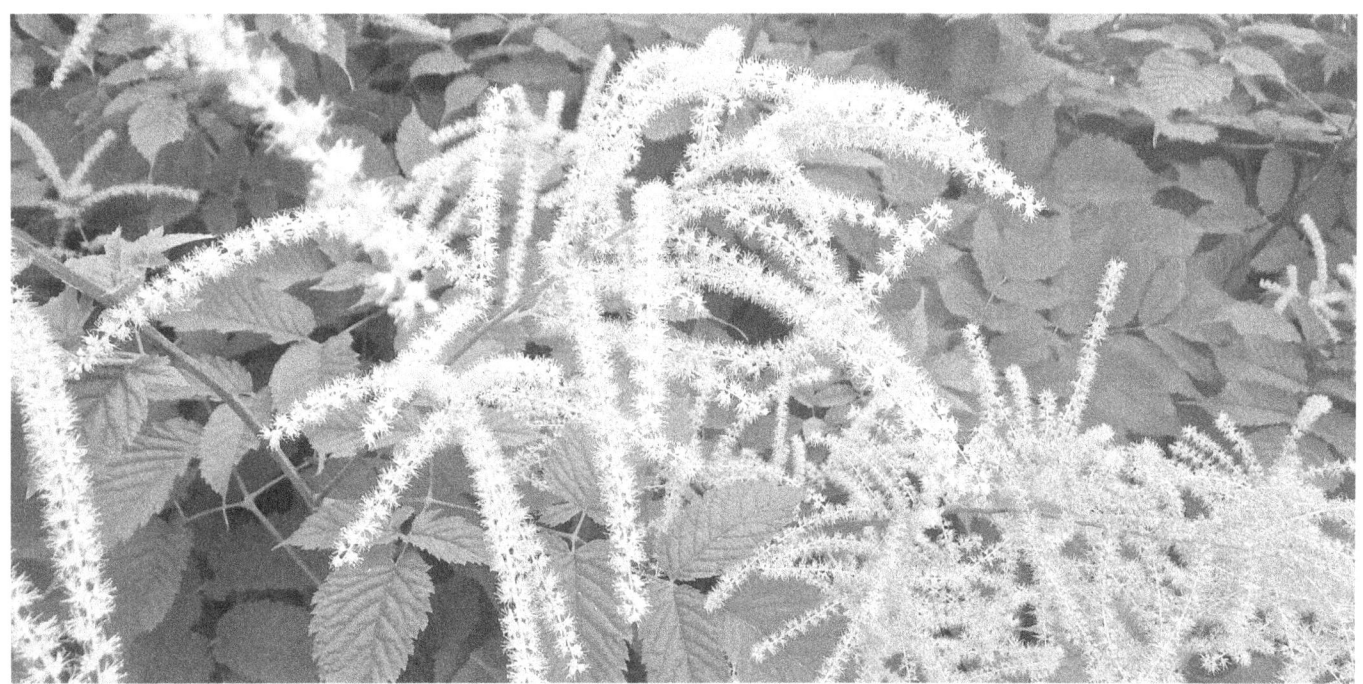

CLOSE UP OF FLOWERS

MEDICINAL

CONSTITUENTS- root- n-coumaric, ferulic and caffeic acids; cofeil-1-beta-D-gluco-pyranose; 1,3,4-tri-O-(E)-caffeoyl-beta-D-glucopyranoside, 1,4-di-O-(E)-caffeoyl-beta-D-glucopyranoside.
Young shoots- aruncins A, C, D, and E, aruncide A-E, cimicifugolide, caffeoylglucose derivatives, prunasin (increases after first green leaves).

An early study by Abraham EP et al, *Nature* 1946 identified an antibiotic compound in the plant.

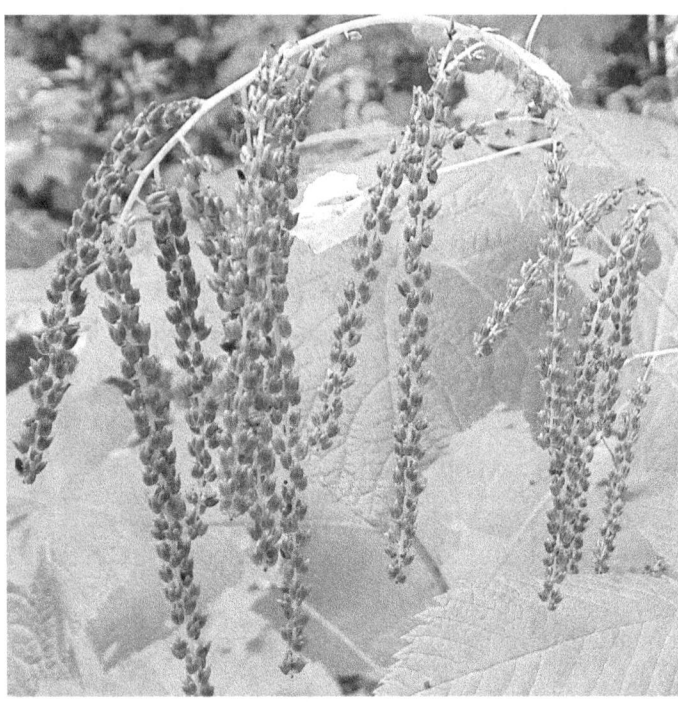

MATURE SEED HEADS

Some of the compounds in young shoots show weak cytotoxicity against human prostate adenocarcinoma cell lines. Granica S et al, *Food Chem* 2017 221: 1851-9.

Alcohol extracts appear to reduce kidney damage associated with ischemia/re-perfusion injury. Baek HS et al, *Prev Nutr Food Sci* 2012 17(2): 101-8.

Aruncin B, identified in this species, has been found to induce apoptosis (self-programmed death) via a novel microtubule damaging pathway. More research on our local species is warranted. Han et al, *Bioorg Med Chem Letters* 2012 22(2): 945-53.

Aruncin B also shows potent cytotoxicity against Jurkat T cells. Jeong SY et al, Bioorg Med Chem Lett 2011 21(11):3252-6.

The roots contain various phenylpropanoid glycosides that exhibit significant free radical scavenging ability, roughly half of ascorbic acid. Que M et al, *J Asian Nat Prod Res* 2014 16(2):158-62.

FLOWER ESSENCE

Goats beard flower essence enables us to see ourselves as calm and relaxed in stressful situations. It activates the thymus gland to deal with stress effectively. This is the remedy of non-action, of resolving tension by creating a state of inner alignment before taking action.

Goats beard reminds us that desires can be fulfilled only when we are willing to balance mental, physical and emotional by pausing in peace. Only then can we be fully able to respond to whatever life presents to us. Rest before activity brings greater fulfillment from the action.

Primarily a remedy for the mental aspect, it is also related to the Small Intestine meridian in Chinese medicine, and assists us with the assimilation of experience. Its connection with the Spleen strengthens the immune system and promotes the production of white blood cells. **PACIFIC**

SPIRITUAL PROPERTIES

"Let me bathe you with my healing white cascade of flowers.
Let me nourish your wei qi. Let me support your immunity.
I am the energy of the goat-sure footed and determined.
I give you the ability of the cat-
To sink down into the ground of being where harmony prevails." **PETTITT**

YELLOW GOAT'S BEARD
WESTERN SALSIFY
(*Tragopogon dubius* Scop.)
(*T. major* Jacq.) not accepted
COMMON SALSIFY
OYSTER PLANT
WHITE SALSIFY
(*T. porrifolius* L.)
MEADOW GOAT'S BEARD
MEADOW SALSIFY
JACK GO TO BED AT NOON
(*T. pratensis* L.)
PARTS USED- roots, flowers

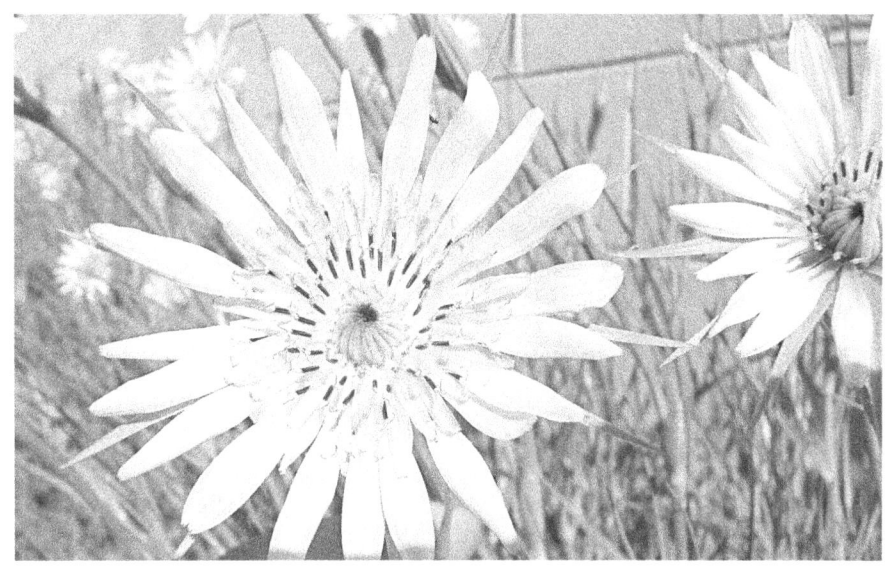
YELLOW GOAT'S BEARD

The Goats beard, which each morn
Abroad goes peep,
But shuts its flower at noon, and goes
To sleep.

ABRAHAM COWLEY

Tragopogon is from the Greek **TRAGOS** meaning Goat; and **POGON** meaning Beard; probably in allusion to the silky pappus. Porrifolius is from the leaves of Leek (*Allium porrium*). Dubius means doubtful, but I'm unsure of what; perhaps its place or origin.

Salsify is a corruption of the Latin **SOLSEQUIUM** from **SOL** the sun, and **SEQUENS**, following. This is probably due to the flowers habit of tracking the sun.

Goat's beard is a fairly common biennial of the prairies that has moved further north with time. It is found in waste spots, along roadsides, and rail tracks.

The lemon yellow flowers close at mid-day, when their long bracts close over the flowers. All open up to seed resembling a large dandelion fluff.

The white, flesh roots of *T. dubius* exude a thick orange substance.

Natives of Alberta used the white sap juice like chewing gum. It was first gathered and rolled up and dried.

Common garden salsify has purple flowers; with a fleshy, white root that is often called "Vegetable Oyster", due to its subtle flavor. It tastes, to me, more like asparagus, with a coconut after taste.

When peeling salsify, plunge it in cold water with some apple cider vinegar or bit of lemon juice to prevent it turning black.

Soil pH should be at 7.0 or slightly higher; light frosts help give the distinctive flavour a boost. They can be harvested in fall, or over wintered for an early spring crop.

It was well known to ancient Greeks and Romans, who gathered the wild roots, and favored them for treating indigestion.

It is used in present day Lebanon to treat cancer and liver dysfunction.

It was introduced into North America in the 17th century, and valued as a diuretic with tonic properties.

The Goat's Beard roots are very bitter, and need proper preparation. They need to be cleaned, scraped and soaked for over an hour in water. Boil until tender and then add to casserole, or deep fry in batter.

Roasted, and ground, the roots make a decent coffee substitute.

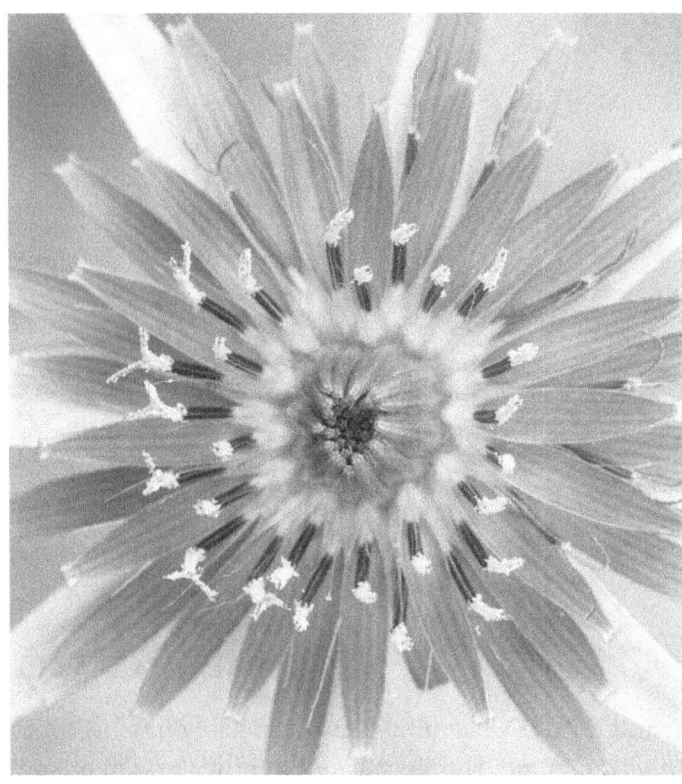

The young shoots, from the second year roots, can be used as an asparagus or artichoke substitute. Cut the crown and young stalk, wash and steam.

John Evelyn, an English herbalist said of the roots... "tho' medicinal, and excellent against the palpitation of the heart, faintings, obstruction of the bowels. etc, are besides a very pleasant sallet."

Meadow Salsify was suggested by Culpepper as, "very good for the heartburn, loss of appetite, disorders of the breast and liver; expels sand and gravel, and even small stones."

Traditionally, the plant tea was taken by humans or given to livestock bitten by rabid coyotes. How often does this come up in your neighborhood?

Historically, the plants are of taxonomic and genetic significance. Linnaeus, in 1759, made the first deliberate and scientifically conceived interspecies cross by hybridizing *T. porrifolius* with *T. pratensis*. This hydridization has been going on ever since. The hybrids are diploid and tend to grow taller with more buds.

WHITE SALSIFY FLOWER

A fungus *Ustilago tragopogi*, sometimes attacks the plants, reducing the flower head to a black powder.

Goat's Beard is often included in floral clocks, which were first devised by Linnaeus, and became quite popular in 19th century England. The plants, of course, all open their petals to release pollen or invite nectar seekers to improve fertilization. In the case of Goat's Beard, if it is cloudy, the flowers open at 5 a.m. and close at 9 p.m.

Otherwise, they open with the sun, and close by noon. Farmers of France and England observed the flowers to determine their lunch break.

The plants indicate gold may be present in the soil, according to some authors.

MEDICINAL

CONSTITUENTS- *T. pratensis-* various tragopogonosides A-I, tormentic acid glucoside ester.
roots- 5 triterpenic glycosides, inulin, inositol, mannitol and plant sterols.
T. porrifolius- root- potassium, calcium, iron, niacin, thiamin, riboflavin, phosphorus and protein, ascorbic acid, tragopogonic acid, three dihydroisocoumarin derivatives, three bibenzyl derivatives.
As a genus, Tragopogon contains vitexin, isovitexin, O-xylosylisovitexin, swertisin, vicenin-1, vicenin-2, orientin, isoorientin, swertiajaponin, lucenin-1, lucenin-2 (C-glycosylflavones).
T. dubius seed- gold

Goat's Beard is not used medicinally as much as past years. It is anti-bilious, diuretic, emollient, expectorant, mild laxative and de-obstructant. That is it is said to liquefy bile that has become too thick.

All three plants relieve heartburn, due to their ability to improve digestion. The root tea is most useful for stimulating urination, and removal of small sand and gravel in the kidneys.

Goat's Beard root has a detoxifying action, stimulating appetite and digestion. Its high inulin content makes it suitable food for diabetics. Inulin is made of fructose, rather than glucose sugars, and does not raise blood glucose levels.

The milky sap can be applied externally to wounds and cuts, or bleeding sores.

172

Tormentic acid appears to irritate inflammatory bowel conditions, suggested the herb be avoided in diets of those suffering colitis, Crohn's disease and IBS.

It may, however, have benefit in the prevention and treatment of atherosclerosis. Wang YL et al, *Mol Med Rep* 2016 14(4):3559-64.

It may also be useful in the treatment of osteoarthritis, based on work by Yang Y et al, *Inflammation* 2016 39(3): 1151-9.

Tormentic acid may offer neuroprotection related to Parkinson's disease, via activation of P13-k/Akt/GSK3beta signaling pathway. Zhao Q et al, *Neurochem Int* 2016 97: 117-23.

Tormentic acid shows higher cytotoxicity against ACHN kidney cancer cell lines than vinblastine. Loizzo MR et al, *Anticancer Agents Med Chem* 2013 13(5):768-76.

The root may be decocted and used as a dental rinse for periodontal disease. Tormentic acid has been shown to reduce inflammation caused by *Porphyromonas gingivalis*, a leading cause of oral disease. Jian CX et al, *Arch Oral Biol* 2015 60(9); 1327-32.

Tormentic acid is also found in various species of Rosa, Potentilla and Agrimony genera.

Meadow Goat's Beard leaves, when young, can be juiced and used to neutralize excessive gall bladder function. The seed heads show activity against *Staphylococcus aureus*. Borchardt et al, *J Med Plants Res* 2008 2:5.

The leaf and stem show activity against J-45.01 human acute T leukemia cell lines, via apoptosis. Wegiera et al, *Acta Pol Pharm* 2012 69(2): 263-8.

The flower phenolics inhibit proliferation of HaCaT cancer cell lines. Kucekova Z et al, *Molecules* 2011 16(11): 9207-17.

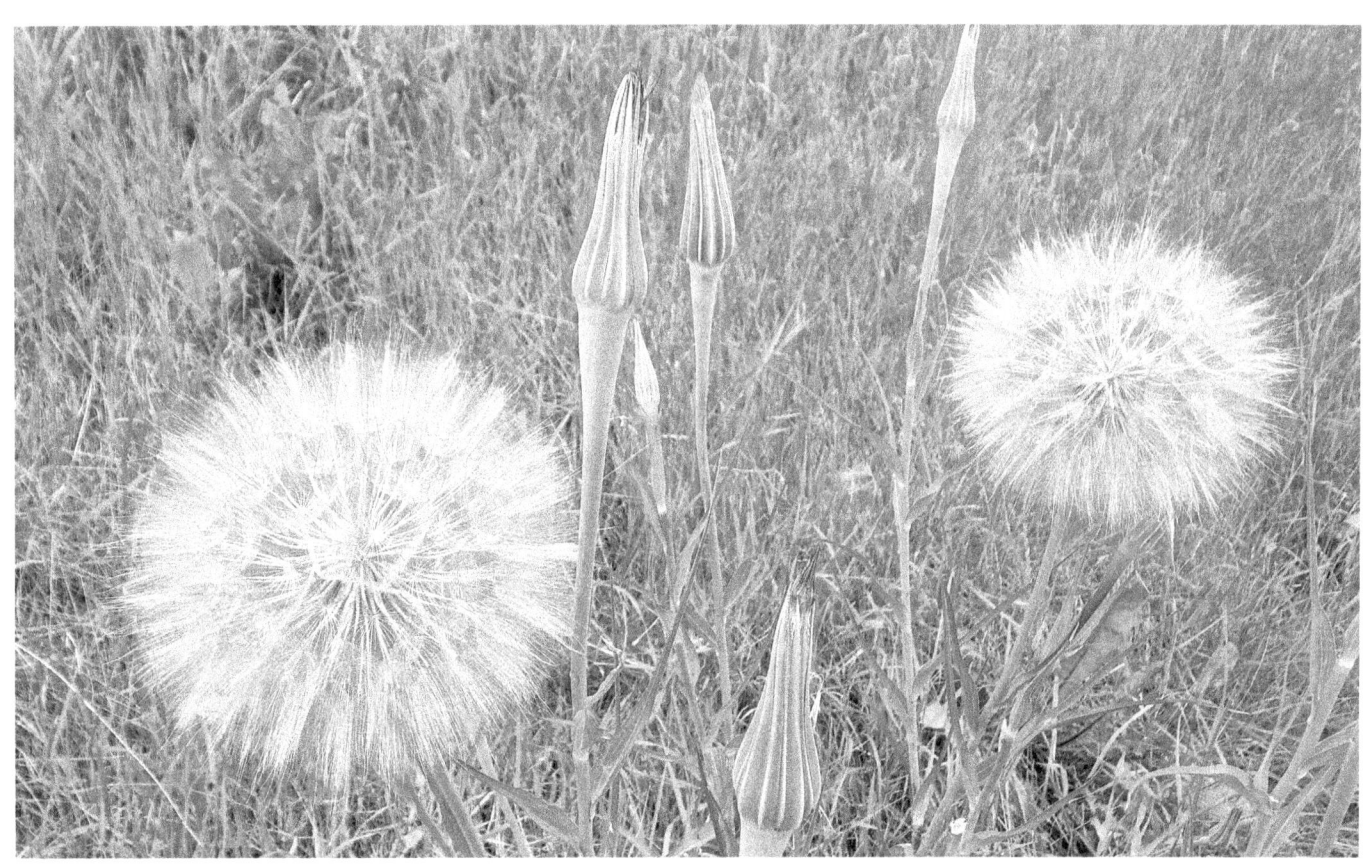

GOAT'S BEARD IN SEED

Salsify root is a common winter food in southern Europe. It is a cleansing plant, and is used to treat arteriosclerosis and high blood pressure.

The root is good for gout, and rheumatoid arthritis. The juice can be applied directly to warts.

It is a rich source of naturally occurring fructooligosaccharides (FOS) that are prebiotic for intestinal microflora.

Studies by Long X et al at the ABA Institute in 1990, found the root to exhibit anti-fatigue and improve resistance in low oxygen environments (anoxia) created in the lab.

The seed tips of *T. dubius* are high in organic gold, which is anti-inflammatory and useful in arthritis.

White Salsify alcohol extracts show activity against KHOS cancer cell lines, reducing total cell count or inducing apoptosis in a drastic manner. Al-Rimawi F et al, *Evid Based Complement Alternat Med* 2016:2016:9612490.

Alcohol extracts show potent liver protection, and activity against MDA-MB-231 human breast cancer and Caco-2 colorectal cancer cell lines. Tenkerian C et al, *Evid Based Complement Alternat Med* 2015;2015:161720.

The root, fed to mice, prolonged their duration of swimming and stick climbing, anti-fatigue and anoxia toleration. Long X and Tian J. *Zhongguo Zhong Yao Za Zhi* 1990 15(12): 741-3.

Water extracts of the aerial parts show evidence of improving lipid profiles and increased short-term satiety, at least in rats. Zeeni N et al, *Appetite* 2014 72:1-7.

Vicenin-2, present in all species, can help inhibit vascular inflammation associated with diabetic complications and atherosclerosis. Ku SK and Bae JS, *Can J Physiol Pharmacol* 2016 94(3): 287-95.

It appears to combine well with docetaxel in the treatment of advanced and metastatic prostate cancer. This compound is also found in Tulsi or Holy Basil. Singhai SS et al, *Biochim Biophys Acta* 2017 1868(1): 167-175.

ESSENTIAL OIL

The aerial parts of white salisfy have been steam distilled and analyzed by GC mass spectrometry. Thirty-eight constituents were found including carbonylic compounds (24.6%), phenols (21.5%) and fatty acids and esters (19.7%). The most abundant compounds were 4-vinyl-guaiacol (19%), hexadecanoic acid (17.9%), hexahydrofarnesylacetone (15.8%) and hentriacontane (10.7%).

HYDROSOL

Meadow Salsify distilled water "gives relief to pleurisy, stitches or pains in the sides".

FLOWER ESSENCES

Yellow Goat's Beard flower essence is for those who have difficulty with life transitions.

It can be a useful remedy in all phases of change, from childhood to puberty, from single to married, from married to divorced or widowed.

It is a special remedy for those who have difficulty with mental and physical energy from 2-4 pm.
PRAIRIE DEVA

Salsify supports us in the maturation process if we have difficulty in bringing a project or some aspect of ourselves to fruition. It is excellent for finding all the vital elements for growth and the expression of our full potential.
DESERT ALCHEMY

Salsify (T. porrifolius) is useful when you feel like you are walking on a tightrope. Purple Salsify creates a transmuting synergy and stable foundation for integrating energies after a soul expansion.
VORTEX ESSENCES

PERSONALITY TRAITS

Goat's beard's nature is such that it is always accustomed to break whatever exists in the same place it resides. So it dashes to pieces whatever is fetid, where it finds it.   **HILDEGARD**

Scientists have recently found that biological clocks exist in plants. Plant physiologist Autar K. Mattoo, from Maryland, has spent considerable time studying these internal clocks.

He found that the clock controls an enzyme that modifies D1, a protein critical to photosynthesis. Binding phosphorus to D1 at a specific threshold provides a plant with a bio-timing signal that tells it to adjust its metabolism to face the onset of the day's brightest light. The plant also puts on its own sunscreen, to protect itself from UVB radiation.

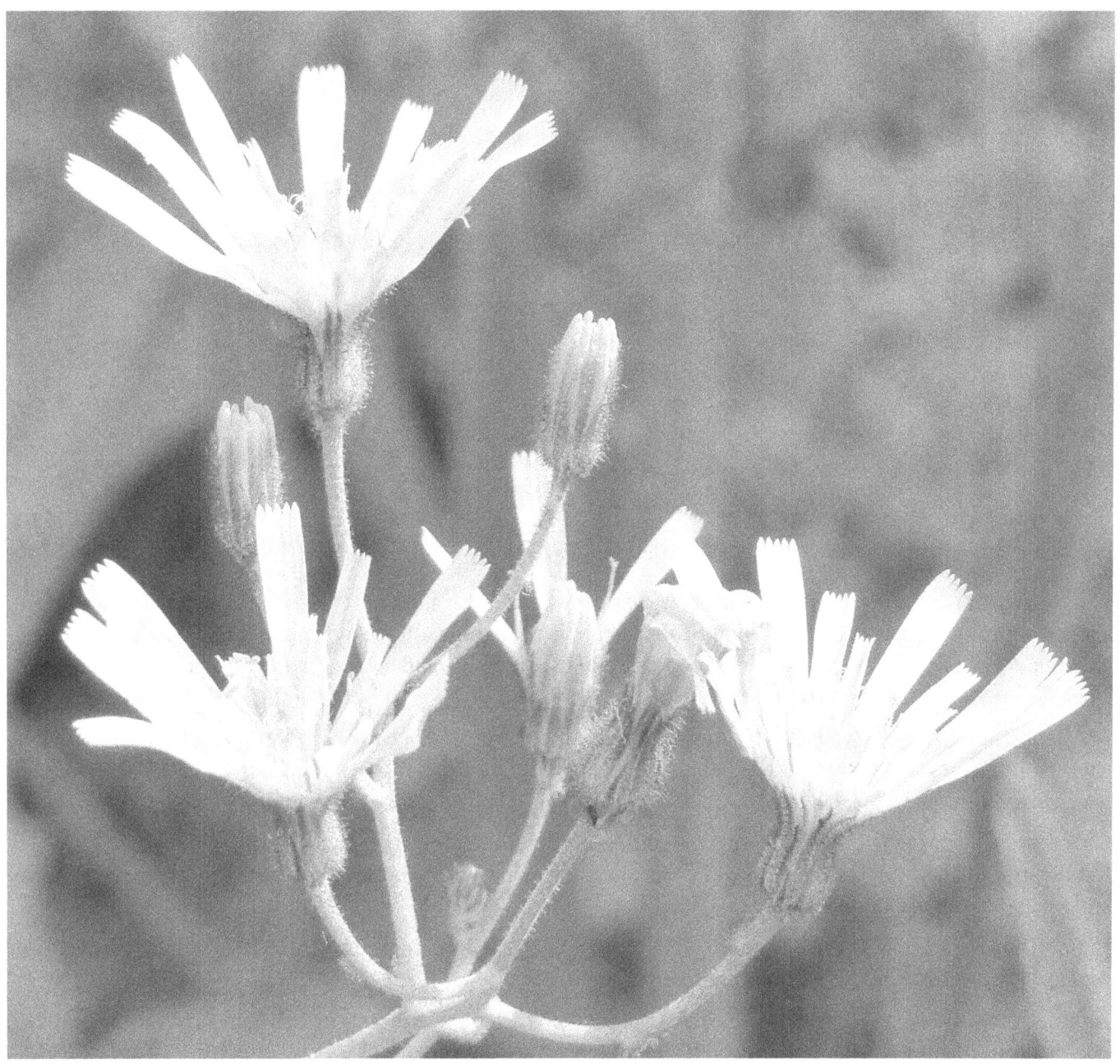

MEADOW GOAT'S BEARD (*T. dubius*)

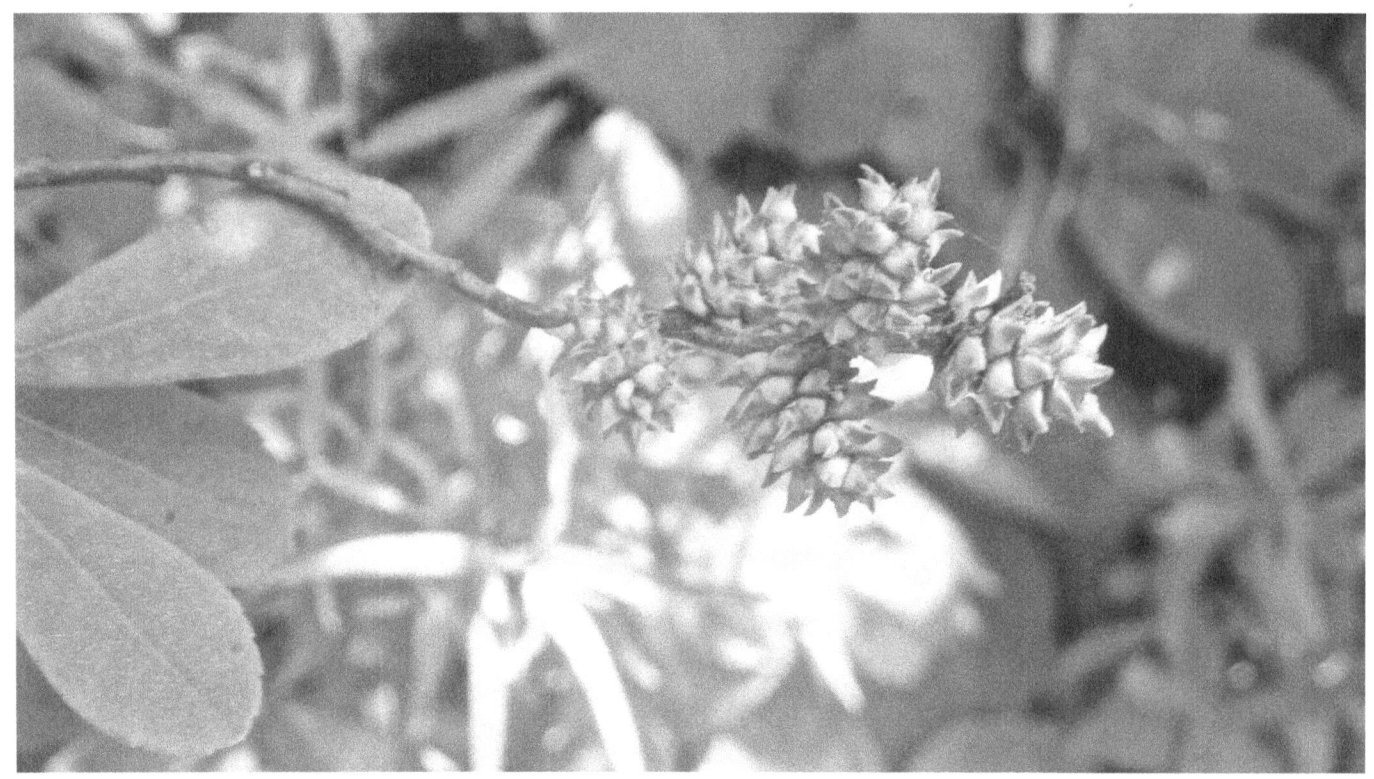

SWEET GALE LEAF AND CATKINS

SWEET GALE
(**Myrica gale** L.)
(**Gale palustris** A. Chev.) not accepted
PARTS USED- leaves, catkins, flowers and buds

I love to go forth ere the dawn to inhale
The health breathing freshness that floats in the gale.

ANON

I found a low-branching shrub frozen into the ice near its edge with a fine spicy scent, somewhat like sweet fern, and a handsome imbricated bud. When I rubbed the dry-looking fruit in my hands, it felt greasy and stained them a permanent yellow, which I could not wash out. It lasted several days and my fingers smelled medicinally.

THOREAU

Myrica is from the Greek **MYRIZEIN** meaning to perfume or from **MURIO** or **MYRO** to flow, because it inhabits river banks, or because it resembles Tamarisk. Myrica may be from the German **MIRTLEBAUM** so-named because it resembled a kind of myrtle.

Gale may be from the Latin **GALEA** meaning helmet, referring to the brown catkins; from **GALL**, in reference to the bitter quality; the German **GAGEL,** or from the Norse **GAYR**, meaning foolish. The last may be closest and related to the use in ale cited below.

In Scotland, sweet gale is the badge of the Campbell Clan. The Vikings used infusions to treat problems of memory, depression and to maintain well-being.

Although common to the Canadian Shield, it occupies only a small northeast corner of Alberta, and a great deal of Northern Manitoba. It tends to inhabit the same type areas as hardhack (*Spiraea*). The Slave call it **DAKONE**, while the Northern Cree call it **NWAKOPAKWAHTIK**.

Decoctions of stem, leaf and catkin are used by the Slave to treat tuberculosis.

The leaves have been connected with money, and putting a leaf in your wallet helps fill it with other green. The wax is used for meditation candles associated with ensuring plenty.

The wax is extracted from the shoots and catkins by soaking them in warm, salted water.

Branches were fixed to the eaves of houses in Scandinavia to repel witches; and even today a bunch is kept for good luck.

An ancient name Flea wood relates to the insect repelling quality of the branches, and use in woven mattresses. The branch bark was used to tan leather.

The Cree used the flower buds of this small shrub to dye their porcupine quills. Known as **MWAKOPAKWATIK** to the Woods Cree, the fragrant catkins were collected in fall, dried, and used as a trap lure.

The male catkins are orange colored and stalk-less, growing in crowded clusters, while the female flowers are on a separate plant, and are red, thicker and shorter than the male. In flower, the plant gives a lovely resinous scent.

The Bella Coola on the west coast, used decoctions of the dried branches as a diuretic, and attempted to cure gonorrhea with it.

The leaf infused by Alaskan natives as a tea for tuberculosis. Switches for the steam bath were made from the whole plant. The northern Dene gargled leaf tea for mouth infections and sore throat, and applied it to skin rashes, and sore eyes.

It is called Monkey Bush, by the Stl'atl'imx tribe, possibly because it was used by Bigfoot, the Sasquatch.

The Mik'maq of Nova Scotia used its close cousin bayberry (*M. cerifera*), as a stimulating beverage made from leaves, berries and bark. Sweet Gale root was reserved for pounding and soaking in hot water to relieve inflammation.

Like Labrador tea, buckbean and sundew, the sweet gale loves its feet in acidic, boggy marsh. Use the aromatic leaves to ward off the mosquitoes and black flies that also love the same area. The leaves have a pleasant odour, that repels moths and ants. Sweet Gale can also be used to lightly scent stored linens.

The fresh leaves make a pleasant and refreshing campfire tea. You can dry the leaves and flavor stews or soups, the dried buds can be crushed and added to venison and poultry dishes.

The tea, taken hot, will often nip a cold or flu. It has a long history of astringent use, for diarrhea and sore throats.

The British and Swedish used sweet gale branches as a hop substitute in beer making.

From the 14th -17th century, sweet gale was used as a source of taxation in Norway. Rent for farms could be paid in sweet gale, or **PORS** as it was known.

It was also used for flavoring ale when juniper, tansy, yarrow or St. John's Wort were not available. Numerous references to the strength of Pors ale, and its narcotic and intoxicating effect, cannot be validated by chemical analysis. Perhaps some unknown constituents combine with the alcohol.

Sweet Gale was commonly used in Ale production throughout Europe through World War II, even into the 1950s in rural parts of Scandinavia.

Gruit Ale, was THE Ale of Europe for over 700 years; and was primarily a combination of three mild to moderately narcotic herbs; sweet gale, yarrow and Labrador tea. It varied, according to the individual producer, who kept it secret.

Stephen Harrod Buhner, in *Sacred and Herbal Healing Beers*, (an excellent book) writes:

"Gruit Ale stimulates the mind, creates euphoria, and enhances sexual drive. The hopped Ale that took its place is quite different. Its effects are sedating and anaphrodisiacal."

Thorleif Bjornsson, in an Icelandic medicinal manuscript of 1475, notes, "its fragrance counteracts the shooting-pains in the head. Sweet gale, crushed, dries boils. The juice of sweet gale dries matter in the ears. Green sweet gale crushed with vinegar stops nosebleed if applied to the flesh; oil of sweet gale give the hair strength to grow more."

Today, the Heather Ale Company in Scotland produces several Sweet Gale Ales, including Fraoch, combined with heather flowers, and Grozet, combined with meadowsweet. They are also experimenting with a bitter vetch beverage. In 2000, this new company used 4,500 litres of pine and spruce shoots, 5,800 litres of sweet gale, and 2000 litres of meadowsweet flowering heads.

Maclays also produces a sweet gale beer called Honey Weizen, with a gingery flavour. Approximately 20 kilograms of leaves are used in a seventy barrel brew.

Plans are underway in Scotland by a company called *Scotia Pharmaceuticals* to increase production from 50 hectares to 5000 hectares by 2013 for essential oil production.

Rafinesque noted that the tincture of the berries with cow parsnip is used for violent flatulent colic cramps.

In parts of France, the peasants believed leaf decoctions would bring on menstruation and even abortions.

The Chinese sipped infusions of sweet gale to settle stomach upsets. Nordic Europeans made very strong decoctions of the leaves for washing itchy skin; and killing lice and fleas. Berry infusions were taken internally as a vermifuge.

The French used the leaves for emmenagogue and abortifacient conditions under the official name **HERBA MYRT RABANTINI**. The dried berries were added to broths and stews for flavour.

It is a good general tonic for farm animals, especially those lacking appetite or as a nerve tonic. Feed one handful several times daily of the fresh or dried leaves.

Sweet gale is also a good hair tonic, and rinsing with a mild decoction after cleansing will give the hair strength.

Various Myrica species have been dried and powdered as snuff, for nasal congestion. Sweet gale was crushed and applied to dry up boils.

The bark gives a yellow dye used traditionally for tanning leather.

The catkins, or cones are boiled in salt water and give a scummy wax used to make candles. The yield is small, but aromatic. The waxy wood is an excellent fire starter.

The catkin wax is more brittle than beeswax and yet combines well for candles, ointments and such.

It combines well with lye or caustic soda in the making of fragrant soap.

In Japan, some pharmaceuticals are stabilized in pastes containing the rubber adhesives from sweet gale leaves.

Myricitrin has been used in Japan as a flavor modifier in snack food, dairy products and beverages. It is considered GRAS by the United States. It inhibits acrylamide toxicity and may protect against colorectal cancer. Deep-fried foods, such as French fries, are significant contributors to this health concern. Chen W et al, *Biomed Res Int* 2013;2013:724183. A creative health food formulator could use this to good advantage in a sauce or "catsup" for the fast food industry.

MEDICINAL

CONSTITUENTS- stem- myricinic acid, c-methylated leaf flavanoids such as kaempferol-3-rhamnoside, myricetin-3-galactoside, myricanol, and quercitins; myricanone, myricitrin, galeon, hydroxygaleon, dihydrochalcones, diarylheptanoids (12-dehydroporson, 12-hydroxymyricanone), catechin, epicatechin, gallocatechin, epigallo-catechin, epigallocatechin-3-0-gallate, and other condensed tannins, and resins. Also contains macrocyclics like geleon and porson.
leaves- high in potassium, and nickel
twigs- high in molybdenum and zinc.
fruit- C-methylated dihydrochalcone, myrigalone B (flavonoid)

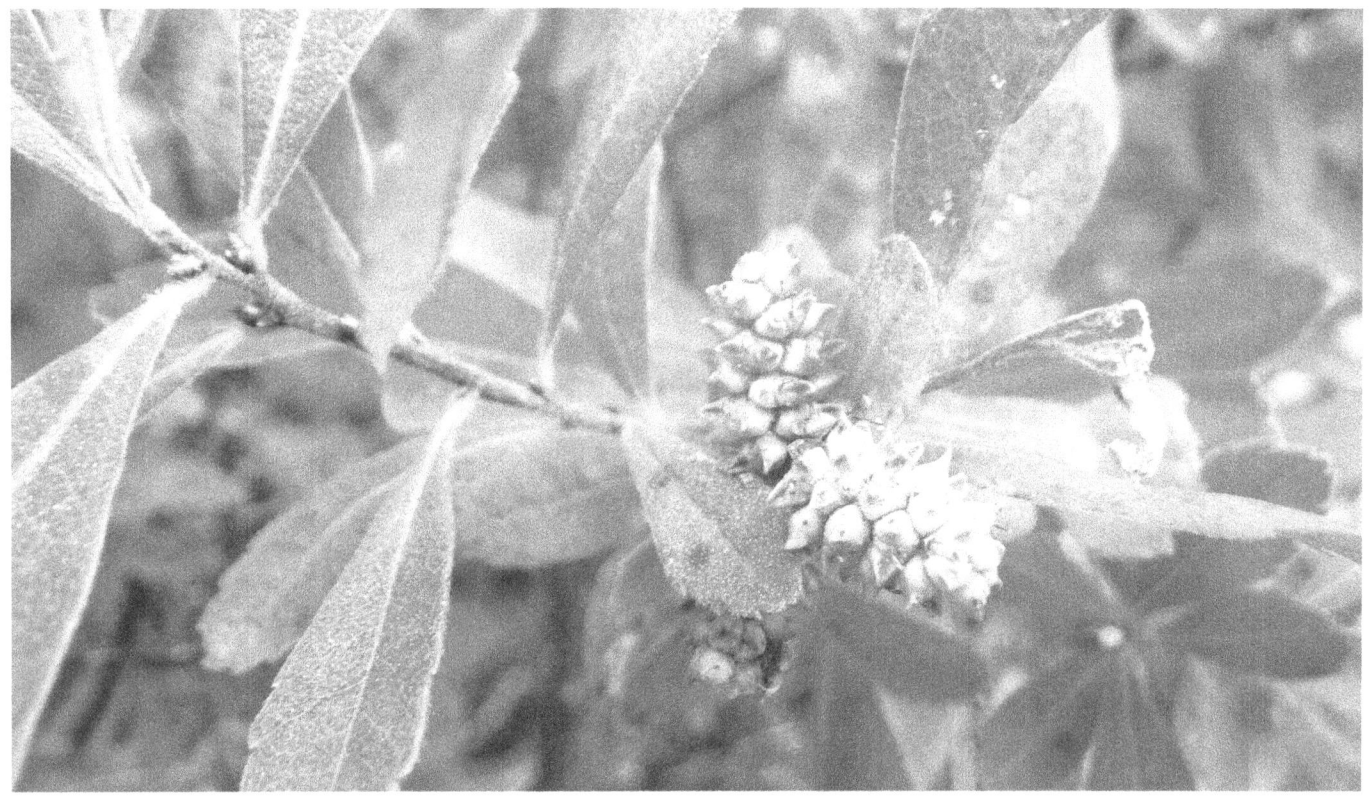

SWEET GALE

It is probable, according to Felter, Millspaugh, and other eclectic herbalists that sweet gale possesses many of the properties of its cousin, bayberry *(M. cerifera)*

The bark is dry, warm, astringent and stimulating; and useful in small doses in the treatment of catarrhal conditions of the digestive system.

The tincture is a good stimulant of the nervous system, as well as aiding digestion, blood formations and nutrition in small doses. In larger doses, it is a gastric stimulant.

Some authors have suggested its use in cases of feeble venous circulation, such as preventing varicose veins. It is a diaphoretic, circulatory stimulant, and therefore useful in cold, deficient conditions.

Fatigue, cold limbs, and mental depression are all indications of its use.

Mild infusions can be used for vaginal discharge, as well as bringing on delayed menstruation aggravated by cold.

The powdered gum is decocted and gargled for tender, spongy and bleeding gums. For ulcerated tonsils, combine with Echinacea or wild indigo, with eyebright for sinusitis with excessive mucous.

The wax from catkins is applied to slow healing skin ulcers.

A study by Iain Stewart, of the *Scottish School of Herbal Medicine*, suggests the herb has use for treating mild depression or stagnating psychological conditions where the patient would benefit from increased motivation.

An interesting study conducted on sweet gale at the University of Maine in 1995, showed that hemoglobin, probably in form of a dimer, was present in high concentrations in the root nodules. This could be of potential use.

Studies from the University of Oslo indicate gram-positive bacteria inhibition from leaf flavonoids. Early work by Bishop and MacDonald, *Can J Botany* 1956 29 found water, alcohol, ether and acetone extracts significantly inhibit *Staphylococcus aureus*.

The root and stems exhibit 93-99% activity against *Mycobacterium tuberculosis*, supporting traditional, indigenous use. Gordieu et al, *Phytother Res* 2009 Oct 13.

Porson exhibits activity against *Mycobacterium tuberculosis*, suggesting its use by Alaskan indigenous groups was well-founded. Ting YC et al, *Phytochemistry* 2014 103:89-98.

The most recent pharmacological studies have focused on myrigalone B, extracted from the fruit (catkin). It is a potent anti-oxidant that inhibits lipid peroxidation and may help protect liver tissue. MyB inhibits copper-induced peroxidation in low-density lipoprotein (LDL) from cholesterol fed humans, indicating a possible role in the prevention of atherosclerosis and a possible role in anti-oxidant and free radical scavenging in humans. Mathiesen et al, *Pharm Toxicol* 1996 78:3.

Sweet Gale was shown to inhibit human lung carcinoma cells. *Phytomed* 2005 12:4.

Matsuda et al, *Biol Pharm Bull* 2001 24:3 found myricanone exhibits 5-alpha reductase inhibition, suggesting use in prostate and other issues associated with testosterone metabolism. Ishida et al, *Biorg Med Chem* 2002 10:10 found the compound possesses significant anti-tumor activity.

Myricitrin shows marked inhibition of neurogenic pain in lab animals, without muscle relaxing or sedative activity. It is also found in hazelnut and black walnut.

Myricitrin suppresses myocardial apoptosis induced by doxorubicin, a widely used anti-neoplastic antibiotic. Sun J et al, *Evid Based Complement Alternat Med* 2016;2016:6093783.

It also attenuates H9c2 cell apoptosis induced by high glucose levels, suggesting benefit in patients with elevated blood sugar and cardiac damage. Zhang B et al, *Molecules* 2016 21(7).

The compound facilitates hippocampal neurogenesis, contributing to its anti-depressant-like effects and atypical anti-psychotic-like profile. Meyer E et al, *Behav Brain Res* 2017 316:59-65.

It appears to be neuroprotective, preventing dopaminergic neuronal degeneration, *in vivo*. Kim HD et al, *J Med Food* 2016 19(4): 374-82.

Myricitrin appears to modulate aromatase CYP19 and luteinizing hormone, suggesting possible benefit in fertility issues. Kassem ME et al, *Pharm Biol* 2016 54(11): 2404-9.

Myricitrin shows activity against Coxsackie A16 viruses, suggesting benefit in treating hand, food and mouth disease. Van Nguyen TH et al, *Nat Prod Commun* 2014 9(5):643-5.

Myricitrin significantly inhibit the inflammatory cytokines IL8 and TNFalpha associated with acne infections.

Myricanol induced apoptosis in HL60 cancer cells via both mitochondrial and death receptor pathways. Zhang J et al, *Chem Biodivers* 2016 13(11):1601-9.

It induced apoptosis in non-small cell lung carcinoma, in work by Dai G et al, *Int J Mol Sci* 2015 16(2): 2717-31.

Myricetin, myricanone and myricanol all appear to inhibit testosterone reductase inhibition and anti-androgenic activity. This suggests benefit in hormone related issues such as polycystic ovary syndrome, prostate enlargement or cancers, etc. Matsuda H et al, *Biol Pharm Bull* 2001 224(3): 259-63.

Myricetin and myricitrin are synergistic, helping induce apoptosis in prostate cancer cell line PC-3. Xu R et al, *Food Chem* 2013 138(1):48-53.

Microcanone induces apoptosis in HepG2 liver cancer cells. Paul A et al, *J Acupunct Meridian Stud* 2013 6(4): 188-98.

The fruit contains a flavonoid, C-methylated dihydrochalcone, a very rare compound in nature. It has anti-microbial and lipoxygenase-inhibiting activity. The above two appear to work well together.

Anti-viral activity was indicated in tincture extractions of sweet gale. Influenza A and *Pseudomonas pyocyanea* were suppressed. Traditional folkloric use of *Myrica gale* in Scandinavia for *Herpes zoster* (shingles) seems supported by this evidence.

A study conducted at the University of Strathclyde in Glasgow, Scotland 1990, showed a flavonoid from sweet gale leaves possessed anti-fungal activity.

Work by Popovici et al, *Nat Prod Res* 2008 22:12 confirmed the anti-fungal activity and its use in beer and as a spice for soups, stews and other foods.

Extracts of sweet gale, Labrador tea and yarrow all showed repellant activity against mosquitoes. Jaenson TG et al, *J Med Entomol* 2006 43(1):113-9.

An adhesive topical pharmaceutical paste containing sweet gale extracts was issued a Japanese patent in 1984.

HOMEOPATHY

Myrica cerifera has marked action on the liver, relieving sleeplessness.

The patient may be despondent, irritable, and gloomy.

There is characteristic dull, heavy aching around the temples and forehead on waking.

Stringy mucous in the mouth and throat; as well as a bitter and nauseous taste is common. There is loss of appetite, and a feeling of fullness in the stomach after a meal.

Accompanied dull pain in the liver region, with jaundice and bronze-yellow skin that itches, and crawls.

The urine may be dark, frothy, highly coloured and biliary.

The sleep is disturbed, with bad dreams and frequent waking.

DOSE- Tincture to the third potency. This is not *Myrica gale*, as it has not been proved, but may be very similar in actions.

ESSENTIAL OIL

CONSTITUENTS- germacrone, alpha pinene (41.3%) alpha phellandrene (6.5-10%), delta and gamma-cadinene, cineole, limonene (6.7-11%), beta-elemenone, 1.8-cineole, beta caryophyllene (9-11%), alpha-bisabolol (5%), para-cymene, nerol, selin-11-en-4-ol (14.6%), mycrene (12-21.9%) and palmitic acid. The yields of germacrone and beta-elemenone tend to diminish as the summer progresses. Carophyllene oxide content increases with length of distillation.
The brownish-yellow essential oil is strongly balsamic and aromatic. The yield is .076% from fresh leaves; and .0203% from the dried. Forty-one compounds were found in a study conducted in 1974, including the presence of selin-11-en-4-ol (14.6%) and alpha bisabolol (5%).
The catkins yield an essential oil (0.4-0.6%) containing alpha and beta pinene, d'alpha phellandrene, cineol, caryophyllene.
The wax yield is 0.5% from leaves and catkins; specific gravity of 0.876, melting point of 47-49 degrees°C; and solid at 12.5 degrees°C.
Recent work in Quebec, carried out by Belanger et al, in the *Journal of Essential Oil Research* 1997 shows a different picture. Sweet gale leaves when steam or hydro-distilled contained mycrene (7-20%), limonene (8-15%), p-mycene (3-10%) and beta-caryophyllene (9-18%).
When a supercritical CO2 extraction was made, limonene was 11%; selin-11-en-4-ol at 25% and nonacosane at 26%.
Sylvestre et al, *J Herb Spice Med Plant* found eudesm-11-en-ol 11.5%, mycrene 11.3%, beta carophyllene 8.4%, alpha phelladrene 7.1% in the Quebec plants.
A microwave assisted hexane extract contained over 71% nonacosane.
Headspace technology revealed even different ratios, with mycrene 32%, limonene 24%, and p-cymene, 19%.

The oil is strongly anti-tumor, anti-catarrhal and mucolytic. It is indicated for use in certain types of cancer (according to Dr. Penoel), and respiratory infections. It is contra-indicated for babies, infants and pregnant women, due to its abortive and neuro-toxic effect.

Work by Sylvestre et al, *Phytomedicine* 2005 12(4): 299-304 examined the anti-cancer activity of the oil against human lung carcinoma cell line A549 and human colon adenocarcinoma cell line DLD-1. Essential oil hydro-distilled for one hour showed activity against both cell lines with an IC50 value of 88 mcg/ml.

In 1994, sweet gale essential oil was found to have strong insect repellant properties that led to an anti-midge product now being produced in the United Kingdom. In an eight person trial for ten minutes, the essential oil applied to the naked arm yielded 13 bites vs. 155 for an unprotected limb.

A company on the Isle of Skye tested the essential oil as a way to control house mites, implicated with asthma. They also found the oil useful for pest control as in aphids and potato blight.

Work by Svoboda et al, in 1995 at the *Scottish Agricultural College*, found sweet gale essential oil very effective against all eight fungal species.

Scientists have recently discovered the oil four times more powerful than tea tree oil for killing bacteria associated with acne.

The oil is active against Gram-positive bacteria, particularly *Bacillus subtilis*. *Journal of Oleo Sci* 2013 62(9): 755-62.

In follow up work in 1998, they found the oil yield in Scotland was 0.11-0.29% from the leaves and 0.97% from flowers; while in Finland, it was 0.4-1.46% in buds, and 0l3-0.69% in flowers.

The main components were alpha pinene at 18-39%, 1,8-cineole (3.7-24%), and either germacrene (0.4-13%) in Scotland, or gamma cadinene (8.4-21%) in Finland.

WAX

The plant has berry like fruit covered with green yellow waxy secretions. The berries can be placed in hot water and when the wax floats to the surface, it can be skimmed off to make fragrant candles, or added to beeswax for an aromatic combination.

HYDROSOL

Sweet Gale floral water is very pleasant, complex and green in nature, the taste being somewhat sweeter, almost floral and yet green.

The pH is 3.7-3.8.

Suzanne Catty uses the hydrosol for lucid dreaming, meditation, group and distance healing, working with crystals and all forms of energy work. She considers this one of the most powerfully energetic of the waters she has tested.

It should be researched for anti-tumor activity, like the oil.

Avoid during pregnancy, lactation and in young children.

FLOWER ESSENCES

Sweet gale helps one identify and release deep emotional pain and tension. It is for the core of our emotional interactions with others, especially male/female relationships.   **ALASKA**

Sweet gale flower essence is for those individuals who are argumentative, and are seduced by emotional, rather than logical discussion. It is important to have a balance between the head and the heart, and it is important to recognize your own belief systems so that new information is not rejected out of hand.   **PRAIRIE DEVA**

Sweet Gale essence helps resolve conflict, and negative feelings by helping identify the process and then disband them.   **MIRIANA**

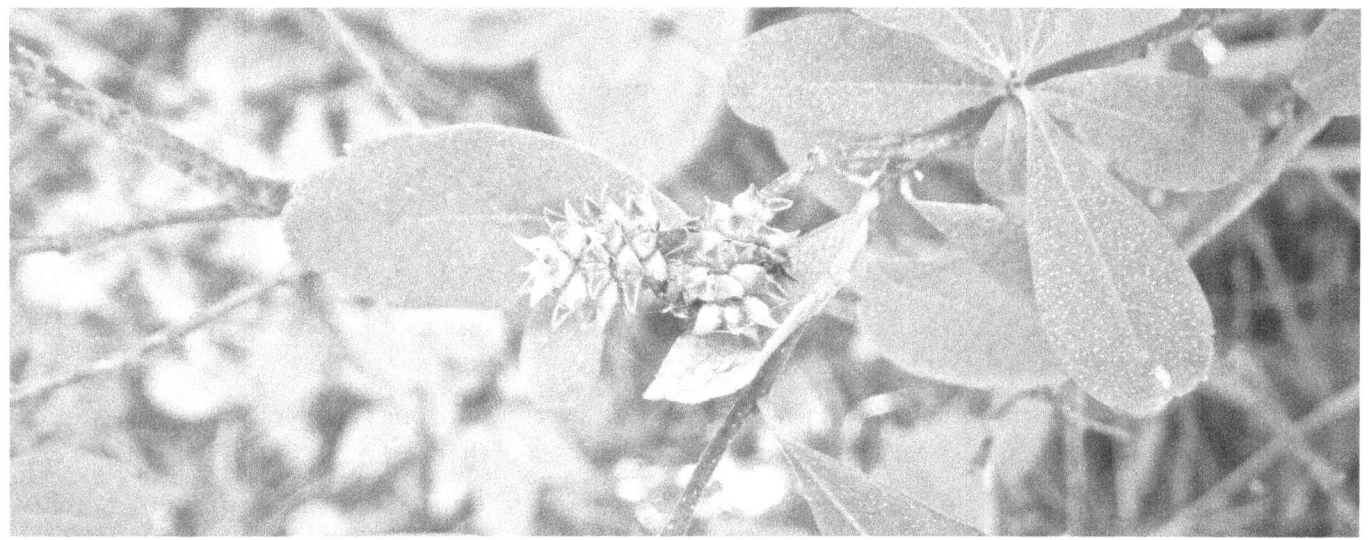

SWEETGALE LEAVES AND CATKINS

PERSONALITY TRAITS

Myricaceae grow in watery places and as such it is especially noteworthy that they affect water balance. There are chemical constituents that are known to go right to the heart of the fluid matter by affecting aldosterone, the hormone that regulates water and mineral salts in the body. **VERMEULEN**

Sweetgale is the wise old grandmother. She's one of the weavers who made this land. Her roots hold the land close like a basket, like a nest, not giving Earth away to the sweeping fingers of the water along shorelines. Her sweet comforting aroma invites us in to sleep safely on her shores.

Like all plants and animals She has a spirit twin. The totemic animal of Sweetgale is the loon…Our consciousness, like the Sweetgale roots are all interlaced underground and underwater. We are one in the collective dream realm.

While our dreams with Her may be more colourful, Her teachings that come to us are black and white, like Loon's markings. Loon's eye, orange like the setting sun, purifies us when we are in the dreamtime. Like Loon's masterful flying underwater, when we drink Sweetgale we have lucidity, we have the ability to move whatever direction we will in our dreams. **STEVEN MARTYN**

MYTHS AND LEGENDS

An eighteen-month old child who was fractious and not thriving, after a resentful beggar woman had cast the evil eye on her, was passed eighteen times through a burning hoop, then taken home and put to bed under a sprig of the bog myrtle, which was left in place for a month. By then, she had significantly improved in both health and temper; six months later she was fully recovered. **TESS DARWIN**

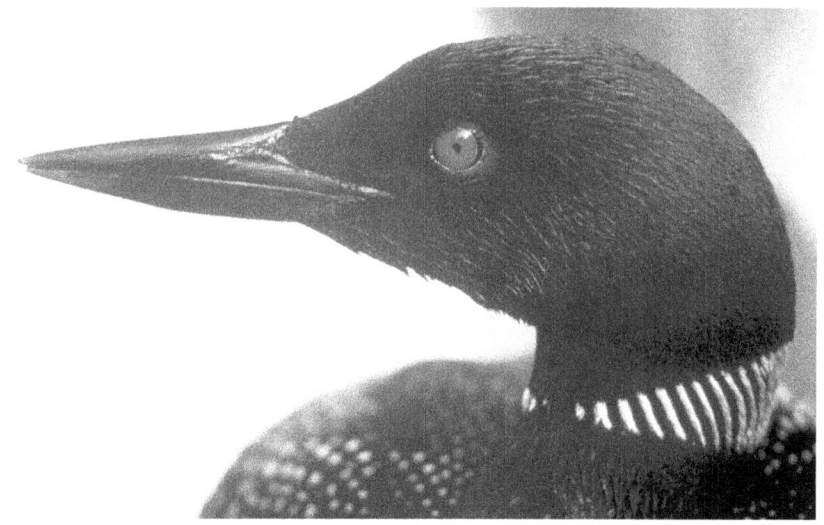

LOON

RECIPES

INFUSION- Lucid Dream Tea is one of my favorites. Steep and drink before bedtime.

DECOCTION- Take one ounce of leaves and catkins to one pint of boiling water. Continue to slowly simmer for thirty minutes. Sweeten if desired.

DOSE- One half cup as needed.

TINCTURE- Use 1:4 ratio of fresh leaves, buds and catkins in 60% alcohol. 10-20 drops as needed.

GRUIT ALE- Heat one gallon of water to 170 F, and pour onto 1¾ pounds of pale malt, and 1½ pounds of CaraPils (crystal malt), enough water to make a stiff mash.

Let stand, covered for three hours. Sparge slowly with this 170° F water until one gallon total liquid is acquired. Boil wort and 1½ grams each of sweet gale, yarrow and labrador tea herb for 90 minutes.

Cool to 70° F and strain. Pour into fermenter and add yeast. Complete fermentation and prime bottles, siphon and cap. Store four months.

MYRICA OR PORS ALE- Malt five pounds of malted barley at 150° F for 90 minutes. Run the rest of four gallons of water through the malt and boil together with two ounces of *Myrica gale*. Strain and cool to 70° F; pour into fermenter and add yeast. Hang two more ounces of herb in muslin bag into the fermenter. Complete fermentation, siphon into bottles, prime with ½ tsp of sugar and cap. Ready in 10-14 days.

CAUTION- Sweet gale leaves have emmenagogue properties and will induce miscarriage.

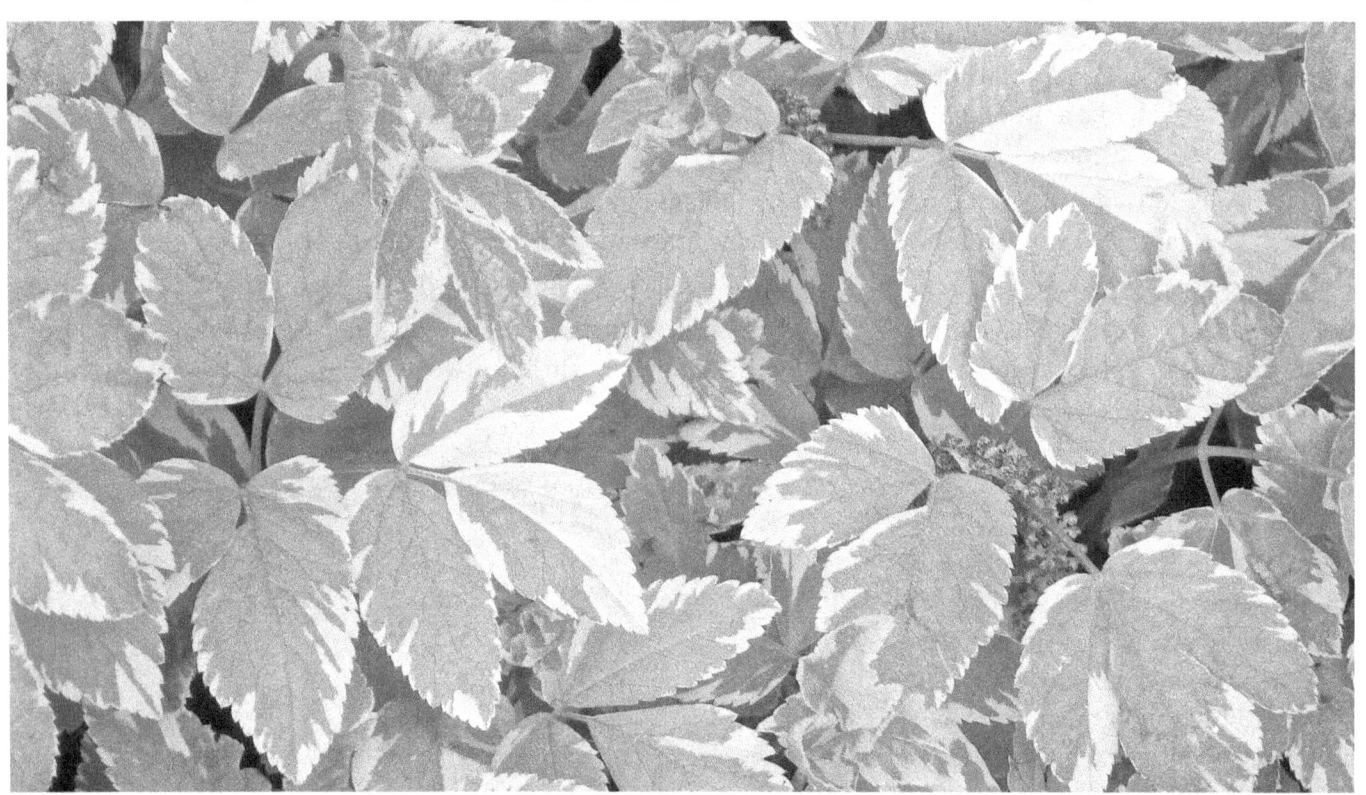

VARIEGATED GOUTWEED

GOUTWEED
GROUND ELDER
(***Aegopodium podagraria*** L.)
PARTS USED- leaf, root

It is the perfect garden weed; beautiful, tough, irrepressible and invasive. Never gives up. Ground-elder rhizomes creep around the edges, find the cracks and infiltrate the root of dormant plants.

He can't shake off this feeling of threat. However hard he tries to get rid of it, there a fragment of that dream inside him, a growing fear of being overtaken by a terrible, impending danger.   **PAUL EVANS**

Goutweed is named for its traditional use in treating this painful, arthritic condition. Gout is from the Latin **GUTTA** meaning "drop" as it was once believed that drops of bad blood or acrid material dropped from the bloodstream into the joints and caused the painful condition. It arrived in English via the French **GOUTTE** around 1290 AD.

Aegopodium is from the Greek **AIGOS**, meaning goat, and **PODOS**, meaning foot. This is for the resemblance of the leaf shape to the foot of a goat.

Podagraria is from the Latin word for gout, **PODAGRA**.

It is called Bishop's Goutweed, or Bishop's Weed or Wort, because it was so frequently found near old ecclesiastical ruins. In the Middle Ages, it was cultivated as a herb by monks and was called Herb St. Gerard, after the saint who was formerly invoked to cure gout. Ground elder arose due to resemblance to elder leaves.

The subspecies "variegatum" is often seen in nursery and sold as a fast growing ground cover, especially under trees and shrubs. It is very aggressive and should not be planted near less hardy individuals. It will revert to its original green leaf, if allowed.

The plant is relished and eaten by pigs when available. An old Anglo-Saxon herbal says:

"To preserve swine from sudden death take the worts, lupin, bishopwort and other, drive the swine to the fold, hang the worts upon the four sides and upon the door."

The rootstock is pungent and aromatic, the leaves are strong and unpleasant in flavor. It was believed at one time that simply carrying the herb in a pocket would prevent gout.

Linnaeus recommended the young leaves could be boiled and eaten as a potherb, or used in a spring salad. The taste is one of personal choice. It is still very popular as both a vegetable and salad in Russia and Lithuania.

The leaves are best before flowering, which can be all summer, if you pinch the tops. The stems are triangular, helping ensure identification to those unfamiliar.

Falcarinol and falcarindiol, from flowers have potential for development of natural nematicides. Try a flower infusion soak in your gardens for nematodes.

MEDICINAL

CONSTITUENTS- leaves- two flavanoid glucosides, hyperoside and isoquercitrin; umbelliferose.
Flowers- polyacetylenes- falcarindiol (88mg/g), falcarinol
Rhizomes- lectin (unusually high Mr- 480000)

Goutweed is a useful diuretic and sedative. According to Grieve, it can be successfully employed internally for aches in the joints, gouty and sciatic pains, and externally as a fomentation for inflamed parts.

The root and leaf can be made into a poultice and applied to the hip for relief from sciatica.

Culpepper writes:

"It is not to be supposed Goutwort hath its name for nothing, but upon experiment to heal the gout and sciatica; as also joint-aches and other cold griefs. The very bearing of it about one eases the pains of the gout and defends him that bears it from the disease".

Gerard, another English herbalist wrote: "with its roots stamped and laid upon members that are troubled or vexed with gout, swageth the paine, and taketh away the swelling and inflammation therof, which occasioned the Germans to give it the name of Podagraria, because of its virtues in curing the gout".

Hildegard de Bingen suggested its use for stomach pains.

There may be scientific validation for this folkloric claim of anti-inflammatory properties. Work by Prior et al, *J Ethnopharm* 2007 113(1):176-8 found the flowers provide significant COX-1 activity, due in large part to content of falcarindiol.

Falcarinol and falcarindiol prevent formation of neoplastic lesions and growth rate of polyps in a rat study, suggesting preventative effect. Kobaek-Larsen M et al, *Food Funct* 2017 Feb 15.

Falcarindiol preferentially kills colon cancer cells, but not normal colon epithelial cells. It also exhibits strong synergy with 5-fluorouracil, and promotes cell death by inducing endoplasmic reticulum stress. Jin HR et al, *Cell Death Dis* 2012 3:e376.

Falcarinol is cytotoxic to human lymphoid leukemia cell lines. Zaini RG et al, *Anticancer Agents Med Chem* 2012 12(6):640-52.

The two polyacetylenes improve glucose uptake in adipocytes, and act as proliferator-activated receptor gamma (PPARgamma) agonists, suggesting anti-diabetic benefit. El-Houri RB et al, *Food Funct* 2015 6(7):2135-44.

Goutweed leaf tincture combined with a low dose of metformin partially increases efficacy of the early diabetic drug in dexamethasone-treated rats. Tovchiga OV, *BMC Complement Altern Med* 2016 16:235.

Falcarinol differentially modulates GABAA receptors, suggesting its benefit as a sedative, and insecticide. Czyzewska MM et al, *J Nat Prod* 2014 77(12): 2671-7.

Falcarindiol inhibits glycogen kinase-3beta, and protected mouse neuroblastoma HT22 cells from glutamate-induced oxidative cell death. This suggest possible use in type 2 diabetes and possible prevention of Alzheimer's disease. Yoshida J et al, *J Agric Food Chem* 2013 61(31): 7515-21.

Falcarindiol induced apoptosis and cell cycle arrest in human colorectal and breast cancer cells. Wang CZ et al, *Phytomedicine* 2013 20(11):999-10006. This compound is also found in Devil's Club (*Oplopanax horridus*), and Cow Parsnip (*Heracleum lanatum*).

Goutweed lectins have been studied; and shown to have polynucleotide:adenosine glycosidase activity. This is based on work by Battelli et al, in Bologna, Italy.

The herb is used internally for eczema, gout and sciatica, externally for hemorrhoids, gout, and burns. Both water and ethanol extracts have tested active against Gram positive bacteria. The plant contains a natural fungicide.

The lectin in rhizome was first isolated from members of Apiaceae family in 1985.

HOMEOPATHY

Goutweed tincture is used for arthritis and rheumatism.

Aversion to company, conversation and consolation. They feel better when alone. They are easily offended and resentful about things that happened in past. They are discontented or indifferent to themselves. Confusion and difficulty in concentrating, and whether things really happened, or were dreamed.

Gloomy and pessimistic, with a desire to dress in black. Very tired, with chilliness and worse from cold, but desire for chocolate, salt and sour food.

Floating sensations as if walking in cotton, vertigo, nausea especially at night or upon waking. The urine is offensive and brown like beer.

DOSE-Mother tincture doses as needed. A proving by Mattisch in Austria in 1989 on six females and five males showed a wide range of symptoms.

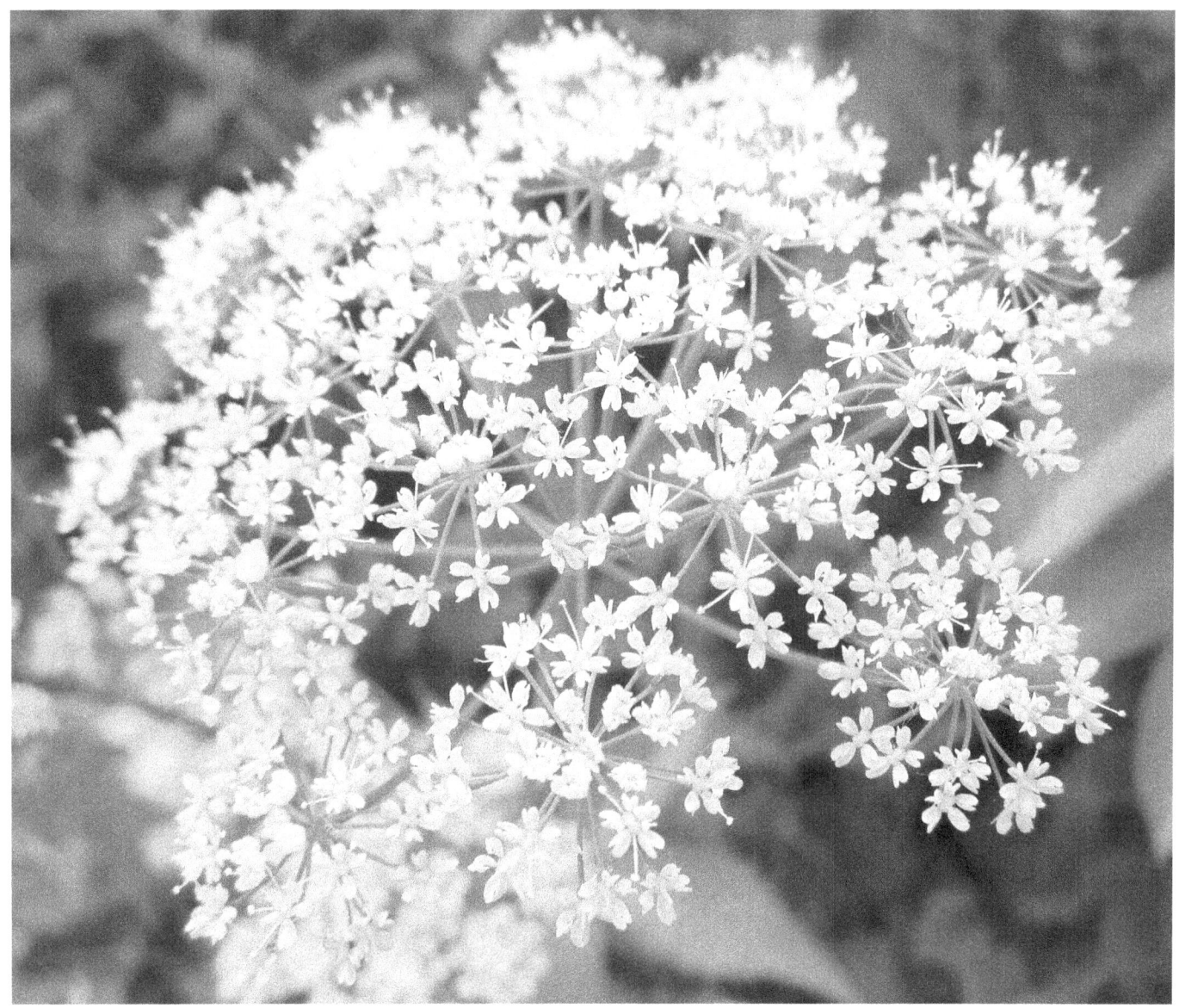

GOUTWEED FLOWERS

ESSENTIAL OIL

Work has been conducted on flowering Goutweed, with more than 20 volatile organic compounds identified so far.

The essential oil is composed mainly of terpenes, with sabinene predominating, and smaller amounts of alpha (13%) and beta pinene, p-cymene (8%) myrcene, alpha geraniol, alpha thujene, and beta phellandrene also present. Minor amounts of citronellol, linalool, isoborneol and terpeneol acetates also present.

The stems contain up to 92 monoterpenes, and the leaves have 43 monoterpenes and 29 sesquiterpenes so far identified. Kapetanos C et al, *Chem Biodivers* 2008 5(1):101-19.

FLOWER ESSENCE

Goutweed essence helps to reduce aggression and issues of self-control. It also assists in addictions.
MIRIANA

187

RECIPES

TINCTURE- 5-20 drops as needed. The fresh root/leaf tincture is prepared at 1:4 in 40% alcohol.

GOUTWEED SOUP- Take one heaping bowl of well-washed goutweed leaf and boil in salted water for 5 minutes. Drain.

Make a white sauce with sautéed onions. Add leaves and simmer for 15 minutes. Blend or puree; and add milk. Return to heat and bring up to simmer. Enjoy.

Note- The smell of the leaves disappears with cooking. Thank goodness.

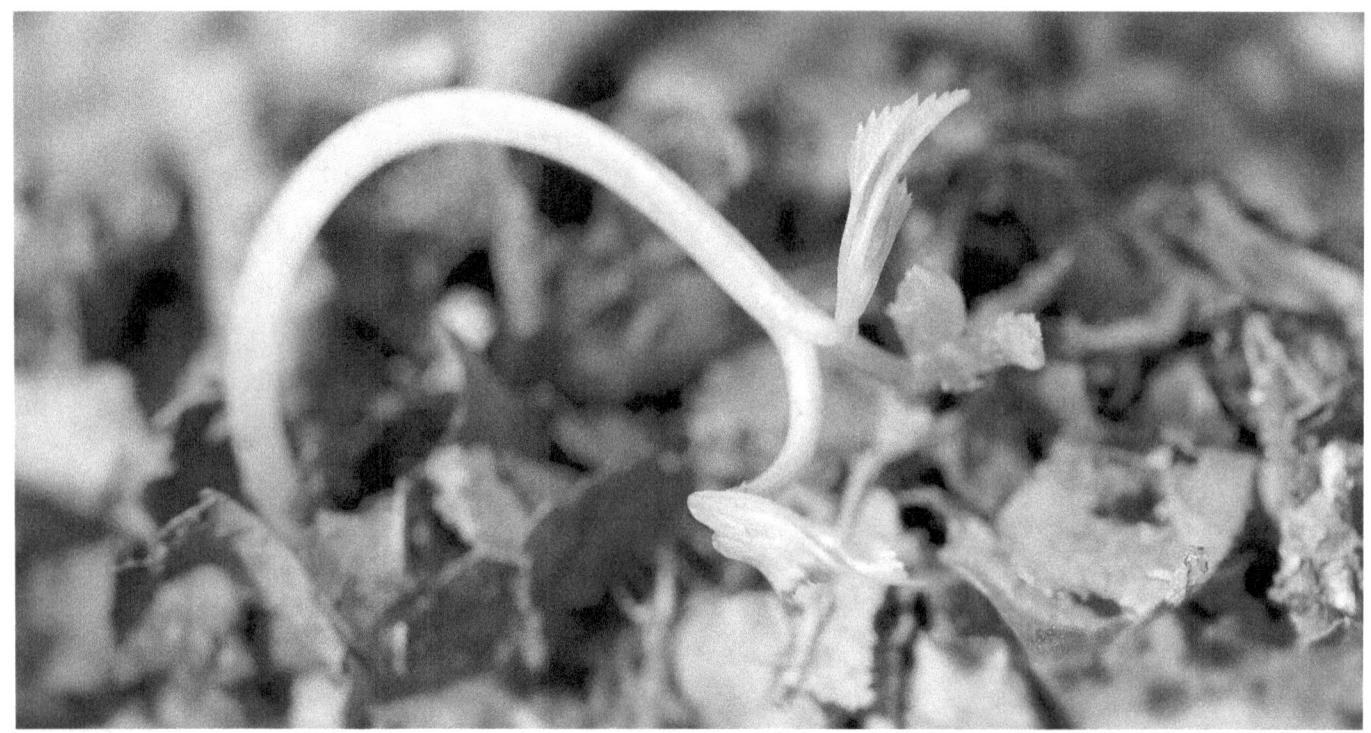

YOUNG GOUTWEED SPROUT

ASSORTED GRASSES, SEDGES AND SUCH

Grass is the forgiveness of Nature-her constant benediction. Fields trampled with battle, saturated with blood, torn with the ruts of cannon, grow green again with grass, and carnage is forgotten. Streets abandoned by traffic become grass grown, like rural lanes, and are obliterated. Forests decay, harvests perish, flowers vanish, but grass is immortal.
ANONYMOUS

Oh, good scholar,I say to myself, how can one help but grow wise with such teachings as these, the untrimmable light of the world, the ocean's shine, the prayers that are made from grass?
MARY OLIVER

Their eyes did fail, because there was no grass.
JEREMIAH 14:6

You ask me to cut grass and make hay and sell it, and be rich like white men! But how can I cut off my Mother's hair?
WANAPAUM CHIEF

The moment one gives close attention to anything, even a blade of grass, it becomes a mysterious, awesome, indescribably magnificent world in itself.
HENRY MILLER

The prairie grass dividing, its special odor breathing.
WALT WHITMAN

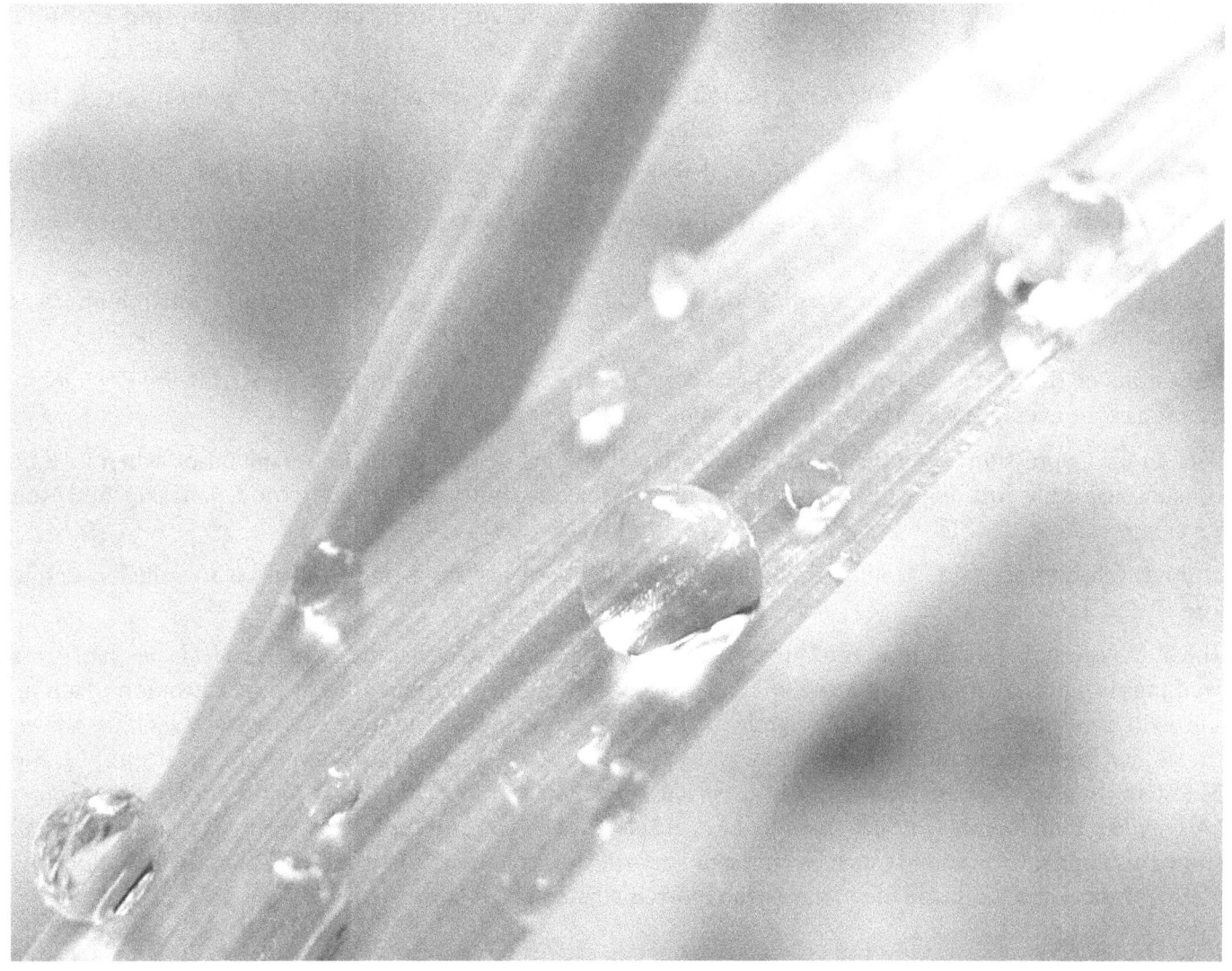

WATERDROPS ON GRASS

You approaching me
With the smell
Of fresh cut
Morning grass:
My nipples turn hard.   **YUKO KAWANO**

Sedges have edges; rushes are round.

Grasses have joints (when the cops aren't around).

Having turned to bow as graciously as water over stone

Sartwell's Sedge and Woolly Sedge simply there with tiny flowers and a triangular stem that the botanist draws in his book

Humble as rain when night is short and night is long and the nightwind's voice is true.   **REAUME**

If the Knotted Rush could dream it would dream rivers summers spent leaning into the wind so go ahead and say it the pure grace of green the lush curve of a stem

O what do we really know though nature can instruct us if we open our hearts to it.   **REAUME**

The grasses are a reflection of the moon, the sun and Mercury, even into their flowering sections.

E. M. KRANICH

Grass is from the ancient Teutonic **GRO**, meaning things that grow, and is the root of grow, green, etc. In turn this may be from the Aryan **GHRA** to grow, with graze from same origin.

According the Doctrine of Signatures, a grass that shakes in the wind is a treatment for chills and fever.

In this chapter is a smorgasbord of various grasses and grass-type vegetation as well as some domesticated grasses, now known as grains.

Grass is one of Nature's richest sources of food nutrition. As well as chlorophyll, the plants contain high levels of vitamins A, B, C and K.

It is estimated that five kilograms of dried grass contains more vitamins than 155 kilos of fruit and vegetables-more than the average person consumes in a whole year.

Back in the Depression of the 1930s, Dr. Charles Schnabel suggested that "the time is not far off when we'll be consuming a daily portion of grass in butter, bread, milkshakes, candy bars, breakfast food, pancakes, and even ice cream and cookies." He was right!

Thomas Edison once said, "Until man duplicates a blade of grass, Nature can laugh at his so-called scientific knowledge." I have to agree!

The biophysicist, E. J. Lund from the University of Texas, demonstrated that the cylindrical leaf sheath of grass seedlings is more electropositive at the tip than the base. This is turn is influenced by phytochrome and auxin, a growth hormone, both of which play a role in plant growth patterns. A number of native grasses have shown the ability to phyto-remediate petrochemical hydrocarbons. Western Wheatgrass (*Agropyron smithii*), Big Bluestem (*A. gerardi*), Little Bluestem (*A. scoparious),* Side Oats Grama (*Bouteloua curtipendula*), Blue Grama (*B. gracilis*), Buffalograss (*Buchloe spp.),* Red Fescue (*Festuca rubra*) and Indiangrass (*Sorghastrum nutans*) all show this ability. Compounds such as chrysene, benzo(a)pyrene, benz(a)anthracene, naphthalene, fluorine, phenanthrene, crude oil, and diesel have been bio-remediated at contaminated sites.

RAZOR GRASS
SEDGES
(*Carex species*)

Over a little steel smooth pond, stand multitudes of thin and withering sedge.

A. LAMPMAN

Carex is from the Latin for sedge, or grass with sharp edges. Sedges have edges!

Carex comes from Greek **KAIRO** meaning to cut in allusion to the sharp edges.

All Carex are edible to humans, although cows may bloat from over-consumption. The plants are easy to recognize, as sedges have edges, and sharp ones at that.

They can be used as an absorbent, like peat moss, or made into padding for walking, hence "shoe grass". It is edible when cooked, particularly the edible, pink root stem.

Razor Sedge (*C. aquatilis,* or *C. stans*) is known as **TLH OGH TSENE**, "Grass that smells", by the Chipewyan.

They used the fragrant root in a medicine to bring on delayed menstruation. It was also added to a compound medicine for intestinal problems.

The white leaf base can be eaten raw, and has a palm heart, nutty taste.

The root of *C. hoodi* is also fragrant, with a distinct spicy pungent odour worthy of a trial steam distillation.

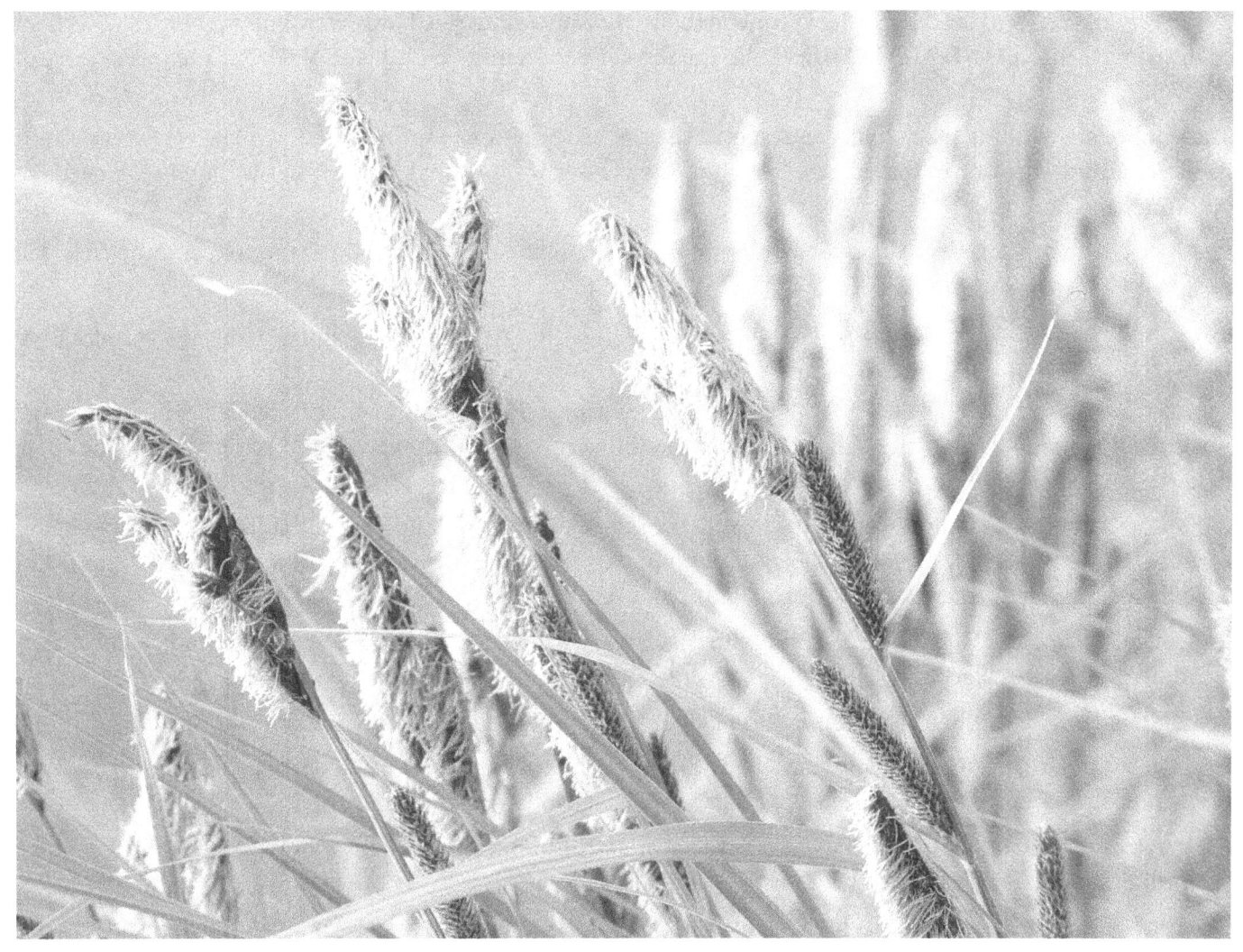

CAREX ACUTIFORMIS

A fungal parasite, *Myriosclerotinia caricis-ampullacea*, is found on this and other sedges. This was known to the Saskatchewan Cree as **MWAKOKOT**, and found on sedge stems. The black, thin sclerotia were used similarly to the ergot of rye for speeding up difficult labor. It was mixed with other herbs as a decoction to expel afterbirth, or to regulate menstruation. The Iroquois used fungi of the related *C. brevior* for the same purpose.

The Slave call Soft leaved Sedge *(C. disperma)*, Moose Brain Grass, or **NEZHI TLHOH.** As the name suggests, the leaves were used to wrap moose brains for making a tanning solution. The bundle was whirled in hot water and repeatedly wrung out until the brain was completely infused in the water, with the sedge retaining the brain membrane.

Brain tanned hides are most flexible and prized, especially when smoked properly. When I lived up North, I wore brain-tanned moose moccasins throughout the winter.

The Iroquois used the roots of *C. vulpinoidea* as part of a compound decoction as a "rooster fighting medicine"; but I'm not sure what that means. The stems of *C. lacustris* can be eaten raw, while the Dene consume the root of *C. gigantea*.

Carex pensylvania was used by the Navaho-Ramah tribe as a cold infusion topically applied to "Eagle infections". It was taken internally whenever there was discomfort associated with over-eating.

Carex nebraskensis was used by the Cheyenne in their Sun Dance and Massaum ceremonies. They call it serpent or dragon plant, **MEHNE-MEHNO?E STSE.** The former used a buffalo skull and the latter the head cavity of the wolf.

The symbolism of filling the buffalo "represented the earth's vegetation, especially that which grows near water; its use continues the prayer that plants, trees, and the grasses will be plentiful, in order to supply the needs of both men and animals.

The Blackfoot used the same Carex tied onto the horns of buffalo during the Sun Dance Ceremony. They call the grass Cut Your Finger, or **SO YOU TOI YIS.**

The Iroquois drank *C. oligosperma* decoctions as an emetic before running or playing lacrosse; the Navaho used C. festival as a ceremonial emetic.

The root of *C. siccata*, or Tall Swamp Sedge, was used for fine basket making by natives of California. The sedge was called **MATSO ZUMP** and the root buried in still warm ashes with water added to make a black color material for weaving.

Other Carex species, including *C. fedia* have been researched in Japan and India for seed oil content and isolation of anti- microbial activity against *Staphylococcus aureus*. One stilbenoid called epsilon-viniferin is similar to the phytolexin in grape leaves and is worthy of further research.

The sedge, known as **BIRODO-SUGE**, contains resveratrol, a powerful anti-oxidant and free radical quencher, found in grapes, and Fleece Flower.

Kobophenol B, a tetastilbene *from Carex pumila and C. kobomugi* has similar structure.

Epsilon-viniferin and whole plant extracts of the former show anti-biofilm activity against *Pseudomonas aeruginosa* and *E. coli* 0157:H7. Cho et al, *J Agric Food Chem* 2013 61(29): 7120-6.

Resveratrol oligomers from *C. folliculata* and *C. gynandra* inhibit the growth of human colon cancer cells. Gonzalez-Sarrias A et al, *J Agric Food Chem* 2011 59(16): 8632-8.

The root of *C. distachya* contains a high quantity of polyphenols, found in grapes and olives, that could be used as a natural source of antioxidants for food processing. Fiorentino et al, *J Ag Food Chem* 2008 56.

Both *C. microglochin and C. macloviana* contain luteolin 7-glucoside in the northern Hemisphere, but is replaced by tricin 5-glucoside in southern populations. *C. curta*, on the other hand, shows no variation in different geographies.

Sand Sedge (*C. arenaria*) is a European species with rhizomes that smell like turpentine. It is widely used for its benefit in rheumatism, gout, inflammation of joints, venereal disease, colic, liver disorders, diabetes, edema, lung tuberculosis, amenorrhea and various metabolic diseases. The root contains essential oils such as 1,8 cineole and methyl salicylate.

It was formerly used as a substitute for sarsaparilla, and known as German sarsaparilla.

Prostate Sedge (*C. chordorrhiza*) is found in fens, and along the edge of shallow water across the boreal forest. The rhizomes of this and other large sedges are soaked, peeled and split for weaving ropes, baskets and such.

Kim et al, in *the Korean Journal of Weed Science* 1993 14:1 studied *C. chordorrhiza* for medicinal activity. They found that the plant showed activity on human leukemia K256 cells, as well as significant broad-spectrum anti-bacterial action.

The related *C. brevicollis* contains beta carboline or norharman, harman, brevicarine and brevicolline.

The latter constituent is a potent vasodilator that inhibits peristalsis and is a uterine contractant. If you look at the chemical structure and remove the indole ring and the 1-methyl group you are left with the molecule nicotine.

Carex rostrata has been found to help remove ammonium and elevated levels of zinc from wetlands, suggesting use in bioremediation. Matthews et al, *Environ Pollut* 2005 134:2.

The related *C. humilis* inhibits COX activity, suggesting anti-inflammatory properties. Work by Lee et al, *Planta Medica* 64:3 found the compound (+)-alpha-viniferin is 3-4 times more powerful than resveratrol.

Bears, in the few months before hibernation, start to eat bearberries to paralyze the bowel and then *Carex* in large amounts, followed by large dung deposits containing long tapeworms. The long coarse grass obviously scrapes the intestine of parasites. Canada Snow Geese do a similar cleansing before migration.

Baikal Sedge (*C. sabulosa*) is a very rare, sand dune loving plant in the Yukon, with only six identified populations.

Seed extracts of C. grayi exhibit activity against *Staphylococcus aureus* and show significant anti-oxidant activity at 19,700 TE/100 grams. Keep in mind that blueberries are only 3,300. Borchardt et al, *J Med Plants Res* 2008 2:4.

Carex folliculata, found in northern United States, contains pallidol, a resveratrol dimer equivalent to that found in red wine. The flavonoid luteolin shows activity against human colon cancer cells and 3-O-methyl quercitin shows activity against MRSA, or methicillin-resistant *Staphylococcus aureus.* Li et al, *J Ag Food Chem* 2009 57:16.

The seeds of *C. vulpinoidea* contains vulpinoideol A and B, that inhibit tyrosinase enzyme activity. Niesen DB et al, *Nat Prod Commun* 2015 10(3): 491-3.

Carex species are plentiful in Alberta, and a thorough examination would probably reveal many with useful medicinal benefit.

FLOWER ESSENCE

Hairy Sedge (*Carex hirta*) flower essence is for poor memory having habitual causes. In such people there is a chronic lack of attention to what is in the present moment.

They are always looking back or forwards and are unwilling to look things straight in the face. Their memory lack is used as an excuse, although somehow they always remember the things for their own benefit. This apparent memory lack is used to reinforce their own beliefs and opinions, and to prevent newness and change in their lives, (which they would find very threatening).   **BAILEY**

PERSONALITY TRAITS

In Lapland, a tradition is to line boots with fine sedge that grows along the edges of marshes. The sedge is beaten and dried, then packed carefully into the boot. With a cozy sedge liner, feet stay warm and comfortable no matter what- which would be impossible with regular socks. If the sedge gets wet, it's removed and simply hung on a stick near a fire to dry out in a few minutes. It can then be reworked and remolded by folding it around the fist and slipping it back into the boot. Thus outfitted, one can continue along the way.

Luxuries aren't always the things we've come to expect- the stately homes, prestigious automobiles, cruise vacations, and costly jewels.

They are the things that cushion our daily walk and give us respite from our troubles. They are simple and plentiful if we know where to look and how to enjoy them. They are the moments of stillness, the kind word given and received, and the pleasure of a good laugh. These offer a renewable, resilient insulation to soften the day.
                                                                                          GINA MOHAMMED

MARSH REED GRASS
BLUE JOINT
(*Calamagrostis canadensis* [Michx.] Beauv.)
PURPLE REED GRASS
(*C. purpurascens* R. Br.)
PINE GRASS
TIMBERGRASS
(*C. rubescens* Buckl.)

Calamagrostis is taken from the Greek **KALAMUS**, meaning reed, and **AGROSTIS**, meaning grass; hence Reed Grass.

Marsh Reed grass is very common to the lakeshores and meadows of northern Canada. Purple Reed grass and Pine Grass are common to the open woods and along riverbanks along the foothills in Alberta, but also into northern Saskatchewan and into Manitoba.

Marsh Reed grass is the most abundant over widespread areas, and known to the Cree as **MASKOSI**. The Slave tribe, further north call it **THLOHGA DITLI** meaning, grass which is blue. Both tribes used it as a mattress stuffing or as lining for food storage pits.

The seeds contain 4.2% oil that has not yet been analyzed. Various reed grasses also contain serotonin.

The hollow stems of purple reed grass were used as drinking straws.

The Natives of the interior of British Columbia used Pine grass, or Timber grass, for various purposes.

The root ends were cut off and the leaves used to whip buffalo berries into a froth.

The Nlaka'pamux, Secwepemc, and others cooked soapberry and poured it onto pine grass mats.

Or the berries were piled on braided grass and dried over a small fire, and then stored for winter attached to the grass. To reconstitute them, the berries with grass attached was soaked in water and mixed by hand. The grass helped whip up the froth, and later floated to the top to discard.

Soaks and insoles of pine grass were used inside moccasins for winter warmth. The grass first had to be worked and softened, or in some cases was twined together with sagebrush bark as a sock. Women would also soften the grass by rubbing it, and using it as a sanitary napkin. Various tribes would use the grass to wash their traps and guns, when they became available.

BROOK GRASS
WATER WHORL GRASS
WATER HAIRBRUSH
(*Catabrosa aquatica* [L.] Beauv.)

Catabrosa is from the Greek, **KATABROSIS** meaning "eating out", in allusion to the torn ends of the glumes.

Brook Grass is a fairly common perennial of streams and wet ground in the prairie region. The Shoshone natives decocted the plant as a stimulant or tonic beverage.

FALSE MELIC
PURPLE OAT GRASS
(*Schizachne purpurascens* [Torr.] Swallen)

The Chipewyan twisted the grass together to make a wick for their grease lamps. The wick was laid across usually a birch bowl with one end sticking out and lit.

The grass is uncommon in the boreal forest, and parkland; and rarely found on the drier southern prairie.

BLUE GRAMA GRASS
(*Bouteloua gracilis* [Kunth] Lag. ex Griffiths)

Blue Grama Grass is a low growing perennial of the dry prairies. It can live over 400 years old, and maybe much longer. Nobody really knows.

Because of its long life, it concentrates large amounts of nitrogen from the interplant zones beneath it. This is important, because dry grassland and deserts are usually deficient in useable nitrogen. The accumulation is slow and steady, but when you live centuries, the result can be significant.

The Navaho Ramah chewed Blue Grama grass roots and spit it on cuts and incisions on castrated colts.

Whole plant decoctions were given as a postpartum medicine, while a cold compound infusion of the root was used externally and internally as a Life Medicine, or to counteract overdoses of other Life Medicine mixtures.

The related Side oats Grama (*B. curtipendula*) was used by the Tewa to make brooms and hairbrushes. The Kiowa wore the feathered grass as an honour for killing enemies in battle.

The hollow stems were used as straws, while the Apache ground the seed with corn as a mush, or baked bread.

The Montana and Blackfoot used the grass to determine the severity of the coming winter. One fruit spike meaning mild and more indicating the degree of severity.

Blue Gamma Grass has been shown to reduce toxic TPH and PAHs in soil.

ALKALI CORD GRASS
(*Spartina gracilis* Trin.)
PRAIRIE CORD GRASS
(*S. pectinata* Link.)

Spartina is from the diminutive Latin **SPARIUM**, meaning broom, or more probably from the Greek meaning cord. Pectinata means in the form of a comb.

The plant length and tough fibre make it ideal for cordage.

Water extracts of *S. pectinata* reveal activity against gram negative bacteria.

More study of Cord grass may reveal additional medicinal benefits. The closely related *S. cynosuroids*, for example contains beta sitosteryl-D-glucoside, beta sitosterol, vanillin and tricin; and exhibits anti-leukemia activity.

Work by Bonilla-Warford and Zedlar, looked at Prairie Cord Grass potential in storm water wetlands, as an alternative to invasive exotic grasses. The ability of the grass to grow well under variable water levels makes it a valuable choice for further research. *Environ Management* 2002 29:3.

RABBITFOOT GRASS
(*Polypogon monspeliensis* [L.] Desf.)

Polypogon is from the Greek **POLY** meaning many, and **POGON**, a beard; hence many beards.

Rabbitfoot Grass is a rare, introduced annual grass found on dry stream banks. The Navaho were quick to integrate the new plant into their materia medica. They would infuse the ashes of the plant for heart palpitations.

In south Australia, the grass has been implicated in corynetoxin poisoning of sheep.

MANY FLOWERED WOODRUSH
(*Luzula multiflora* [Ehrh.] Lej.)
FIELD WOOD RUSH
(*L. campestris* [L.] DC.)

CONSTITUENTS- luteolin-7-glucoside

195

Luzula is derived from the Italian word for a glowworm, **LUCCIOLA.** This is due to the appearance of woodrushes, shining after a rain, or covered with morning dew. It may also be from the Latin **LUZULA**, meaning light.

Acetone extracts of Wood Rush indicate activity against gram positive bacteria.

Field Wood Rush rhizomes are utilized in decoction form in India, as a diuretic.

The related *L. luzuloides* exhibits anti-inflammatory activity. Toth B et al, *Fitoterapia* 2017 116: 131-8.

TIMOTHY
MEADOW CAT'S TAIL
(*Phleum pratense* L.)
(*P. nodosum*)

CONSTITUENTS- taurine, caffeic acid, 4- and 5-caffeolylquinic acids, isoflavonoid derivatives like genistein, biochanin, formononetin, and daidzein; chlorogenic acid.

I find my dry cows like timothy grasses. They seem to calve so much easier on that field that's got timothy in it.
WEST LANCASHIRE DAIRY FARMER

Timothy is named after the American agriculturist, Timothy Hanson, who felt it would make a good forage grass. When he introduced it the Carolina, it was known as Timothy's seed, then timothy grass and finally shortened to its present name.

Timothy is an introduced hay crop. When first recognized, the Cree named it **MASKOSEYA**, or a grass grown for hay, **KA ASAMASTIMIWEHK MASKO-SEYA KOHPIKIHTAHK.**

Timothy is so highly prized for horse feed that a whole industry has developed around the Cremona area of Alberta. The perfect combination of growing environment and sufficient but not overly plentiful moisture has led to a significant opportunity. The high quality bales are shipped to Japan and elsewhere for racehorse forage.

Water extracts of the flowers, leaves and root show activity against both gram positive and mycobacterium.

This may be due, in part, to the presence of ferulic acid, which additionally is antifungal, anti-yeast, anti-tumor, and anti-hepatotoxic.

Ferulic acid stimulates phagocystosis, and is a serotonin antagonist.

The seeds have been studied and found to contain both trypsin and chymotrypsin enzyme inhibitors.

Timothy seed has been used traditionally to reduce the inflammation of appendicitis. Take a cup of seed and cover with one litre of boiling water, sweeten and drink hot if possible. It may be taken cold if necessary.

Several patents exist from the United States, Britain and Germany for the preparation of desensitizing agents for treating allergies caused by timothy pollen; and related cross reacting allergens.

One US patent from 1963, involved extraction of hypocholesterolemic agents from timothy grass.

Timothy pollen was traditionally, one of eight pollens in Cernilton, a well-known formulation for treating prostate problems. I react strongly to the pollen in season, with itchy eyes, nasal congestion and fullness in head.

The epicuticular wax contains hexacosanol.

Work by Sarker et al, *Chem Nat Compounds* 41:3 found the seeds, which contain caffeic acid decyl ester, have a higher anti-oxidant level than trolox.

FLOWER ESSENCES

As a plant essence, Timothy Grass works on the heart chakra and is the perfect remedy for helping you to love yourself and to enable you to love others. It is especially useful for healing the intestines, stomach and bowels.
OLIVE

Timothy essence is for helping balance opposing poles, for contradictions and summoning new energy.
MARIANA

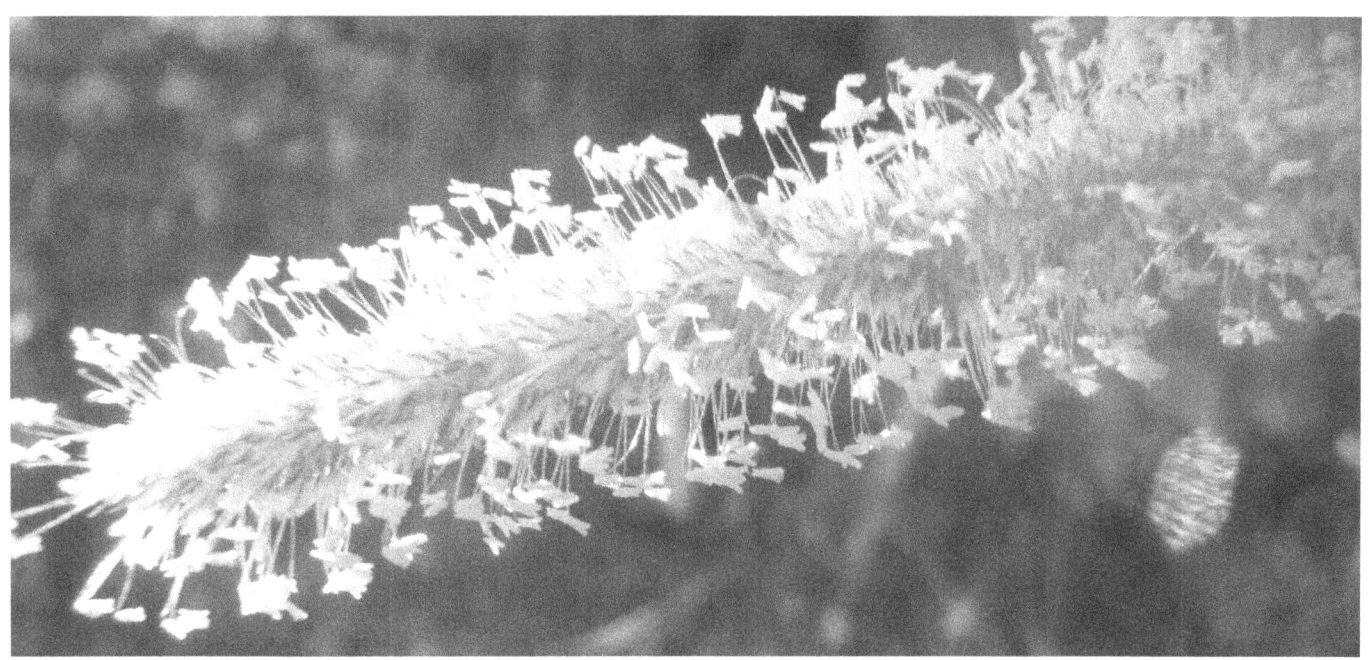

TIMOTHY SEED HEAD IN FLOWER

MANNA GRASS
(*Glyceria species*)

Glyceria is from the Greek **GLYKEROS**, meaning to have a sweet flavour, as in glycerine.

This is probably due to the spikes of some species being covered with a sweet substance. The seeds of some species are sweet and prized in Europe to thicken soups and even make bread.

Linnaeus said that geese fattened faster on manna seed than any other grain. During the 1700s the seeds were an item of commerce in Germany and Sweden.

Tall Manna Grass (*G. grandis*) and Graceful Manna Grass (*G. pulchella*) are fairly common across the northern prairies.

The former has seeds that have been tested and show activity against *Staphylococcus aureus*, and are significant source of anti-oxidant potential. Work by Borchardt et al, *J Med Plants Res* 2008 2:4 found seeds exhibit activity of 70,940 TE/100 grams, some 20 times more powerful than blueberries.

Northern Manna Grass (*Glyceria borealis*) contains 0.6 grams of protein, and small amounts of calcium and phosphorus per 100 grams of fresh weight. The leaves will not retain moisture, with water simply beading and running off.

The seed heads can be eaten, although fresh Fowl Manna Grass (*G. striata*) leaves may be high in cyanogenetic potential and toxic to grazing animals. The dried hay is fine.

The plant has been investigated for medicinal properties. Ethanol extracts of the whole plant reveal activity against gram-positive bacteria.

Sweet manna grass (*G. fluitans*) was used by the Crow, Montana and other natives as a substitute for Sweet grass. The true Sweet grass (*Hierachloe odorata*) was more prized when available, but for incense and ceremonies this manna grass was a good substitute.

The ergot of Sweet manna grass does not contain alkaloids.

Rattlesnake Grass root (*C. canadensis*) was utilized by the Flambeau (Ojibwa) as a remedy for female problems.

WOOD BLUE GRASS
(*Poa nemoralis* L.)
(*P. nemoralis* L. *interior* [Rydb.] Butters & Abbe.) not accepted
FOWL BLUE GRASS
(*P. palustris* L.)
KENTUCKY BLUE GRASS
(*P. pratensis* L.)
ANNUAL BLUE GRASS
(*P. annua* L.)

CONSTITUENTS- *P. annua-* mannitol, tannins, luteolin-6-C-mannosyl glucoside, orientin, isoorientin, friedelinol, oxalic acid, tricin.

Poa is from the Greek meaning grass, or may be related to the Po river of northern Italy. A native of Europe, it was renamed Kentucky Blue Grass. In 1936, Florence Graham, found of Elizabeth Arden, named a new classic perfume, Blue Grass.

Fowl Blue Grass or Swamp Meadow Grass was utilized by the Chipewyan. It is called **TLH'OGH** and the seed heads were gathered and boiled by women as a hair rinse, to make it grow thicker and longer. The Cree call it **SIPHIHKWASKOSIYA**.

Fowl Blue Grass leaves make up 50% of the American Coot's diet.

The stem base and seeds of various blue grass were used by Natives for food.

All three grasses have been tested for biological activity, and all exhibit activity against gram-positive bacteria. Kentucky Blue Grass was also active against gram negative bacteria.

Kentucky Blue Grass is reported to have estrogenic activity; and the seed is both a trypsin and chymotrypsin enzyme inhibitor.

Bluegrass pollen is used to make hay fever vaccines. It may be useful in phyto-remediation of manganese. Padmavathiamma et al, *Int J Phytoremed* 11:6.

Annual Bluegrass odor is repellant to the Colorado Potato beetle.

It bio-accumulates lead in the shoots and could be used for bioremediation of mine and other contaminated heavy metal sites.

FLOWER ESSENCE

Annual Blue Grass essence helps to smooth away to inner peace and harmony.   **MARIANA**

BIG BLUESTEM
RED HAY
(*Andropogon gerardii* Vitman)
LITTLE BLUESTEM
(*A. scoparius* Michx.)
(*Schizachyrium scoparium* [Michx.] Nash)

If it's flat and smooth, it's little bluestem.
If it's flat and fuzzy, it's big bluestem.
If it's round and smooth, it's switch grass
If it's round and fuzzy, it's Indian grass.   **SCHULENBERG**

Andropogon is from the Greek **ANDROS** meaning men, and **POGON** meaning beard. Schizachyrium may be from the Latin **SCHIZO** meaning "to cut or cleave", and the Old English **CYRNE**, meaning grain. Cyrne, and then churn, finally became corn.

Both of these grasses are common to the alkaline dry soils of the southern prairies. Big Bluestem can be up to 150 cm in height, while its little brother will only be half that. Both have flattened oval culms, in reference to the ditty above.

Big Bluestem was traditionally used by the Fox and other native tribes for treating a wound with accompanied fever. The grass was then applied directly to the cut.

The Chippewa decocted the root of **MUCKODE'KANES**, meaning "small prairie", for indigestion, and analgesic for stomach pain; or in combination with Snowberry (*Symphoricarpus albus*) for stoppage of urine.

The Omaha decocted the leaves as a wash in fevers, and internally for general debility and languor. Both the Omaha and Ponca call it **HADE ZHIDE**, meaning Red Hay. They used the thick jointed stems on poles to support the earth covering their lodges. The little boys of several tribes used the stems for their arrows in play. They would insert a Hawthorn spike on one end, and shoot frogs for practice.

The lower blades were chopped fine and decocted for general weakness by the Oto, and taken internally or added to baths in cases of fever.

The Kiowa Apache call it Red Grass.

A single Big Bluestem plant may have up to 25 miles of root, seeking out valuable nutrients from below. One acre of Big Bluestem produces a quarter ton of raw organic matter a year for the top six inches. Each year, eight miles of root will die and be reborn, with this underground fiber acting as food for thousands of insects, worms, bacteria and mold. In turn this creates new healthy, humus-laden soil, and makes dissolved nutrients available to the new thirsty roots.

Little Bluestem is nutritious when young and prized for grazing.

Native people would rub the grass into softness and used it like fur insulation in their moccasins in winter.

The Comanche used bundles or stems as switches for their sweat lodge. The stems were burned and the ash applied to syphilitic sores.

The Kiowa Apache switched their arms, neck and shoulders to cure aches and pains, and drive away evil spirits.

Little Bluestem has been analyzed for its epicuticular wax, which is 0.6% of its dry weight.

It contains over two-thirds tritriacontane-12, 14-dione, 29% hentriacontane-10,12-dione and other assorted and related compounds.

The Houma used an unspecified species of Bluestem leaf as a decoction for pregnant women, to give both mother and child strength.

Both grasses received US patents in 1984, for a process involving hydrogen peroxide under controlled pH to produce a non-toxic ruminant feed.

BARNYARD GRASS
(*Echinochloa crus-galli* [L.] Beauv.)
(*E. pungens* [Poir.] Rydb.) not accepted
JAPANESE BARNYARD MILLET
(*E. crus-galli var. frumentacea* [Link] W.F. Wright) not accepted
(*E. frumentacea* Link.)

Crus is Latin for leg or shank, Galli is from the Latin **GALLUS**, for cock or rooster. Linnaeus probably saw the cockspur resemblance in the awns of the seed.

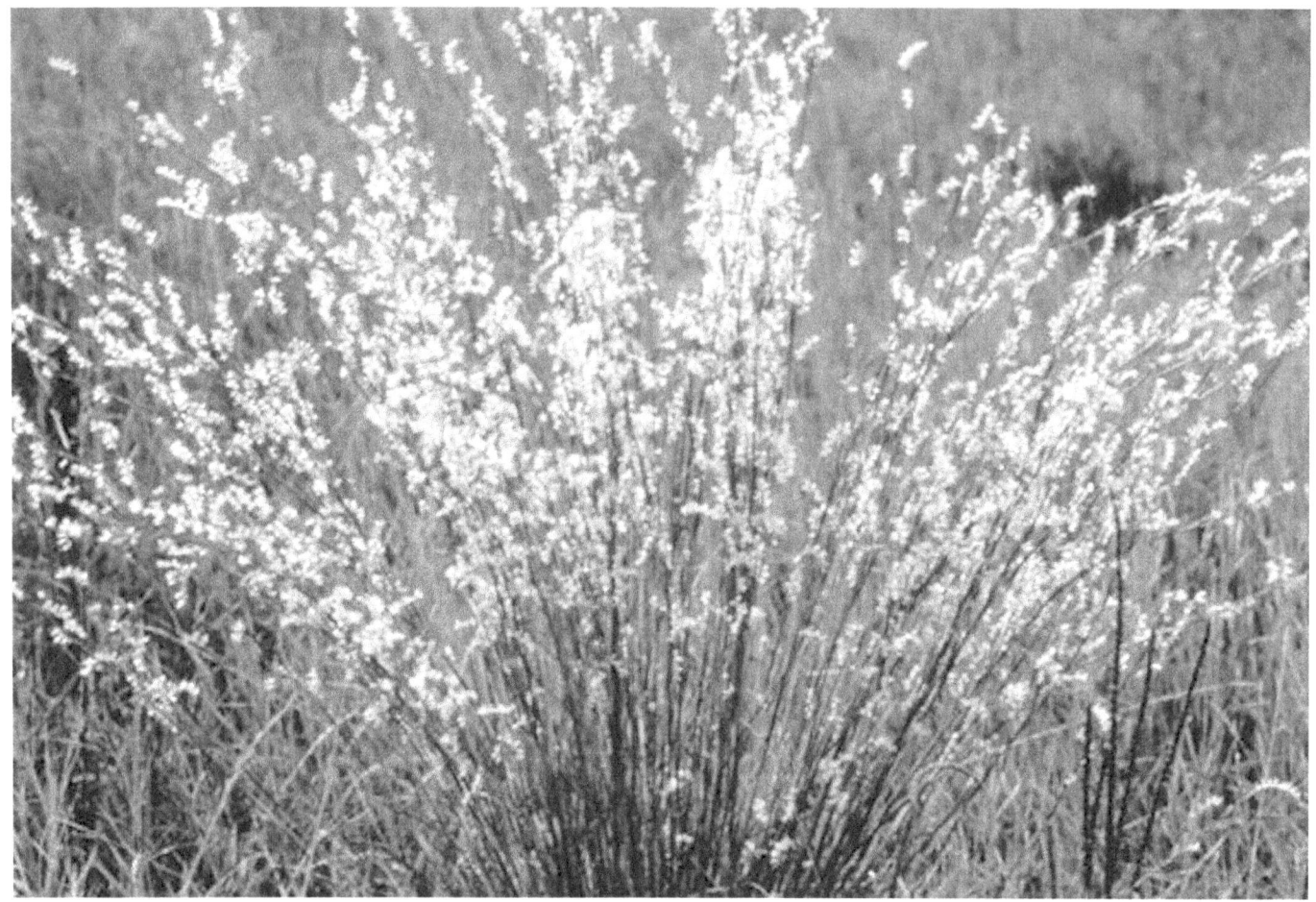

LITTLE BLUESTEM

Echinos, from both the Greek and Latin, means prickly or spiny. Chloa is Greek for grass or young herbage. Frumentum is from the Latin for grain.

Barnyard grass is native to Eurasia, and migrated into North America without much documentation.

The grass has fairly large seeds that were used as food by Native peoples. The seeds were dried or parched and then ground into a meal or flour. This was mixed with water, or milk, and baked into cakes, or mush.

To use in soups, stews, or legume dishes, simply cut the entire seed cluster in late summer, and put into a paper bag. Then spread on a newspaper, to fully dry.

A variety of Barnyard grass, var. *frumentaceae* (Japanese Millet) was advertised and sold by American seedmen as "Billion Dollar Grass", for forage. It has some forage value but requires considerable water to do well, and is too succulent for hay.

It produces edible seed, which can be ground into flour, or meal; and made into breads and mush. One plant can produce up to a million seeds, and as many as 2.25 million under optimal conditions.

In Japan, over 120 cultivars are grown at the Tohoku Agricultural Experimental Station. The protein content is nearly twice that of polished rice, and is often cooked in the ratio of 3:7 with rice. The true Japanese Millet (*E. esculenta*) is widely grown in Asia.

The seeds contain vitamins such as thiamin 0.33mg, riboflavin 0.10 mg and niacin 4.0 mg per 100 grams.

In tropical Asia and Africa, it is cultivated for its seeds that are eaten.

MEDICINAL

CONSTITUENTS- epicuticular wax (0.06%), trans-aconitic acid, crusgallin.

Barnyard grass has been investigated for anti-fertility activity. Research conducted by Saxena et al in 1988, indicates that the roots and leaves have a slight, but significant effect on sperm production. This would be worthy of further investigation.

The seeds have been found by Sushil et al, to show relatively high inhibition against *E. coli, Bacillus subtilis, Pseudomonas cichorii* and *Salmonella typhimurium. International Journal of Pharmacognosy* 1997 35:3.

Barnyard Grass (*E. crus-galli*) is a geo-botanical indicator of lead in soil. It tolerates high levels of this heavy metal and could be used as part of a bioremediation project.

Japanese Millet is used in Ayurvedic Medicine, for its drying effect. **SYAMAKA**, therefore, aggravates vata and alleviates kapha and pitta conditions.

The prolamin fraction of Japanese Millet (*E. esculenta*) ameliorates type 2 diabetes. Nishizawa et al, *Biosci Biotech Biochem* 73:2.

Acacetin in this grain induces apoptosis and cytoprotective autophagy in Jurkat T cells simultaneously. Lee JY et al, *J Microbiol Biotechnol* 2016 Nov 4.

SEED OIL

The seeds of Barnyard grass yield about 6.7% oil, composed of 68% linoleic acid, 20% oleic acid, and 7.7% palmitic acid. Traces of stearic and linolenic acid are present.

ORCHARD GRASS
COCKSFOOT
(*Dactylis glomerata* L.)

CONSTITUENTS- palmitic, linoleic and alpha linolenic acid, beta sitosterol and glucoside, dactylin, calciferol, citrulline, isovitexin, isoorientin, 5,7-dihydroxy-3',4',5'-trimethoxyflavone; and small amounts (3.05 micromoles/gram) of phospholipids composed of 35.5% each of phosphatydl choline, hydroxycinnamates, flavonoids, and glycerol.

Dactylis is from the Greek **DACTYLON**, meaning finger. Glomerata is from the Latin **GLOMERATUS**, to make into a ball or sphere; hence clustered.

Cocksfoot, or Orchard grass contains a wax composed mainly of n-hexaconsanol, and less than 1% tetraconsanol, with a melting point of 79.5 degrees C.

The leaf, stem and flower of Orchard grass are all reported to have estrogenic activity.

In France, the herb is used as a substitute for Couch Grass, as a soothing diuretic for the urinary tract. It is used in Turkey for similar purpose.

The hydroxycinnamate content is from 2.6-4.0 kilos per hectare. It has an anti-oxidant activity comparable to trolox. Hauck B et al, *J Agric Food Chem* 2014 62(2): 468-75.

Ergot growing on *D. glomerata* contains predominantly ergocristine, ergosine, and ergometrine.

Orchard grass contains significant levels of fatty acids, 51.8 mg/g^{-1}, especially alpha linolenic acid at 34.7 during the first harvest.

Where dense, the plant is a good source of seed that makes good eating and is easier to de-husk than tall fescue.

SEASIDE ARROW GRASS
GOOSEGRASS
(*Triglochinin maritima* L.)
SLENDER ARROW GRASS
MARSH ARROW GRASS
(*T. palustris* L.)

CONSTITUENTS- *T. maritima* flowers and seedlings- taxiphyllin, triglochinin and iso-triglochinin. Aerial parts- 10-20% proline
T. palustris- same as above.

Triglochinin is derived from the Latin **TRI**, meaning three, and **GLOCHIS**, a point. This refers to the 3-pointed fruit of some species. Maritima means, "of the water", and palustris means, "marsh-loving".

Seaside Arrow grass is a perennial herb of the marshes that is circumpolar.

It has unique, spike-like clusters of green flowers with pink stigmas. These later form easily recognized seedpods. It is not a true grass, but belongs to the Arrow Grass family (Juncaginaceae), a rather primitive group, like Horsetail.

The whole plant produces hydrocyanic acid, with plants in water up to 10 times less toxic to cattle and sheep than those growing on dry land. The green leaves are very high in hydrocyanic acid and should be avoided.

Triglochinin, the source of the acid, is found in several medicinal plants like California poppy, and Columbine *(A. vulgaris).* Up to 20% free proline has been found in dry land plants.

The Cree call it **MINAHIKOS,** which means "Little Spruce".

Traditionally, native people would gather the leaf base in late spring as a mild, sweet vegetable, like cucumber.

The seeds can be gathered later in the year, and roasted and ground as a coffee substitute.

The whole plant was boiled and the decoction taken to treat diarrhea with blood in stool.

Dr. Jones, an Eclectic physician from Colorado, reported *T. maritimum* to be an active diuretic and of considerable value in kidney and bladder affections as a hot and then drunk, when cooled, infusion.

Taxiphyllan shows mild activity against *Staphylococcus aureus.*

CAUTION- Arrow Grass contains cyanogenic glycosides that have caused cyanide poisoning in cattle. Boiling destroys nearly all or most cyanide. Taxiphyllan, a cyanogenic glycoside, is also present in raw bamboo shoots. There are reports in the literature of deaths caused by pickled bamboo shoots.

JAPANESE BROMEGRASS
JAPANESE CHESS
(*Bromus japonicus* Thunb. ex Murray)
SMOOTH BROMEGRASS
AWNLESS BROMEGRASS
(*B. inermis* Lyess.)
FRINGED BROMEGRASS
(*B. ciliatus* L.)
(*B. richardsonii* Link.)
DOWNY BROMEGRASS

JUNEGRASS
MORMON OATS
CHEATGRASS
(*B. tectorum* L.)
CALIFORNIA BROME
(*B. carinatus* Hook. & Arn.)
(*B. marginatus* Nees ex Steud.)
RYE BROMEGRASS
(*B. secalinus* L.)
PARTS USED-seeds, stem, leaves

Bromus is from the Greek **BROMOS**, for a kind of Oat, and **BROMA**, which means food. Tectorum is from the Latin **TECTOR**, which means one who overlays, and **TECTUM**, which means roof.

Bromegrass is common in the prairie provinces, some are native, some introduced.

Natives have long consumed the fiber-rich brome seeds.

The Araucano natives of Chile made a unleavened bread and chicha, a fermented drink from the seeds of the closely related *B. mango*.

The Cree of Northern Alberta called it Brome Grass or Bone Grass, **OSKANASKOSIY.**

The seeds can be roasted as a coffee substitute, or ground up and made into beer, as you would use malt barley.

Hay yields from Smooth Bromegrass have exceeded 2.5 tons/acre. It is very invasive of natural habitats, and should not be used for restoration work.

The Iroquois used Fringed Bromegrass as a decoction for soaking corn, possibly to hasten germination. The Navaho used infusions of Downy Bromegrass *(B. tectorum)* as a face wash for God-Impersonators.

In Tibet, **JUKU** *(B. tectorum)* is ground into a paste and applied to the chest to relieve pain.

Cheatgrass has been shown to increase species richness of fungi and invertebrates, abundance of active bacteria, generalist pathogenic fungi and numbers of non-mycorrhizal fungi, as well as decrease specialist pathogenic fungi.

This leads functionally to a decrease in nitrogen mineralization rates and de-nitrification enzyme activity.

California Brome seeds can be collected and eaten.

Fringed Brome is recommended by the Alberta Research Council in Vegreville as an effective erosion control. It has relatively large seed (300,000/kg), produced in the second year.

It is excellent forage for both wild ungulates and livestock, with a protein level of 20% in June. By July, this is 9%, and only 3% by October.

As a sole source of fodder for horses, however, it appears to cause gastric ulcers. A study by Nadeau et al, University of Tennessee, *Am J of Vet Res* 2000 61:7 found horses fed bromegrass hay induced squamous gastric lesions, compared to the higher pH alfalfa hay-grain rations. It requires 40 centimeters of annual precipitation to thrive.

Rye Bromegrass has been used in Sweden as source of flour, sheep fodder, a green dye, and in brewing of beer.

MEDICINAL

CONSTITUENTS- *B. inermis*- beta-carotene (51 mg/kg), 4-hydroxycinnamic acid, and ferulic acid.
B. tectorum- esterase, glutamate-oxalate transaminase, acid phosphatase, and peroxidase, 11-15% protein, 4% lignans, 27-30% cellulose, 0.64% calcium.

Fringed Bromegrass (*B. ciliatus*) leaves are an efficient relaxant purgative, according to Dr. Cook. Infusions are mild, and yet act promptly to secure evacuation of the gall ducts and lubrication of the intestinal tract. The leaves are slightly stimulating, but not griping like some laxatives.

The infusion also promotes expectoration, and is mildly influential upon the uterus.

The taste is faint and rather pleasant bitter. Take two ounces of hot infusion every two hours for cathartic purpose, or one ounce every four hours for delayed menstruation.

Awn-less Bromegrass flowers, leaves, roots and stems have been tested for activity using water extracts. The plant shows activity against both gram positive and mycobacterium.

Downy Brome seeds contain 7.32% protein, and 5.5% minerals.

FLOWER ESSENCE

Wild Oat flower essence is for those individuals who have not yet discovered their own true vocation. Because of this they are confused and indecisive about life direction, and try many activities that end up in lack of commitment, focus or chronically dissatisfying.   **BACH**

Wild Oat (*Bromus ramosus*) flower essence is one of Dr. Bach's 38 English Flower Essences. The grass is not grown locally, but could be easily introduced into garden plots for essence production.

RECIPES

INFUSION- One ounce of fresh or dried leaf to one pint of hot water.

FESCUE
(*Festuca species*)
PARTS USED- seed, stem

Fescue is from the Latin **FESTUCA**, meaning straw or "a mere nothing".

Fescues are a native grass, originally part of the short-grass prairie that has now virtually disappeared. An introduced Fescue, called Blue Fescue (*F. ovina var. glauca*) is planted as an ornamental.

Creeping Red Fescue is grown in the Spirit River region of Alberta as a seed crop. The Peace River Seed Co-op in Rycroft has an 8 million pound storage capacity for cleaning processing and storing turf and forage seed, and two new production lines that can process up to 3000 pounds of seed per hour.

Red Fescue is a two-year crop that can be planted with a cover crop or a nurse crop like barley, canola or peas. The second year, it produces valuable seed, and the straw can even be used for feed. Buffalo ranchers use it for feed.

The grass appears to concentrate copper in its rhizomes, suggesting phyto-remediation potential. Padmavathiamma et al, *Int J Phytoremed* 11:6.

A local company, AgraFibre set up a plant to make particleboard from the straw previously considered waste. It produced a product useful for furniture and kitchen cabinets. Unfortunately, on October 29 1999 the plant was ordered into receivership.

Native tribes of the southern prairie ate the seeds of Sheep Fescue (*F. ovina*) and others; unaware of the various alkaloids they contained.

Nodding Fescue (*F. obtusa*) root decoctions were used by Iroquois, for heart disease. They used the root as part of a combination known as Corn medicine.

Rough Fescue (*F. scabrella*) was designated the official native grass of Alberta in the spring of 2003.

Several Fescues are recommended by Alberta Research Council for reclamation and range rehabilitation, including *F. hallii, F. campestris, F. altaica, F. idahoensis, F. saximontana,* and *F. brachphylla*.

A new Fescue called Hi Mag, has been developed that has 20% more magnesium than other plants. Developed from Tall Fescue, the advantage of palatable magnesium rich forage is a reduction of grass tetany, caused by grazed on pastures overloaded with high potassium fertilizers or potassium rich manures.

The seed was first made available to plant breeders in the summer of 1999.

Acute Fescue poisoning can be sometimes spotted in animals that want to continue standing in cold running water. *Secale cornutum* (ergot from rye) in low homeopathic potencies can often prevent deaths.

Tall Fescue *(F. arundinacea)* has been shown to be an efficient boron accumulator, in a study by Banuelos published in 1995. It helps degrade recalcitrant PAHs, and pyrene in soils. Red Fescue degrades both PAH and TPHs.

Various fescues, including *F. rubra, F. pratensis* and *F. arundinacea* can become infested with mycotoxins.

The seeds are difficult to parch and de-husk, but they are found in such amounts and are so rich in nutritional benefit that they make an attractive survival food.

Red Fescue, for example, can attract *Epichloe festucae* that produces alkaloids such as ergovaline; while Meadow Fescue (*F. pratensis*) is more susceptible to *Neotyphodium uncinatum* that produces lolines up to 56 milligrams per gram of dry weight.

Tall Fescue may be contaminated with *N. coenophialum* that produces ergovaline, creating toxicosis of an ergot-like nature. See below. Tall Fescue contains harmane and other MAO inhibiting beta carbolines.

It also contains GABA like compounds. Kagan et al, *J Ag Food Chem* 2008 56:14.

Fescue Seed producers will sometimes use Roundup to ensure even ripening of seed. The remaining straw is baled and sold as livestock forage, for bison, a very suspect trail of herbicide residue that may migrate into tissue of feed animals.

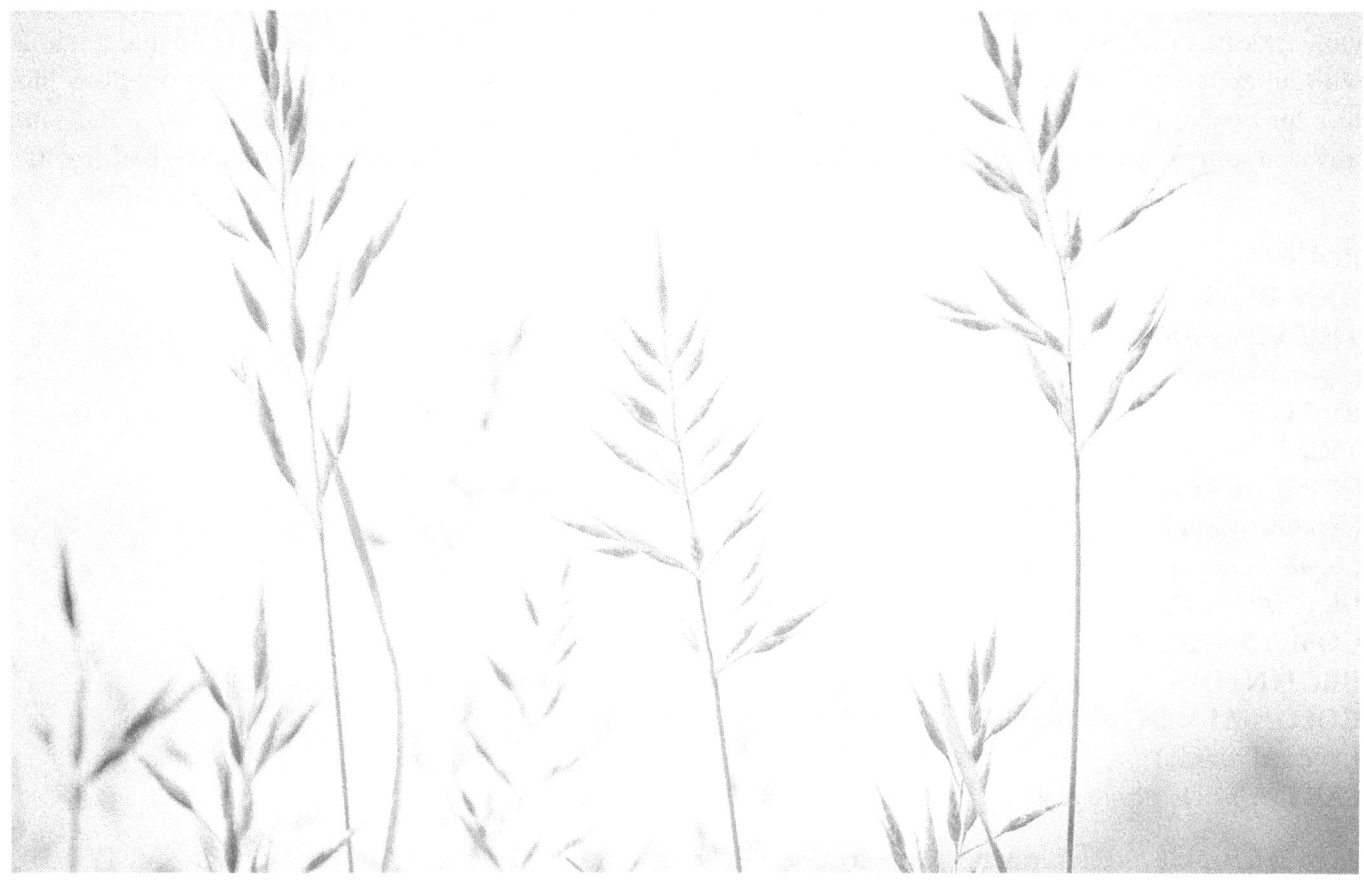

MEADOW FESCUE (*F. pratensis*)

MEDICINAL

CONSTITUENTS- *F. elatior-* carotene <0.01%, ferulic and coumaric acid, perloline, leaf xanthophylls 0.02%, 2E-hexenal
F. ovina or *F. saximontana-* epicuticular wax (1.2% of dry plant), abcisic, caffeic and coumaric acid.
F. arundinacea- melatonin

The grains of various Fescue are prone to infection by a toxic fungus, *Anguina agrostis,* which makes them inedible.

Ergovaline is a fungus that causes constriction of blood vessels to the extremities, leading to foot rot, frostbite, and dry gangrene.

Epichloe typhina, isolated from tall fescue also produces ergot alkaloids like ergosine, ergosinine and chanoclavine.

Outside of Claviceps and Balansia, this is the only other fungi capable of producing alkaloids that are N peptide substituted amides of lysergic acid.

Leaf extracts from *F. ovina* reveal activity against gram-positive bacteria.

Transgenic Tall Fescue (*F. arundinacea*) experiments are ongoing including the introduction of sucrose phosphate synthase cDNA from corn.

Tall Fescue contains 43.5 mg/g^{-1} of fatty acids on first cut, suggesting a good source for creation of CLA in meat and milk products as forage.

Work by de Medeiros et al, *J of Ethnopharmacology* 2000 72 157-65 found extracts from *F. jubata* exhibiting anti-thrombin activity of higher than 78%.

FLOWER ESSENCE

Focum (*F. elatior*) floral essence helps remove violent traumas from this life and past lives. It works on the cleaning and purifying of the supra-physical residues that certain people carry, due to traumas of violent deaths suffered in past lives. This floral essence is indicated for babies that are agitated and anxious without apparent motive, because they still carry, in their memory, some trauma from their previous life. It is for people who cannot drive a car due to fear, generally unfounded, on the conscious level. It cleans physical and rotten supra-physical residues, therefore being indicated for people who have bad breath.

FLORIAS DE SAINT GERMAIN

ROUGH HAIR GRASS
HAIR BENT GRASS
TICKLE GRASS
(*Agrostis scabra* Willd.)
REDTOP
TICKLE GRASS
CREEPING BENT GRASS
(*A. stolonifera* L.)
(*A. alba* L.) not accepted
(*A. palustris* Huds.) not accepted
COMMON BENT
BROWNTOP
COLONIAL BENT GRASS
(*A. capillaris* L.)
PARTS USED- whole plant

Agro is from the Greek meaning field, earth or soil. From both the Greek and Latin comes Agrostis, a kind of grass. Agrostology is a branch of botany that deals with grass.

Scabra means rough or scurfy, and refers to the feel of the stems and leaves. It is from the Latin meaning scabies.

Tickle Grass is self-obvious, for those who have walked through the tall plant. The Slave call it Mountain Boss, and observe that caribou, and moose frequently eat it.

Redtop is an introduced species, often used as part of lawn turf grass seed. Work by Li et al, *Plant Physiol* 2005 July 1 found the Crs-1 locus in creeping bentgrass is undergoing gene loss within the plant species. The implications are unknown.

It is found in moist areas of the southern Boreal forest.

Also known as Fiorin Grass, the identity of this plant has long been discussed in Ireland. It is said to be the cause, once stepped on, of violent hunger, abnormal craving, and a cure for diabetes. In Monaghan it was traditionally used in combination with other roots for a particular sore or boil found on toes and fingers. It has been known as Fear Gorta, or fairgurtha.

The related *A. castellana* hyper-accumulates heavy metals such as arsenic, lead, zinc, manganese and aluminum and has application for bioremediation of toxic soils.

Common bent grass is used for golf fairways, but is also a valuable fodder. It appears to hyper-accumulate lead, or at least has acquired resistance and will grow where other grasses cannot. Rodriguez-Seijo A et al, *Environ Sci Pollut Res Int* 2016 23(2): 1312-23.

HOMEOPATHY

Agrostis acts like Aconite in cases of fever and inflammation. That is, at the 30th potency, it helps to alleviate the acute, sudden and violent invasion of fever.

This is often accompanied by a state of fear, anxiety, and anguish in the mind and body.

DOSE- Sixth to 30th potency. The mother tincture is made from the whole, fresh plant of Redtop (*A. stolonifera*).

Agrostis capillaris may be helpful for anorexia. It helps eating disorders, desire to be thin, disgust when seeing others eat. Bulemia in evening and nausea next day.

Suicide in family history, with depression, feelings of guilt, self-reproach. Vision, taste and smell very acute. Laughing over serious matters. Aversion to breakfast or bread. Disgusted by alcohol, butter, oil, vinegar, but desire for yogurt, peach and strawberries.

DOSE- LM1-LM6 up to 200 and 1M. Proving by Hans Eberle and Fredrich Richter with 23 provers in 1997. Also clinical observation by same in over 100 cases between 1997 and 2008.

FLOWER ESSENCE

Hair Grass flower essence helps in healing depression.   **CHOMING**

WATER FOXTAIL
(*Alopecurus aequalis* Sobol.)
MEADOW FOXTAIL
(*A. pratensis* L.)
SLENDER FOXTAIL
HUNGRY GRASS
(*A. agrestis*)

CONSTITUENTS- *A. aequalis*- various triterpenoids, cylindrin, alpha and beta amyrin and their methyl ether, arundoin, friedelin, glutinone, fernenol, miliacin.

There's many feet on the moor tonight,
And they fall so light as they turn and pass,
So light and true, that they shake no dew,
From the Featherfew and the Hungry Grass.   **THE FAIRY MUSIC**

Alopecurus is from the Greek **ALOPEX**, meaning Fox, and **CURTUS** from the Latin meaning curt, or short, and the same root as curtail, curtain, etc.

Curtal came to mean a horse with a docked tail. Some authors believe it is from **OURA** meaning tail, hence Foxtail.

Water Foxtail contains some interesting compounds including arundoin, alpha- and beta amyrin and their methyl ethers, cylindrin, friedelin, glutinone, fernenol, and miliacin.

Friedelin inhibits the complement system. Fernenol shows selective cytotoxicity against human acute monocytic leukemia cell line (THP-1).

Both of these compounds are found in lingonberry leaves. Miliacin has been found to reduce the intensity of toxemia in mice given Salmonella infection.

It has been found effective in the biological control of root knot nematodes in a greenhouse environment.

In Traditional Chinese Medicine, Water Foxtail grass is called **GAN MAI NIANG**.

Its sweet, neutral properties are used as a diuretic, and anti-inflammatory; or to help mature chicken pox.

Meadow foxtail was used by school children in England to give their classmates a "Chinese haircut". The flowers were stripped off the stalk and this was twiddled into the hair of the child in front of them.

The pollen of *A. pratensis* causes immediate allergic response in the nostrils, throat and mouth. Work by Blackley in 1873 rubbed the pollen in the nose and caused violent attacks of sneezing, and profuse discharge of serum that continued for hours.

One swift tug quickly removed all the attached hair in a very painful manner.

Symbolically, the Foxtail genus means, "sporting".

The related *A. geniculatus* gathers ergot composed mainly of ergosine, ergocristine, and ergotamine.

TOAD RUSH
(***Juncus bufonius*** L.)
(***J. sphaerocarpus*** Nees)
WIREGRASS
WIRERUSH
ARCTIC RUSH
(***J. arcticus*** Willd. ***ssp. balticus*** [Willd.] Hyl.) not accepted
(***J. balticus*** Willd.)
SLENDER RUSH
(***J. tenuis*** Willd.)
SOFT RUSH
(***J. effusus*** L.)
WOOD RUSH
SWORDLEAF RUSH
(***J. ensifolius*** Wikstr.)
IRIS LEAF RUSH
(***J. xiphioides*** E. Mey.)

CONSTITUENTS- *J. effusus-* juncosides 1-5 (triterpenes), flavonoids, including luteolin-7-glucoside, juncusol, effusol, dehydroeffusol, luteolinidin, oxalic acid, cynaroside, tripeptide, r-glutamyl-valyl-glutamic acid, apigenin, juglandic acid, juglonone, barium, coumarins including daphnetin, daucosterol steroid, beta sitosterol, beta bisabolene (sesquiterpene), linalool, luteolin, luteolin-glucoside, fatty acids including oleic, palmitic, myristic, lauric and linoleic; protein, xylan, and arabic gum. Also contains volatile oils including alpha and beta ionone, p-cresol, eugenol, beta- bisabolene, vanillin and alpha cyperone.
Significant numbers of phenanthrene derivatives have been found, as well as capric, lauric and myristic acid; mono-p-coumaroylglyceride, alpha tocopherol, and amino acids including norvaline, glutamic acid, and beta alanine.

Wantons, light of heart,
Tickle the senseless Rushes with their heels.   **SHAKESPEARE**

Green grow the Rushes, oh!
Green grow the Rushes, oh!
The sweetest hours that e'er I spent
Were spent among the lasses, oh!
Fair lady, rest till morning blushes,
I'll strew for thee a bed of rushes.
All haile to Hymen and his marriage day,
Strew rushes, and quickly come away:
Strew rushes, maides; and ever as you strew,
Think one day, maides, like will be done for you.   **ENGLISH SAYING 1615**

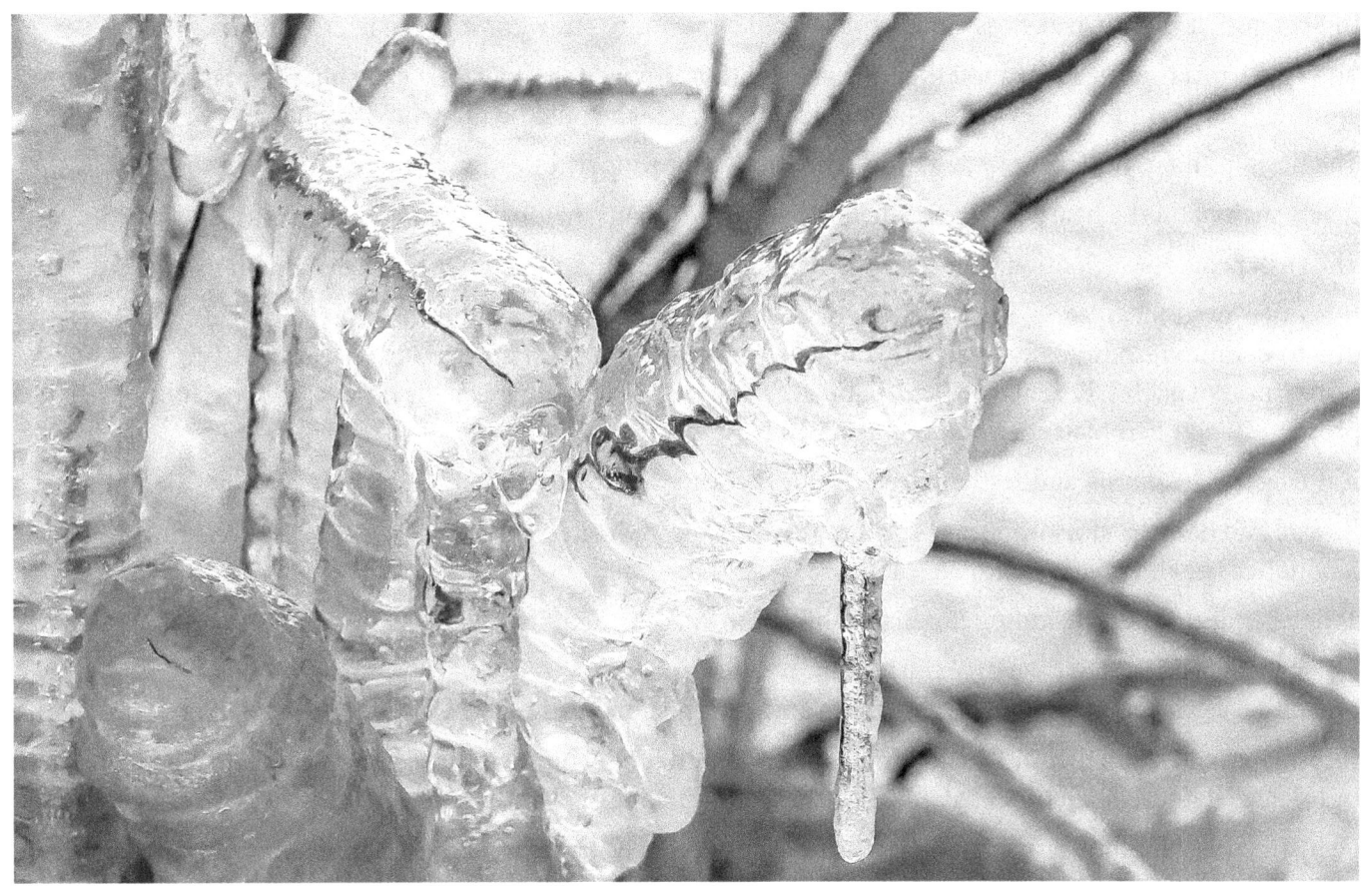

FROZEN JUNCUS EFFUSUS

Juncus is from the Latin **JUNGO**, meaning to bind or join, as in conjunction, referring to the traditional use for weaving baskets. Effusus means "vast or extensive", in reference to the large tussocks. Bufonis is from the Latin, meaning "living in damp places", or "of the toad."

The rush, according to Homer and Greek mythology, was formed when Polyphemus (the one-eyed Cyclop) discovered the beautiful Galatea in the arms of Acris, a shepherd. The Cyclop killed Acris with a rock, and as Galactea mourned over his body, she changed his blood into water that would flow forever. As the water cleared, the body of the shepherd appeared. Gradually his arms lengthened and sprouted green blades. Soon the whole brook was lined with rushes.

Soft Rush has come to symbolize music, and the birth date of February 22nd.

Rushes stand for docility in the language of flowers. The old saying "sweet and tractable as a rush", originated from a time when the pliant stalks were used for domestic purpose.

Soft Rush is a circumpolar perennial rush, used by various native tribes to weave baskets, mats, bags and even clothing. The Ojibwa know it as **KIZAEBUNUSHKOON**.

The Chumash used *J. effusus* or possibly *J. acutus* stems for various purposes. They did not cut the stems but pulled them one by one and used them fresh for twined baskets. They caulked their water baskets with asphaltum to make them water-tight. Meshed baskets were used to leach acorn meal.

The dried stem pith is used in Traditional Chinese Medicine. The Rush is known as **TENG HSIN TSAO**, or **DENG XIN CAO**, so named because the pith was used as a lamp wick in ancient times. Other names are **WU KU TS'AO** meaning five-grain grass, and **LUNG HSU TS'AO**, or Dragon's Beard Grass. In Japan, it is used to make tatami, the split rush flooring.

In Scotland, it is known as floss, and is considered superior to straw for making narrow ropes.

The epidermis is peeled away and then the dried pith is dipped in tallow for a slow burning candle. These rush lights are very fragile so they were stored in rush bark, which could be hung on the wall.

The dried pith has a slightly sweet flavor, with mild, cold properties.

It acts mainly on the heart, lung and small intestine meridians, helping eliminate dampness, and heat.

The rush promotes urination, and clears urinary tract infections, with or without sexually transmitted disease.

It is often used for dysuria, anuria, strangury, water retention, postpartum diarrhea and insomnia, the latter due to definite tranquilizing effect. This may be put to good use in quieting incessant nighttime crying and restlessness of babies. Recent work has found the compound dehydroeffusol to possess anti-anxiety and sedative properties. You Jiao Liao et al, *Planta Med* 2010 Nov 23.

It is used for insomnia and restless sleep due to excessive heart fire, and kidney yin deficiency.

Effusol and dehydroeffusol appear to act on GABA A receptor sites, suggesting sedative and relaxing influence. Singhuber J et al, *Planta Medica* 78:5 455-458.

Two phenanthrenes, including juncusin, show anti-anxiety activity. Wang Y et al, *Nat Prod Commun* 2014 9(8):1177-8.

The pith was placed upon a mother's nipples and administered to a nursing child for the relief of night crying.

Effusol, juncusol, juncuenin B, dehydrojuncuenin B and juncuenin D induce caspase-3 mediated cytotoxicity in HT22 cell lines. Ishiuchi K et al, *J Nat Med* 2015 69(3): 421-6.

Dehydroeffusol inhibits gastric cancer cell growth by selectively inducing a robust tumor suppressive endoplasmic reticulum stress response and moderate apoptosis. Zhang B et al, *Biochem Pharmacol* 2016 104:8-18; Liu W et al, *Toxicol Appl Pharmacol* 2015 287(2): 98-110.

Dehydroeffusol exhibits anti-spasmodic activity in gastrointestinal models. Di F et al, *Planta Medica* 2014 80(12): 978-83.

Work by Ma W et al, *Arch Pharm Res* 2016 39(2):154-60 looked at ethanol extracts of *J. effusus*, and their cytotoxic effect against five human cancer cell lines. Earlier work by author found effususin B exhibits moderate to strong anti-cancer activity.

Both juncusol and effusol show activity against methicillin resistant and methicillin sensitive *Staphylococcus aureus* and *Candida albicans*. The anti-microbial activity is enhanced with ultraviolet A light.

Various species, including *J. alpinoarticulatus*, *J. tenuis* and *J. filiformis* show mild to strong inhibition against MRSA, methicillin-resistant *S. aureus*.

Juncusol is toxic to estuary fish and is lethal within 36 hours at 2 ppm.

The rush is used in several forms, including raw for jaundice, nausea and vomiting. It is stir fried until carbonized for sore throat due to wind heat, and for application to open sores, to stop bleeding.

Indigo and Cinnabar processed pith are also used, but these are prone to toxicity in the hands of those not possessing considerable knowledge.

The uncooked is white, the cinnabar is red, the indigo is blue and the carbonized is black. The latter is carbonized in a tin can without oxygen. This makes the herb more efficient at cooling blood and stopping bleeding.

The root bark of *J. effusus* appears to protect the salivary glands against the serious side-effects of platinum-based chemotherapy. Xerostomia (dry mouth) is often a consequence of this treatment, and it appears this herb improves the life of patients undergoing chemotherapy. Mukudai Y et al, *Oncol Rep* 2013 30(6):2665-71.

The dose is 2-3 grams of fresh or dried pith in decoction. Do not give to patients with spleen or stomach cold and deficient conditions. As suggested in one medical text, "its nature specifically unblocks and facilitates- it is not appropriate for extremely deficient people, and should not be consumed by those with cold in the middle or urinary incontinence."

Topically, it has a calcine preserving nature, simply ground and sprinkle on, or use as a laryngeal insufflation, the powder blown into the throat.

Toad Rush was drunk by Iroquois as part of a compound decoction taken as both an emetic and to wash the entire body. It was also part of a decoction to "give strength to runners and other athletes".

A handful of the plant was steeped in a pail of water, with about two quarts drunk to induce vomiting, and then a second time to vomit again.

This was done about three times during the week before a race.

They used Wiregrass decoctions or infusions as both a wash and emetic for lacrosse players.

Plant infusions were given to young horses that had too much feed.

Wire Grass was used by the Cherokee to "dislodge spoiled saliva". An infusion of the grass was used as a wash to give babies strength, and given orally with plantain to prevent lameness, and other walking problems in children.

Wiregrass or Wire rush stems were cut and soaked in water by the Paiute. Known as **PAWAHAVE**, or **SINA-VA** the top of the sweet plant was soaked for several hours, and then put into jugs. It was sometimes used to boil food due to its mild sweetness, but mainly drunk as liquor by both men and women, without a hangover. The Owens Valley Paiute called this sweet candy **PAWAHAVIHAVI**, or **SINAHAVIHAVI**.

Gathering the plants was often a communal effect, usually in morning, and by noon the jugs were filled. It was even drunk on the way home, causing some to stagger with intoxication. The effect does not last very long, if at all.

Baltic Rush was used for baskets, waterfowl decoys, and insulation. The sheath leaves were used for a yellow pattern in baskets. The small seeds were eaten as well as the stems.

The Chumash call this rush **TASH** and preferred it for coiled baskets used mainly for seed storage.

Arctic Rush flowers produce a pink dye when chopped and boiled for several hours. The used of alum or cream of tartar produces a green dye.

The Blackfoot of Alberta obtained a brownish-green dye from the stems.

The Cheyenne of Montana gave it a name meaning "for robe ornamenting", as well as basket weaving. The fine rootlets were sewn in patterns on robes and other leather items.

Arctic Rush is used in Traditional Chinese Medicine, and known as **SHI LONG CHU**, **LONG XU**, meaning Dragon's Beard, or **CAO XU DUAN**, Herbaceous Dipsacus.

The whole herb is bitter and slightly cold, and used mainly to treat qi deficiency of the heart and abdomen, inhibition of urination, or dribbling or urine, as well as damp wind conditions. Taken over time it is said to sharpen the eyes and ears and prolong life.

Wood Rush (*J. ensifolius*) bulbs were eaten by the Swinomish. The tender new shoots were given to barren women to chew as a fertility aid.

HOMEOPATHY

Common Rush (*J. effusus*) is a diuretic, and used for urinary affections, such as dysuria, strangury and lachuria. It gives relief to asthma symptoms in hemorrhoid patients.

Bubbling sensations, and abdominal flatulence are noted.

Arthritis and liathisis conditions may be present. It is helpful in cases of spinal irritability, with cramped tightness in the arms and legs, as well as headache.

Anxiety in morning during a partial slumber, like orgasm of blood with frequent palpitation. Dreams of hunting, of jests, laughs aloud in sleep. Dreams that his abdomen is covered with warts and ulcers to which he is indifferent.

DOSE- Tincture and 1st potency. The mother tincture is prepared from the fresh rush before flowering. First proving by Wahle as self-experiment with tincture of root around 1840.

FLOWER ESSENCES

Soft Rush Grass (*J. effusus*) essence helps with finding new directions and purpose in life. Positive energy helps to increase cross energy to help with the healing process, making it ideals for sufferers of chronic arthritis and rheumatism.   **OLIVE**

Common Rush (*J. effusus*) flower essence facilitates grounding and stability. It clears foggy headedness and out of body sensation to help you think more clearly.   **TREE FROG**

Soft Rush essence is for issues of realism, for those who have been fooled by false promises or impossible promises.   **MARIANA**

SCRATCH GRASS
(***Muhlenbergia asperifolia*** [Nees & Mey.] Parodi)

Muehlenbergia is named after the American botanist, G. H. E. Muehlinberg.

The grains of Scratch Grass were collected and stored as food by a number of Native tribes. Also known as Muhly grass, the Navaho made a compound decoction of *M. dubia* roots to make sheep blood coagulate.

The related *M. filipes or M. capillaries* is known as Sweetgrass in parts of the southeastern United States. It is used as material for constructing African coiled baskets, a three-century tradition passed down over time. This is often interwoven with pine needles and *Juncus* species for design.

SAND DROPSEED
(***Sporobolus cryptandrus*** [Torr.] A. Gray)
PRAIRIE DROPSEED
NORTHERN DROPSEED
(***S. heterolepis*** [A. Gray.] A. Gray)
NEGLECTED DROPSEED
(***S. neglectus*** Nash.)

Sporobolus is from the Greek **SPORA**, meaning seed, and **BALLO** meaning to throw; in reference to the free grains.

Both Dropseed species are scarce natives of the prairies, the former on sandy, dry sites in aspen park land, and the smaller, slimmer Prairie Dropseed from Manitoba.

The poor, neglected Dropseed has been found around Edmonton.

All grains of these species were gathered and eaten by various Natives. Like other small grains and seeds, they were generally parched, ground and made into mush. Although small, the seeds were easily removed from the husk.

The flowers smell like sunflower seeds, or buttered popcorn.

The Navaho Ramah used cold infusions of Sand Dropseed on sores or bruises on horse's legs.

Prairie Dropseed was utilized by the Ojibwa as an emetic, the root decocted for moving bile. The fresh, crushed root of **NAPO GUSH-KUNS** was utilized as a poultice for skin sores.

The related *S. festivus* root is chewed in Africa for stomach complaints, while *S. indicus* is used in childbirth. The root is chewed and applied to the inflamed navel of infants, and a root infusion is drunk for depressed fontanelle in babies.

For whooping cough, the roots are ground and mixed with plant salt and water and taken as a drink.

SPIRITUAL PROPERTIES

Dropseed (*S. capillaris*) represents humility related to being adorable in its simplicity.   **THE MOTHER**

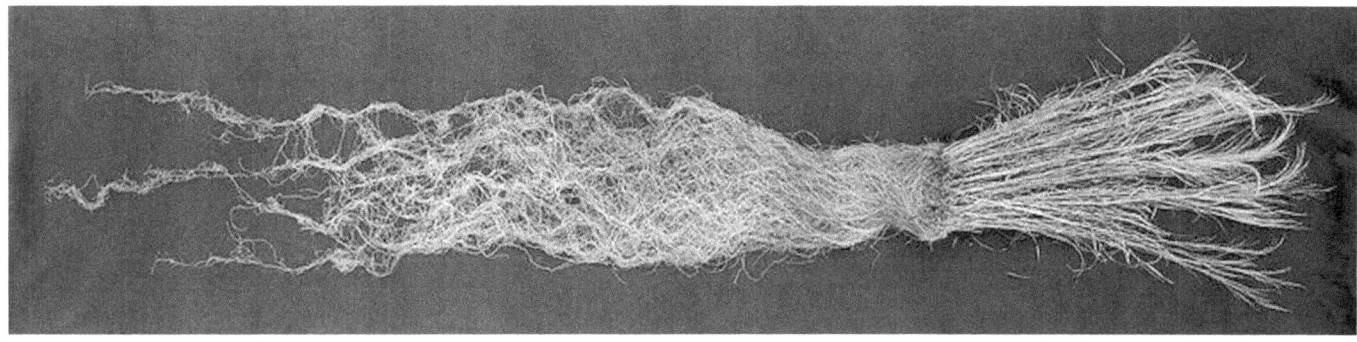

SWITCHGRASS

PANIC GRASS
WITCH GRASS
(***Panicum capillare*** L.)
SAND MILLET
(***P. wilcoxianum*** [Vasey] Gould & C. A. Clark) not accepted
(***Dichanthelium wilcoxianum*** [Vasey] Freckmann)
(***D. oligosanthes***)
SWITCHGRASS
(***P. virgatum*** L.)
BROOMCORN MILLET
PROSO
(***P. milaceum*** L.)

Panicum is from the Latin **PANIS**, meaning bread, or **PANUS** meaning panicle.

The grains of Witch Grass were widely used by Native tribes of North America as a source of cereal. It was formerly eaten in parts of Europe, but considered by Hildegard de Bingen to have very little strength when eaten. She suggested mixing panic grass in warm wine to break a burning fever.

The Mahuma infused the plant and took it as an aid for reducing weight.

The Mi'kmaq of Eastern Canada used Witch Grass as a spring tonic. The grass was simply steeped as an infusion and drunk as a tea to help regenerate the body "after a long hard winter".

Panic Grass may have a role to play in bio-remediation of atrazine contaminated soils. Work by Anderson et al, 1995 found mineralized ^{14}C-atrazine in microbial rich rhizosphere soils around the root of *P. capillare* growing in highly contaminated areas. More study is needed.

Sand Millet was used by the Navaho Ramah as a decoction used ceremonially for snake infections.

Other tribes like Creek, made warm leaf infusions for reducing fevers. One tribe bathed in the infusion for "gopher-tortoise sickness" which had symptoms of a dry throat and noisy cough.

Research on *P. bisulcatum* extracts indicates anti-blebbing activity in human chronic leukemia K562 cell lines.

Switchgrass (*P. virgatum*) is a native North American perennial, and one of the three major grasses of the tall grass prairies.

It is very hardy and produces enormous amounts of fibre that is a great potential source for pulp. Work by Goel et al, reported at the 84th annual meeting of the *Canadian Pulp and Paper Association* concluded that spring harvest offers advantage to both farmers and pulp mills.

Switchgrass can be easily pulped with a total yield of about 49% at a kappa number of 13, and could replace 20% of hardwood kraft pulp in production of fine paper.

Full report can be accessed at www.reap-canada.com/reports/switchgrass .

Another study looked at Switchgrass as a biofuel source. An acre of grass delivers enough material to produce as much energy as 12 barrels of oil. Even after production, chopping, pelleting and delivery, a net gain of 11 barrels of oil energy per acre is derived. This compares to 1.5 barrels for corn ethanol. In wood pellet stoves, the efficiency rate was 82-84%. It does create more ash, but all in all, this is a great fuel option that will grow on extremely poor soil.

Switchgrass ethanol can generate 500% more energy that was needed to produce it. On one test farm, the greenhouse gases were 94% lower than for comparable energy from gasoline.

The grass enhances degradation of PAHs in contaminated soils. For phytoremediation of lead and zinc, application of BAP (growth regulator) and citric acid, improve the work.

SPIRITUAL PROPERTIES

The leaves can be harvested anytime and braided for a specific purpose. You can gather the fresh leaves and, as you braid them, think about what you want to create.

For help with your love life, bind a bunch of Witch Grass with a golden cord and place it under your bed. It will increase your sexual pleasure and make sure your mate doesn't stray.   **S. GRIGG**

SPIKE RUSH
(*Eleocharis ssp.*)

Common to wet places, Spike Rush is usually found tufted or in solitary clumps. The Cheyenne of Montana wove baskets from the grass, the smaller for dishes for serving food and larger for shades for baby's cradles.

There are nine species common to the prairies, and yet none have been studied for constituents.

Beaked Spike Rush was used as a ceremonial emetic by the Navaho-Ramah.

The perennial Meadow Spike Rush (*E. palustris*) contains a sugar sap that was enjoyed by the Paiute. They call it **PAMASIB.**

In China, the closely related *E. plantaginea* is used for medicine. Known as **PO-CH'I**, or **CH'IH-SHAO**, the whole plant is used for its slightly cooling properties, and sour/bitter taste. It is said to purge liver fire, and resolve bruises and clots.

It is used mainly for pain in abdomen and haunches, malnutrition due to parasites, anemia, hernia and gassy stomach, inflamed swellings, pink eye and amenorrhea. Use 5-10 grams of the dried herb in decoction.

The related *E. dulcis* is used in Zimbabwe to make salt, and is known as **MASUNGU.**

SLOUGHGRASS
(*Beckmannia syzigachne* [Steud.] Fern.)

Beckmannia is named after Professor Johann Beckmann, a late 18th century botanist from Germany.

The seeds of Sloughgrass have been collected and used for gruels, meals and porridge all over the world.

In Alberta, various native tribes would first parch the grain and then either boil as a porridge or grind into a flour.

The seeds are relatively large and easily collected.

NEEDLEGRASS
(*Stipa species*)

Stipa is from the Latin **STIPE**, meaning stem.

Needle grass is a perennial common to the prairies, in isolated spots. It is frequently infected with an *Acremonium* endophyte that yields various alkaloids.

Lysergic acid amide (ergine- 20 mcg/mg dry weight) is the largest component, leading to the common name Sleepy grass. When eaten by horses, they become stupored for several days. Closely related to LSD, the hallucinogenic drug, ingestion of this alkaloid only results in sleepiness and drowsiness.

Also present is isolysergic amide (8 mcg), 8-hydroxy-lysergic acid (0.3 mcg), ergonovine (7 mcg), chanoclavine-I (15 mcg) and N-formylloline (18 mcg).

Green Needle Grass (*S. viridula*) hybridizes with Indian Rice Grass below to form a sterile combination *Stipa viridula X Stiporyzopsis caduca*.

The related Porcupine or Sleepy Grass (*S. vaseyi*) has been used traditionally in the American Southwest to make brooms, by binding the stalks together.

The roots have been decocted as a tea for kidney problems, in both humans and animals.

Because of its connection with brooms, the New Mexican Spanish associate it with witches. The plant is used as part of protection ceremonies.

INDIAN RICE GRASS
(*Oryzopsis hymenoides* [R. & S.] Ricker)

Oryxopsis is from the Greek **ORYZA**, meaning rice, and **OPSIS,** meaning like.

Indian Rice Grass, as the name suggests, has abundant seeds that readily fall to the ground when ripe. They can be cooked as a cereal or gruel, or ground into flour.

The Paiute call it **WY**. The tops were cut off with a stone knife and piled in large heaps. A fire was built nearby to dry the plants so the seeds fall off. These are gathered and winnowed. Then they are cracked and winnowed a second time to separate the black husks from the seed. They are then made into flour for mush or soup.

It was considered a good food when one suffered a bellyache, colic or aching bones, taken alone.

The seeds were traditionally stored in pits lined with willow and sagebrush bark.

COMMON VELVET GRASS
YORKSHIRE FOG
(*Holcus lanatus* L.)

Holcus is from the Greek, meaning millet; and lanatus means woolly. Fog is from the old Norse **FOGG**, meaning a long, lax, damp grass.

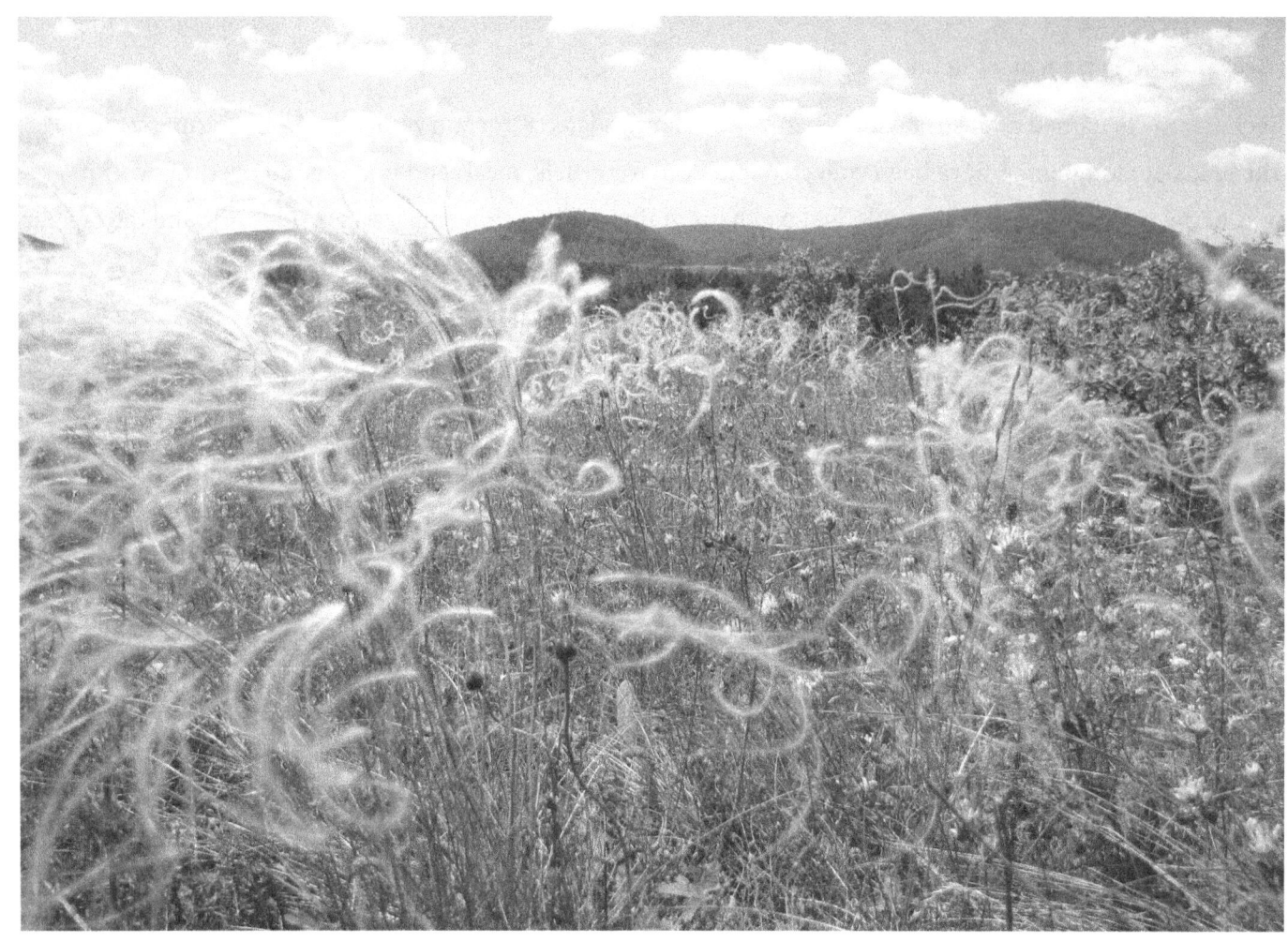

RIPE STIPA GRASS

Velvet Grass is an introduced perennial meadow grass from Europe. In 1940, it was found in a plot of Reed Canary Grass growing at the Beaverlodge Research Station in Alberta.

It is considered only somewhat hardy, but I have seen it in my hometown of Edmonton.

Velvet Grass is able to survive on low nutrient soils, and the young shoots are more digestible than perennial rye.

Compared to other grasses, it has a low, dry matter content, and the ability to absorb large amounts of minerals. It is quite tolerant of heavy metals such as copper, zinc, lead and arsenic, found in mine tailings.

Protein ranges from 4.5-11% and fiber content of 23-34%. The grass contains trans-aconitic acid. This compound exhibits significant anti-oedema properties. Garcia Ede F et al, *Phytomedicine* 2010 18(1): 80-6.

WESTERN DITCH GRASS
(*Ruppia maritima* L.)
(*R. occidentalis* S. Watson) not accepted

Western Ditch Grass is a native perennial often found in saline sloughs, and covered in water. It contains 0.2% sterols by dry weight, consisting of 47% beta sitosterol, 31% stigmasterol, and 22% campesterol.

TUFTED HAIRGRASS
(*Deschampsia caespitosa* [L.] Beauv.)
(*Aira caespitosa* Muhl.) not accepted

Deschampia is named after the French physician and botanist, J. C. Deschamps.

The introduced grass grows in tall tufts throughout the prairies, usually in good, and moist soils.

The seeds were eaten by various native groups all over North America.

The seeds are small but the protein is concentrated in the aleurone layer just below the surface, and thus a higher ratio of protein to carbohydrate the smaller the seed. It is easy to de-husk.

The grass contains up to 4.5% silica; while the seeds contain 43.6% linoleic acid, 25% palmitic and hexadecenoic acids; 24.1% linolenic acid, 4.9% oleic acid, 1.5% stearic acid, and 0.9% myristic acid.

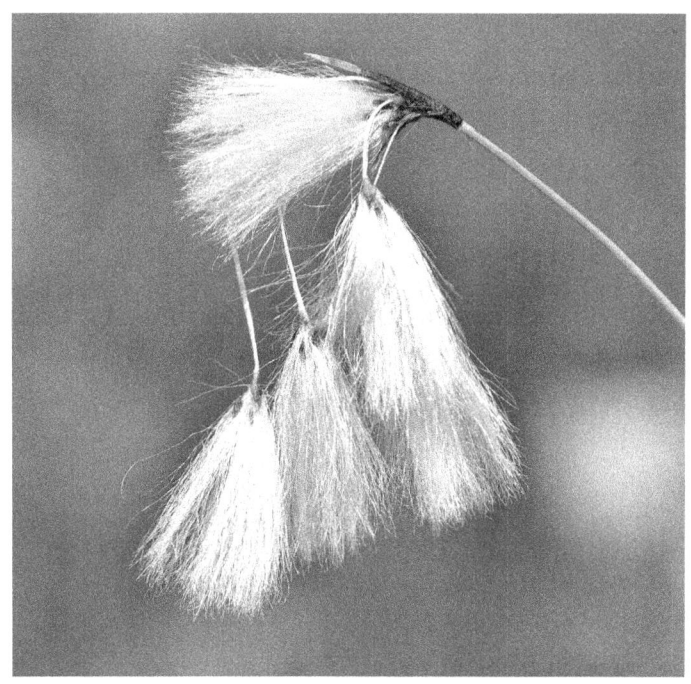

DESCHAMPSIA LITTORALIS

GOLDEN OAT GRASS
YELLOW OAT
(*Trisetum flavescens* [L.] P. Beauv.)

Tristeum is from the Greek **TREIS**, meaning three, and **OSTEON** meaning bone, and referring to the hard seeds.

Golden Oat Grass is an introduced species, and other *Trisetum* species have been noted by ranchers to cause enzootic calcinosis in pasturing animals.

The increasing calcium phosphate levels in blood serum, accompanied by low magnesium levels can prove fatal to horses and cattle by affected cardiovascular health.

Young plants have more effect.

In addition to vitamin D3 it also contains a much more effective, glycosidal bound, steroid hormone 1,25-didhydroxy-vitamin D3. The amount is sufficient to cause heavy calcification.

However, the plants contain water-soluble levels of a vitamin D glycoside with calcinogenic effect that may be extracted for natural product formulation.

The compound 1,25(OH) 2D3 has a vitamin D like activity, and is found in levels of 12,000 IU per kilogram. Vitamin D2 from mushrooms and D3 from lanolin are present alternatives to sunlight on skin for this valuable vitamin.

SALT GRASS
(*Distichlis stricta* [Torr.] Rydb.)

Distichlis may be from the Greek **DIS**, meaning double, and **STICHOS** meaning to walk or go.

Salt Grass is found around saline sloughs of the prairies. It is a low perennial with creeping rhizomes, and rather innocuous to all but the keenest taxonomist.

The grass has an interesting role to play in the reproductive cycle of montane voles. As the salt grass in their diet begins to flower and die back, it releases two phenolic acids in high amounts. These phenols actually reduce reproductive response, and the following spring another compound in the grass stimulates the breeding cycle.

This is classic example of nature aligning food supply with reproduction.

The closely related *D. spicata* is known as **ONGAVI** by the Paiute of Owens Valley. The leaves have a salty deposit that can be scraped off with sticks while dew is on the grass. This is formed into balls and cooked in ash as a salt supplement.

The Yurok put the tiny, black salty specks in hot water and boiled until a dark, red brown gum.

The Kawaiisu used the salt in a drink as a laxative and to help slow the heart. The southern Paiute used the grass for sandals, baskets, matting, etc.

SKUNK GRASS
STINK GRASS
(*Eragrostis cilianensis* [Bellardi] Vignolo ex Janch.)

Eragrostis is from the Greek **EROS**, meaning love, and **AGROSTIS**, the name of a grass; hence Love Grass. The name was created by Bauhin, after *Briza media*, or "amourette".

Skunk Grass is a rare, introduced annual found along roadsides and waste areas of the prairies. The grains are small but edible.

In Africa, root decoctions are taken during flu epidemics. It is a close relative of Teff (*E. tef*) a cultivated grain from Ethiopia.

MELIC GRASS
(*Melica smithii* [Porter] Vasey)
ONION GRASS
(*M. spectabilis* Scribn.)
ALASKA ONION GRASS
(*M. subulata* [Griseb.] Scribn.)

Melic Grass is a perennial confined to the mountain woodlands.

It may be infected with the fungus *Acremonium*, which causes a staggers condition similar to that caused by perennial ryegrass (*Lolium perenne*) infected by another related species. The fungus is intracellular within the tissue of the grass. The related *M. decumbens* is known in South Africa as Dronk Grass.

SPIRITUAL PROPERTIES

To arrive at a true picture of grasses it is not enough to look at the individual plants. The full picture, the reality, emerges when we take into consideration the fact that grasses form swards. The whole earth is thus clad as if in a vegetable fur. The single stalks can thus be likened to the hairs of animal and human organisms.

Rudolf Steiner often used this comparison in order to show that the plant, separated from the earth organism, is just as inexplicable as a hair without the organism of which it is a part.

That the connection with the earth is much stronger in the case of grasses than with other plants is very obvious.

Legends and fairy tales recount that grasses and cereals have had to renounce the highest, most beautiful and crowning glory of the plant's development-namely the colourful blossom.

Grasses are pollinated by the wind, a function of the earth as a whole, and no animal has a part in this important process. From whatever angle we look, the grasses are pure vegetative in every respect. **GROHMANN**

SLENDER BEAK RUSH
(*Rhynchospora capillacea* Torr.)

Rhynchospora is from the Greek, meaning snout seed, in reference to the beaked seed. Capillacea means slender in the hair, in reference to the thin foliage.

Slender Beak Rush is a relatively rare plant, found in calcareous bogs and wet sands of the boreal forest.

I can find no record of aboriginal use. The closely related *R. cyperoides* is boiled and used to treat toothache pain in Puerto Rico.

The same plant is called Wild Quinine, in the Dominican Republic, and used for fevers.

Brown Beak Rush *(R. fusca)* is found on the south shore of Lake Athabasca.

CRABGRASS
(*Digitaria sanguinalis* [L.] Scop.)

Digitaria is from the Latin **DIGITUS**, meaning finger, in reference to the ways the spikes group together.

The genus is infamous for "crabgrass" that ruins perfect suburban lawns.

The seeds are edible and were prized by the Slavs. It was cultivated at one time in Poland as a cereal plant.

The related White Fonio (*D. exilis*) and Black Fonio (*D. iburna*) are indigenous, annual grasses of West Africa. Some species produce grain after six weeks. It is one of that continent's oldest cereals. It is grown commercially on a small scale and marketed in North America.

DROOPING WOOD REED
(*Cinna latifolia* [Trev.] Griseb.)

Wood Reed seeds were eaten by various Native groups of western North America.

The related *C. arundinacea*, or Stout Wood Reed, was used as part of a decoction for sugar diabetes.

GAMA GRASS
(*Tripsacum dactyloides* [L.] L)

Tripsacum is from the Greek **TRIBÔ** meaning to rub or grind. The seeds are edible, and in fact, this relative of corn may provide opportunity for perennial grain domestication.

Preliminary work at the Land Institute found this plant one of four promising candidates for further research as a food crop.

WESTERN GROMWELL

WESTERN GROMWELL
WOOLLY GROMWELL
LEMONWEED
YELLOW PUCCOON
(**Lithospermum ruderale** Douglas ex Lehm.)
(**L. pilosum** Nutt.) not accepted
HOARY PUCCOON
ALKANET ROOT
(**L. canescens** [Michx.] Lehm.)
FIELD GROMWELL
BIRD MILLET
(**L. arvense** L.) not accepted
(**Buglossoides arvensis** [L.] I. M. Johnst.)
YELLOW GROMWELL
YELLOW STONESEED
NARROW-LEAFED PUCCOON
FRINGED PUCCOON
STONESEED
LONG FLOWERING STONESEED
(**L. linearifolium** Goldie) not accepted
(**L. incisum** Lehm.)
(**L. angustifolium** Michx.) not accepted

GROMWELL
EUROPEAN STONESEED
(**L. officinale** L.)
AMERICAN GROMWELL
AMERICAN STONESEED
(**L. latifolium** Michx.)
FALSE GROMWELL
MARBLESEED
WESTERN FALSE GROMWELL
SOFT HAIR MARBLESEED
(**Onosmodium molle** var. **occidentale**) not accepted
(**O. bejariense** var. **occidentale** [Mack.] B. L. Turner)
SOFT HAIRED FALSE GROMWELL
(**O. hispidissimum**) not accepted
(**O. bejariense** var. **hispidissimum** [Mack.] B. L. Turner)
EASTERN FALSE GROMWELL
WILD JOB'S TEARS
(**O. virginianum** [L.] A. DC.)
PARTS USED- seeds, roots, plant

LITHOS means stone, and **SPERMA** a seed; referring to the nutlets that are indeed as hard as little stones, or porcelain hearts. Incisum refers to the fringed margins of the petals.

Gromwell is from the old French, **GROMIL** in turn from the Latin **GRUINUM MILIUM** or "crane's millet".

Ruderale is from the Latin **RUDIS** for wild or rustic, growing among rubbish. Onosmodium is from the Greek **ONOS**, "ass", **OSME**, "smell", **DI**, "two", and **UM** meaning, umbels. This is a most unpleasant description of a very useful plant.

Puccoon may come from the Algonquin word for dye plants. Onosmodium is probably from the related Onosma, another genus of the same family. Molle is from the Latin for soft, occidentale means western. Bejariense is derived from **BEJAR**, the former name of San Antonio, Texas.

Gromwells are common to the dry slopes and grassland of southwestern Alberta, as well as British Columbia, Saskatchewan, Manitoba and south.

Gromwells long, thick roots were used for food by various First Nations. They produced a red dye used for staining the skins of animal bows and faces. Native people throughout North America used the gromwell seeds for their diuretic and dissolving effect in kidney gravel and calculi, gouty conditions and urine retention.

Gromwell was used by native people as a natural contraceptive in the form of cold infusions of the pounded root. Today, it is still used by native women as a daily cold water infusion for a period of up to six months, the time required to ensure infertility.

A powder of the leaves and stems was wetted and applied to rheumatic pains, and soreness by the Cheyenne.

The Thompson call it **PANAWE UXTEN**, "fluffy on the root" or **SCHWO'OPA** "bushy stem or bushy on the bottom."

The plant was sometimes used to inflict bad luck or sickness by putting it on the person or in their clothes or bedding. Even today, many natives will not touch the plant, believing it a mystery plant. Some tribes, like the Okanagan used the plant as a charm to make it rain.

The plant was used for itching hemorrhoids in an unspecified manner.

The Flathead of Montana used Yellow Puccoon root in decoction for diarrhea. The dried root has been found at the ancient Lodaisha site, near Denver, indicating traditional use dating back 10-14 thousand years.

The Assiniboine tribes used the root tea for suppressed menstruation.

The Crow of southern Montana called it miscarriage plant, or **ELDOCXABIO**.

The Blackfoot used the tops and seeds of Stoneseed (*L. linearifolium*) and Narrow-leaved Puccoon, or Yellow Gromwell (*L. incisum*) as incense in medicinal ceremonies.

The former was known as *PONO-KAN-SINNI*, or Elk Food.

Red dyes were obtained from the roots of all Lithospermum species, changing to violet with time. The color was fixed with the fresh and heated pads of prickly pear, or from hot animal fats, and rubbed onto the skinned hides.

The dried, pounded roots were boiled in fat broth.

When used green, the leaves were wrapped in cloth crushed with the teeth and rubbed on.

The Lakota used the plant for hemorrhaging of the lungs, while the Cheyenne ground the dried leaves, roots and stems to treat paralysis. They named it **HOH'AHEA NO IS'TUT**, meaning Paralysis or Lame Medicine, and when rubbed into the affected area it acted as a counterirritant causing a prickly sensation.

If a person were delirious, they would make a whole plant tea and rub it into the patient's head and face.

For insomnia, the medicine man would chew gromwell, spits it on the patient's face and rubs it into the heart.

The Thompson tribe prayed over the root and put it on enemies to "inflict sickness or bad luck". New fishing lines were drawn through a handful of the herb by the Okanagan to mask human scent. They call it **TIKTIK'ESE** or "root paint".

Root powder was sprinkled on chest wounds. A tea of the root and seeds was used for a liniment to heal swelling on horses. The Okanagan drank hot infusions of the roots to stop internal bleeding; and as part of charms to make it rain. Children made the little nutlets into necklaces.

Sucking nectar from the bottom of the yellow flower tube was another treat.

False Gromwell is a somewhat rare perennial in Alberta; but more common in Saskatchewan, at the edge of bluffs, and into southern Manitoba.

False gromwell seeds were used by the Cheyenne. Cree and others to attract worldly goods, as love charms and as incense.

A tea of the leaves was used as a laxative. The Cheyenne smashed the leaves and stems into fat and rubbed this on the back for lumbago and numbness. They call it **MAK ESK O WA NI'A**, meaning big rough medicine.

The Lakota have two names, at least, for the plant; **POI'PIYE**, meaning something to fix swelling with, or **SUNKCAN' KANHUIPIJE**, meaning horse spine cure. As the names suggest, the root and seeds were made into a tea as well as salve, the first internally for horses, and the latter rubbed into human swellings.

The Shuswap decocted the dried root "to clean the germs off the body".

Further east, the Chippewa know the plant as **MI'GISENS'IBUG**, meaning Little Shell Leaf.

The related *L. officinale*, in fruiting stage, is decocted in Northern Spain as a social drink that is taken after meals for digestive, heartburn and stomach problems. It is known as White Tea, or Te Blanco.

The leaves were at one time used as a substitute for black tea, and known as Croatian or Bohemian Tea.

This species is introduced from Europe, but now found growing wild in parts of south-eastern Manitoba and further south.

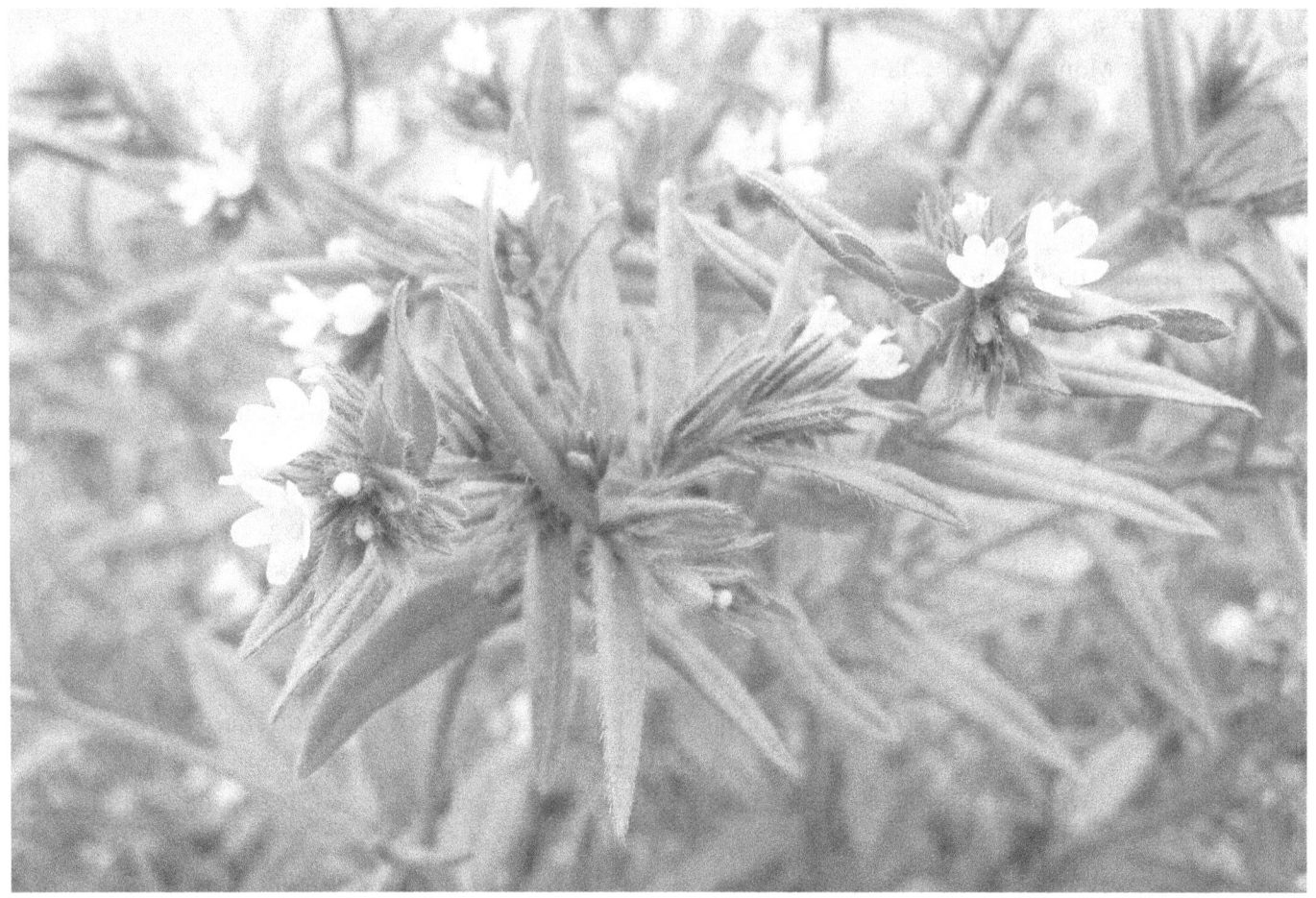

FIELD GROMWELL

Nutlets from *L. officinale* have been found in archeological gravesite dating back to early Bronze Age, 1750-1600 BC. They were found ringing a tub mouth in a piece of pottery dating back to the same time period in China.

Hoary Puccoon and Field Gromwell are common my home province of Alberta.

The former herb was taken by the Menominee in a compound infusion to quiet convulsions.

The latter leaf infusion was used to treat urinary complaints.

Interestingly, practitioners of TCM use gromwell root (*L. erythororhizon*) internally and externally for excessive skin rashes, or to bring out the rash.

The herb lubricates the bowels with slight laxative effect, and is an effective douche for leucorrhea, herpes and genital itching. In Traditional Chinese Medicine it is called **ZIA CAO**, while in Kampo, the Japanese form, it is called **SHISO**.

The roots are most potent in September; and remain active for up to four years after harvest.

A red dye, for medicine and coloring lipstick is commercially produced in Japan from *L. erythrorhizon* cells in culture. In fact, shikonin was the first secondary metabolite commercially produced in cell culture.

Hairy cells cultures produce a yield of five milligrams per day from a two-litre airlift fermenter over a 220-day period. Shikonin is anti-bacterial, and stimulates tissue granulation, as well as its cosmetic applications.

The related False Gromwell (*O. virginianum*) root is considered a diuretic with some stone-dissolving capacity, but mainly to relieve sub-acute and chronic irritations of the kidney and bladder.

MEDICINAL

CONSTITUENTS- *Lithospermum ruderale* root- 7-hydroxycoumaran, rosmarinic acid, rutin, allantoin, chlorogenic and succinic acid, lithospermic acid (3% of dried root), an inositol derivative and polyphenolic carboxylic acid; and salts of D-3-(3,4-dihydroxyphenyl) lactic acid and family of its oligomeric polyesters. The red pigment is probably shikonin.
Leaf- rutin, bornesite, phlobotannins, carbonic acid, phytoestrogens, and lithospermic acid.
L. canescens root- acetylshikonin, isobutyrylshikonin, canescine, canescenine, traces of 7 different pyrrolizidine alkaloids.
L. officinale root- caffeic acid, chlorogenic acid, ellagic acid, lithospermic acid, rosmarinic acid, rutin.

Gromwell and False Gromwell both possess diuretic properties in the seeds, flowers and root. The principle activity is in the roots, although the flowers and seeds are potent as well. The stems contain almost no activity.

Acute and chronic cystitis, accompanied by sand or gravel is a good indication for using these herbs.

Experiments in Germany confirm gromwell's (*L. officinale*) hormonal action. It contains anti-gonadotrophic properties, suggesting use as a contraceptive. It inhibits the production of luteinizing hormone by the anterior pituitary, and may have direct action on the hypothalamus.

Aqueous extract from the leaves show equal activity as the root; and interestingly the same compounds as bugleweed, and motherwort.

Gromwell could be thought of as an herbal Lupron, a drug used for prostate and breast cancers. By shutting down the reproductive hormonal output, it is believed that estrogen and androgenic sensitive tissues may have the opportunity to normalize.

Studies have shown water extracts of *Lithospermum* contain oxytocin, control uterine contractions and reduce blood pressure.

Numerous studies on mice have shown anti-estrus and impaired development of secondary sex organs.

Human studies conducted showed daily intake of 240 mg of freeze-dried *L. officinale* caused no overt adverse effects after eight weeks.

The production of both prolactin and thyroid stimulating hormone are reduced as well, so caution must be exerted. Sourgens H et al, *Planta Medica* 1982 45(2): 78-82.

That is, unless you are consciously trying to reduce overproduction of TSH associated with hyperthyroidism or goiter with hypothyroid symptoms.

Here is a summary to present. The species *L. latifolium*, *L. arvense*, *L. officinale* and *L. ruderale* all increased pregnant mare's serum gonadotropin, in early work by Graham et al, *Endocrin* 1955:56.

Only the latter two have influence on chorionic gonadotrophin, luteinizing hormone (LH), follicle stimulating hormone (FSH), prolactin, and thyroid stimulating hormone.

Only *L. officinale* has been studied for effects on Grave's IgG, iodide pump, adenylate cyclase, T4, T3, iodothyronine deiodinase and other factors involving thyroid health.

While gromwell may not replace the "pill", it has been shown to be a gentle herb. There is no dramatic, instant contraceptive effect- and yet there is no evidence of the numerous side effects produced by the various commercial synthetic products.

In laboratory tests, 400 mg tops/kg body weight and 364mg roots/kg daily was found to effective dose in both male and female rats.

An equivalent dose in a 70 kg human would be 25-28 grams daily. This is a lot, but it must be remembered that Native Americans used cold-water infusions of the root over six months with apparently good results. I am not recommending this method of birth control, simply noting its traditional use.

In one study, a human female at dose of 20-40 grams of dry herb daily for one month exhibited luteinizing hormone inhibition. Weisner et al, *Nature* 1952 170.

Shikonin derivatives, including acetylshikonin, show potential for the treatment of medullary thyroid carcinoma, resistant to chemotherapy and radiation. Hasenoehri C et al, *Endocr Connect* 2017 6(2):53-62.

Alkanet root (Hoary Puccoon) shows significant anti-tumor activity against MDA-MB-231 human breast cancer cell lines. Mazzio E et al, *Phytother Res* 2014 28(6): 856-67.

The acetylshikonins, isolated from root, inhibit cutaneous angiogenesis induced by L-1 sarcoma cells. Pietrosiuk A et al, *Acta Pol Pharm* 2004 61(5): 379-82.

It may be helpful for treating obesity and non-alcoholic fatty liver disease. Su ML et al, *Molecules* 2016 21(8).

It induces endoplasmic reticulum stress, a prerequisite for apoptosis of hepatitis B virus X protein in liver cancer cells. Moon J et al, *Eur J Pharmacol* 2014 735:132-40.

Both acetylshikonin and isobutyrylshikonin, isolated from roots show immune modulation on cellular and humoral immunity. Pietrosiuk A et al, *Pharmazie* 2004 59(8): 640-2.

Isobutyrylshikonin, and other derivatives of shikonin possess anti-leukemia activity. Zhao Q et al, *Oncotarget* 2015 6(36): 38934-51.

They appear to work synergistically with eroltinib in the treatment of human glioma cells. Zhao Q et al, *Int J Cancer* 2015 137(6): 1446-56.

Acetylshikonin suppresses fertility in rats by decreasing serum FSH and LH levels by suppressing secretions of gonadotropic hormone. He Y et al, *Biochem Biophys Res Commun* 2016 476(4): 560-5.

It may be promising for the treatment of pancreatic cancer. Work in Korea by Cho SC and Choi BY, *Biomol Ther* 2015 23(5): 428-33 found the compound inhibits pancreatic PANC-1 cancer cell proliferation by suppressing NFkappaB activity.

Our native *L. ruderale* can be considered to possess activity like Chasteberry or Vitex, helping to promote regular menstrual rhythm, when used sparingly in the luteal phase. It may also be used during the full cycle to suppress elevated estrogen levels.

Lithospermic acid, derived from water extracts, inhibit luteinizing hormone. Findley WE et al, *Biol Reprod* 1985 33(2): 309-15.

It significantly attenuates neurotoxicity by blocking neuronal apoptosis and neuro-inflammatory pathways, suggesting benefit as a novel intervention in Parkinson's disease. Lin YL et al, *J Biomed Sci* 2015 22:37.

It shows a preventative effect on the development of diabetic retinopathy, in an animal model. Insulin resistance and glucose intolerance were significantly improved, due to anti-oxidative and anti-inflammatory effects. Jin CJ et al, *PLoS One* 2014 9(6):e98232.

It is worth noting that monardic acids, from Wild Bergamot (*M. fistulosa*) are diastereomers of lithospermic acids. Moderate hyaluronidase and histamine release inhibition is noted. Murata T et al, *Fitoterapia* 2013 91:51-9.

Lithospermic acid exhibits strong cytotoxicity against MCF-7 breast cancer cell lines, including adriamycin-resistant strains. Berdowska I et al, *Food Chem* 2013 141(2): 1313-21.

Intestinal ischemia can occur for a number of reasons, including complications associated with long-lasting surgery. Lithospermic acid appears to attenuate issues associated with this clinical issue. Ozturk H et al, *Adv Clin Exp Med* 2012 21(4): 433-9.

The flowers and seeds are more potent than roots and leaves. Stems have almost no activity. Roots harvested in September are more potent than those pulled in August.

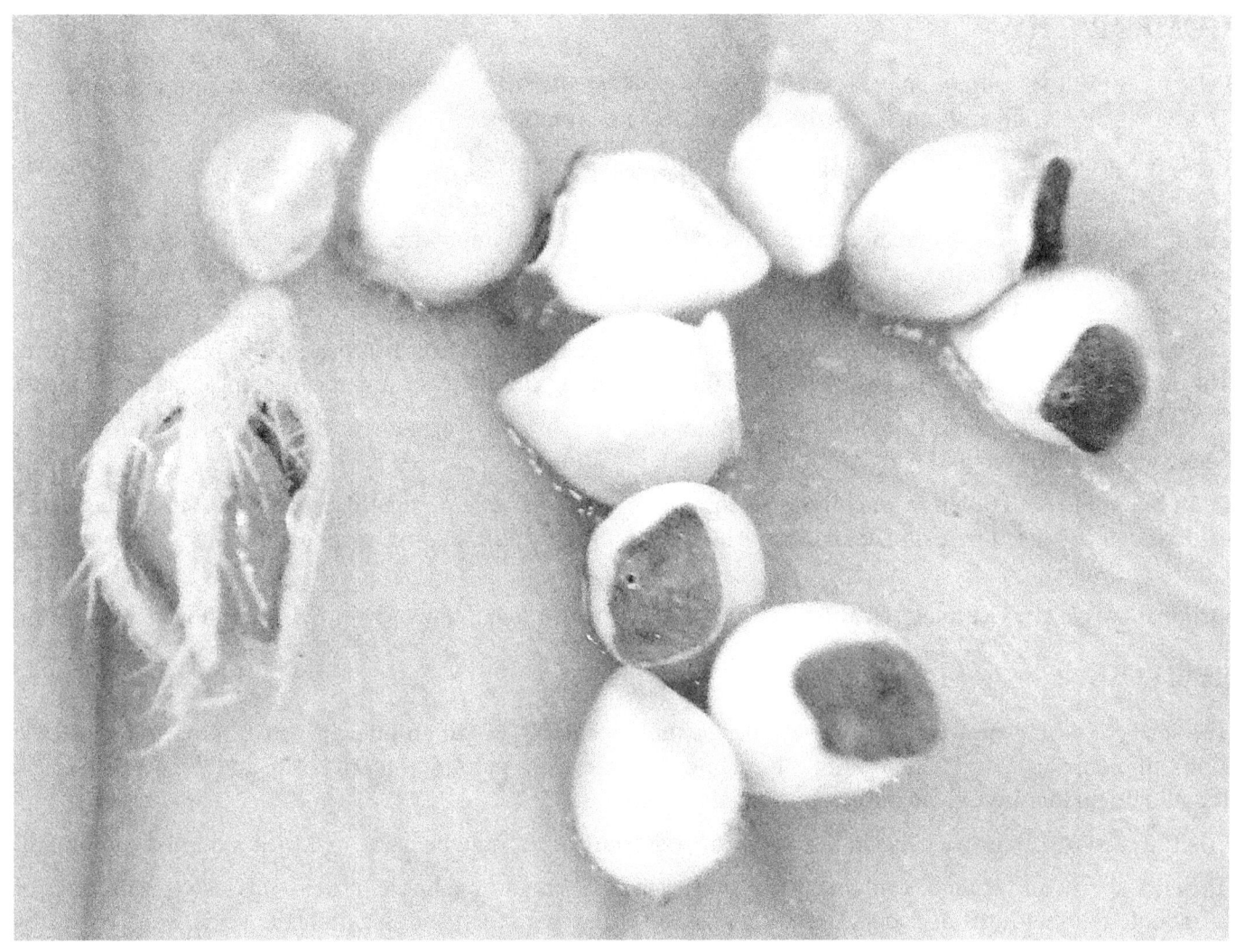

WESTERN GROMWELL SEEDS

The dried root is useful for diarrhea and the fresh root is more useful to aid menopausal transition.

It reduces enlarged prostate gland due to inactivation of luteinizing hormone. Use a combination of fresh flower/leaf and root tincture.

Field Gromwell (*B. arvensis*) seeds have been found non-toxic in mice studies and possess androgenic and aphrodisiac activity. Ilarionov et al, *Eksp Med Morfol* 1989 28(1): 28-33. The LD50 was over 3000mg/kg, suggesting very low toxicity.

The plant contains acetylshikonin that is a novel CYP2J2 inhibitor, and is cytotoxic against HepG2 liver carcinoma cell lines. Park SH et al, *Phytomedicine* 2017 24: 134-40.

Hoary Puccoon root contains compounds with anti-microbial activity. Pietrosiuk et al, *Herba Polonica* 2003 49.

Acetylshikonin inhibits the growth of oral squamous cell carcinoma by inducing apoptosis. A gargle of root decoctions may be a useful treatment or adjunct for this problematic condition. Kim DJ et al, *Arch Oral Biol* 2016 70:149-157.

This species is widely found throughout eastern Saskatchewan and down through southern Manitoba.

Obviously, much greater efforts on researching our native species should be undertaken.

HOMEOPATHY

False Gromwell (*O. virginianum*) is useful for those who suffer from lack of concentration and coordination. There may be vertigo and muscle weakness, tiredness and weariness.

It is for migraines, especially related to sexual tiredness, in both sexes. The eyes have blurred vision and tightness around the ocular muscles.

The male is in constant sexual excitement, but with psychological impotence. This can lead to loss of desire or insufficient erection, or in some cases to premature ejaculation. There is cold feeling in penis, with complete loss of sexual function.

The female may have her sexual desire completely destroyed. There is uterine soreness, with a bearing down pain. The breasts ache, the nipples itch. Days between the menstrual cycles are short, and the bleeding cycle is prolonged.

Symptoms are exaggerated from motion and tight clothing, humid, warm air, and darkness. The patient feels better when undressed and lying on back, from rest, or eating.

DOSE- Sixth to 30th potency. The migraines sometimes respond better to the third potency. The closely related *O. occidentale* is used in a similar manner. The mother tincture is made from the whole fresh above ground plant in flower.

Original proving by Green on self and woman with tincture in 1884, followed by proving on four males in 1885.

SEED OIL

The seeds of false gromwell (*O. molle var. occidentale*) yield 16-18% of an interesting oil composed of 25.8% alpha-linolenic acid, and 22.9% gamma-linolenic acid; as well as palmitic, stearic, oleic and docosenoic acids. It could be further investigated for commercial potential.

The 100 seed weight is twice that of flax and brown mustard, and could be harvested with modified equipment.

The endosperm and embryo contain 60% oil, of which 22.5% is gamma linolenic acid. It is also a rich source of tetraenoic acid, setting it in a very interesting position with regard to major essential fatty acids. More correctly, it is also known as eicosa-5, 8, 11, 14-tetraenoic acid.

Tetraenoic fatty acid inhibits proliferation and induces apoptosis in human liver cancer cells. Mondal A et al, *Int J Mol Sci* 2016 17(10).

Various tetraenoic acids can be synthesized, and act as endocannabinoid analogues, with high affinity for the CB1 cannabinoid receptor. Papahatjis DP et al, *Chemistry* 2010 16(3): 4091-9.

American Gromwell (*L. latifolium*) seeds contain up to 23.9% GLA, or gamma linolenic acid.

HYDROSOL

Gromwell water is distilled from the leaves. It is good for stone and gravel.   **BRUNSCHWIG**

FLOWER ESSENCES

False Gromwell flower essence is related to the soul qualities of fertility and sexuality. The qualities of abundance are universal in nature and difficulties regarding sexuality can permeate into the material world.

The essence is useful for those women who feel they can conceive by merely thinking about sex; or conversely, by those women who wish they did not have to deal with a monthly cycle.

It is for the man who suffers premature ejaculation, and yet cannot stop thinking about sex. It can be taken by couples that desire a healthier sex life.   **PRAIRIE DEVA**

Yellow Gromwell flower essence is for those who keep trying to make the dysfunctional family more "normal"; the fixers.   **ROCKY MOUNTAIN**

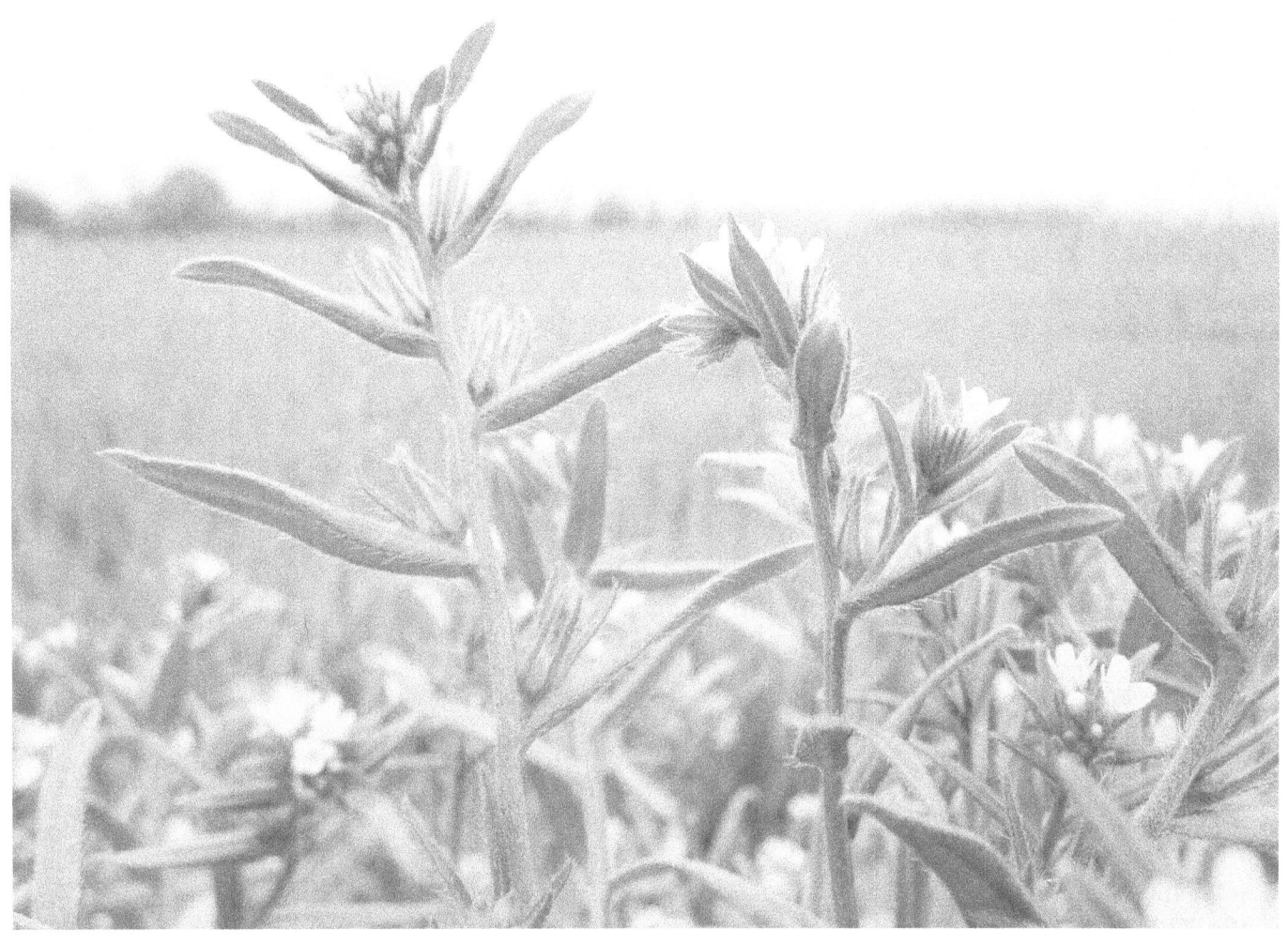

FIELD GROMWELL

PERSONALITY TRAITS

Where there is courage, there is also cowardice. Where there is boldness there is also timidity. Onosmodium's lack of confidence and mental weakness makes him wonder about whether he is doing the right thing or not. Clarke says: "Feeling as if something terrible was going to happen and that she was powerless to help it". Both Onosmodium and Symphytum are timid about appearing in public. The feelings of inadequacy are, in part, a representation of the waste ground that serves as the home for a good many of the species.   VERMEULEN

RECIPES

COLD INFUSION- Take one ounce of gromwell root to one pint of water. Steep overnight and gently warm in morning. Take one tablespoon every three hours for bladder complaints. One cup once a day is used for fertility control (theoretical).

September harvested roots are best, in my part of world.

SEEDS- powdered. Take one-half teaspoon every 4-5 hours for diuretic effect. One dose daily for fertility control (theoretical).

TINCTURE- fresh roots are cut and pounded and covered with 60% alcohol at 1:4 ratio. Use 10 drops for menstrual and menopausal issues, up to 40 drops in cold water for thyroid issues, including Grave's disease. The fresh flower/leaf tincture is very potent and made in season with same ratios.

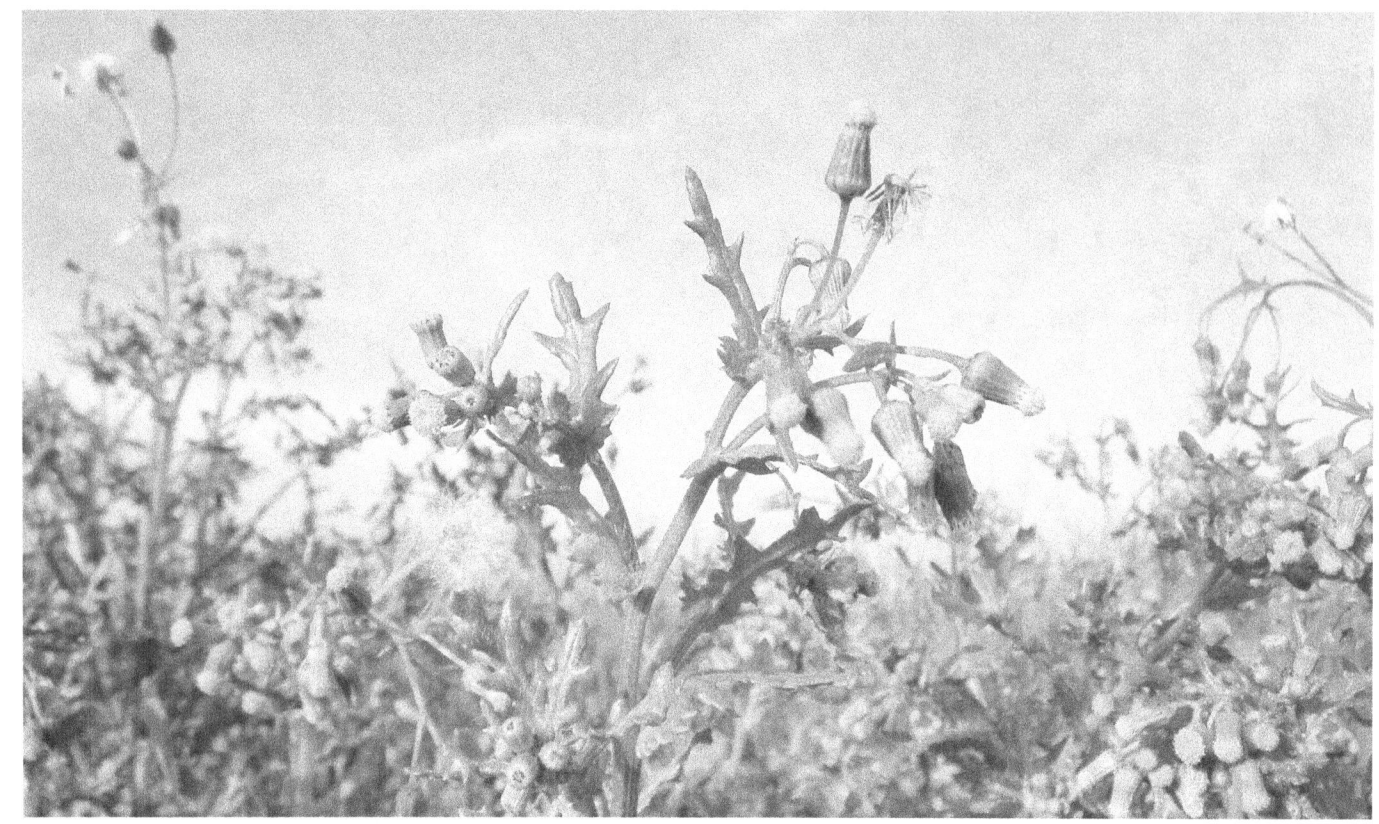

COMMON GROUNDSEL

GROUNDSEL
RAGWORT
(*Senecio vulgaris* L.)
GOLDEN RAGWORT
LIFEROOT
FALSE VALERIAN
STREAMBANK BUTTERWEED
(*S. aureus* L.) not accepted
(*S. gracilis* Pursh) not accepted
(*Packera aurea* [L.] A.& D. Löve)
MARSH RAGWORT
MASTODON FLOWER
(*Tephroseris palustris* [L.] Reichenbach)
(*S. congestus* [R. Br.] DC.) not accepted
(*S. palustris* [L.] Hook.) not accepted
(*Cineraria congesta*) not accepted
TANSY RAGWORT
RAGWORT
JACOB'S GROUNDSEL
(*S. jacobaea* L.) not accepted
(*Jacobaea vulgaris* Gaertn.)
LAMB'S TONGUE GROUNDSEL
(*S. integerrimus* Nutt.)

BLACK TIP GROUNDSEL
(*S. lugens* Richardson)
BALSAM GROUNDSEL
CANADIAN BUTTERWEED
(*S. pauperculus* Michx.)
(*Packera paupercula* [Michx.] A. Löve & D. Löve)
STINKING COTTON
STICKY GROUNDSEL
(*S. viscosus* L.)
ARROW-LEAVED GROUNDSEL
(*S. triangularis* Hook.)
ROCKY MTN BUTTERWEED
(*S. streptanthifolios* Greene) not accepted
(*P. streptanthifolia* [Greene] W. A. Weber & A. Love)
DUSTY MILLER
SILVER RAGWORT
(*S. cineraria* DC.) not accepted
(*S. bicolor* [Willd.] Todaro) not accepted
(*Jacobaea maritima* [L.] Peiser & Meijden)
PARTS USED- leaves, root

With venerable locks the Groundsel grows:
Hard care more quick than years
white head-gear shows.

ANON

A single tree cut down makes no greater a gap, and is no more missed, than when one pulls up a stalk of groundsel.

RICHARD SPRUCE

Let Warlocks grim, an' wither'd Hags
Tell how wi' you [Devil] pm ragweed nags
They skim the muirs an' dizzy crags
Wi' wicked speed.

ROBBIE BURNS

Decking rude spots with beautys manifold
That without thee were dreary to behold
Sunburnt & bare—the meadow bank the baulk
That leads a waggonway through the mellow field.

JOHN CLARE

Senecio is from the Latin **SENEX** meaning, old man, and referring to the fluffy white seed heads. It is derived from the same source as senile.

Balsam is either related to balmy, as in good weather, or to en-balm, as in Balsam fir. Packera is named after Canadian taxonomist John G. Packer.

Ragwort derives from the long use of Senecio species for menstrual issues.

Cineraria means "ashy gray", hence dusty. The color is supposed to resemble the dusty white wings of the miller moth; that in turn was named after the dusty clothing worn by grain millers.

Speaking of moths brings to mind the Tiger moth. Both the winged adult and younger larvae feed voraciously on *Senecio* spp. flowers, helping store toxic alkaloids in their flesh as a defense against predators. These moth larvae eat all in their path, save those plants with low pyrrolizidine alkaloids (PA) that the aphids (*Aphis jacobaeae*) graze on. They are no threat to the caterpillars, but the ants (*Lasius niger*) that keep the aphids company and enjoy the honeydew protect them jealously and will not allow even hungry caterpillars to attack them.

These low PA plants enjoy protection from the caterpillars because the low level of PA attracts aphids, which produce honeydew that is not too bitter for ants. A complex and yet workable arrangement.

Groundsel is derived from the Anglo Saxon, **GRUNDESWYLIGE** meaning ground swallower or glutton; referring to the rapid way it spreads or swallows the ground. Or it may be the name was transcribed to **GUNDESWEIGE**, from **GUND**, meaning matter discharged from the eyes, and **SWEIGE**, meaning swallower; thus Pus Absorber.

This developed into **GROWDYSWYLI** in the 15th century, when it was grown in monastery gardens.

Groundsel is associated with water and Venus. Carried as an amulet against toothache, it was believed to keep teeth healthy. St. James, the patron saint of horses, is the origin of the species name Jacobaea given to Tansy Ragwort.

At one time it was believed a cure for staggers that affects the nervous system of horses. The Saint's day, July 25, was believed to be its flowering day.

Tansy Ragwort is associated with the 19th Nordic Rune, Ehwaz. In Scotland, it is said that the fairies took shelter beside ragwort in stormy weather and road astride the plant from island to island. The stem was used to make wicker baskets, and a switch for livestock and mis-behaving children.

Because Senecio is a bio-accumulator of selenium, it is generally not used in medicine. Alberta has very few sites of selenium rich soil, but in other western regions it can vary greatly. Senecio species have been observed to rhizo-degrade crude oil.

Groundsel can go through a life cycle, from seed to flower to seed in just six weeks.

Groundsel (*S. vulgaris*) is an introduced annual that has been around so long we think of it as a common plant. It probably crept into grain sacks from Europe, and since one plant can lead to one million in a single year, it hasn't looked back.

Goats and pigs love it, while cows, sheep and horses avoid it if there's anything else in their field. Rabbits also love it, especially those raised in pens. Early German settlers cooked rabbit with Groundsel and milk as a favorite dish. The seeds are a popular food for canaries.

Ragwort is known in parts of Ireland as Fairy's Horse, as it was believed that fairy or witches rode on the stems of Ragwort.

One Gaelic name **AM BUALAN**, means the remedy.

It was said beloved by Leprechauns, or Clauricanes, the little fairy cobblers, who were sometimes seen singing or whistling over their work on a tiny shoe.

It was believed that every Leprechaun kept a buried treasure under a Ragwort, and if he is captured, he will show you where to dig.

Yellow Groundsel was believed to grow where a witch had paused to urinate. Burning the plant was a way to drive evil from the house, and get rid of vermin in clothing and bedding.

Pliny claimed it relieved toothache, but in a manner reserved to magic: "If a line is traced around Groundsel with an iron tool before it is dug up, and if one touches the painful tooth with the plant three times, spitting after each touch, and replaces it into its original ground so as to keep it alive, it is said that the tooth will never cause pain thereafter".

Dioscorides, from ancient Greece, was a little more scientific writing "that with the fine powder of frankincense it healeth wound in the sinues. The like operation hath the downe of the floures mixed with vinegar".

Gerard wrote, "The leaves of Groundsel boiled in wine or water, and drunke, heale the paine and ach of the stomacke that proceeds of Choler (cholera). Boiled in ale with a little hony and vinegar, it provoketh vomit, especially if you adde thereto a few root of wild ginger."

He added, "the leaves stamped and strained into milke and drunke, and helps the red gums and frets in Children."

Culpepper jumped into the fray and recommended the juice in wine to provoke urine and expel "the gravel in the reins and kidneys."

He recommended a poultice with salt for dissolving "knots and kernals in any part of the body", and infusions for "horses suffering botworms."

In Germany, the herb infusion was widely given to children as a vermifuge.

Infusions were recommended for sore throats, and pounded with lard for application to the pain of gout.

It combines well with ivy as a green burn salve, or with various mallow flowers for inflamed swellings.

The herb was used to soften water, by pouring hot water over the herb and letting it sit.

An old German recipe calls for boiling two handfuls of leaves in two quarts of white wine; drunk morning and evening to encourage delayed menses.

Freshly pulped groundsel combined with barley flour and a little rose oil, was laid over swellings of the private parts to get rid of inflammation. Groundsel and ground ivy are a traditional poultice for reducing skin tumors and overgrowth of keloid tissue.

Like Chrysanthemum, it attracts the marguerite fly, which lays its eggs on the leaves in spring. By acting as an early trap, it can be gathered and destroyed, helping save your cultivated garden plants in the Compositae family.

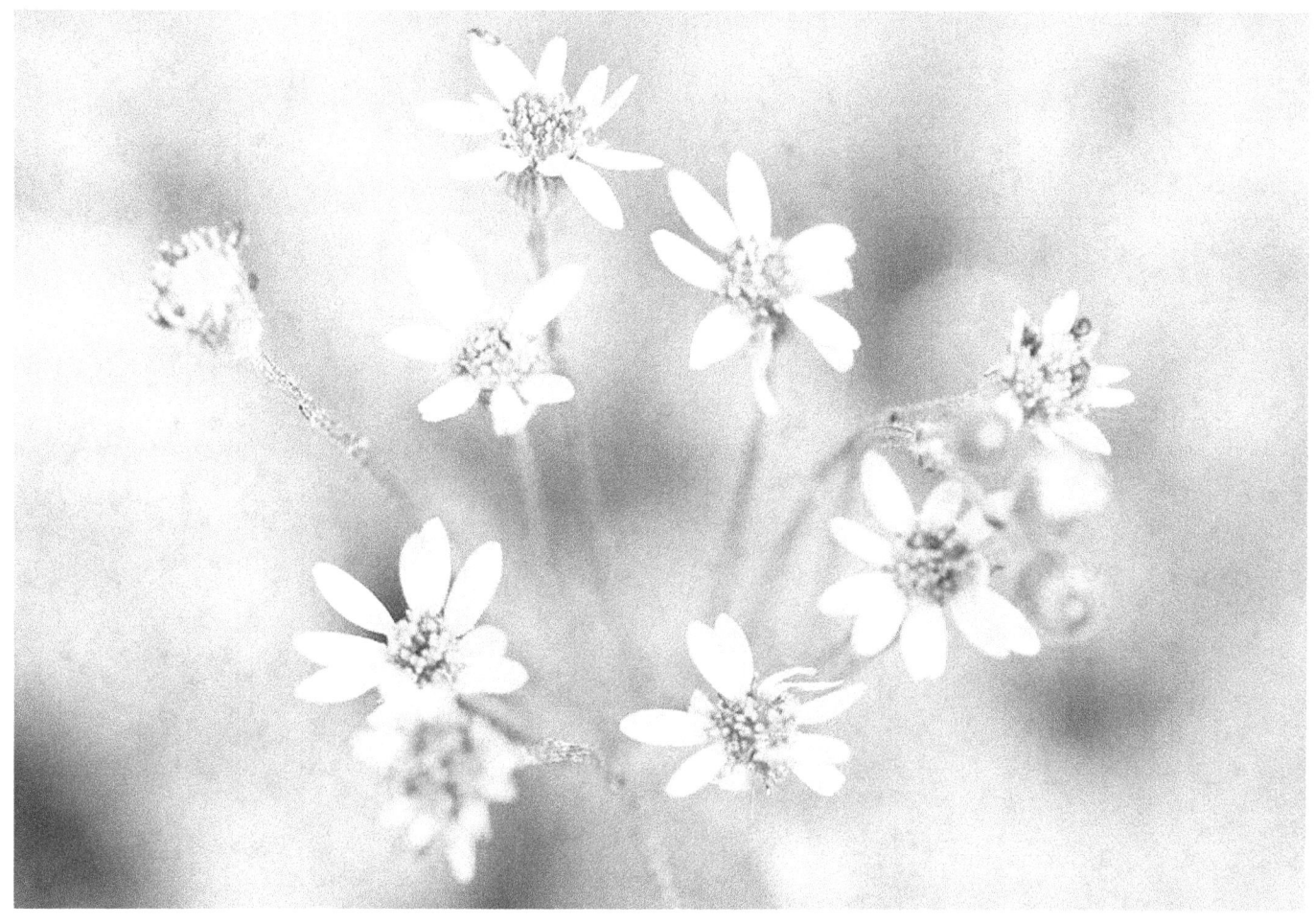

LIFEROOT

Chickens love the plant, and will seek it out as a tonic if allowed to free range, probably due in part to its iron content.

In Africa, the plant is macerated and rubbed onto affected hemorrhoids, chronic mastitis and gout.

The introduced plant is known in China as German Ivy, **QIAN LI GUANG**.

The aerial parts are prepared into an ointment for swellings and hemorrhoids.

Over 120 semi-synthetic compounds have been developed and investigated pharmacologically from Senecio species. The range of activity is from hypotensive, local anesthetic, ganglion blocking, neuromuscular blocking and antispasmodic activity. Work by Atal in the July-August 1978 issue of *Lloydia* gives additional information.

Golden Ragwort or Liferoot (*P. aurea*) is a native perennial long associated with assisting female reproductive problems, and used by various indigenous tribes. Names like unkum, waw weed and squaw weed speak to its use for menstrual issues.

It was used to speed up labor, but was also taken to prevent conception.

The Cherokee called it **DA LO NI GE I**, or Gold, and used it in formulas to prevent pregnancy.

They infused the plant for heart troubles, while the Iroquois used the roots as a diaphoretic, and a rosette infusion for children with fevers.

Nineteenth century herbalists believed it a menstrual regulator, and used it for treating vaginal discharge, and irregularities associated with menopause. It is still an ingredient, along with Black Cohosh and Fenugreek, in Lydia Pinkham's herbal formula for menstrual problems.

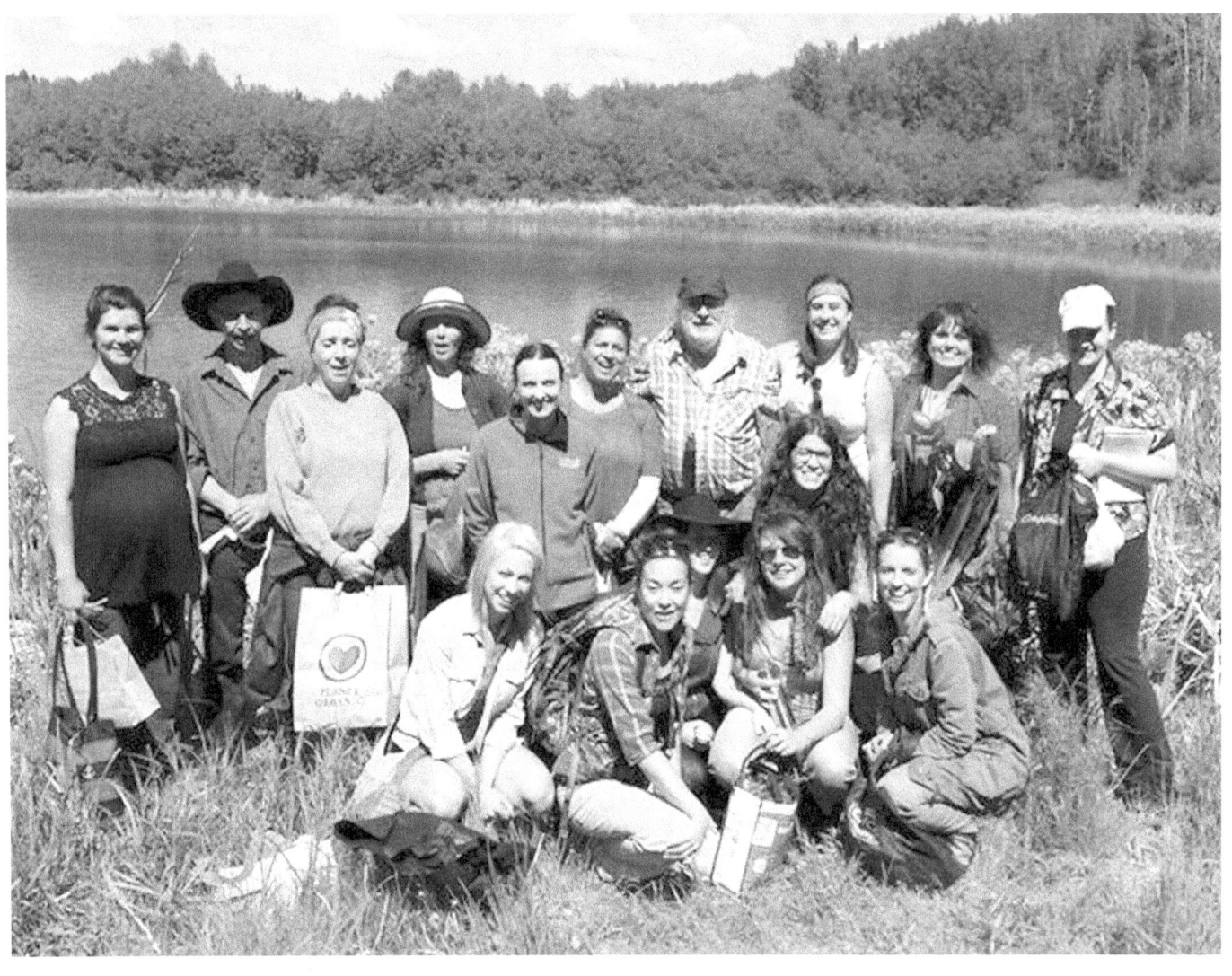

NORTHERN STAR STUDENTS AND MARSH RAGWORT

Dr. King believed, "Senecio often cures leucorrhea when associated with weakness of the vaginal walls, allowing uterine displacements, and accompanied with vascular engorgement and pelvic weight.

Senecio is of value in many genital disorders of the male, the indications being pelvic weight, and full, tardy, or difficult urination and sensation of dragging in the testicles."

Frederick Peterson wrote, in 1905. "Its special action is on the reproductive organs of both sexes, but especially the female. A tonic to the nervous and muscular structure of the reproductive organs of the female, with a tendency to bring about normal action, and therefore applicable alike to amenorrhea, metrorrhagia, menorrhagia, or dysmenorrhea. We think of it in a relaxed condition of the uterus and its appendages, relaxed condition of the support of the uterus resulting in displacements."

It is "of value in capillary hemorrhage, hematuria in large doses, albuminaria, especially during pregnancy, leucorrhea, chlorosis [kidney anemia]."

Professor O. Phelps Brown believed, "it exerts a very powerful and peculiar influence upon the reproductive organs of females. This has given it the name of Female Regulator. Combined with the Lily, and other native and foreign plants, it is one of the most certain cures in the world for aggravated cases of leucorrhea; also in cases of menstrual suppression."

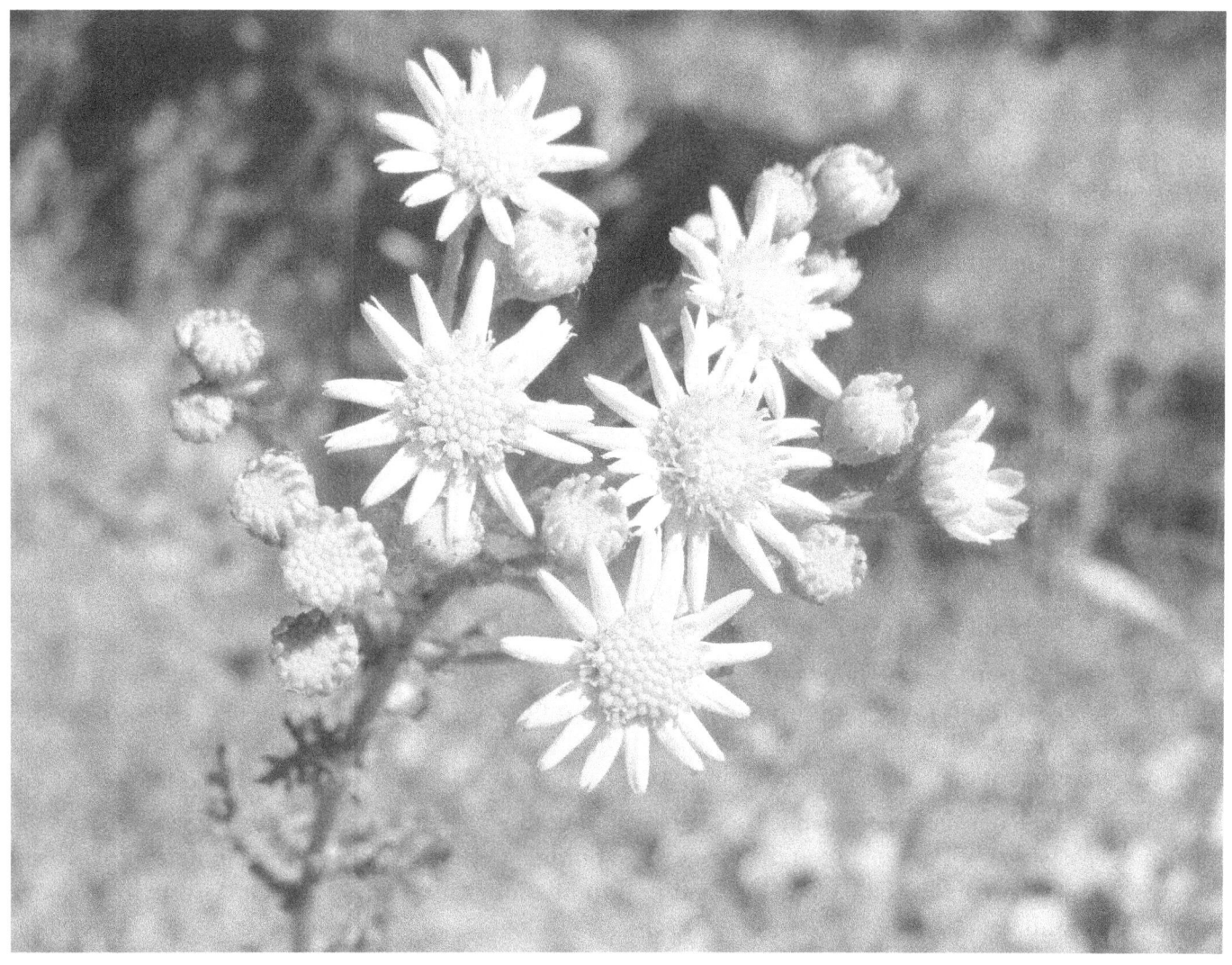

TANSY RAGWORT

It was believed useful in the very early stages of tuberculosis, a teaspoon of fluid extract in water acting as a tonic.

Golden Ragwort has been utilized for urinary problems including kidney stones, with dubious effect.

One study from Spain, reported the death of a man from sub-acute portal hypertension after consuming several cups of tea daily for two years.

Marsh Ragwort (*S. congestus*) was considered traditionally, to be poisonous by Western Arctic Eskimos. This is not true, as the young leaves and flowering stems can be eaten raw, or steamed as a potherb.

However, Marsh Ragwort is found in ditches, ponds, and marshes that may be polluted, either with herbicide or pesticide residues, or even excessive nitrites from fertilizer run off.

It can be considered an emergency food, but is really not that tasty.

Triangle leaved Groundsel (*S. triangularis*) roots and leaves were infused and given as a sedative for chest pains by Cheyenne of Montana. It was known as yellow medicine.

Black Tip Groundsel has come to be a symbol of mourning for the Inuit. The black tips of the involucral bracts are considered to symbolize the massacre at Bloody Falls on the Coppermine River, by a party headed by Samuel Hearne in 1771.

The Slave name is **NOGEOE NAYDI**, meaning Fox Medicine.

The introduced annual *S. viscosus* is known as Stinking Cotton, no doubt attributable to its odorous nature.

It was formerly used in Europe for both carminative and emetic properties.

Culpepper wrote, "this has been praised in fluxes of the belly, and the dysentery; it has the power of ipecac, but in a less degree, and not so agreeable a manner, it is very good in hysteric complaints. The leaves are carminative, and may be used in poultices, fomentations, and baths, but more especially the flowers..\. Inwardly, an infusion will expel wind, strengthen the stomach and stop vomiting."

Dusty Miller is a perennial in its native Mediterranean climate, but on the prairies is grown as an annual.

Its silver gray foliage makes a nice contrast in both rock gardens and more formal arrangements. It is often propagated from cuttings 8-10 weeks before last frost. The plant represents A Star, and birth date of January 25th.

Tansy Ragwort is found on disturbed soil, in warmer parts of British Columbia, such as the lower Fraser Valley and southern Vancouver Island. It has recently migrated to Edmonton's river valley (zone 3), and is considered a prohibited, noxious weed.

In Ireland, it is referred to as Fairie's Horse, and if you tread on them after sunset a horse will rise from the injured root and gallop away with you.

The expression "as rank a witch as ever rode on ragwort" stems from this belief.

Gerard says, "the country people doe call it Stagger-wort, and also Rag-wort". The name Staggerwort alludes to its use as a remedy for "staggers", which affects horses. It is probably the cause as well. In Scotland, the plant is known as stinking Billy, due to its unpleasant scent when bruised. Billy was William, Duke of Cumberland who was victorious at the Battle of Culloden in 1746.

Gerard also noted "It is much commended, and not without cause, to helpe old aches and paines in the armes, hips, and legs, boiled in hog's grease in the forme of an ointment. Moreover, the decoction hereof gargarised is much set by as a remedy against swellings and impostumations of the throat, which it wasteth away and thoroughly health...".

In regions where common, it is found to cause bizarre behaviour in horses confined to pastures with nothing else to eat. Liver function and structural changes occur, and abate themselves with time when new pasture is found.

The chronic lethal dose of Tansy Ragwort is 3.6% of body weight in horses.

Cattle can tolerate up to 1.5%, but die after twenty days at 2% or more in diet. Sheep are able to consume up to 20 times more Senecio compared to cattle due to different bacterial detoxification. The plant exceeds nutrient requirements for sheep in both protein and digestibility.

Larvae of the Cinnabar Moth (*Tyria jacobaea*) will graze on the plant until it is completely defoliated.

The alkaloids obtained, are retained through metamorphosis.

Tansy Ragwort roots are infused in Nepal for indigestion. In the Hebrides, the green, flowerless plant was said to have a smell that deters mice and rats, and sprinkled around grain bins and other food storage areas.

The plant was cut up with fresh butter and applied to tumors or boils to help them ripen; and to women's breasts that are hard or swollen.

The juice is astringent and used for burns, eye inflammation, sores and cancerous ulcers, and gargle for sore and ulcerated throat. Poultices were traditionally applied to sciatica, gout and rheumatic muscles.

The plant is a bio-monitor of iron, manganese, and zinc, and particular useful for monitoring manganese in aerial fallout.

MEDICINAL

CONSTITUENTS- *P. aurea*- aerial- florosenine, otosenine, and floridanin are pyrrolizidine alkaloids; ligularenolide, dehydrofukinone, (E)-9-oxofurano-ere-mophilane, 8alpha-ethoxy-10alphaH-eremophilane, tetra-hydro-ligularenolide, trans-9-oxo-furanoere-mophilane, cacalol, volatile oils, senecine, tannins, resins, rutin and other quercetin derivatives including kaempferol-3-0-glucosyl acetate and quercitin-3-0-glucosyl acetate.
shoot- senecifoline, senecine, senecionine.
S. integerrimus- senecionine, integerrimine.
S. congestus- senecionine, platyphylline, neoplatyphylline, undecene, tridecene.
S. vulgaris- up to 0.16% pyrrolizidine alkaloids including senecionine, senecionine-N-oxide, seneciphylline, integerrimine, retrorsine, spartioidine, usaramine, essential oils, and flavonoids including isorhamnetin-3-0-glucosides, isohamnetin-3-0-rutinosides, isorham-netin-3-monosulphate; and volatile oils.
S. triangularis- 7-0-angelyl; 9-0-angelyl- and 7-0-angelyl-9-0-sarracinylretronecine; as well as 9-0-acetyl-7-0-angelyl-retronecine; senecionine, senecionine N-oxide.
From 60-80% of the pyrrolizidine alkaloids are found in the flowers.
S. pseudaureus- retrorsine, senecionine.
S. strepthanthifolios- as above
J. maritima- several chemotypes that contain pyrrolizidine alkaloids (0.1-0.9%) one containing jacobine, jacozine, jaconine, jacoline, and senecionine; and another containing erudufoline and 0-acetyllerucifoline; as well as volatile oils.
S. viscoscus- senecionine, squalidine, pachypodol.

Groundsel, through its cholinergic activity, is a uterine sedative. It is used in amenorrhea in women with blood vacuity, anemia or low estrogen levels. It should not be used over a long time, due to the danger of liver toxicity.

Groundsel also has action on the parasympathetic nervous system, and is astringent, expectorant and emollient.

In Germany, the expressed juice was a popular de-wormer for children, while in France, Groundsel tea is believed to regulate and induce menstruation.

The plant juice is cooling, and acts like plantain on insect bites, and is a styptic like yarrow for bleeding wounds.

As a warm poultice, it draws boils and brings abscesses to a head, but for inflamed breasts a cold poultice is preferred.

Chapped hands can be soothed, by soaking them in warm Groundsel infusions.

Senecionine possesses spasmolytic activity. Litvinchuk MD et al, *Farmakol Toksikol* 1979 42(5): 509-11.

Seneciphylline has hypotensive action.

Work by Loizzo et al, *Phyto Res* 18:9 found hexane extracts of the plant active against *Trichophyton tonsurans*.

Liferoot, or Golden Ragwort, has been used by indigenous healers to treat various gynecological problems. It is particularly noted for relieving labor pains after delivery. Two to five drops in warm water every half hour as needed.

Atonic, spastic and congestive conditions of the uterus, and other pelvic organs, is where it is most helpful. The herb may be combined with motherwort, or cramp bark as required.

Note that senecionine, mentioned above, is plentiful in the shoots, and is anti-spasmodic.

Scanty, late painful periods are helped, as are early, excessive bleeding conditions.

This action also applies to painful, spasmodic urination or in cases of urinary incontinence when cold damp conditions are present in the body.

If used for preparing for childbirth, use only 10-20 drops once a day, about ten days before due date.

A plant decoction, strained and cooled, can be used for excessive vaginal discharge. It is an ingredient in the famous Lydia Pinkham's herbal for urogential problems.

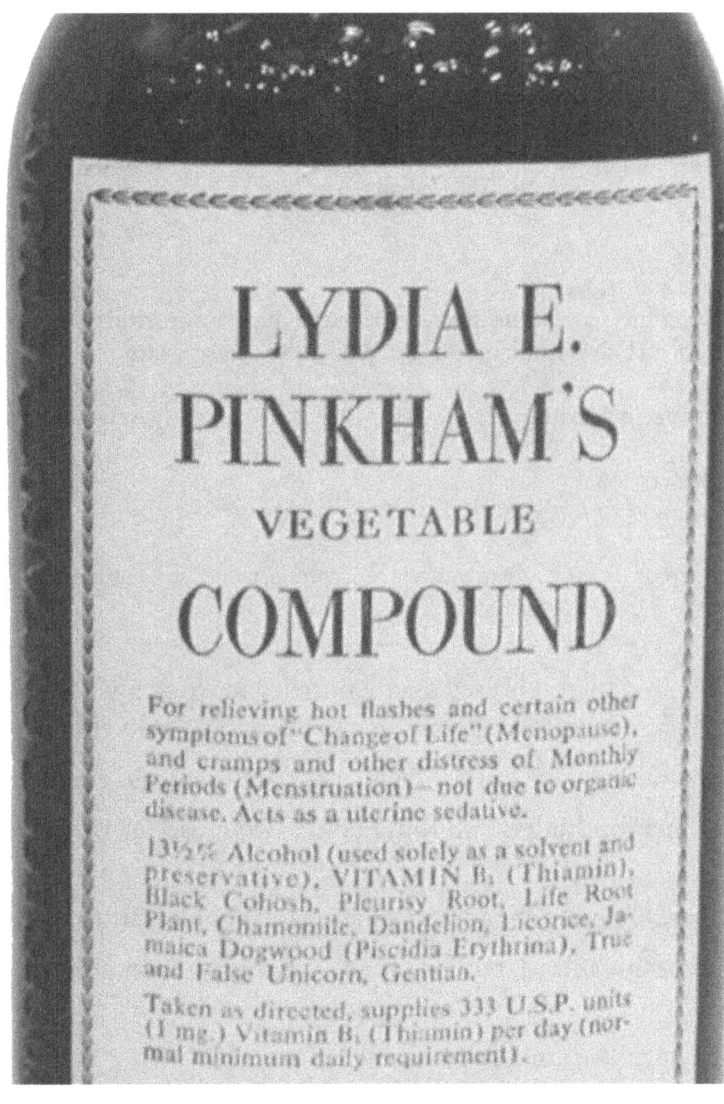

LIFE ROOT IN LYDIA PINKHAM'S
VEGETABLE COMPOUND

Various Eclectic physicians, especially Dr. King considered it one of the valuable remedies in the treatment of female disease.

Ovarian or uterine atony, including prolapse, sterility, dysmenorrhea and amenorrhea are all relieved. Dr. Bastyr suggested the herb to treat lax uterine ligaments in women, caused by numerous deliveries.

In cases of chronic leucorrhea, combine life root with white pond lily root as both a vaginal douche and infusion.

A very definite relationship has been traced between the nose and female sexual organs. Jacobson's organ, or vomeronasal organ is found in small pits of the nasal passage, and has direct links to a more primal aspect of self. It responds to scents in a completely different manner to our olfactory nerves.

Senecio is indicated when nasal catarrh takes the place of menses, when suppressed from any cause. The menses may be early and profuse, or late and absent.

For menorrhagia, Liferoot combines well with raspberry leaves and cinnamon. For suppressed menstruation, combine with Motherwort, and with Green flowering Oats for menopausal relief.

Cacalol, a sesquiterpene, induces apoptosis in breast cancer cells, and is synergistic with taxol and cyclophosphamide, helping overcome chemo-resistance. Liu W et al, *Breast Cancer Res Treat* 2011 128(1): 57-68.

The compound blocks K(ATP) channels in a manner similar to glibenclamide in lowering plasma glucose levels. Campos MG et al, *J Ethnopharm* 2009 123(3): 489-93.

It also possesses anti-inflammatory activity. Jimenez-Estrada M et al, *J Ethnopharm* 2006 105(1-2): 34-8.

And it is a potent anti-oxidant and neuro-protective compound that could guard neuronal cells from L-glutamate toxicity. Shindo K et al, *Biosci Biotechnol Biochem* 2004 68(6): 1393-4.

King believed the plant useful for male genital disorders with pelvic congestion, tardy or difficult urination, and dragging of the testicles. Add to this, the use of the herb in benign prostatic hypertrophy, keeping in mind the herb should not be taken long term.

Capillary hemorrhage, or bloody urine also call for its use, and in combination with other diuretics was considered specific in strangury.

In pulmonary and hepatic affections, it can be quite useful, the remedy bringing slow effect in chronic disorders.

For asthmatic spasms, use equal parts of life root, Cudweed *(Gnaphalium uliginosum),* and Wormwood as an inhalation steam. See below.

Dr. William Cook believed it useful for old and debilitated coughs, and suggested that some physicians prefer it to goldenseal root for sub-acute and chronic dysentery.

"It is only be remembering it tonic and nervine qualities, that the true character of its action can well be understood".

David Hoffman suggests combining Life Root with St. John's wort, Green-flowering Oats or Pulsatilla for menopausal symptoms.

There are probably safer ways to induce menstrual periods or to relieve menopausal symptoms. Using the flowering tops and leaves in tincture is best. It is best during the luteal phase of menstrual cycle. Like all senecio species, the plants are most toxic when young shoots. The combination of PAs and other alkaloids in this species are at the lower end of toxicity.

CAUTION- Most of the herb products available on the market under this name are *S. vulgaris*, even though they don't look similar, nor have the same constituents.

Today, decoctions or tinctures of Tansy Ragwort are used for their detergent and diaphoretic effects, in the treatment of coughs, colds, catarrh, and to relieve sciatica, rheumatism and gouty pains. The plant is also used as a gargle for relaxed throats.

Tansy Ragwort combines well with *Lobelia inflata*, St. John's Wort and *Pyrola rotundifolia* for lotions to relieve arthritis, rheumatism, muscular pain and sciatica. Regulations in Britain restrict Ragwort use externally to 10% dilutions.

Work by Hol et al, *J Chem Ecol* 2002 28:9 found the pyrrolizidine alkaloids (PA) of Tansy Ragwort were efficient inhibitors of fungal growth.

Dusty Miller (*J. maritima*) is native to the Caribbean and used for the treatment of senile cataract, conjunctivitis, or when vision is generally weak, especially after serious acute illness. The mechanism appears related to some form of lymphatic drainage from the eye.

Seneciphylline has been found to have hypotensive properties.

Marsh Ragwort (*S. congestus*) contains platyphilline, a hypotensive agent.

Senecio triangularis contains tumor inhibitors. Kupchan SM & MI Suffness, *J Pharm Sci* 1967 56(4): 541-3.

Senecio pauciflorus, sometimes known as *Packera pauciflora*, is a familiar moist alpine and subalpine meadow plant.

Work by Shavarda et al, *Rastitel'nye- Resursy* 1998 34:2 found anti-oxidant properties in the aerial parts of the plant.

Dutch research in 1994 showed Ragwort plants have significantly lower levels of pyrrolizidine alkaloids, when growing in areas of reduced sunlight.

It is worth noting that although various senecio toxins are cumulative and may cause Budd-Chiari syndrome and progressive liver cirrhosis, small doses for a short period of time appear to reduce cancerous growths.

Senecio campestris, for example, contains alkaloids that inhibit sarcoma 180 cell lines.

Chachacoma (*S. graveolens*/*S. nutans*) found in the Andes Mountains, contains compounds active against various breast cancer cell lines, including ZR-75-1, MCF-7 and MDA-MB-231. Echiburu-Chau C et al, *Int J Oncol* 2014 44(4): 1357-64.

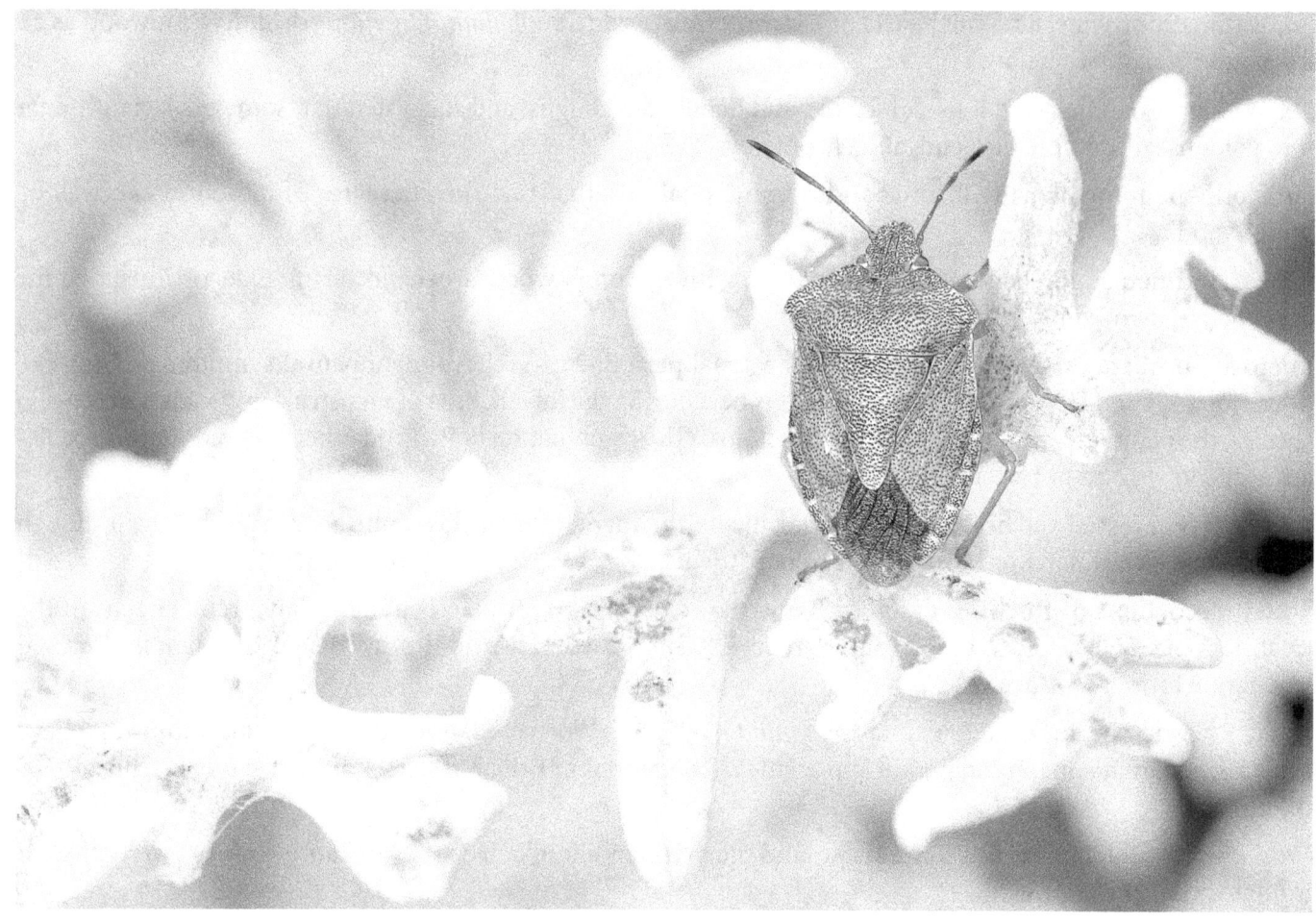

SHIELD BUG ON DUSTY MILLER

HOMEOPATHY

Dusty Miller- *Cineraria maritima* is an unproved remedy but is said to have proved its worth in glaucoma and corneal opacity. In such conditions, generally the pure juice of the plant is dropped into the eye externally and the treatment continued for some months.

However, internal use is also said to be successful, especially where the formation of glaucoma follows injury, or in corneal opacity or even senile glaucoma. Thus in cases where there is no strict indication for surgery, it is recommended to attempt treatment for cataracts. I personally observed great benefit in early stage cataracts in clinical practice.

DOSE- Tincture- 4-5 drops, diluted in pure water in eyecup, in each eye daily. The mother tincture is prepared from the whole fresh plant, gathered before flowering.

Golden Ragwort (*S. aureus*) is used for cases of exhaustion and lassitude in displacement of the uterus. It is used in pulmonary catarrhs with blood streaked expectoration and tendency to hemorrhage.

Sharp pain in teeth and headaches on the left side, as well as dry throat and burning in pharynx.

Urine is scanty, bloody and with constant urging and great heat.

Males may suffer from enlarged prostate, hard and swollen to touch, involuntary seminal emissions and sexual dreams, or a dull heavy pain in the spermatic cord, extending to testes.

For women, the menses are suppressed with functional amenorrhea in young girls with dropsy tendency. Inflammation of the throat, chest or bladder can occur before menses and disappear afterwards.

Anemic dysmenorrhea with urinary disturbances can occur.

Nasal congestion in the place of menses can also occur.

Talcott regards this remedy to be midway between the pugilistic state of Belladonna, and the tearful state of Pulsatilla. An apt description.

DOSE- Tincture to 3rd potency. The mother tincture is prepared from the fresh plant during flowering. First proving by Small on self and other male with tincture in 1865. Jones also self-experimented in same year. Additional clinical observations in Hering and by Phatak. Useful case studies in *Plants Volume One* by Vermeulen & Johnston pages 794-800.

Tansy Ragwort (*S. jacobaea*) is for cerebro-spinal irritation, rigid muscles chiefly of the shoulders and neck. It is also used in some cancers. Observations by Cooper found it causes a very depressed state of mind and body and incoherent talking, loss of memory, exhaustion in the back of the head and a feeling of rigidity of the neck and shoulders; also diarrhea and enuresis.

DOSE- Tincture to 3rd potency. The mother tincture is prepared from the fresh plant in flower.

Cooper added this case: A man, 68, many years apoplectically inclined, had constant twitchings at night with vascular deafness of right ear, loss of memory, pressure and heat of head: after a dose of *Senecio jacobaea* Ø he remained comfortable for three months and hearing improved.

ESSENTIAL OILS

The flowering tops of Common Groundsel (*S. vulgaris*) consist of 26% alcohols and phenols, 37% aldehydes and ketones, and about 10% esters.

The leaf and stems are much richer in alcohol and phenols (37%), with smaller amounts of aldehydes and ketones (11%) and less than 7% esters.

The roots contain nearly 30% alcohol and phenols, nearly 9% aldehydes and ketones and less than 3% esters.

Beta caryophyllene is the main component, with mycrene, alpha copaene, beta farnesine and germacrene D also present.

The essential oil from the plant consists of (Z)-3-hexen-1-ol, 3-methylhexan-1-ol, alpha terpineol and decanol, 2-methylbenzyl alcohol, benzyl alcohol, furfuryl acetate, methyl palmitate, and 6,10,14-trimethylpentadecan-2-one.

Tansy Ragwort (*S. jacobaea*) contains essential oils consisting of germacrene D, and 1-undecene as major components, and 1-nonene, myrcene, trans-ocimene, and beta caryophyllene. Small amounts of alpha pinene, beta phellandrene, cis-beta-ocimene, damascenone, cerany-lactone, trans-beta-farnesene, humulene, gamma cadinene, calacorene, and lauric acid also present.

The oil could be used externally in an ointment of lotion for the relief of rheumatic pain, and myalgia.

The essential oil of Marsh Ragwort *(S. congestus)* is rich in 1-tridecene, some lauric acid, and traces of 1-nonene, 1-undecene, alpha cedrene and trans-beta-farnesene.

The essential oil of the closely related *S. graveolens* shows activity against *Micrococcus luteus* ATCC 9341, oxacillin-sensitive and oxacillin-resistant *Staphylococcus aureus*, as well as anti-fungal activity on *Candida albicans*.

Dusty Miller (*S. cineraria*) has been steam distilled and reveals 32 components, mainly composed of alpha pinene (27.8%), camphene (22.9%) and borneol (7.39%).

From the leaves, dihydroquercetin, aginenin 7-0-glucoside, luteolin 7-0-glucoside were isolated.

Xanthtoxin, isopimpinellin, marmesin, aesculetin, alpha amyrin, beta amyrin, stigmasterol and beta sitosterol were isolated from the roots.

HYDROSOLS

The distilled water performs everything that can be expected from its virtues, especially for inflammations or watering of the eyes.

CULPEPPER

Sauer, in his Compendious Herbal wrote, "the distilled water of groundsel is useful for treating blockage of the liver and for getting rid of jaundice, when taken in a half gill dose with Succory (chicory) water in the morning before breakfast".

FLOWER ESSENCES

Golden Ragwort (*S. aureus*) flower essence is for uprooting rage and earthing the Creative Self. The Flowering Soul surrenders in reality and one's Life roots in the Earth.

naturasSacredplay

Tansy Ragwort (*S. jacobaea*) flower essence is for those fearing to give of self, as in fear of commitment; being afraid you can't love; the inability to make friends with much insecurity and inferiority complex.

In the positive, there is greater security of the inner and outer self. Being successful, achieving loving relationships, and intimacy.

NEW ZEALAND

Ragwort (*S. jacobaea*) helps to build respect for our body's natural wisdom. It calms an emotionally confused and mentally overactive mind.

HAREBELL

Tansy Ragwort (*S. jacobaea*) essence helps us get back to the roots of development and puts technical achievements in relative importance.

MIRIANA

Groundsel (*S. integerrimus*) essence stimulates the nervous system into receptivity to be in connection with all of life around you and recognize that there is a safe and meaningful pattern to all of life.

This is a grounding essence and operates on the first, second and third chakras to bring the physical body into a state of openness, acceptance and relaxation. The gentle calmative quality of this essence is much like the kind of energy you might get from grandparents tucking you into bed.

HIGH SIERRA

SPIRITUAL PROPERTIES

Senecio is associated with observation and prolonging attention in order to see better.

THE MOTHER

RECIPES

INFUSION- One tbsp. of dried herb to one cup of hot water. Steep 10 minutes. Drink three times daily.

TINCTURE- 1-15 drops 3 times daily. For speeding childbirth and re-establishing stopped labour, take 10-15 drops of the fresh plant tincture every half hour. Tincture of *S. aureus* dried plant is made at 1:5, fresh at 1:2 with 50% alcohol. Use only the flowers and leaves. Do not use for an extended period of time.

INHALATION STEAM FOR ASTHMA- Combine equal parts liferoot, wormwood and marsh cudweed (one ounce of each to quart of water. Simmer for ten minutes and remove from heat. Cover head and pot with towel and inhale for one half hour as needed. In mild attacks, combine with hot mustard footbath.

All Senecio species are potentially tetragenic and contra-indicated during pregnancy and breastfeeding. A recent animal study look at toxicity of PAs in comfrey, *Petasites hybridus*, *Senecio vernalis*, and comfrey.

Contrary to previous reports in the literature for PAs exposure, no hepatic and biliary toxic effects were observed after 28 days. Seremet OC et al, *Rom J Morph Embryol* 2016 57(3): 1017-23.

The plants are most toxic when young. Studies of Tansy Ragwort (*S. jacobaea*) indicate hepatotoxicity is potentiated by copper.

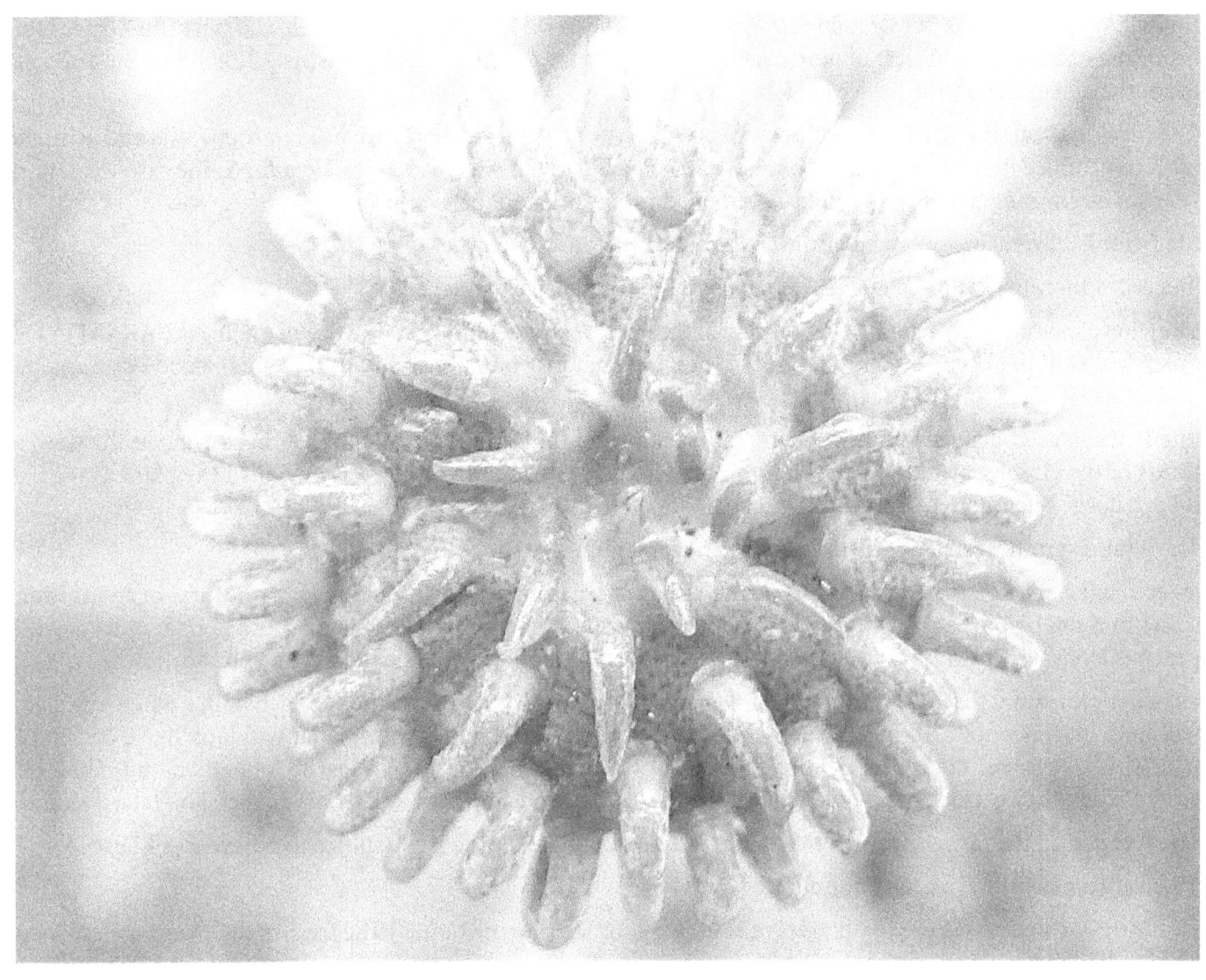

GUMWEED RESIN ON UNOPENED FLOWER BUD

GUMWEED
ROSINWEED
(**Grindelia squarrosa** [Pursh] Dunal)
PARTS USED- flowers and leaves

Grindelia is named after the 19th century Latvian botanist David Grindel. Squarrosa is from the Latin **SQUARROSE** meaning rough with scales, or parts spreading to a right angle, or re-curved.

Gumweed is native to the drier plains of the prairie, and plentiful in certain locations. The name comes from the resinous and sticky exudations of the plant and from where the medicinal properties come. The resin protects the plant from solar radiation and water loss. The early French voyageurs noted the resinous quality and called it **EPINETTE DE PRAIRIE**.

The Cree call it **KAH-PUS-KUN-ASKIK**, **KAPASAKWASK MASKIHKIH** or **KAPIKIYOWAPAKWANI**.

They use the entire plant, with pineapple weed, for kidney pain and buds and flowers only for gonorrhea. The aerial plant was ingested by women in an unspecified manner, to prevent pregnancy.

241

Russell Willier, a northern Cree healer, calls it Gum flower. He has patients inhale the burning flowers for headaches. Some Cree healers of Northern Alberta use it for treating venereal disease. The indigenous people of southern Alberta used a flower tea for migraines.

The Blackfoot call it **AKS-PEIS** or "sticky weed". The resinous, upper parts are used in bronchitis and asthma, both to produce more mucous and to relieve spasms. The plant was made into a tea for kidney troubles, and later for attempting to control syphilis. The boiled root was eaten for liver problems.

Many tonic beverages contained gumweed for its cleansing action.

The self-adhering flowers can be stuck on wounds like adhesive bandage.

The Cheyenne rubbed the gum on the outside of the eyes for snow-blindness. The Pawnee name is **BAKSKITITS**, or sticky head; the Dakota name is **PTE ICHIYUHA** for curly buffalo, and both the Omaha and Ponca name of **PEZHE WASEK** means, "strong herb".

The Pawnee used decoctions to wash the saddle sores on their horses, while the Flathead rubbed the flower heads of the closely related *G. howellii* into horse hooves to strengthen them. They boiled the plant as tea for tuberculosis, pneumonia, bronchitis, and asthma.

The young, gummy flowers can be used as a chewing gum.

Josephine Peters, a Karuk elder, suggests grindelia aerial parts for settling the stomach in the form of an infusion thirty minutes before eating. For cancer patients, drink about half a cup, then wait half and hour and drink wild peach (*Oemieria cerasiformis*) leaf tea. Grindelia settles the stomach so the wild peach will stay down.

Take both for about three weeks. After taking grindelia for two to three days, the stomach lining, when expelled, will look like coconut. "All of a sudden you'll get really sick, and you'll vomit what will look like a bunch of hair. This is fevers of the cancer coming out. A lot of patients will only take it just so long, then quit. They get scared when they get sick. But you take it three weeks, then you stop for a week or two, then you take it again."

The Crow used the flowers in a tea to soothe postpartum pain, or as a hot poultice to relieve swellings.

The leaf-less stems have been bound for brooms.

Hot baths, or steams are used by natives of southwest for "cold in the bones". The fresh green plants are crushed and applied to rheumatic pains.

Traditionally, *G. squarrosa* was used to treat the intermittent fevers associated with infections like malaria. It was used for spleen enlargement, associated with liver congestion. This was accompanied by indigestion, a sense of fullness and pain in the left hypochondrium, weakness, lethargy, and a pallid, sallow complexion.

The herb entered the modern *Materia Medica* when James Steele presented a monograph to the *American Pharmaceutical Association* in 1875. It was official in the *USP* from 1882-1926 and the *National Formulary* from 1926 until 1960. *Grindelia robusta* and *G. integrifolia* are practically inter-changeable.

Frederick Petersen wrote in his *Materia Medica & Clinical Therapeutics* 1905.

"Interruption of respiration takes place, so that it can sometimes only be carried on by will power. It is the remedy for chronic or old cases of malaria, malarial cachexia, splenic hypertrophy, stomach troubles, neuralgia, irritable coughs with nervous erethism, the results of malaria."

Plant patents exist for gumweed related to hydrocarbon extraction, food preservative, and freeze-resistant latex paint.

It grows well in a community of Tasselflower, Penstemon and Mullein. In southeastern Alberta it seems to enjoy the company of *Artemisia* species.

Gumweed may be useful in treating asthma or kennel cough in dogs, combining well with coltsfoot, mullein and wild cherry bark.

The buds may be added to cheap white wine to produce a Retsina-type drink.

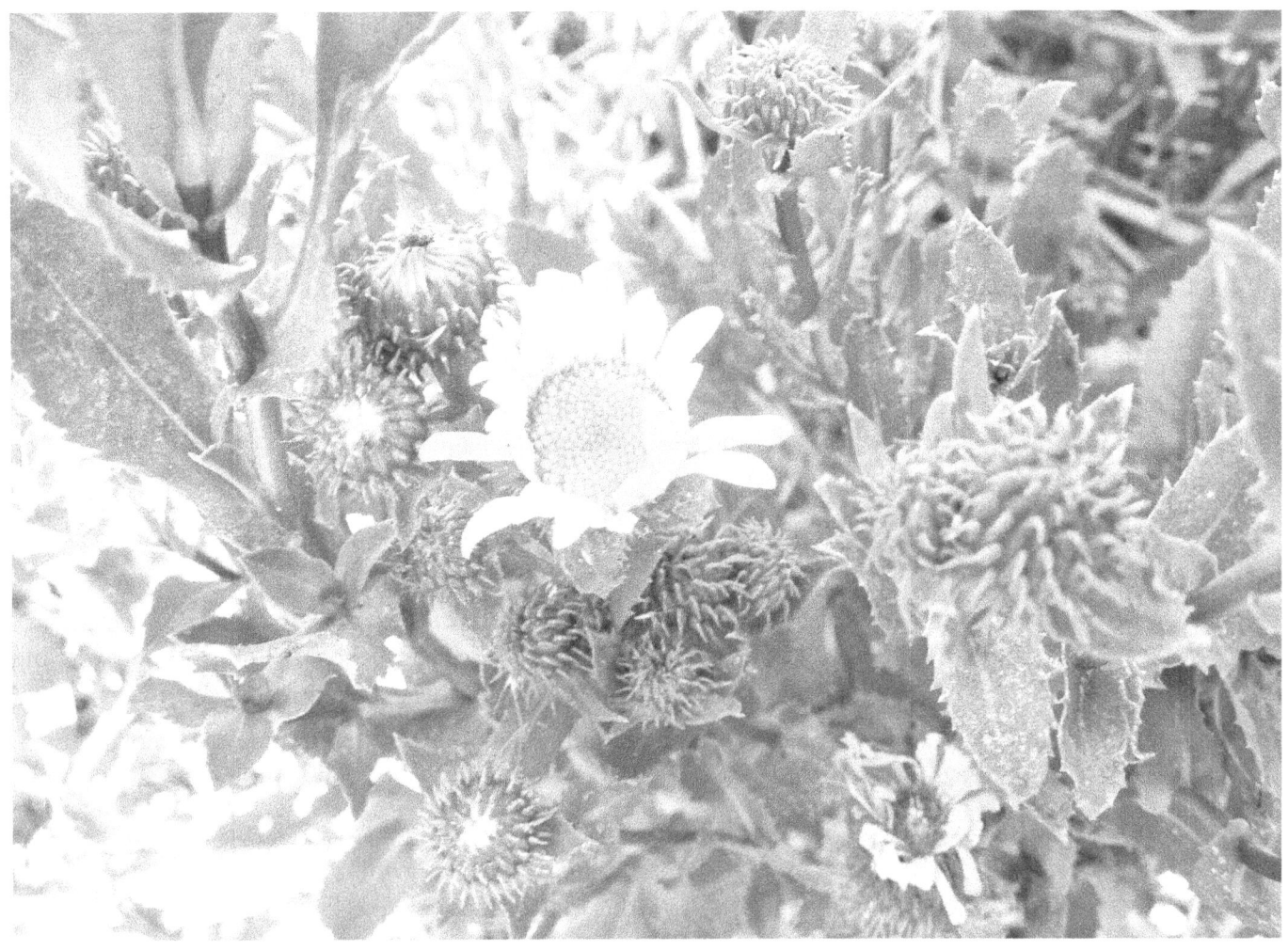

GUMWEED FLOWERS AND STICKY BUDS

MEDICINAL

CONSTITUENTS- leaves- 10-16% resin, grindelic acid, 13-iso-grindelic acid, 17-grindeloxygrindelic acid; various flavonoids: acacetin, kumatakenin, and quercitin, grindelia sapogenin (a triterpenoid lactone), oleanolic acid, bayogenin, phytosterin, matricarianol and its acetate, matricianol, laevoglucose and tannins.
flowers- 16% resins, various flavonoids including quercetol, 3-methyl-quercetol, 3, 3'-dimethylquercetol, apigenin methyl ether, 3-methylkaempferol, 3,7-dimethyl-kaempferol, chrysoeriol 7-glucuronide and luteolin; hentriacontane, eryl alcohol, palmitic acid, saponins, phytosterol, and grindelol, a phytosterol glycoside. Phenolic acids in flowers are 6.81 mg/g, and leaves 6.59 mg/g.
G. integrifolia- aerial parts, tarapacol, tarapacanol A, grindelic acid, methyl grindeloate, 3beta-hydroxygrindelic acid, and manoyl-alpha-arabinopyranoside diterpenoids.

Gumweed is a circulatory regulator and respiratory relaxant, or anti-spasmodic.

Gumweed relaxes the smooth and swollen bronchials as well as heart muscle. This makes it invaluable in asthmatic and bronchial conditions where there is rapid heart beat and nervous response. Gumweed combines well with sundew for whooping cough, or whenever increased expectoration is called for.

One of the key symptoms is the dry, spasmodic coughing, but also in excessive thick and sticky phlegm that is difficult to remove.

It softens and moisturizes the bronchi, increasing mucolytic activity. A strong hot infusion of half cider and half water helps loosen a cough and relax the lungs. It helps to desensitize nerve ending in the bronchial tree and slow heart rate.

For Gumweed think of constricted and labored breathing along with dry cough and sore, raw, irritated membranes.

It is useful for acute and chronic bronchitis, with thick, viscous and unproductive mucus.

For asthma, combine with mullein leaf and small amount of lobelia. For dry, irritating cough, and dry asthma combine with sundew.

The dried heads can be combined with lobelia as an herbal smoke for acute asthma attacks. It is no cure, but relieves the spasms and constriction.

Kumatakenin exhibits inhibition of *Mycobacterium tuberculosis*, suggesting possible benefit in this serious health condition. Villaflores OB et al, *Pharmacogn Mag* 2010 6(24): 339-44. The compound is also present in flower bud of *Artemisia scoparia*.

Eclectic symptoms include plethoric or excessive individuals, with dirty brown tongue and pale mucus membranes in the mouth. The skin is sallow and pale, and the face is dusky and flushed.

There may be dull, heavy headaches with dizziness, nausea and lassitude.

Cool water infusions are more useful for stomach indigestion and settling the stomach due in part to a mild aromatic bitter sensation.

Gumweed is relaxing to the heart and pulse rate, thereby reducing blood pressure; after an initial rise. It combines well with lily of the valley in cases of pulmonary edema, or left-sided heart congestion, as both are good draining diuretics. Use with caution in cases of bradycardia, as the herb can slow heart rate.

Because gumweed leaves a bitter, acrid sensation in the mouth, the flow of saliva continues for a considerable time. It can irritate the kidneys, which explains its diuretic effect, but it does treat bladder and urethral infections effectively.

Nasal congestion and sore throats respond well to steaming and gargling with gumweed.

Splenic enlargement due to congestion; or sluggishness is due to poor digestion will benefit from a short duration of gumweed.

Ellingwood wrote in 1915. "Dr. Webster is the authority for the statement that *Grindelia squarrosa* is specific in its anti-malarial properties. He is very positive concerning its influence upon headaches and especially those of malarial origin. Headache present where there are masked intermittent symptoms, headache accompanied with dizziness and some nausea, where the subject walks with the sensation that he is going to stagger.

It seems as though his equilibrium were uncertain, or where there is mild staggering and irregular gait, where the head feels light and dizzy all the time. In this form, *Grindelia squarrosa* is a positive and specific remedy, decided and satisfactory in its action.

Another form of headache this agent will cure is one that seems to follow and depend upon slow autointoxication.

It is persistent, day after day, and there is dullness, drowsiness and dizziness. There is apt to be torpor of the liver and spleen in these cases. There is lassitude and the patient tires easily. A dull headache is present when he awakes in the morning and with some exacerbations continues all day.

This form is quickly cured with this remedy. A tincture made by covering the fresh plant with 98% alcohol is required to relieve this headache. Give from ten to fifteen drops of this tincture every two or three hours."

The saponin fractions have shown strong hemolytic activity in German studies.

Michael Moore suggested the herb may be worthwhile trying in some cases of apnea.

He wrote of its use in cases of cystitis from food or fungal infections.

"The tincture is especially useful for bladder or urethra infections…Calendula has a major reputation as a tissue-healing agent, but in all respects Grindelia is its equal, stimulating epithelial regeneration, increasing surface blood supply with its rubifacient oils, its flavones limiting unwanted inflammation, and in general possessing some rather efficient antimicrobial activity.

Externally, the resins are useful in lotions, to soothe poison ivy, old chronic ulcers and vesicular eczema, burns, insect bites, and rashes; impetigo, as well as fungal infections such as tinea, athlete's foot or nail fungus. It will give relief to *herpes zoster*, or shingle irritation and nerve pain when applied externally. Hair lice can be treated with external application."

Eczema and asthma are often alternating or related symptoms, making gumweed useful in both acute and chronic states.

In my own clinical practice over 18 years, I witnessed at least 800 cases of young children treated for atopic eczema with cortisone creams that later developed asthma symptoms, before their sixth birthday. Coincidence, I think not!

It has anti-bacterial activity, but the most active compound has yet to be identified. It is probably due to the resin fraction, at least in part. Methanol extracts have been found effective against both Gram positive and negative bacteria, and the fungus *Trichophyton mentagrophytes*. Bayogenin is found in English Daisy (*Bellis perennis*), and Goldenrod (*Solidago canadensis*) as a sapogenin.

Grindelic acid derivatives exhibit activity against five human solid tumor cell lines. Reta GF et al, *Eur J Med Chem* 2013 67:28-38.

Phytosterin ameliorates 4-nitrophenol induced oxidative stress on testicular function in rats. This suggests possible protection and prevention of apoptosis in germ cells. Human implication is unknown. Zhang Y et al, *Environ Sci Pollut Res Int* 2016 23(13): 13035-46.

Hentraicontane, in flower buds, exhibits anti-inflammatory, anti-tumor and anti-microbial activity. It is a potent suppressor of inflammatory cytokines and has a regulatory effect on NF-kappaB. Khajuria V et al, *Biomed Pharmacother* 2017 23(92): 175-86. The compound is also found in flowers of *Salvia miltiorrhiza*, an important TCM herb.

An animal model of ulcerative colitis, found the compound attenuated weight loss, colon shortening and levels of IL-6 inflammatory mechanisms. Kim SJ et al, *Am J Chin Med* 2011 39(5): 957-69. Other work by authors, confirm its anti-inflammatory nature.

The essential oil *of Lonicera japonica* flower buds contains up to 20% hentraicontane.

The Japanese fermented soybean product Natto contains high levels of this compound. Work by Takahashi C et al, *Carcinogenesis* 1995 16(3): 471-6 found it highly protective against tumor formation, with effect on gap junctional intercellular communication.

Gumweed tincture works well on tinea infections and acne as a topical preparation.

The flavonoids, 3-methylquercitin and 3,3'-dimethylquercitin, exhibit anti-viral activity, *in vivo* and *in vitro*.

For Legionnaire's disease, combine one part gumweed, with 8 parts each of echinacea and pleurisy root tincture, and add to decocted fenugreek seed tea.

For *Chlamydia pneumoniae* consider a mixture of gumweed, elecampane, yarrow and thyme.

Apigenin methyl ether inhibits mast-cell histamine release, while quercetin, kaempferol and their glycosides have anti-spasmodic activity against histamine-induced contractions. This helps explain its use in hay fever and other allergic respiratory conditions.

Water extracts show anti-inflammatory activity. Mascolo, et al, *Phytotherapy Research* 1987 1:1. Quercitin-3-methylether, a flavonoid from related *G. robusta* inhibits neutrophil elastase and possesses anti-inflammatory activity. Kreen et al, *Fitoterapia* 80:5. The flower heads have some sedative activity.

HOMEOPATHY

Grindelia robusta (Rosin wood) is useful in asthmatic and chronic bronchitis conditions, where the mucous is tough and difficult to detach from the lungs.

The patient stops breathing when falling asleep, or awakes with a start and gasps for breath. It is effective antidote to poison ivy- both internally and externally.

Herpes zoster (shingles) pain, erythema and pruritis are relieved; as well as other rashes that burn and itch. It may help iritis, headaches and pain in the eyeball.

Grindelia squarrosa is similar but more useful for spleen conditions with dullness and fullness associated with malaria. There may be cutting pains in the spleen radiating to left hip.

Apnea, respiratory arrest, at moment of falling asleep; respiration resumed when awakened by feeling of suffocation.

The spleen may be enlarged, due to mononucleosis. It is considered a specific for spleen cancer.

DOSE- Tincture and lower potencies. One to 15 drops as needed. The mother tincture is prepared from the dried green parts, gathered in unexpanded flower stage. Externally, the tincture is diluted 10:1 for application. Proving by Bundy with tincture in 1877.

ESSENTIAL OIL

CONSTITUENTS- over 100 compounds. Alpha- pinene (25.53%) is a major compound of *G. squarrosa*, followed by limonene. Other constituents include borneol, terpineol, beta-pinene; and a group of labdane diterpene acids including grindelic acid. The flower heads have more grindelic acid and less of the epoxide and 6-oxo-grindelic acid present than the in rest of plant. Limonene is highest in the leaves. Kaltenbach et al, *J Essential Oil Res* 1993 5.

Essential oil of grindelia is not, at present, produced commercially on the prairies.

Grindelia produces an oleoresin that is very valuable in aromatherapy and the perfume industry. This thick, dark brown mass is solid at room temperature and is washed with alcohol to produce a suitable vehicle for blends. It is collected by boiling the fresh gummy flower buds and boiling them, or dissolving them in a alcohol solvent. Gumweed provides a deep, balsamic, earthy base note for perfume work.

Sun infusions can be made of the gummy resin and used for shingle pain, or with other oils for various skin problems.

A potential commercial market should also be mentioned. Naval stores is a generic term for a large class of chemicals including turpentine, fatty acids and rosins recovered from pine trees and stumps.

Over one billion pounds of rosin are used in the USA market every year. High quality wood rosin from pine stumps is quite exhausted, and the hand labour of tapping living trees is expensive.

Gumweed contains grindelane diterpene acids very similar to those in wood rosin and is an economic, renewable crop. They can be used for food, rubber coatings, textiles and polymers.

FLOWER OIL

Take one part un-opened flower buds to five parts vegetable oil. Sun infuse for two weeks shaking daily. Strain and keep cool. Excellent for poison ivy, insect bites and dry eczema. In cooler climate use a crockpot at lowest setting for 4-6 hours.

SEED OIL

The seeds produce 20% oil that is 0.6% saturates and up to 61% of octadecadienoic acid.

FLOWER ESSENCES

Gumweed (*G. squarrosa*) flower essence is related to the soul qualities of the dream state. These individuals are so afraid of the messages from the sub-conscious that they wake themselves.

What they fear is that they are not following their life's work, and do not feel up to drastic life changes.

Gumweed flower essence works at allowing them more comfort in the face of inevitable change. Gurdjieff suggested that we must challenge ourselves with small shocks, or the universe will give us a big one. The flower essence helps us understand the difference between searching and running. **PRAIRIE DEVA**

Gum Plant (*Grindelia* spp.) flower essence can enhance the communication between individuals to share deeper levels of truth and spiritual purpose without over-philosophizing. It can draw together, connect and enhance relationships.

It can greatly enhance step-parent/step child relationships at the soul level. It increases intuition, inspirational writing, astral projection, and the dream state. It also aids in schizophrenia, and balances the astral body. **PEGASUS**

PERSONALITY TRAITS

The gumweed person is lethargic and weak. They have difficulty breathing when lying down, or they stop breathing when falling asleep; awaking with a start.

In the negative state, the gumweed person has a long history of bronchial and respiratory troubles. Perhaps they suffered asthma as a child, which they "outgrew". Perhaps they had unresolved chicken pox as a child that comes out later in life as herpes zoster. Or they have spleen problems, perhaps dating back to mononucleosis as a teenager.

In the positive state, the gumweed person assists the body to control various viral infection. Their energy rebounds, and the apnea subsides. **PRAIRIE DEVA**

RECIPES

TINCTURE- 2-3 ml daily. The tincture is a 1:5 concentration from the dried plant at 60-80% alcohol. The fresh flowering tops are best at 1:3 at 95%. The aerial parts are collected before the sticky buds open, the exception to the rule.

OIL- Fill large glass jar half way with fresh gumweed buds. Cover with canola oil in a 1:5 ratio and set in sun for ten days. Strain. In colder climates use a low temperature crockpot.

CAUTION- Grindelia has the capacity to take up and store selenium from the soil. Many parts of the northern plains are selenium deficient, but in large doses selenium is toxic, even the organic type. Since the active principles are excreted through the kidneys, it will initially raise blood pressure and heart rate, and then lower them. Use recommended doses.

Large amounts of tincture can cause mild symptoms of exhaustion, according to Michael Moore. I guess I have never reached that limit, but will take his word over many others. Do not use during pregnancy, or those with weak hearts. Excessive dosage irritates the kidneys.

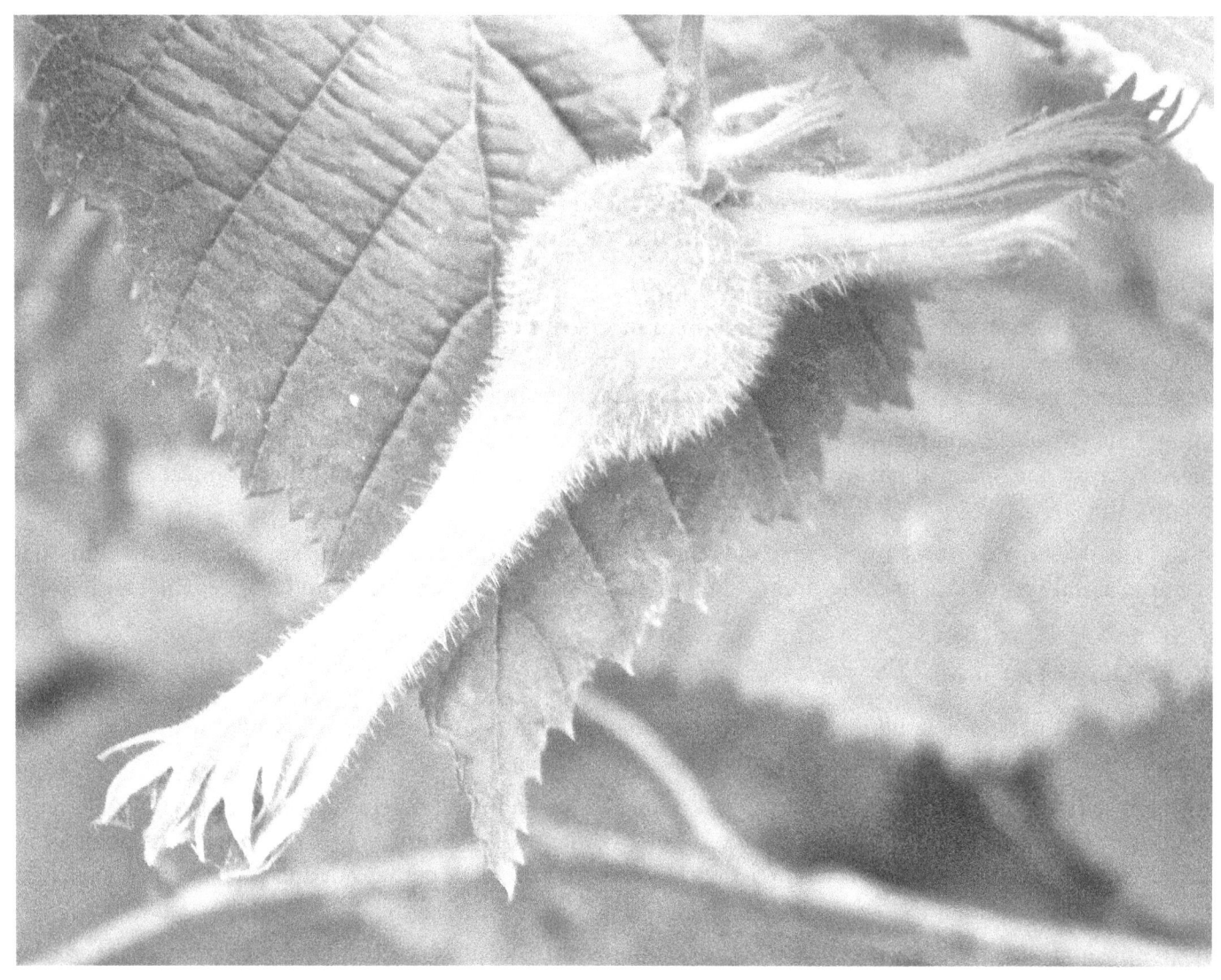

UNRIPE HAZEL HUSK

HAZELNUT
(***Corylus cornuta*** Marsh.)
(***C. rostrata*** Aiton) not accepted
CONTORTED HAZEL
CRAZY FILBERT
(***C. avellana*** "*contorta*")
EUROPEAN FILBERT
(***C. avellana*** L.)
AMERICAN FILBERT
(***C. americana*** Walt)
PURPLE HAZEL
(***C. maxima purpurea***)
PARTS USED- nuts, husk, buds, stems, roots and leaves.

The hazelnut is a symbol of happy marriages, because the nuts grow united in pairs. **ANON**

Thou wilt quarrel with a man for cracking nuts,
Having no other reason, but thou hast hazel eyes. **SHAKESPEARE**

248

The hazel blooms in threads of crimson hue. Peep through the swelling buds and look for Spring.

JOHN CLARE

O sland'rous world! Kate like the hazel-twig
Is straight and slender, and as brown in hue
As hazel-nuts, and sweeter than the kernels.

SHAKESPEARE

Hazel is from the Anglo Saxon **HAESEL** meaning headdress or bonnet. Corylus is from the Greek **KORYS** or helmet, and cornuta from **CORNUS** meaning horned or beaked.

Hazel is associated with hazy, from the Syrian **HAZEH**. Hazing rituals may stem from the same root. It may stem from the German **HAES**, meaning a command, from the ancient use of sticks and switches to keep slaves and livestock in control. The Anglo-Saxon name **HAESEL** means, "hood".

The closely related Filbert, is the emblem of St. Philibert, whose feast day is August 22.

He was a Benedictine monk who founded the Abbey of Jumieges in 684 AD. Maybe. Philbert is a Norman French word from the 13th century.

Filbert is from the German **VOLLBART**, meaning full-beard. An old British slang term Gilbert Filbert is derived from the song Gilbert the Filbert, Colonel of the Nuts. Ah, nothing like English humour!

Generally speaking, the hazel is reserved for the wild grown nut, and filbert for the cultivated.

Pliny, the ancient Greek author, mentions, "filberts put more fat on the body than one would think at all likely."

The Greeks dedicated hazel to Mercury; and in Ireland, it was a wand of hazel that St. Patrick used to drive the snakes into the sea. The winged hazel rod, entwined with two serpents is still today the symbol of communication, reconciliation and commerce; as well as the Caduceus, the symbol of healing arts.

Chinese manuscripts over 5000 years old, mention the hazelnut. Cultivation began in southern Europe, and then eastward into Turkey.

Hazel is associated with the number nine, the number of muses, and the sacred number of Gaia.

Hazel is the ninth month of the Celtic tree calendar, and considered the Tree of Wisdom. From the Hazel, fell the nine poetic nuts of knowledge, into a pool of sacred salmon. The metaphor of salmon returning to the sea and back for spawning is related to the passing of wisdom from one generation to the next.

It is the letter C (Coll) in the Druid tree alphabet.

Druid masters were said to chew hazelnuts as a way of focusing the mind to compose satirical poems that carry curses or to obtain knowledge of things hidden or lost. In Scotland, the tree was sacred to the Celtic sea god Manannan.

In Sweden, hazelnut twigs were woven into crowns, and worn by those wishing to become invisible. In Wales, twig caps were worn to bring good dreams and wisdom. To fall asleep under hazel will give you prophetic dreams.

It was believed that hazelnut pins driven into the beams protected the building from fire, and made it immune to damage from lightning, as hazel was the handle of the hammer of Thor, and Donar, the God of thunder, war and strength.

A protective wall of hazel was planted around the Goetheanum to ward off evil spirits.

Charcoal made from hazel wood was combined with sulphur and saltpetre to make gunpowder.

In Bohemia, the presence of a large number of hazel nuts foretells the birth of many illegitimate children.

D. H. Lawrence, in *Women in Love*, had the hero explain to a lady admirer the function of the "long danglers", and the "little red flames" of the female flower.

Hildegard de Bingen, some six centuries earlier, suggested that hazel represents lasciviousness.

She suggested to, "take the shoots, that is, the parts where the flowers first bud. Dry them in the sun and reduce them to a powder. Put this powder where there is scrofula on a person, and he will be healed."

She also recommended hazel shoots, stonecrop along with goat liver and fatty pork as a stew for men with immature sperm.

The expression to "go into the hazelwood" meant to have sex in the woods. A hazel wand was given to "easy" girls on May Day. An old Swiss folk song goes: "Anneli, with the red breast, come, we'll wend our way into the hazelwood".

In Scotland, "burning the nuts" was a ritual of lovers to see if they were well matched. Two hazelnuts were placed on embers, and if they burned steadily side-by-side, they were true lovers. If, however, they sputtered and one jumped away, they were ill matched. This may be the source of its symbolic meaning of reconciliation. In the middle ages, hazel was considered the tree of seduction.

Hazel shoots were hung over the bed of infertile couples.

The plant is related to the birth date of April 29th while the nut itself is related to October 20th.

Caledonia, the Gallic name for Scotland is derived from the Cal Dun, or Hill of Hazel. The Gallic term for wisdom, Cnocach, also stems from the word for hazelnut, CNO.

Hallow's Eve, October 31st, is known as Nutcrack Night, a night when hazelnuts were cracked, accompanied with fortune telling in some traditions.

The forked branches are used for divining water or gold. This was called **RHABDOMANCY**, from the Greek **RHABDOS** for rod, and **MANTEIA**, divination. In the Bible (Hosea IV:12) hazel rods are mentioned for finding concealed objects. The Cornish attributed this power to the influence of pixies.

Ancient Etruscans used hazel wands to find buried springs, and Chinese feng shui masters used them, five millennium ago to detect the flow of "dragon lines" (ley lines?) in the earth.

Forked hazel wands are best cut on Midsummer's Eve.

This stems (sorry, I couldn't resist) from the Celtic God of love, *Aengus mac in Oic*, who carried a hazel wand that predicted success or failure in courting.

The lovers placed two hazelnuts in water, and if they remained close, all would be well. Any drifting apart indicated the same. Two nuts joined together was called St. John's Nut in Scotland, and considered a good omen to carry and protect oneself against the evil eye.

The air surrounding hazel is believed charged with the quicksilver energy of exhilaration and inspiration. It is said that two hazel trees growing together near water form a bridge to the fairy kingdom, and passing through can lead to this other world.

It was believed hazel energy can change weather.

Hazel rods make excellent walking sticks, after seasoning with the peel on for a good six months. Oetzie, the Ice Man used hazel for the U shape spar of his pack frame and as a quiver stiffener.

The shrubs grow from one to three metres tall, and produce paired nuts that are quickly gathered by squirrels, crows, blue jays, and even bears that love the taste.

Thoreau put it well. "There is not a hazel bush but some squirrel has his eye on its fruit, and he will be pretty sure to anticipate you; for you only think of it between whiles, but he thinks of it all the while. As we say, "The tools to those who can use them," so we may say, "The nuts to those who can get them."

In front of my cabin on Lesser Slave Lake, the hazelnuts were variable from year to year. Gloves are a must in harvesting, due to the rough husk; but if your skin is irritated simply rub fresh leaves on the inflamed area. This green husk is quite salty when chewed, indicating another possible source of landlocked sodium salts from plant ash.

The smaller, immature nuts still in the milky stage are soft and sweet. I like them this way, before the squirrels start to gather them.

The Cree call the bush **PAKANÂHTIHK**, and the nut **PAKAN**. They used the twig tea for treating heart disease.

Some native people buried the harvested nuts until the husks rotted, by filling the hole with wet mud for up to ten days. After removing the husks, they were shelled and eaten, or stored for later use.

The Lakes people of British Columbia made a special type of relish with hazelnuts.

They would crush the nuts and mix them with bear fat and berries, and then form the mixture into cakes to dry or stuffed into an animal's intestine like a sausage.

Ancient archeological sites on Colonsay, off the west coast of Scotland reveal shallow depressions where hazelnuts were placed, covered with sand and then subjected to a top fire. This cooking process turns the hard to digest food into a starchy delight that can be eaten in the hundreds at one sitting.

The cooking also preserves them for future use.

Young, straight shoots were prepared by natives of the Canadian prairies for arrows, snowshoes and drumming sticks.

They twisted the peeled shoots to break the fibre and used them as plied rope for lashing and tying.

Spoons were carved from the wood, as they did not have a strong flavour.

A blue dye, used to colour baskets, was made from the buds or root when scraped and exposed to air. It could then be rubbed on, or a decoction was made from soaking either part in water.

One modern member of the Thompson says that chewing the buds of hazelnut will help make one a good singer.

The Iroquois used decoctions of the bark, as part of mixtures to induce vomiting. Smaller amounts of the stem tea, combined with Horsetail (*Equisetum arvense*) root were given to help ease teething pain in children.

The Chippewa used root infusions to stop hemorrhage of the lungs. The Ojibwa made medicine from the hairs of the husks to expel intestinal worms.

Hazelnut leaves can be made into a poultice, for headaches, skin conditions, as well as tendonitis and other sore muscle pains. The bark, leaves and twigs were boiled together and crushed into poultices for treating skin tumours and ulcers.

Several Algonquian tribes boiled the leaves and twigs for rheumatism, heart disease and intestinal disorders, and the bark to reduce fevers, and relieve hives. The Eastern Cree made a tea of the branch tips to cure heart troubles.

The twigs are good chewing sticks, for maintaining dental health; the astringent bitter properties helping dry and heal bleeding or inflamed gums.

Rousseau mentions that the Mohawk cut the stalk into pieces to make a collar used by babies suffering teething.

According to Midred Fielder, author of Plant Medicine and Folklore, the inner bark of hazelnut acts as a binder to cement the virtues of various tonic herbs together, a property first reported by Smith in 1923.

Various native tribes boiled the nuts and skimmed oil off the top to flavour food, and for soothing toothaches.

Hazelnut oil is also a good mosquito repellant and insecticide, and when rancid can still be used for industrial purposes.

Poultices of the bark were used to promote healing wounds, tumours and skin cancer.

The ripe nuts were burned for divination, to enable visionary prophecy by medicine men and women.

A necklace of the young branches was put around teething babies.

In European folk medicine, the nuts were used to treat hypotension and parotid tumours. Dr. Crato, a 16th century German physician, said that many people were cured of stone and gravel by eating 9-10 hazelnuts before both midday and evening meals.

Culpepper believed "the dried husks and shells, to the weight of two drams, taken in red wine, stays lasks and women's courses, and so doth the red skin that covers the kernels, which is more effectual to stay women's courses".

The wood is in demand for small pieces of turned furniture, walking sticks, barrel hoops, and as a source of charcoal made into gunpowder.

The leaves have been used for smoking like tobacco.

The shelled nuts can be rubbed on articles of wood to polish and oil them. They were also slightly scorched and ground into a powder as a medicine for kidneys and promoting labour.

Crushed and broken shells and husks are burned as fuel.

The bark and leaves have been used for tanning of leather, the boiled bark making a reddish dye for moose hide. The nuts boiled for an hour give a green dye. From the roots and inner bark a blue dye was obtained to colour baskets.

The plant is associated with the Air element, and Mercury. Stringing the nuts together and hanging them in the house was considered good luck. Given to a new bride is a way of wishing her good fortune. Amulets made from the hazelnuts imparted the wearer wisdom.

It was believed that, eaten, the hazelnut imparted wisdom and increased fertility. As the nuts are rich in essential fatty oils and Vitamin E, there is scientific truth to this belief.

While living in Spain, I had the good fortune to taste Salsa Romesco, a sauce of hazelnuts and peppers used with shellfish and salads. Delicious! The Italian liqueur Frangelico is made from hazelnuts.

The fine flour, from freshly ground nuts, is used in cleansing face masks.

A cure for bedwetting in Spain is to eat 12 nuts just before going to sleep. It seems to work!

Proteolytic enzymes from the nuts improve the flavour of cheese, through better aging.

Ancient herbalists like Pliny recommended hazelnuts for catarrh and chronic coughs. Culpepper suggested powdering and mixing hazelnuts with honey water for the same purpose.

Hazel wood decoctions were used in veterinary medicine to cure fever in cattle; while the foliage was fed to cows to increase butterfat content in milk production.

Contorted Hazel, is a domesticated from for the garden, that is a series of curls and twisted branches, that are used by florists. It rarely produces hazelnuts, but the squirrels usually get them first.

In winter, the bare branches are eerie and silly, the perfect addition to the backyard collection of the unusual.

European and American Filbert as well as Purple leafed Hazel (*C. maxima* 'Purpurea') are fully hardy to the Edmonton region (zone 3). American Filbert is found throughout southern Manitoba but introduced further west.

Healthy specimens are found at the George Pegg Historic Garden near Glenevis, Alberta.

Hybrid hazelnuts from tissue culture cloning, are creating new crop opportunities in Minnesota and Nebraska. Growers plant their hazel rows on eight or ten foot centers for a machine-harvested crop. More information may be obtained from Philip Rutter at badgersett.com.

Dr. Bob Bors at the U of Saskatchewan has developed hybrid hazelnuts suitable for the Canadian prairies. The first cultivars were available in 2004. Contact bob.bors@usask.ca.

Hazelnut is the second most plentiful nut in the world, so markets are already well developed. Annual production is some 600,000 tons.

Most exciting is the inoculation of hazelnut roots with mycorrhizal truffle cultivation.

The hard, inedible shells have high heating value when burned.

German artist, Wolfgang Laib, makes sculptures from small piles of hazelnut pollen. He prefers working with natural substances like milk, beeswax, and various pollens, including buttercup and hazelnut. Since each catkin contains up to four million grains of pollen, and each bush up to several thousand catkins, there is a lot of pollen.

A Turkish hazel, *C. colurna* var. *jacquemontii*, has a chromosome number that is quite variable, making it a good choice for breeders wishing to produce vigorous northern hybrids.

Pure Hazelwood is a Quebec-based company that makes necklaces, bracelets as well as ointments and lotions. Testimonials proclaim benefits for acid reflux, skin conditions, arthritis, etc from simply wearing the jewelry. It is a stretch!

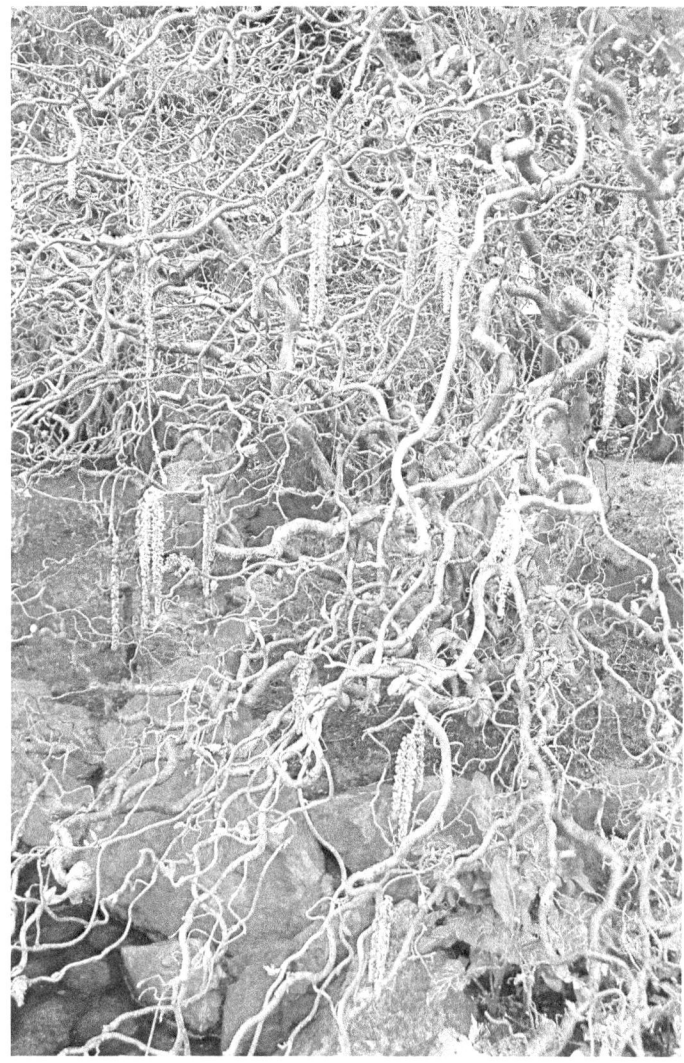

CONTORTED HAZEL

MEDICINAL

CONSTITUENTS leaves- up to 5% tannins including catechins, flavonoids, 2.58%; including myricitrin 1.35%, and quercitrin, 0.3-0.4%; taraxerol, b-sitosterol, essential oils, glycosides, ferric oxide and sugars. Leaf protein is over 14%, with a nitrogen/sulphur ratio of 14:1; iron (118 ppm), moderate zinc, calcium and boron, and very high manganese content (373 ppm). Italian hazel leaves contain up to 237mcg/gram dry weight of alpha tocopherol, as well as the giffonins found in male flowers; quinic acid, and flavanoid and citric acid derivatives.
kernal- 60% fatty oils, protein , vitamin E, B1, B2, B3, B5, B6, carotene, phosphorus, magnesium, potassium, and copper, gallic acid, p-hydroxyl benzoic acid, caffeic acid (epicatechin) sinapic acid, non-tocopherol, enzymes and quercetin, boron as calcium fructoborate, ellagic acid, 121 mg/100 grams of phytosterols, composed mainly of beta sitosterol in levels similar to ground flaxseed.
Hull/shell- protocatechuic acids, neolignans such as balanophonin, a diaryheptanoid, lawsonicin, cedrusin, C-veratroylglycol, beta hydroxypropiovanillone.
bark- lignoceryl alcohol, betulin, and sitosterol; tannins and organic acids; as well as various flavonoids including kaempferol, quercitin, myricetin, afzelin, quercitrin, and myricitrin,
pollen- guanosine ($C10N13N5O5$) and n-triacosan.
Male flowers (catkins)- giffonins Q-U (diarylheptanoids).

Hazelnut milk is very good for those suffering from coughs and colds. The Chinese use hazelnut milk for those with weak spleen or stomach, frequent diarrhea, loss of weight, and who tire easily.

Eating hazelnuts before bedtime helps ease restlessness, irritability, anxiety and insomnia, due to the rich stores of calcium, magnesium and phosphorus.

Studies by Yuritas et al, in the *Journal of Food Science* 2000 65:2 indicate hazelnuts contain non-tocopherol phenolics with anti-oxidant activity. Oliveira et al, *Food Chem Tox* 2008 46:5 found extracts exhibit anti-oxidant and anti-bacterial properties against gram positive bacteria such as *Staphylococcus aureus* and *Bacillus species.*

Ethanol extracts of the seed clusters and leaves show activity against *S. aureus.* Borchardt et al, *J Med Plants Res* 2008 2:5.

Shahidi et al, *J Ag Food Chem* 2007 55 found antioxidant activity in skin, hard shell, green leafy cover and tree leaves all higher than the kernel itself, suggesting great byproduct potential.

Hazelnuts are a rich source of vitamin E, necessary for reproductive health.

Hazelnuts are also the perfect heart food, helping ensure that the blood vessels remain flexible and blood pressure is reduced.

Nine studies of 425 participants found hazelnuts in diet decrease LDL and total cholesterol levels. Perna S et al, *Nutrients* 2016 8(12).

Circulation is improved, helping those who suffer from cold hands and feet.

Hazelnuts are high in protein and fasts, and low in starch and sugar, making them useful for those suffering blood sugar problems.

Hazelnut kernel skins show activity against *Candida albicans.* Piccinelli AL et al, *J Agric Food Chem* 2016 64(3): 585-95. The skin extracts improved lipid profile and reduced lithocholic/deoxycholic bile acid faecal ratio, a risk factor for colon cancer, albeit in a hamster study. Caimari A et al, *Food Chem* 2015 167:138-44.

The nuts are also extremely rich in boron, at 2.72 mg/100 grams. Boron is a very important mineral in the prevention and treatment of osteoporosis, by playing a key role in controlling calcium excretion and retention.

Hazelnuts are rich in copper, a key mineral in the creation of superoxide dismutase that disarms free radicals that damage cholesterol and other fats. One ounce of hazelnuts supplies 41% of RDI of copper.

Calcium fructoborate, the organic form present in hazelnuts, helps reduce pain associated with osteoarthritis and bone health in general. It is available as an odorless soluble white powder that can be used in beverages, nutritional food bars and meal replacement products. VDF Futureceuticals have a patented form, FruiteX-B, on the market.

According to their literature, the product "increases blood levels of vitamin D in individuals suffering from a deficiency, optimizes calcium, magnesium and phosphorus metabolism and improves mental functions such as eye-hand coordination, attention, perception and memory".

A 50/50 mixture of defatted hazelnut and pea flour possesses protein quality similar to casein from milk.

An animal study found hazelnut supplementation ameliorates neuroinflammation and apoptosis caused by amyloid beta, suggesting a healthy dietary supplement for healthy aging and prevention and/or treatment of Alzheimer's disease. Bahaeddin Z et al, *Nutr Neurosci* 2016 January 25.

Hazelnuts contain up to 66 mg/100 gram of ellagic acid. Ellagic acid prevents the activation of carcinogenic substances into cellular toxins, which lose their ability to react with DNA and induce mutations capable of triggering cancer growth. It increases the cells' capacity to defend itself from toxic aggression by activating its own detoxifying action. It has recently been found to inhibit VEGF and PDGF, two proteins associated with inhibiting angiogenesis, thus denying cancer cells the blood supply they require to survive.

The leaves are diuretic and useful for varicose veins and circulatory problems, usually as a hot infusion, or fluid extract. The hot leaves can be poulticed as a vein tonic, the astringency helping to shrink the tissues.

Externally, the leaves can be decocted and added to baths for hemorrhoids and slow healing wounds.

Studies conducted in Sweden in 1995, indicated that hazelnut plant water extracts exhibited both prostaglandin inhibition and platelet activating factor; proving that the traditional usage for anti-inflammatory activity has a basis in scientific fact.

Anti-oxidant and strong free radical scavenger activity was isolated from flavonoids in related hazel leaves (*C. colurna*). In the study, conducted by Benov and colleagues in Bulgaria, the leaf flavonoids were found to be strong inhibitors of ischeameia/reperfusion-induced peroxidation in both the brain and liver.

This combined with low toxicity and easily isolated flavonoids, makes further study important and essential.

Hazel leaves, standardized for proanthocyanidin content, may be used in a manner similar to pine bark. Leaf and bark extracts are used for varicose veins and phlebitis.

Afzelin, from bark, may be useful for its inhibition of aldose reductase, associated with diabetic complications. Kim SB et al, *Int J Mol Sci* 2017 18(2).

The bark extract, containing afzelin, may be useful for promoting melanin production in the skin, helping protect against UVA radiation. Jung E et al, *Chem Biol Interact* 2016 254: 167-72.

Further work by Rusu et al, *Phytotherapy Research* 1999 13 2 found leaves of Hazelnut (*C. avellana*) provide hepatoprotective effect against acetominophen-induced liver damage and toxicosis in lab studies.

This appears to confirm some of the traditional usage of the leaf fluid extract for vaso-constriction.

Hazelnut hull extracts possess anti-oxidant activity similar to synthetics such as BHT and BHA. Moure et al, *J Ag Food Chem* 2000 48:9.

The burrs or husks can be infused and the water used as a retention enema for hemorrhoids.

Hazel pollen is one of the original eight plant pollens in a well-known prostate health product called Cernilton.

Dr. Larry Daley, in the Department of Horticulture at Oregon State University has been exploring the potential of taxol in hazelnuts.

Paclitaxel is the active ingredient in the anticancer drug Taxol, a taxane fround in yew trees of the *Taxus* species. Taxol, as a drug, has been approved for the treatment of ovarian and breast cancers, as well as non-small cell lung cancer.

It may also be of possible benefit in psoriasis, polycystic kidney disease, Multiple sclerosis, and Alzheimers disease.

Recent research of the St. Michael's Hospital in Toronto indicates that paclitaxel may also have application in the treatment of multiple sclerosis.

Micellar paclitaxel, which is a soluble form, appears to curb an enzyme that damages the myelin sheath. When damaged, it is harder for nerves to transmit signals to the rest of the body. No tests have been conducted on hazelnut twig extracts, but considering the relative safety would be worth a trial.

Hazelnut contains paxlitaxel in both the twigs and leaves; as well as kernels and shells of the nut.

Alcohol leaf and stem extracts (not taxol or taxanes) show activity against cervical cancer, hepatocarcinoma and to lesser extent, breast cancer cell lines. Gellego A et al, *Biomed Pharmacother* 2017 89:565-72.

Hazelnut shell extracts induce apoptosis through caspase-3 activation in both human melanoma (SK-Mel-28) and human cervical cancer (HeLa) cell lines. Esposito T et al, *Int J Mol Sci* 2017 18(2): pii: E392. Balanophonin and cedrusin appear are most cyctotoxic.

The former compound also inhibits protein tyrosine phosphatase 1B. It also appears to increase UMR 106 osteoblast-like cells. Xu MM et al, *Zhongguo Zhong Yao Za Zhi* 2014 39(14): 2684-8.

Various fungal endophytes isolated from the leaves and bark are able to produce paclitaxel, setting the stage for cell culture.

What I find most exciting is another natural product that could be part of preventative herbal teas or products, growing wild all across northern Canada.

The recovery of paclitaxel from hazelnut tissues is 10% or less than Pacific yew, but without the toxic components in the latter.

The discovery of taxanes in differentiated and undifferentiated hazelnut tissue, is leading to new sources of paciltaxel. Miele et al, *Phytochem Reviews* 2012 11:1.

Zobel and Schellenberger, *Pharmaceutical Biology* 2000 38:3 found that paclitaxel, when combined with coumarin could be used in much higher amounts for treating cancer, without extreme clastogenic effects.

This raises some interesting possibilities in the herbal world, combining hazelnut paxitaxel with coumarin rich plants such as angelica root, cow parsnip, caraway, dill, lomatium, or sweet cicely.

Ottaggio et al, *J Nat Prod* 2008 71:1 identified different taxanes in the leaf and shell, including paclitaxel, 10-deacetylbaccatin III, baccatin III, paclitaxel C and 7-epipaclitaxel. Leaf extracts are highest in content of taxanes that inhibit metaphase to anaphase in human tumor cell lines.

As a general rule, the bark is best for fevers, the leaf as a depurative and the catkin as a sudorific.

The catkins contain giffonin U that is anti-microbial against *Bacillus cereus, Staphylococcus aureus, E. coli* and *Pseudomonas aeruginosa.* Cerulli A et al, *J Nat Prod* 2017 May 18.

CAUTION- Hazelnut and soybean allergies may play a role in night-time bedwetting in children, based on a recent British study.

Hazelnut pollen creates acute allergic response in some individuals. Data suggests the intake of gastric anti-ulcer drugs may lead to induction of immediate type food hypersensitivity toward hazelnut.

GEMMOTHERAPY

Hazelnut tree bud (*C. avellana*)

The new, spring buds are first and foremost anti-fibrotic; and restore elasticity to the lungs. This makes them useful in treating emphysema and pulmonary fibrosis.

The buds also have a pronounced effect on liver tissue, and are indicated in more severe hepatic insufficiency, and the arthritis that can accompany it.

It is useful for circulatory insufficiency and cases of neuro-vegetative imbalance.

DOSE- 1D of glycerin macerate. Twenty to thirty drops up to three times daily.

NUT OIL

CONSTITUENTS- 70-84% oleic, and minor amounts of linoleic (10-20%), palmitic (3-8%), stearic (1-4%), alpha linolenic (<1.5%), and myristic fatty acids, corylin, melibiose, raffinose, and stachyose. The nuts contain over 56% oil; of which 4.8-8.4% is saturated fatty acids.

Cold pressed hazelnut oil is believed first extracted during the Bronze Age. It has the lowest fat content of any nut and contains sizable quantities of Vitamin E.

After pressing, the oil is left in vats for one week, to allow sediment to settle. One litre is produced from 2.5 kilos of nuts. The seed meal (19% protein) left over can be substituted up to 40% for soybean meal in egg laying feed for hens.

Like canola oil, it contains a large percentage of mono-saturated fats, and low levels of saturated fats.

When rabbits were fed a high cholesterol diet all the risk factors began to present, and when hazelnut oil was added to the diet, not only did the levels of oxidized lipids, LDL, and VLDL drop, so did the number of atherosclerotic lesions that had formed in their aortas.

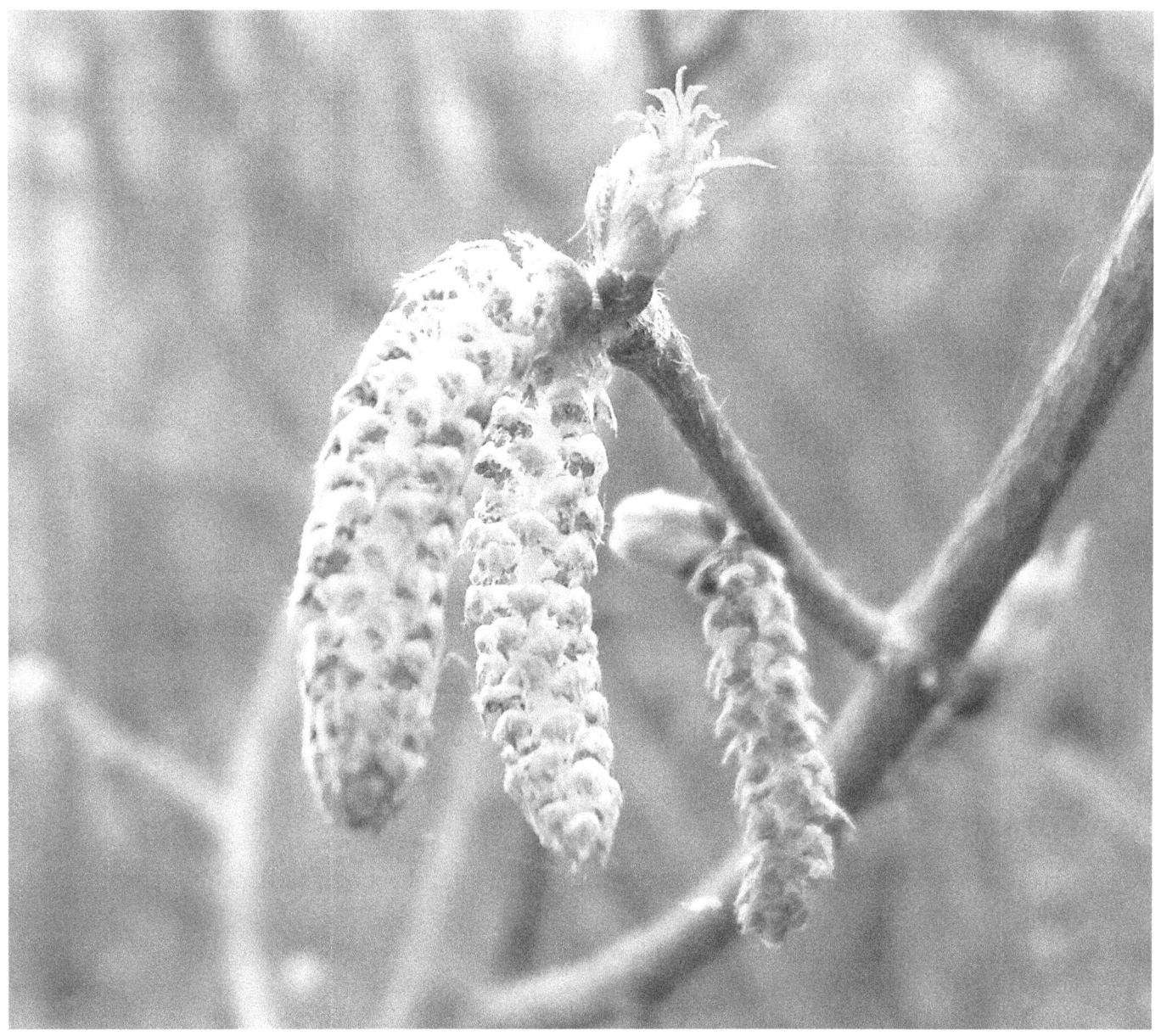

MALE CATKINS AND RED FEMALE FLOWER

Its true value in cooking is for salad dressings and sauces; as well as nutty cakes. This oil will give your popcorn a buttery taste without the butter.

The oil is very gentle, but effective, in cases of threadworm or pinworm in babies and young children. It is used in Quebec to this day for toothache.

The oil is slightly astringent, and perfect for oily or combination skin in cosmetic care. It also helps acne, dermatitis and seborrheic eczema.

Hazelnut is more easily absorbed than most oils, making it ideal for facial application, as well as a carrier for varicose vein treatment.

Hazelnut oil is used in perfumes and making of soaps; and when rancid for machine lubrication and old watch springs.

Culpepper suggested its use for cold afflictions of the nerves, and gout of the knees.

Hazelnut oil can be modified into structured lipids for use as a human milk fat substitute in baby formulas. Sahin et al, *J Ag Food Chem* 2005 53.

Corylin possesses anti-inflammatory, and immunosuppressive activity that may be useful for sepsis and septic shock. Hung YL et al, *Sci Rep* 2017 7:46299. Earlier work found the compound inhibits IL-6 inflammatory response. Lee SW et al, *Planta Med* 2012 78(9): 903-6.

From 1971-1982, over 1075 hectares of hazelnut plantations were established in Russia. New hybrids have greater hardiness, earlier maturity and higher yields. There is economic potential in the northern plains that is largely ignored at present.

Specific gravity of the oil is 0.917, with a saponification value of 190-197, and iodine value of 84-90.

ESSENTIAL OIL

Dry Hazelnut (*C. avellana*) leaves are steam distilled and yield .0425% of spicy, odorous oil. It contains about 18% palmitic acid and paraffin that melts at 50 degrees C.

Hazelnut absolute is made from the nut by solvent extraction. It is useful in the food and beverage industry, finding a place in baked goods, candies and liqueurs.

Early German settlers used the oil distilled from small hazel branches as a remedy for falling evil (epilepsy), by taking a few drops in linden blossom water. A few drops of oil on some cotton was also used for toothaches; while a few drops in several tablespoons of centaury water was said to kill worms and drive them out with the stool.

HYDROSOL

The young soft shells are trampled and distilled on mid-summers day and anointed on hands and arms when they are scabbed.

BRUNSCHWIG

HOMEOPATHY

Hazelnut (*C. avellana*) is indicated for calming influence in stressful situations, particularly when important decisions have to be made.

Indolence, desire to be lazy, thirst for action, delusion of being old, irritability about trifles, dreams of cats, tigers, erotic, forest or being watched.

It is for those who have trouble with criticism, who bear pain in heart from always being found at fault.

To rekindle the spark crushed by the rat race of ambition and competition. Remedy for children who are under pressure at school.

Toothache as if from electricity. Allergic reaction to animal dander.

DOSE- 30C potency. Proving reported in the *New Materia Medica* by Colin Griffith. Peter Alex proved six females and eight males at 12c, 30c, and 200c in 2004. A meditative proving by Evans is also included.

FLOWER ESSENCES

Hazelnut flower essence is the antidote for loneliness. Spiritually, there is often need for a time of aloneness and solitude.

Many individuals isolate themselves, in attempts to protect their fragile hold on reality.

Hazelnut flower essence strengthens one's desire to be part of the world, and protect one from the need to succumb to the influence of other people who need to "show the way".

The road less traveled does make all the difference.

PRAIRIE DEVA

Crazy Filbert (*C. avellana 'contorta'*) essence assists us in releasing a dislike and helps us see that there is no need to hold on to negative emotion. The essence also brings us understanding of the underlying emotion that may create this dislike.   **FALLING LEAF**

Davy Filbert (*C. avellana "daviana"*) essence is for those who are obsessive about improving their physical appearance with makeup, beauty treatments, cosmetic surgery, exercise programs, etc. The essence releases the underlying self-rejection that drives this obsession.   **FALLING LEAF**

Hazel flower essence is for intuitive or creative blockage; or when you need to concentrate on your gifts and talents. It helps bring ideas to the surface through meditation, poetry and divination.   O**GAM**

Essence of Hazel flowers is used to assist "the flowering of skills". It aids the ability to receive, process and communicate wisdom, and the ability to take in information and helps all forms of study, bringing stability and focus to the integration of useful information. This debris is released from the soles of feet, so when taking it, try walking barefoot in the grass…to release it back into nature.   **OLIVE**

Hazel flower essence is for helping reconnect with skill of old ways, and renewing ancient ways. It helps to ground the skill and idea.   **BRYNEHERB**

PERSONALITY TRAITS

The Gods took pity and sent the two sons of Zeus (Jupiter), Apollo and Mercury (Hermes) down to the earth with gifts. Mercury gave Apollo a tortoise shell from which to make a lyre, and received in exchange a hazel rod which had the power to inspire with a love of virtue, and to reconcile hearts divided by hatred and envy.

Apollo sang of eternal wisdom and the gentle influence of charity towards all men. Then Mercury touched all with the wand given to him by Apollo. He set free their tongues and taught them to express thought in words. He told them that nothing could be obtained from the earth without mutual aid. This hazel wand, decorated with two light wings and surrounded by serpents, is the Caduceus, still the symbol of healing, given to the god of eloquence by the god of harmony to bring peace and reconciliation.   **POWELL**

The Haselwurm, a white serpent with a golden crown, was believed to live under a very old hazel tree…This mysterious serpent is connected to the archaic brain stem, including the entire limbic system, which appears in the minds of those deep in meditation (the crowned snake-head). The instincts are anchored here in this most ancient part of the nervous system. Sexuality, fertility, premonitions and emotions have the physiological basis here as well. The hazel is able to transmit subtle impulses to the center.   **MULLER-EBELING**

There are wood of the same family that are infected with a fungus that persuades the Corylus species to produce taxanes, an anticancer drug of immense importance in breast cancer and other reproductive cancer treatment.   **BERESFORD-KROEGER**

MYTHS AND LEGENDS

A man sat on the shore of a lake cracking hazelnuts. He cracked them with a small stone on a big stone. He found a little nut that was hard to hold and as he struck it, it bounded off into the sand. He picked it up and struck it again, and a second time it sprang away. "You are brave", said the man as he picked it up. "but I'll break you anyway." This time the nut leaped far into a grassy hollow and the man couldn't find it.

Some nights later a little Indian boy was searching in the moonlight for his guardian spirit. He heard a tiny voice from the grass say, "Boy, look at me." The boy separated the grass at his feet and there was a little hazelnut. "I am your guardian spirit", said the nut, " and I can give you strength. Do as I bid you and you will have my power. An enemy may catch and try to hold you but you can spring from his grasp and disappear." The boy told no one. But he carried the nut in his pocket and listened to its directions. Soon the Indians noticed that he had strange powers. In time he became chief of his tribe and a great warrior with the help of the hazelnut.   **GUILLET**

In olden days the shepherds picked long, leafy branches of hazelnut trees in spring. They held these up or tied them around their faces to make disguises. Then, on White Friday (nine days before Easter) they went to church and tried to fool their sweethearts.

The branches were blessed and after the leaves had dried and fallen off, the shepherds used the sticks to prod and guide their sheep for the remainder of the year. The next spring they repeated the process.

PALLOWSKI

MacColl, which means "son of the hazel", was one of three brothers, the last of the godlike race, the Tuatha De Danaan, who once ruled Old Ireland. MacColl and MacCeacht, son of the plow, and Mac Greine, son of the sun, were married to three ancient goddesses, Banbha, Eire, and Fodhla. The great Irish hero, Finn MacColl, also bears the name of the sacred tree. Legend tells that his Druid master captured the Salmon of Wisdom and planned to eat it to gain knowledge of all that was happening in Ireland.

While preparing the dish for his master, Finn burst a blister on the side of the cooking salmon with his thumb. To soothe the pain, he put his burned thumb in his mouth and thus Finn received the fish's gift in place of his master.

GIFFORD

RECIPES

HAZELNUT EYEWASH- Take 6 large fresh leaves and cover with one litre of water. Bring to boil, turn down to simmer for twenty minutes. Remove from heat, strain and cool. Refrigerate, and use within one week in a sterile eyecup.

Freeze as ice cubes, to store for longer.

HAZELNUT MILK- Take 500 grams of kernels, equal sugar and one litre of water. Grind into a pulp and then simmer. Drink two large soupspoons full morning and evening.

HEARTBURN TEA- Combine one part coltsfoot leaf with four part hazelnut catkins and two parts pineapple weed. Steep in boiling water when still warm, and drink after meals.

LEAF TINCTURE- 1:5 at 40% alcohol. 20 drops twice daily.

DECOCTION- 1:20 for 15 minutes of dry husks and twigs. One cup daily. Strain well.

LOW SPERM COUNT- Take hazel catkins, a third as much stonecrop, a fourth as much bindweed as stonecrop, and a bit of common pepper.

HILDEGARD

DIVINING- To look for hidden water, grip a fork in each hand and pull them apart until you feel pressure. Focus your intent on water (or whatever you are searching for), and you will feel the stick bend back and turn as you pass over the source. Buried treasure, and various mineral sources can also be divined, and up to the 17th century, was used in England to determine guilt in cases of murder and theft.

COLD PRESSED OIL- Take one tablespoon every morning on an empty stomach for 15 days; for intestinal worms.

HEDGE NETTLE, MARSH
WOUNDWORT
CLOWN WOUNDWORT
(*Stachys palustris* L.)
(*S. palustris ssp. pilosa* [Nutt.] Epling) not accepted
WOOD BETONY
(*S. officinalis* [L.] Trevis.)
(*Betonica officinalis* L.) not accepted

LAMB'S EAR
HEDGE NETTLE, WOOLLY
(*S. byzantine* K. Koch)
BIG BETONY
(*S. grandiflora* [Stephan ex Willd.] Benth.) not accepted
(*S. macrantha* [K. Koch] Stearn)
CHINESE ARTICHOKE
JAPANESE ARTICHOKE
CROSNE
(*S. sieboldii* Miq.)
(*S. affinis* Bunge) not accepted
PARTS USED- flowers, leaves, root

Wood Betony is in its prime in May,
In June and July does its bloom display,
A fine, bright red does this grand plant adorn,
To gather it for drink I think no scorn;
I'll make a conserve of its fragrant flowers,
Cephalick virtues in this herb remain,
To chase each dire disorder from the brain.
Delirious persons here a cure may find
To stem the phrensy, and to calm the mind.   **J. CHAMBERS**

"Wood Betony preserves the liver and bodies of men from infectious diseases."   **ANTONIUS MUSA**

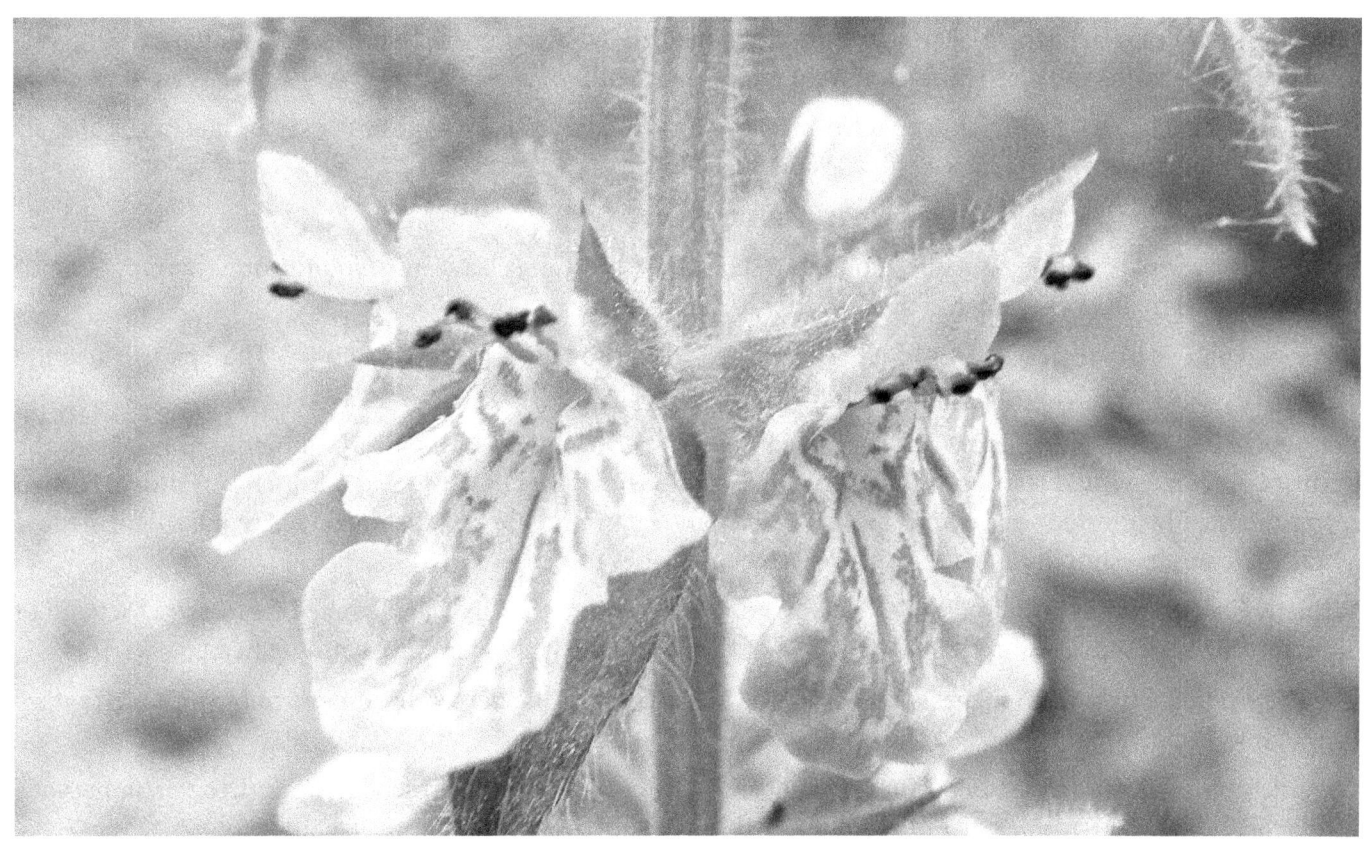

HEDGE NETTLE

Stachys is from the Greek, "a spike", as in an ear of grain, and refers to the flower; or derived from **STACHUS**, meaning a bunch, due to the arrangement of flowers.

Palustris means of the marsh, or swamp.

Betony, according to Pliny, is named after the Latin Betonica, a variation from Vettonica, a plant of the Vettones, an Iberian, or Spanish tribe. Or perhaps it is from the Celtic **BEW** head and **TON**, meaning good, in allusion to the herb's use in problems of the head. Wood probably reflects its forest home.

In Slavonic languages the genus name translates as **CHISTETS**, cleanser or woundwort.

Byzantina means of Byzanthium, or Istanbul. Pilosa refers to the tiny soft hairs on the leaf and stem.

All plants are perennials, native to Europe, and Asia, with Marsh Hedge Nettle long naturalized throughout the prairies. Wood Betony is frequently found in herbal gardens, and is an occasional escapee. Lambs Ear and Big Betony are common garden perennials. All are hardy to zone 2-3, with Wood Betony requiring added protection in winters with light snow cover.

Dioscorides called Wood Betony **KESTRON**, while other Greek physicians called it **PSYCHOTROPHON** meaning, "soul nourisher". Kestron refers to the sharp nature of the flowers.

Antonius Musa, the Roman physician to Ceasar Augustus, wrote an entire book on the medicinal virtues of Wood Betony, or Vettonica, as it was known, listing 47 treatable conditions.

In the 9th century, Walahfrid Strabo wrote of the herb in his Garden Poem (*Hortulus Sanitatis*), and in the 11th century Odo Magdunensis devotes a long chapter on the herb in his *Macer floridus*.

The Old English Herbarium, translated into Anglo Saxon over a thousand years ago, says that "it is good for one's soul and one's body; it protects a person from dreadful nightmares and from terrifying visions and dreams".

In the 17th century, the German pharmacist Schroeder states "there is almost no bodily ailment for which it cannot prove of especial benefit". An early German name **ZEHRKRAUT**, which means "wasting herb", suggests its use for diseases concerning significant weight loss and debility.

Betony was believed to shield the sleeper from visions and dreams, and was one of the six amulet herbs of early herbal medicine, worn to drive away "devils and despair".

The others were Vervain, Peony, Yarrow, Plantain and Rose.

In the Slavic language, the genus name adopted is **CHISTETS** meaning cleanser or woundwort. This corresponds with one of the main uses, namely skin diseases.

Betony's value is expressed in an old Italian proverb "Sell your coat and buy Betony". The Spanish use the expression, "He has as many virtues as Betony".

Betony means, "head herb", and was a traditional remedy for problems of the head. In medieval England, the herb was recommended to cure "monstrous nocturnal visions, devils, despair and lunacy". Hildegard also recommended betony "for one who is foolish or silly and lacks knowledge…if someone is regularly tormented by false dreams, he should have betony leaves …when he goes to bed."

William Coles wrote that Betony is "especially good for the brain". This was deduced from the Doctrine of Signatures, which somehow explained hairiness of the root signifying an affinity with the head.

The Old English Herbarium suggests decocting the plant in wine "if a person becomes tired from much riding or much walking."

The British snuffed the leaves along with eyebright and coltsfoot in Rowley's British Herb Snuff, to relieve nervous headache. It was used in England and France as a tobacco substitute to help one give up smoking.

The leaves are a good substitute for black tea, the infusion tasting similar; but caffeine free.

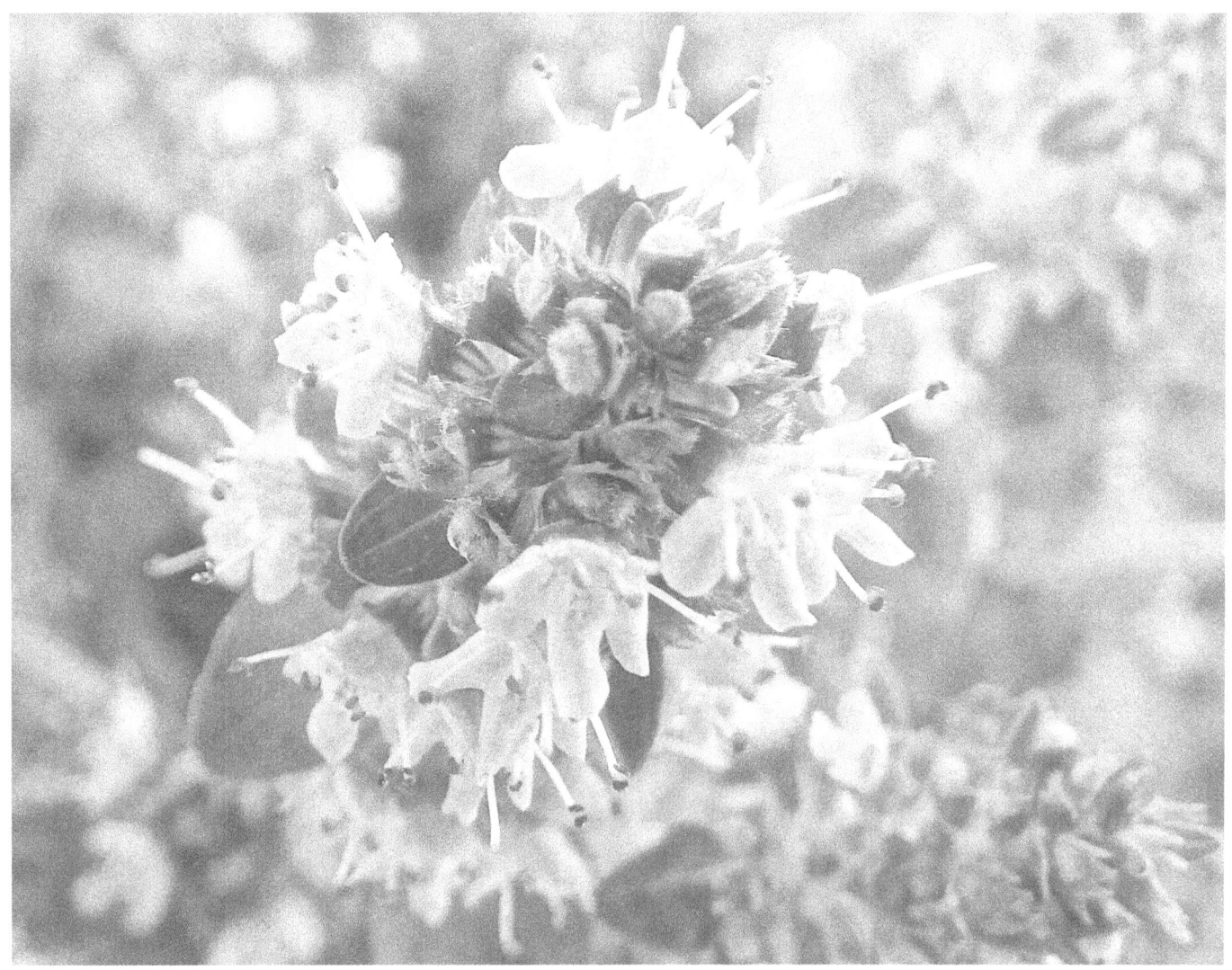

WOOD BETONY FLOWER HEAD

The French recommended the leaves of **BETEINE** for liver, gall bladder, spleen and lung affections. In Italy, the entire plant is used for healing varicose veins, ulcers and infective sores. An infusion of the root is used to aid gastro-intestinal disturbances.

Woundwort received its name for stopping bleeding, promoting healing, and drawing out boils and splinters. In Serbia, it is known as **RANILIST** or **RANJENIK**.

During the medieval times, it was widely used for "all fresh and green wounds- for staunching blood flows- to dry up fluxes-the humours of old and fretting ulcers- and rotting and corroding cankers."

The juice, in the form of syrup, was regarded as second to none for "inward wounds- the breaking of veins-vomitings-the spittings of blood- and ruptures".

For the latter, a poultice of the plant was applied in place.

The tuberous root were boiled and eaten; the unpleasant tasting leaves usually avoided.

Marsh Hedge Nettle is a circumpolar plant that the Chippewa put to good use, naming it **ANDE' GOBUG**, meaning Crow Leaf. Hot infusions of the fresh or dried leaves were taken for sudden colic. The Delaware made a compound containing the root in attempts to treat venereal disease. Despite being a member of the Mint family, Marsh Hedge Nettle, when bruised, has a rather unusual fishy smell, not mint-like at all!

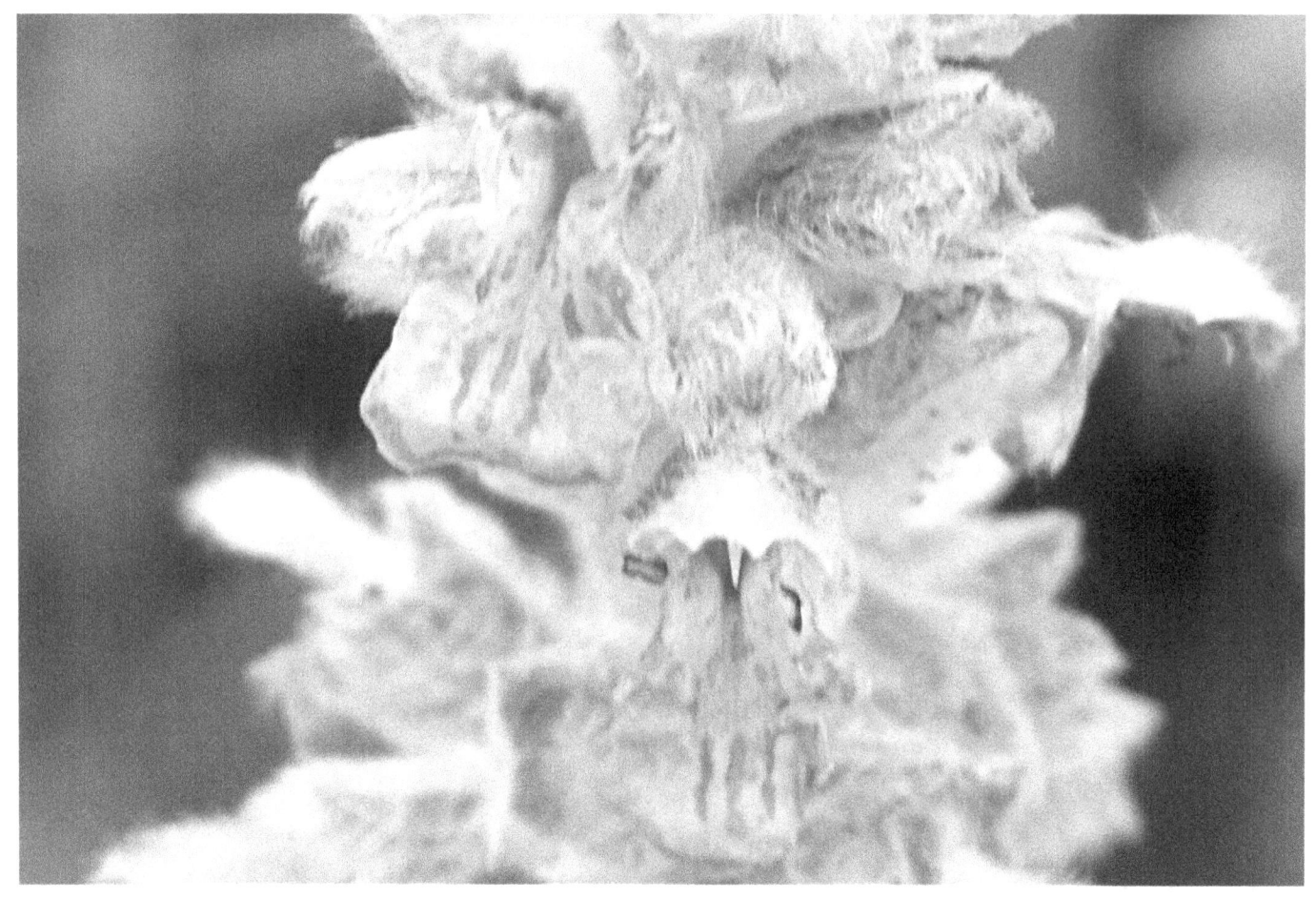

LAMB'S EARS

Kahlee Keane suggests the plant's scent has to do with habitat. "The whole plant may have a minty, rhubarb-like aroma, or may have an unpleasant smell. I have found that they have a wonderful scent when growing in an unpolluted area; otherwise, the plant seems to react by emitting a somewhat less desirable odour." Interesting.

Some tribes ate the seeds, and the tasty roots collected in fall were eaten raw, baked, boiled or dried for later use. They were then ground into flour and used to make a type of bread.

Hildegard de Bingen, the 12th century Abbess, recommended warmed poultices for skin ulcers, but cautioned its use in sword wounds. "Woundwort rapidly heals the skin's exterior surface, but drives the corrupt matter inward."

In traditional medicine, it has been used as an antiseptic, hemostat, emetic, emmenagogue, expectorant, nervine, sedative, tonic and vulenary. It has been widely used in gout, cramps and joint pain.

The famous 16th century English herbalist John Gerard was nearby one day when a farmer cut his leg to the bone with a scythe. He offered his help for free, but with the blood gushing out, the farmer said he would take care of it himself. Gerard said he had never heard such a clownish answer, and dubbed the plant Clown's Woundwort.

He watched skeptically, as the farmer tore off his shirt and tied pieces of the plant to the large open wound.

He applied fresh poultices every day for a week and to Gerard's amazement, it was healed! He then became a staunch believer in the plant and came to recommend it to those injured in tavern brawls, and such. An old gypsy recipe is found below.

The whole plant yields yellow and blue colors for dyeing, and red when used with silverweed and other *Potentilla* roots.

Lambs Ears, on the other hand, makes a pleasant tasting tea. They can be steamed, but may be too fuzzy for some people's palates.

They are a favorite garden plant of children, and my wife, Laurie. She loves the soft, furry texture; so soothing to a cat person.

This hairy covering helps protect plants from excessive heat, cold and sunlight. A German scientist, G. Haberlandt, conducted an experiment in 1918, in which he removed the hairy coating from the upper leaf surface. He found that transpiration doubled when the hairs were removed. Too much spare time,I would say! They were formerly used to bandage wounds, and used instead of lint as a surgical dressing.

Chinese Artichoke (*S. sieboldi*), also known by the Japanese name, **CHOROGI**, is used as a vegetable. Phillip Franz van Siebold was an early 1800s German physician who collected plants in Japan and introduced them to Europe.

Chinese Artichoke is often sold under the French name, **CROSNE**, after the small village southwest of Paris, where it was first grown commercially. It is an odd looking vegetable, with underground tubers that look like a dirty string of pearls, or a snail. They look and taste somewhat like Jerusalem Artichokes, with a delicate, nutty flavor.

It has medicinal benefit, and is widely used in Russia.

In China, the tuber is used in medicine, and is known as **GAN LU ZI** meaning Sweet Dew seed. Other names include Cutworm, Treasure Pagoda Vegetable, Earth Bull, Arhat Vegetable and Grass Stone Silkworm.

MEDICINAL

CONSTITUENTS- *S. palustris* benzoic acid (3.2% flowers, 4.7% leaves); various flavonoids (1.8% flowers, 3.7% leaves), including palustrinoside, palustrin, acetyl palustaside, luteolin, stachyosides, stachydrine (cabadine) O.62%, stachyrene, stachynone, stachone, stacylone, annuanone, scutellarein, cinnamic acid derivatives including caffeic, 1 and 4 caffeylquinic acids, chlorogenic acid, neo-chlorogenic acid, alpha amyrin, beta sitosterol, 4-methoxy-scutellarein, allantoin, betaine, hydroxycoumarins, ursolic acid (0.37%), ascorbic acid (leaf- 46.2 mg%), oxalic, citric, tartaric, malic and succinic acids, and high level of tannins. Also contains glycosides verbascoside and echinacoside, isoscutellarein derivatives, harpagide, 8-O-acetyl-harpagide, and monomelittoside.
S. officinalis- stachydrine (0.49-2.42%), betaine (0.5%), 4',7-dimethoxy apigenin, orientin, anthocyanins (flowers), ascorbic acid (leaf 135mg%), beta-carotene, alpha chlorophyll, various alkaloids (-) betonicine, stachydrin, trigonellin, and turicin, tannins (15%), bitters, various caffeic acids (0.5%), p-coumaric acid, chlorogenic, isochlorogenic and neochlorogenic acid, 12 phenylethanoid glycosides named betonyosides A-F, acetoside, acetoside isomer, campneosides II, forsythoside B, and leucosceptoside B; iridoids glycosides such as allobetonicoside and 6-0-acetyl mioporoside, harpagide, ajugoside, aucubin, acetyl harpagide, betolide, betonidolide, betonicosides A-D, hydrocinnamic acids, saponins, choline, trans-phytol, various flavonoids including apigenin, 4',5'-dihydroxy-3'5',7-trimethoxy-flavone, 7-methoxy-tricin, and scutullarein 7-glucoside; and essential oils. Fifteen amino acids compose 0.42%.
root- betonicosides A-D, diterpenoids, and betonicolide, stachyose
S. byzantina- tannins (5%), resins, organic acids, Vitamin K and C.
S. lanata- stachydrine, vitamins K & C, 30 known compounds including stachysosides E-H, phytol nonadecanoate, manoyl oxide, 13-epi-manoyl oxide.
S. grandiflora- ledol, tartessol, myrtenyl acetate.
S. sieboldii- tubers- acetoside, verbascoside, stachysosides A-C, stachyose, succinic acid, phenylethanoid and iridoid glycosides including leucosceptoside; 37% carbohydrates, 2.36% potassium.

Wood Betony and Marsh Hedge Nettle contain several, similar constituents, and are used medicinally for a few of the same conditions. They are different, of course, but can be used interchangeably for a number of purposes.

They act principally on the nervous system, as restoratives and relaxants. In this way, the plants are somewhat similar to Skullcap.

But they are more complex in a number of ways, addressing the pain of deep-seated nerve damage, as well as the toxemia related to arthritis, or rheumatism. Stachydrine, also found in yarrow, decreases rheumatic pain, and is a systolic depressant. (-)Betonicine, likewise found in yarrow, is anti-inflammatory.

Small amounts are astringent in relieving diarrhea, probably due to the tannins, while larger amounts are laxative.

Matthew Wood, in his excellent "*The Book of Herbal Wisdom*", cites Wood Betony as the herb to strengthen the solar plexus and help people feel more grounded.

The solar plexus is one of the more significant nerve centers of the body, acting as a switchboard for digestive functions and gut level instinct and reaction.

It is the brain of the stomach, if you will, coordinating the secretion of saliva, and the peristaltic action of the stomach, release of gall bladder, and intestinal peristalsis.

It is worth noting that trigonellin, one of its constituents, is found in fenugreek, as well, and is believed to play a role in lowering blood sugar levels. Instinctive wisdom, gut feelings, groundedness and self-confidence are all affected by Wood Betony.

A very interesting book, *The Second Brain*, by Michael D. Gershon, MD, explains in great detail the nervous system of the gut, or enteric nervous system. Various neurotransmitters, including serotonin, are produced in the intestine. Although well researched, the idea of a second brain in the stomach and intestine is not widely known or recognized for its significance. It does explain the phrase "you are what you eat" in a convincing manner, however.

A wide range of problems are due, to weakness of the solar plexus. Various nervous and muscular tensions arise, creating high blood pressure, migraines and neuralgias throughout the body.

Early work by Zinchenko & Fefer, *Farmatsevt Zhurnal* 1962 17:3 found glycosides in Wood Betony possess hypotensive ability.

Wood Betony both relaxes and strengthens, so that one can better deal with stress and tension. It combines well with Linden as a sedative, or mild hypotensive agent; and with Calamus Root and Scullcap as a digestive tonic and stomachic.

Wood Betony nourishes the pineal gland, according to Dr. Lepore. He believes that degeneration of the pineal can cause insanity, and vitiligo, the loss of skin pigmentation resulting in white patches. Flouridation appears to crystallize the pineal gland, suggesting alternate sources of water may be indicated.

Wood Betony, on a daily basis, can take months before any improvement is note. It is first noticed in the centre of the patch, where it will fade to look like a doughnut and finally disappear.

Betaine, in studies on animals, has shown anti-convulsive effect.

It can be used in vertigo, memory loss, or difficulty comprehending. It is one of the best remedies for headaches that require vascular dilation, combining well with St. John's Wort, Scullcap (*S. laterifolia*) or Vervain for tension headaches. Dr. Christopher believed Wood Betony an "excellent remedy for all head and face pains, and for nervous troubles."

It has a similar action to Ginkgo, and combines well with Wild Bergamot, and/or Ginkgo itself for warming and activating circulation and memory.

Menzies Trull, an English physio-medicalist, suggests betony with scullcap or valerian for nervous headaches, with elderflower for headache from chills, with milk thistle for memory, and with black cohosh and scullcap for sciatica.

It strengthens the lungs, in cases of wasting disease and weakness such as acute or chronic bronchitis, copious white or yellow phlegm accompanied with blood.

Work by Fitzpatrick, *Antibiotics and Chemotherapy* 1954 4:5 showed Wood Betony active against tuberculosis, *in vitro*.

It combines well with Linden flowers for sinus headaches and congestion.

Wood Betony increases urination, strengthens the kidneys and reduces edema.

It improves the circulation and health of the uterus, and has been used traditionally for uterine prolapse, menstrual pain, weak labor and excessive bleeding. It combines well with yarrow in the treatment of nosebleeds.

However, in the hands of a skilled herbalist, the plant can actually help improve contractions during childbirth.

It can be considered a specific for head injury, and has been combined with yarrow in cases of brain aneurism. It will give temporary relief in cases of temporal arteritis.

The root has a stronger effect on the liver, and is therefore better for stimulating the liver and bowel in treating jaundice and constipation.

Because it is stronger, use half doses, as excessive doses of either leaf or root can cause severe gastrointestinal discomfort, nausea and diarrhea.

In Russia, work by Kobzar, Zinchenko and Fefer points to the herb's anti-inflammatory, cholagogue and blood pressure lowering activity. Stachydrine, in particular, shows systolic depressant properties.

Infusions, or tincture in water, can be helpful in healing bleeding or infected gums, or mouth sores, due to the plants astringent and hemostatic activity.

The fresh plant can be slowly heated in unsalted butter, for a salve that reduces skin inflammation, cuts and sores.

Wood Betony helps anchor consciousness back into the physical body, according to Sean Donahue. "A traditional herb of exorcism, Wood Betony can also offer a degree of protection if a person is experiencing other entities trying to come into her body or trying to pull her out of her body."

In some cases, Wood Betony and Marsh Hedge Nettle can be used inter-changeably. The biased toward Wood Betony is the more extensive research, especially from Europe. When using the flowering tops of Wood Betony remember to include the basal leaves; which are richest in betaine, caffeic derivatives and flavonoids.

Marsh Hedge Nettle treats a variety of menstrual problems including dysmenorrhea, amenorrhea, ovaritis, metritis, and liver depression associated with menopause.

It is used for visceral spasms from over-stimulated nerves and is helpful for treating hypertension. Stachydrine, a pyrrolidine alkaloid in Wood Betony, and Marsh Hedge Nettle, as well as Yarrow (*A. millefolium*), and Motherwort is a systolic blood pressure depressant.

It also inhibits production of nitric oxide and secretion of IL-10, suggestive of reducing inflammation. It may also protect against beta-adrenergic receptor and act somewhat like a calcium channel blocker for heart conditions. Zhang C et al, *BMC Complement Altern Med* 2014 14:474.

Michael Moore believes Marsh Hedge Nettle useful for internal inflammations of all kinds. It helps migraines, hangover headaches, headaches from eyestrain, with the eyes inflamed and sore.

It helps relieve the pain of urethritis and cystitis, and eases menstrual cramps.

Marsh Hedge Nettle is astringent and antiseptic, and can be used for stopping bleeding and promoting the healing of wounds. It also lessens the pain and inflammation, especially when used externally as a glycerin tincture.

It is used to treat vertigo, of unspecified origin.

For sprains and joint inflammations, it can be taken both internally and externally. Verbascoside is found in many Labiateae family plants, and exerts anti-oxidant, anti-inflammatory and anti-cancer properties. Venditti A et al, *Chem Biodivers* 2014 11:245.

Echinacoside is well-known compound in various Echinacea species.

The two isoscutellarein derivatives are anti-oxidant and exert neuroprotective effects in Alzheimer's disease. Uriate-Pueyo I et al, *Food Chem* 2010 120:679.

Early work with stachyrene on 49 patients with obstructive jaundice before and after the operation, found the majority of patients experienced more rapid homeostasis. Voltenko GN et al, *Klin Khir* 1990(11):26-7.

Chlorogenic acid is a common phenolic acid with anti-oxidant properties, and shows ability to slow the release of glucose into the bloodstream, after a meal. Johnston KL et al, *Am J Clin Nutr* 2003 78:728.

Harpagide and its derivatives are found in various figwort species, as well as Devil's Claw from Namibia, and proven useful in various arthritic conditions.

A poultice of the mashed roots is the most effective form, but tea, tinctures and even glycerine preparations are all useful.

For headaches, try applying the herb to the forehead. For sore throats, the fresh root can be chewed or the tea or tincture in water gargled.

The ethanol extracts inhibit xanthine oxidase, suggesting benefit in gout.

See the recipe below for abrasions, contusions, sprains, cuts, etc. The plant is hemostatic, astringent, disinfectant, and lessens the pain and inflammation. It combines well with Skullcap, Vervain or Valerian for nervousness, irritability, and insomnia in those with sensory oversensitivity.

The preparation **PALUSTAKHIN** made from *S. palustris* possesses anti-hepatotoxic action.

The stem extract of *S. palustris* shows inhibition of HeLa cervix adenocarcinoma cell lines. The stem, leaf and flower show activity against MCF7 breast cancer cell lines. Haznagy-Radnai et al, *Fitoterapia* 2008 79. The stems of Lambs Ears (below) showed activity against MCF7, HeLa and A431 cancer cell lines in the same study.

CAUTION- Because they are mildly uterine stimulating, both Wood Betony and Marsh Hedge Nettle are contraindicated in pregnancy.

Lambs Ears or Woolly Betony is not usually thought of as a medicinal plant. However, both liquid and alcoholic extracts of *S. lanata* have been recommended and used for the treatment of hypotonic disease, and cardiac neuroses. Like its two cousins above, it contains stachydrine (cadabine), which is a systolic depressant.

It both energetically and on a physical plane helps assist the healing process around heart attacks, arrhythmia and strokes. Place the moistened leaves between cotton cloth and place on the chest for 20 minutes. Repeat as desired. On the top of the head, this same poultice may assist seizure activity.

Work by Khanavi et al, *J Ethnopharm* 2005 97:3 463-8 found the aerial parts inhibit pain and inflammation.

Activity against *C. albicans, Aspergillus niger, E. coli, Klebsiella pneumoniae,* and *Pseudomonas aeruginosa* has been noted, in several studies.

The related *S. lavandulifolia* was utilized in a randomized clinical trail of 66 women with polycystic ovary syndrome, and suffering abnormal uterine bleeding. They were given 5 grams of the aerial herb for three months, or medroxyprogesterone acetate. Results were similar, with less adverse effect in drug group. Jililian N et al, *Phytother Res* 2013 27(11): 1708-13.

The related Chinese Artichoke, or Woundwort (*S. sieboldii*) contains acetoside, a promising constituent for the prevention of glomerulonephritis.

This may explain, in part, its use in treating kidney pain.

One part of Wood Ear mushrooms and six parts Chinese Artichokes are simmered, sweetened and given for hollow coughs, and asthma. For tuberculosis with blood, one part watermelon seed is simmered with two parts artichoke roots.

Acetoside is present in Wood Betony as well. Work initiated by Hayashi et al, *Japan Journal of Pharmacology* 1996 70:2 on acetosides should be continued. He found that the anti-nephritic action of acetoside is due to inhibition of intra-glomerular accumulation of leukocytes through prevention of the up-regulation of intracellular adhesion molecule-1.

The tuber, extracted with ethanol, efficiently protects human cells Caco-2, SHSY-5Y and K562 against induced oxidative damage. Venditti A et al, *Food Chem* 2017 221:473-81.

Various *Stachys* species roots contain stachyose, also found in *Lupinus luteus* and *Fraxinus ornus.* The compound is anti-bacterial. Chiba et al, *Bioorg Med Chem Lett* 17:9.

An extract of the tuber was compared with Ginkgo biloba leaf extract in a mouse study on neurotoxicity. Both were found to protect against learning and memory dysfunction associated with ischemic brain injury. Harada S et al, *J Nutr Sci Vitaminol* (Tokyo) 2015 61(2): 167-74.

The optimal extraction is 95 degrees Celsius for 2.5 hours 1:16 ratio of herb to water, repeated three times. Feng K et al, *Carbohydr Polym* 2015 125: 45-52.

HOMEOPATHY

Betonica (Betony Wood) should therefore be considered in stitches in the right temple (gall bladder?), and the inability to concentrate the mind.

Dizziness in forehead, made worse from bending down. Frequent sneezing going from indoors to open air.

There may be pains in the abdomen, hepatic region and of the transverse colon. Also in the gall bladder, inguinal region and spermatic cords.

There may be shooting pain in the back of both wrist joints, or pain in the right groin, hamstring and down the leg, which feels paralyzed or lame.

It is also beneficial for catarrhal colds. There may be profuse, drenching perspiration in bed, almost entirely limited to head, neck and chest.

DOSE- The mother tincture is prepared from the fresh, flowering herb *Stachys officinalis*. Use 5 drops as needed. Berridge used four provers with tincture in 1869.

ESSENTIAL OILS

The amount of essential oil from the aerial parts of various Stachys species range from 0.008-0.83%.

Wood Betony contains aldehydes of an undefined type, plus iridoids such as harpagide and harpagide 8-acetate. The essential oil is a mixture of 32 compounds, including cadinene, phthalate and phytol, the only ones identified by GC and GC-MS.

One study found various monoterpenes, sesquiterpenes, germacrene 42.8%, gamma-cadinene 6.3%, delta-cadinene 5%, alpha amorphene 3.9%, alpha cadinol 2.3%, alpha bergamotene, beta borbonene. Grujic-Javanovic, *Flav Fragr J* 2004 19 139-144.

A more recent study found germacrene D (20%), beta caryophyllene (14%), alpha humulene (7.5%). Work by Lazarevic JS et al, *Chem Biodivers* 2013 10:1335 found activity against *Aspergillus niger* and *Candida albicans.*

Guiliani C et al, separated leaves and flowers and did separate distillations. (E)-carophyllene (20.1%), (E)-nerolidol (14.3%), caryophyllene oxide (6.1%) and gamma-cadinene (5.&%) were main consitituents in leaf volatiles, while caryophyllene oxide (16.5%), (E)-nerolidol (15.4%), humulene epoxide II (9.2%) and alpha pinene (7%) were main compounds in flower fraction. *Nat Prod Res* 2017 31(9):1006-13.

Marsh Hedge Nettle contains iridoids and up to 25% carbonylic compounds.

The essential oil from aerial parts of *Stachys palustris* from Southern Italy, was characterized mainly by carbonylic compounds (25.4%), fatty acids and their esters (24.2%), along with sesquiterpenoidic compounds (16.0%) and phenols (11.2%). The yield is small (0.02-0.05%)

The major components were determined to be caryophylleneoxide, hexahydrofarnesyl acetone, hexadecanoic acid, (Z, Z, Z)-9, 12, 15-octadecatrienoic acid, (Z)-phytol, thymol, p-methoxyacetophenone, 4-vinylguiacole, tetradecanoic acid, (E)-caryophyllene, b-ionone and b-damascenone.

Work by Vendetti A et al, *Chem Biodivers* 2017 14 e:1600401, looked at aerial essential oils from Hungary and France. The former contains 48.8% (E) phytol, 13% hexadecanoic acid and 12% hexahydrofarnesyl actone, and minor amounts of n-alkanes including n-nonacosane and n-heptacosane, caryophyllene oxide, (E)-beta-ionone and n-untriacontane. Essential oil from France was composed mainly of fatty acids including hexadecanoic, linoleic and linolenic acid.

The essential oil has been found to inhibit ACHN renal cell adenocarcinoma by 77%. Conforti et al, *Food Chem* 2009 116:4.

Work by Duarte et al, *J Ethnopharm* 2005 97:2 found Lamb's Ears essential oil active against *Candida albicans*.

Khanaui et al, *Z Naturforsch* 59 identified alpha copaene 16%, spathulenol 16% and beta caryophyllene 14% in the essential oil. Other work found cembrene, phytol, manoyl oxide and 13-epi-manoyl oxide, as well as 3alpha-hydroxy manool.

The leaf contains up to 37% germacrene D and 12% valeranone in one study. The stem yielded 58% nerolidol and 19% thymol in same study.

Activity against a number of bacterium and fungi is noted in descending order: *Enterococcus faecalis, Pseudomonas aeruginosa, Klebsiella pneumoniae, Bacillus subtilis, Candida albicans, Staphylococcus aureus* and *E. coli*.

Two related plants, *S. candida* and *S. chrysantha,* from southern Greece have been analyzed with 42 constituents found in the two oils. The major components are alpha cadinol, manoyl oxide, caryophyllene oxide, epi-alpha-muurolol, and (E)-caryophyllene.

These two oils tested positive against six gram positive and negative bacteria, one of them exhibiting significant anti-bacterial activity.

Stachys recta aerial parts have been steam distilled, but contain only 0.014% essential oil. Thirty-two compounds, mainly alcohols and oxides were found, the major constituent being 1-octen-3-ol at just under 20%. Other minor constituents are caryophyllene oxide, humulene oxide and nerolidol at around 3-4% each.

HYDROSOLS

Several spoonfuls of distilled water of Betony, taken often according to one's disposition, will strengthen a cold, weak, phlegmatic stomach, mollify it unwillingness to accept food, open obstructions of the liver and spleen, prevent dropsy and jaundice, and cleanse the kidneys and bladder of grit, sand and stones.

Furthermore, it will help those who are afflicted with cold piss or dripping urine, warm chills of the matrix, cleanse the chest and lungs of phlegm and pus, ease fits of coughing, and strengthen and warm a head weakened by cold. Likewise, Betony Water will prevent apoplexy and falling sickness.   **SAUER**

The distilled water of Betony is very good for such as are pained in their heads, it prevails against the dropsy and all sorts of fevers, it succours the liver and spleen, and helps want of digestion and evil disposition of the body thence arising; it hastens travail in women with child, and is excellent against the bitings of venomous beasts.   **CULPEPPER**

Betony water is distilled from the plant in flower. It is good for pain in the head from cold, stone in the bladder, old coughs, delayed menses, pain in hips, kidney and bladder.   **BRUNSCHWIG**

SEED OIL

The seeds of Wood Betony and Woundwort contain from 24-44% fatty oils. These include triaclglycerols derived from palmitic, stearic, oleic (20-30%), linoleic (60-70%) and linolenic acids.

FLOWER ESSENCES

Wood Betony flower essence brings inner serenity to the sexual energy flow of a person.
RUNNING FOX FARM

Wood Betony flower essence is an enhancer, working primarily in balancing attitudes in the conflict of sexual energy and the desire for higher principles.

This essence enhances the higher philosophies and the necessary sacrifices that transpire with abstinence. Celibacy should be abstainment and inner calmness, rather than an agonizing struggle and suppression of sexual desires.

A person embracing tantric practices in which the sexual energies are channeled into higher philosophies could use this essence. It helps some oversexed people exert more self-control. Wood Betony also helps people who have certain types of diseases such as herpes in the genitals to adjust to being celibate.

The pineal is also enhanced. This is generally the only part of the physical body that is affected by this essence.

Transits of any planets through Scorpio will have some of their energies increased. **GURUDAS**

Wood Betony (*S. officinalis*) stimulates the higher functioning of the psyche. In addition, Wood Betony stimulates the feeling of clarity regarding the self and its expression in the world. Energetically, there is a mild stimulation of the crown chakra which, in turn, stimulates the pineal gland. This enhances the higher functioning of the brain.
DALTON

As a flower essence, Betony relaxes the mind and triggers awareness of where true healing may lie or be required. It is powerfully restorative, but using it may mean that you reveal more to yourself and to others than you would like to admit. In my practice, this essence is commonly chosen by clients before an energy treatment, and certainly helps them to relax and talk about their concerns. **OLIVE**

Lambs Ear essence may help a low thyroid, tone the male reproductive system, and heal energy surrounding cancers. It may also assist in the recovery from rape and sexual violence and the ensuing disconnection.
AVENSARO

Marsh Woundwort (*S. palustris*) is for the tendency to worry and fret unnecessarily. It is for letting go of the distress from unmet needs in the past and being content in the present. **HAREBELL**

SPIRITUAL PROPERTIES

Ancient and traditional medical systems placed a strong emphasis on the solar plexus and its attendant physical structures. Ayurvedic medicine visualizes the duodenum as the seat of the *AGNI*, the primal fire of the body. The same idea is found in Western Alchemy. Paracelsus said the "Archeus", or innate intelligence of the body dwells in the stomach. A hundred years later, J.B. Von Helmont believed that the "sensitive animated soul" had its residence in the pyloric sphincter. Samuel Thompson thought the stomach was the residence of vital force.

He visualized it like a stove in which a fire of heat and vital force burned, radiating in all directions, warming and vitalizing the body. In Traditional Chinese Medicine (TCM), many of the physical problems described would be classified as "stomach chi deficiency", or " deficient chi of the gall bladder".

The stomach is not given as much credit as a psychological center in the official Chinese medicine of today, but there are different strains of thought, some of which value the stomach more highly. In Taoist folklore, the image of the round bellied, jovial little wise man reflects the idea that the belly is the seat of basic, down to earth wisdom.
WOOD

In calling on the spirit of [Lambs Ear], an elderly male form appears out of the ethers. He is surrounded by penetrating rays of yellow light. His white hair embraces the wrinkles on his tender face, part of which is covered by the beard that he has grown for many years. He wears a modest cloak; for he likes to travel lightly as he has much healing work to do. Every time there is a request for healing from the plant, he makes a journey to answer its prayers. As he nears this sacred shrub, there, protecting it, is a beautiful baby lamb with large and sparkling eyes and brilliant white coat. He guards the plant and all of the prayers that are made in honor of its name.

AVENSARO

PERSONALITY TRAITS

Our Betony grows in a neat clump, close to the earth, the leaves radiating forth from the ground. After it has established itself securely, it sends up long, slender flower stalks.

This is the signature: Wood Betony is a remedy which helps establish rootedness, connectedness, earthiness, and grounded-ness. It is a plant for people who are cut off from the earth or their bodies. It strengthens the solar plexus- the place which helps us feel connected- and through the solar plexus it strengthens the stomach and the rest of the nervous system, including the brain.

WOOD

Wood Betany's (sic) key word is discernment. Wood Betany (sic) carries with it the qualities of insight, perspicacity, and intuition. It is useful for times of making important choices as it gathers and synthesizes all the information. It helps us to stay emotionally detached; to observe the situation in an objective fashion for clear decision-making.

EVELYN MULDERS

Stachys byzantina, the ubiquitous lamb's lugs, is surely the most furry of plants. In our house it is known as the 'ticky plant'.

Both daughters used it as a comforter when they were very young, detaching a leaf and tickling their noses with it in a state of pure ecstasy. The woolliness of the whole plant is created by thousands of tiny hairs, developed to protect the leaf cuticle from the searing sun of its high Middle Eastern home. In the garden its soft, dense clumps belie these tough-guy characteristics.

CAROL KLEIN

Wood Betony affirms mental and emotional equanimity.

CRUDEN

RECIPES

INFUSION- leaf and flower- One tsp of dried to one pint of water. Drink three cups daily. Take three ounces 3-4 times daily for intestinal worms. When drying the flowering tops, use shade and keep cool, as close to 5 degrees Celsius as possible.

TINCTURE- leaf- 10- 15 drops three times daily

root- 5-10 drops 1-3 times daily. To make a fresh plant tincture, take one part plant to two parts pure alcohol. To make a dry plant tincture use one part aerial plant, to five parts liquid that is 50% alcohol. Small amounts are astringent, larger amounts can be laxative.

OINTMENT (sort of). Take one part of fresh plant to two-thirds vegetable glycerine, and one-third 95% alcohol. Mix together in blender and store in covered jar for two weeks. Then pour off the liquid, and use salve (?) as needed for topical injury.

HEDGE NETTLE WINE- Combine a handful each of finely cut hedge nettle root and leaf to one quart of wine. Simmer for 15 minutes and steep five more. Pour over a half handful of chamomile flowers. Allow to cool and strain. Apply as needed to wounds after all infection is cleared.

CAUTION- Marsh Hedge Nettle contains an alkaloid that can paralyze the nervous system in very large doses. Do not overuse. Wood Betony and Marsh Hedge Nettle are contraindicated during pregnancy due to uterine stimulation.

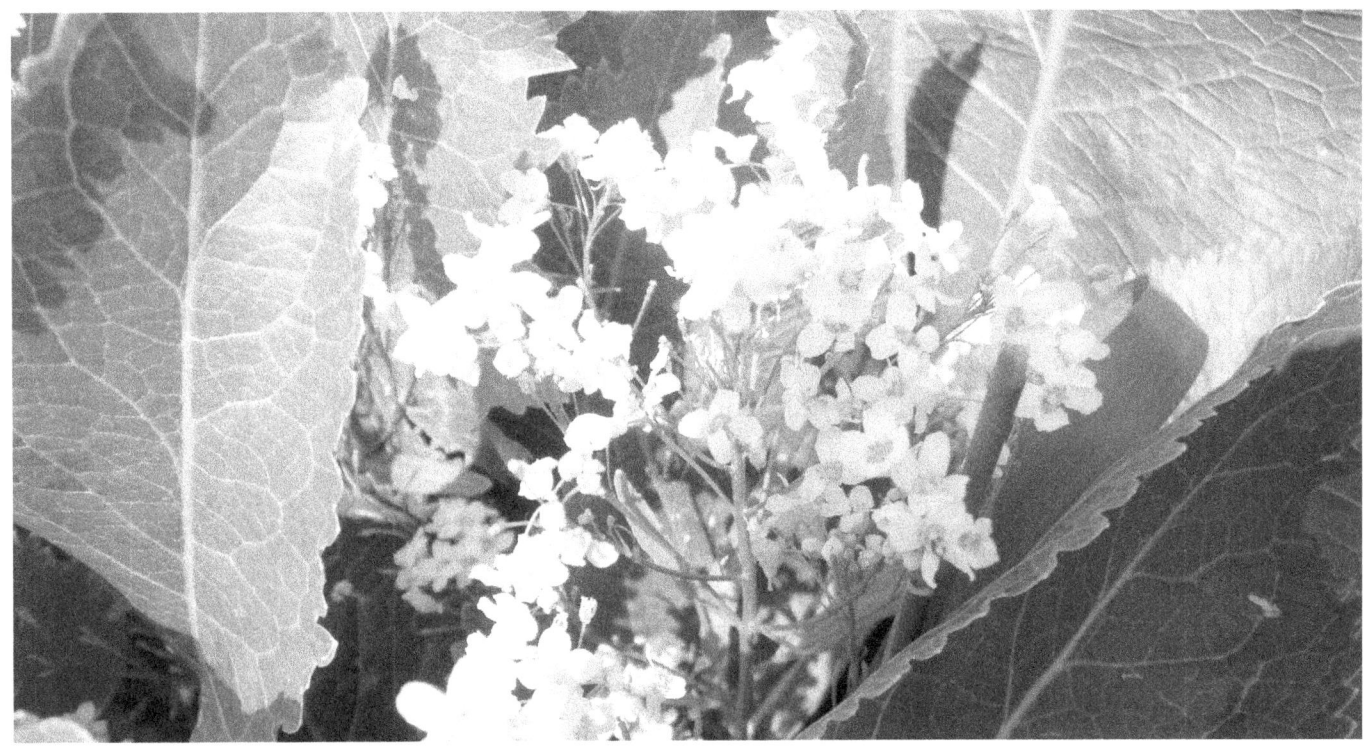

HORSERADISH LEAVES AND FLOWERS

BOTANICA POETICA

Here's an herb with history
Can make a wicked spirit flee
The Middle Ages sang its praise
In the Renaissance, 'twas the craze
A precious herb with virtues dear
Can soul and body make more clear
Wood Betony, a leafy mint
On sandy slopes it makes its print
A tonic for the nervous system
Can relax and bring sedation
Use for headache and for sprain
Ailments where there's nerve like pain
Apply to joints and ulceration
A poultice for the situation
Hysteria and neuralgic grief
Will calm the nerves and bring relief
It's supportive if you're frail
Boosts your strength if it should fail
If you're quitting an addiction
Need more grounding, fact not fiction
Try this tincture or the tea
There might be magic in the leaf!

SYLVIA CHATROUX MD

HORSERADISH
(*Armoracia rusticana* Gaertn. B Mey & Scherb)
(*A. lapathifolia* Gilib.) not accepted
(*Cochlearia armoracia* L.) not accepted
(*Nasturtium armoracia* [L.] Fr.) not accepted
(*Rorippa rusticana* [L.] Hitch.) not accepted
PARTS USED- roots, leaves

Nasturtium is from the Latin words **NASUS** and **TORTUS**, meaning a sharp smell that wrinkles the nose.

Armoracia is Latin for **AREMORICA**, from the ancient Armorica (Brittany) where the plant was once cultivated. It may be from **AR**, near, and **MOR**, the sea, due to its favourite location. Rusticana comes from the root word meaning rustic, or of the country.

Cochlearia is from **COCHLEARE**, an old fashioned spoon leaves are supposed to look like. Or were used like! The Germans called it Sea Radish, or **MEERRETTICH**. This became, through mis-translation, the English Mahre, an old horse, then Mare Radish, to finally, Horse Radish.

Apollo was said told by the Oracle at Delphi that horseradish was worth its weight in gold. Beet was considered worthy of silver, and the lowly Radish, only lead.

Horseradish is an English name suggesting coarse radish to differentiate it from edible radish. Horse was often used in this manner, such as Horse Mint, Horse Chestnut, etc. Some authors suggest it derives from using horses to stomp on and tenderize before grating. This is a bit of a stretch.

In England of the 1500s, it was known as Red Cole, or *Raphanus rusticanus*.

Horseradish is both naturalized and planted with deliberation throughout the Canadian prairies. It is thought to originate from southern Russia and Ukraine. The ancient Slavic name **CHREN** and derivations, are common throughout Europe.

It will produce numerous small white flowers, and round seedpods that usually do not produce seed, at least in my own experience around northern Alberta.

The lack of seed production, or sterility, is indirectly related, some believe, to eating the leaves three times daily to induce an abortion.

Horseradish is a perennial, cultivated for its hot, peppery root. Commercially in the United States, it is grown as an annual or biennial, as older roots become woody.

Root division every 2-3 years helps invigorate the crop. Americans consume around 6,000,000 gallons of horseradish sauce annually, enough to generously season sandwiches to circle the planet twelve times. The city of Collinsville, Illinois hosts an annual International Horseradish Festival to solidify their claim as horseradish capital of the world. I might have to add that to my bucket list!

Horseradish requires cool weather to bring out its pungent best, something the prairies can offer much of the year.

Horseradish has become the condiment of choice with prime rib, and is often used to adulterate wasabi, the hot green condiment served in Japanese restaurants.

In fact, Sakai Spice of Lethbridge, Alberta is a subsidiary of Arashiya Shiro. They process "Wasabi" from horseradish and yellow mustard for the Japanese export market. True Japanese Upland Horseradish (*Wasabia japonica/Entrema wasabi*) is a perennial that grows naturally by streams and has a bright green root. It will grow on coastal BC under very controlled conditions. Real wasabi is served in only the best sushi restaurants. The green color in "fake" wasabi comes from addition of spinach, or spirulina powder.

Horseradish is one of the five bitter herbs eaten during Hebrew Passover.

It first appeared in the Passover *seder* as *maror* in the 13th century as Jews migrated north and east into colder climates. The other four, for the curious, are coriander, horehound, lettuce, and nettles.

The Germans and Slavs were amongst the first people to grate the root for sauces and pickles.

The Germans love their horseradish, and have countless recipes for various sauces including lemon, beer, bread, whipped cream and sour green apples.

The expression **STARIY KHREN**, or "old horseradish" denotes a mean old man, while **KHRENOVO** "feelinghorseradishy" means that life could be better.

Early Ukrainian settlers to Alberta decocted two pounds of root in a gallon of water for one hour. One cup was taken daily for gallbladder pain or stones until improvement.

In Norway, a sauce called **PEPPERROTSAUS** is served with cold salmon. The Danes freeze creamed horseradish and serve it like sherbet.

A favorite Polish condiment called **CHRZAN** is grated beets and horseradish, served with ham. Horseradish soup is a popular Christmas day lunch in that country.

The Greeks wrote of *Raphnos agrios*, or wild radish as a medicinal plant, and this may well have been horseradish.

During the middle ages, the fresh root became popularized for treating rheumatism, gout, asthma, bronchitis, facial neuralgia and sciatica. Like mustard, the plant contains oils that irritate and act as a rubefacient; a poultice of the fresh root can be used as a plaster.

When infused in wine, it was used for its diaphoretic and stimulating action, while in cider, it is used for diuretic and diaphoretic activity, especially in cases of dropsy. If no cider is available, you can always decoct the fresh root with some juniper berries, in a good natural beer. In Russia, **HREN** is made into a decoction with honey for liver detoxification.

Horseradish ale was a popular drink in England, and elsewhere, before hops were introduced. Horseradish ale is mentioned, by Samuel Pepys in his diary.

In Finland, the sex of an unborn baby was determined by placing a piece of root under each of the couple's pillows. If the husband's turned black first, then the expected child was a boy and vice-versa.

The leaves were used to treat nettle stings. The fresh, young leaves have a mild pleasant taste that goes well in a sandwich, or salad, some say especially with smoked mackerel. When the new shoots are freshly steamed, they resemble watercress, and combine well with nettles as a springtime treat. The large leaves are edible when cooked. They taste a bit like cabbage, but are more bitter and pungent.

Large amounts are abortifacient, however, and in parts of England, three leaves a day for an extended time were used to induce miscarriage.

Herbalists of 17th century England, including William Coles, considered horseradish effective for parasites, especially in children. Syrups are still widely used for coughs and sore throats.

In Poland, juice from the fresh root was added to milk in summer to prevent souring too quickly. The large, waxy leaves were used to wrap and preserve butter longer.

Dr. Vogel tells a story about the preservative effects of horseradish, in which he placed one teaspoon of grated root into a litre bottle of freshly made apple juice. This was sealed with a second teaspoon, wrapped in gauze, to act as a stopper. This juice will keep for about a year without fermentation, due to the herb's inhibition of yeast growth.

Various native tribes took quick advantage of the introduced root, especially the Cherokee, who used it for gravel, rheumatism, asthma, colds and obstructed menses. They used infusions as a gargle for sore throats, and to increase appetite and aid digestion.

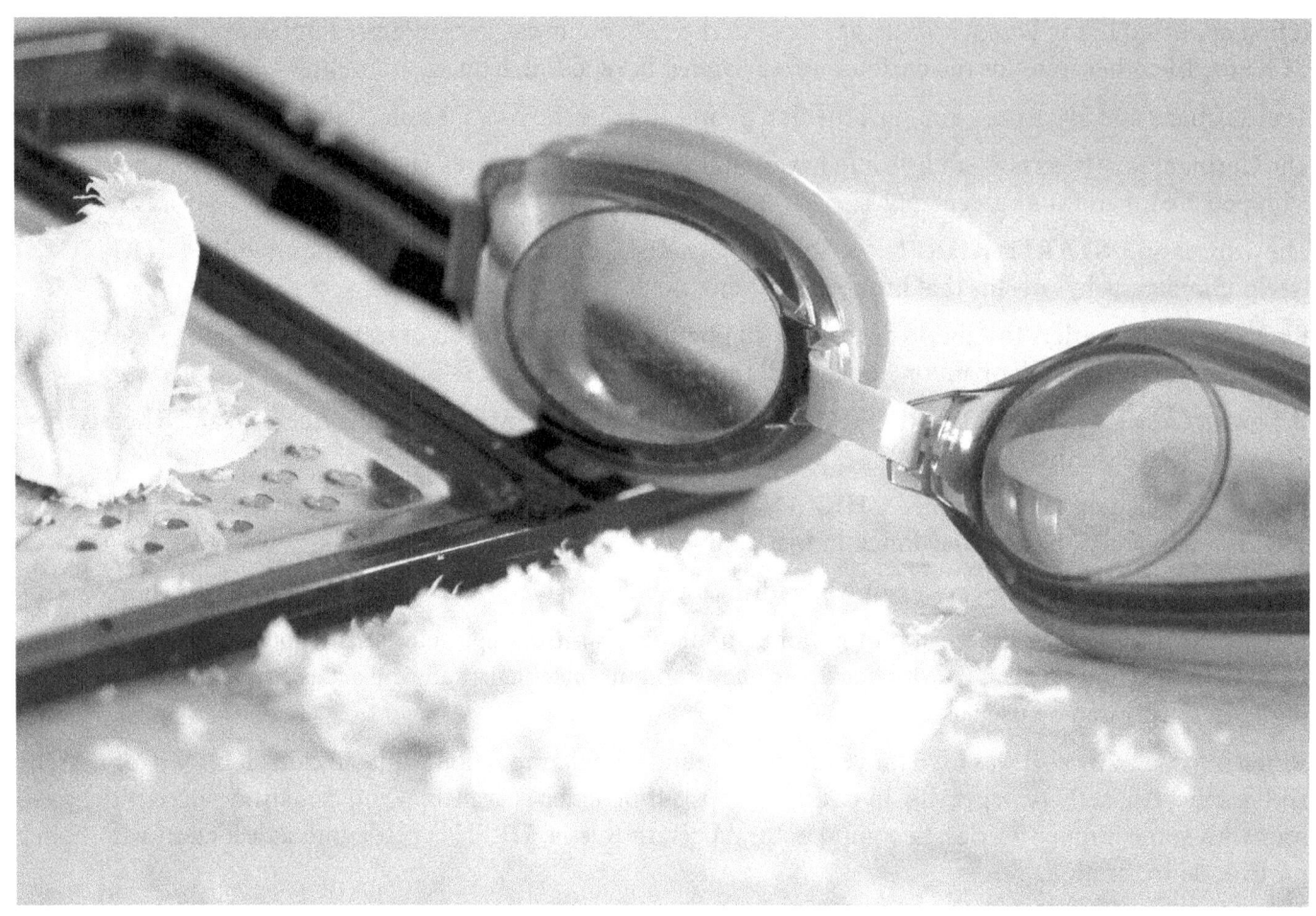

FRESH GRATED HORSERADISH IS VERY POTENT

The Delaware used leaf poultices to relieve neuralgia pain, while the Mohegan used the same for tooth pain.

The Iroquois used the plant for diabetes, in an unspecified manner.

The root can be quite effective in treating hypothermia. Take 2-4 fresh roots, chop into smaller pieces and juice. Combine with apple cider vinegar and a little salt, and take one half teaspoon three times daily between meals.

The wilted leaves make a poultice for facial neuralgia, and placed in the bottom of shoes relieve hot, tired feet.

Veterinarians mix the grated root, or leaf with wheat bran as a worm or kidney treatment for livestock. Chop and add to dog food to dispel worms and improve body tone.

In Germany, Walther Schoenenberger, famous for his fresh plant juices, found the woody root of horseradish does not lend itself to liquefying. He solved the problem by producing a distillate (see below).

The fresh root product will stay fresh for months in a refrigerator. Distillate of horseradish exerts a strong effect on all mucous membranes and general body metabolism.

Over time, it strengthens the peristaltic action of the intestine, relieving gas and flatulence. The distillate is used externally for rheumatism, rubbed directly onto the affected area as a rubefacient.

It stimulates and dilates the capillary system, creating better blood and lymph circulation.

The root is best harvested after the first frost. Some of the most potent root is produced commercially near Tuli Lakes, California, where there is frost every month of the year.

It is said to protect potatoes from the Colorado beetle when planted at the corners of the field. Root infusions can be sprayed on apple trees to avoid brown rot, or *Monilia*. The fall root extract is toxic to mosquito larvae, while the leaf powder kills tick larvae in 18 minutes.

Allyl isothiocynate from horseradish discourages pest infestation of food crops including grain, and may be a healthy alternative to methyl bromide and phosphine. Wu et al, *Pest Manage Sci* 2009 65:9.

Horseradish extracts are used in hair tonics to help promote hair growth.

Horseradish peroxidase enzyme has important industrial application. Work by Xu and Bhandari at Kansas State University found phenols, which are soil and groundwater pollutants, can be polymerized by the enzyme, and then bound to soil or water aquifer solids. This polymerization and binding of phenols can produce large reductions in contaminant bioavailability, due to the low water solubility of the product.

This could lead to a whole new approach to cleaning up contaminated soils and water systems. Full study is available in *J Agric Food Chem* 2003 51.

Horseradish hairy root cultures phyto-remediate 100% of acetominophen, in just 8 days. Kotyza et al, *Int J Phytoremed* 2010 12:3.

About 11 million kilograms of root are processed, for food, annually in the USA.

MEDICINAL

CONSTITUENTS- root- various coumarins (aesculetin and scopoletin) caffeic and hydroxycinnamic acid, sinigrin, sulphur glycoside, myrosin, asparagin, peroxidase enzymes, resin, essential oil, arginin, oxydase, peroxydase enzymes, starch, sugars, thiocyanate, allyl and 2-phenethyl-isothiocyanate, 5-phenylpentyl isothiocyanate, plastoquinone-9, 6-0-acyl-beta-D-glucosyl-beta-sitosterol, 1,2-dilinolenoyl-syl-glycerol, vitamins B, C (81 mg/100g) and K (564 mg/100 g) and minerals including iodine, and calcium (140 mg/100 g); organic germanium.
leaf- quercitin, kaempferol, 3-0-beta-D-glucoside of kaempferol and quercitin, and 3-0-beta-D-xyloside of kaempferol and quercitin, caffeic and hydroxycinnamic acid

Horseradish root is useful in cases of sluggish circulation, with damp mucous and phlegmatic conditions. As well, it is both anodyne (pain relieving) and antiseptic, meaning it will fight infections and inflammation.

In cases of obstructed or difficult urination, horseradish root acts as an effective diuretic and Gram positive and negative bactericide. Work by Schindler et al, *Arzneim Forsch* 1961 10 found horseradish roots useful in urinary tract infections.

The mustard oils, responsible for the roots activity, are formed by fermentation of mustard oil glycosides. These are rapidly absorbed into the small intestine and excreted as mercapturic acid via the kidneys after binding with glutathione.

Horseradish has been used to relieve pain, expel afterbirth, anthelmintic and diuretic. It is antiseptic and has stimulating digestive power, similar to radish seed, in clearing microbial toxicosis, fermentation and putrefaction of the intestinal tract.

Horseradish extracts show anti-cholinesterase activity. Leiner et al, *J Physio* 1980 305 171-95.

Allyl isothiocyanate (ITC) plays a role in both chemoprevention and in the suppression of tumour growth. An organically-bound cyanide, it is non-toxic to all cells, save cancer cells. Peroxidase is an enzyme that reverses cell degeneration and is a potent anti-cancer compound. Studies show this enzyme controls the growth of breast and bladder cancer cell lines. ITC shows strong affinity for colon and lung cancer cells.

The related 5-phenylpentyl isothiocyanate is a significant anti-spasmodic with studies on rat distal colon suggesting it is 100 times more potent than papaverine. It is cytotoxic to HeLa cancer cell lines. Dekic MS et al, *Food Chem* 2017 232: 329-339.

Horseradish contains ten fold higher amounts of glucosinolates than broccoli.

Horseradish is a circulatory stimulant with warming effect, useful for feeble or low circulation, low blood pressure, hypothermia, frostbite and chilblains. In large amounts, it will induce perspiration, and should not be given to those already suffering night sweats.

It is very stimulating and invigorating for lack of stomach acids in the elderly, sometimes working better than bitters when there is an element of chill. Horseradish invigorates the liver, spleen and pancreas, but is contraindicated in low thyroid function.

This knowledge can be put to good use in treating hyperthyroidism, combining well with bugleweed, lemon balm and corn silk.

It is useful in both high and low blood sugar, due to its restorative effect on the pancreas.

Use for dropsy following fevers or when albuminaria is present, combining well with juniper berries. It is a potent herbal diuretic, sometimes combined with mustard seed either in decoction or white wine.

For respiratory hoarseness combine one teaspoon of the fresh juice in honey as a cough syrup. In advanced cases of bronchitis and asthma with hyper-secretion and dilatation of the bronchial tubes, it is most useful. Other herbs, like pine needle and angelica root perform similar function as warming expectorants.

For coughs, neuritis or rheumatic joints use the freshly grated root as a counter-irritant and rubefacient, being careful not to burn or blister the skin.

A slice of fresh root applied on boils, quickly resolves them. Some individuals have found relief from the pain and itch of poison ivy using grated horseradish and lard compresses.

The grated root helps relieve chilblains, and in Russia is applied to calves of both legs for insomnia.

For the onset of the common cold, flu or fever, take one cup of horseradish root tea every two to three hours.

It combines well with echinacea in both liquid and powdered capsules forms. Horseradish has been shown both *in vitro* and *in vivo* to reduce the severity of the influenza virus. Esanu et al, *Virologie* 1985 36:2.

When there are purulent wounds, use the cooled decoction of the roots as a frequent lotion. The root has bacteriostatic action, especially against gram-negative bacteria, in lung and urinary infections. Kienholz et al, *Arnzeim Forsch* 1961:10.

The crushed root volatiles inhibit *E. coli* and *Mycobacterium tuberculosis* var. *hominis*, associated with human tuberculosis.

Horseradish is grown to extract the enzyme peroxidase, used for the diagnosis of the AIDS virus. It is used for some chemical tests for blood glucose and cholesterol and as a molecular probe in joint disorders. It is used to see if hormone levels in the body are influenced by environmental toxins, and chemicals.

It takes several tons of roots to produce one kilo of peroxidase worth $75,000. At the present time, a bio-processing plant in Winnipeg is purifying this product.

The University of Manitoba has experimented with horseradish oil on regular butcher's paper between ground beef patties; killing almost all the *E. coli* 0157:H7 bacteria. Other work at the *Department of Food Science* is a whey film with natural additives that kills salmonella and other bacteria associated with chicken and fish.

Horseradish has been used for centuries for its digestive aid and relieving flatulence and bloating associated with incomplete digestion.

Dr. William Mitchell, the late, naturopathic physician, teacher and former student of Dr. Bastyr, used horseradish in an anti-depressive formula, along with black cohosh, licorice root and other herbs.

The activating enzymes (isothiocyanates) play a key role in inhibiting certain types of carcinogens, known to mutate healthy cells into cancers.

Vinegar of the freshly grated root can be used externally for acne. According to Maria Treben, the horseradish takes away the sharpness of vinegar, and the vinegar the hotness of the root, to make it easily tolerated by the facial skin.

For cosmetic purpose, the root is best soaked one part to four in fresh milk for one hour.

Weiss mentioned that horseradish is one of the most powerful anti-bacterial herbs against lung, skin and bladder infections.

Horseradish root contains several compounds that inhibit COX-1 enzymes, and the proliferation of colon and lung cancer cells. Weil et al, *J Ag Food Chem* 2005 53.

Research at MIT shows horseradish components may be helpful in replaced current microbial treatment to remove toxic pollutants such as amines and phenols, and make them insoluble. A combination of horseradish juice and hydrogen peroxide is used to solidify deadly chemicals such as PCBs (polychlorinated biphenyls).

Taken internally, about 2 tablespoons of each in water, it forms a long chain that is eliminated via the bowels. This is based on work of Alexander Kilbanov who discovered this combination in the 1980s.

Internally, water extracts of horseradish protect human lymphocytes against oxidative damage caused by hydrogen peroxide. Gafrikova M et al, *Molecules* 2014 19:3.

A popular herbal combination in Germany containing horseradish and nasturium is called Angocin Anti-Infekt N.

Several studies suggest its benefit in bronchitis, ear infections, *E. coli* and *Staphylococcus aureus* illness of the intestine, Hemophilus flu in children under five, pneumonia, sinusitis, strep throat, and other *Streptococcus pyogenes* illness, as well as cellulitis, impetigo and scarlet fever, and urinary tract infections.

One study involving 858 children and teenagers in 65 centers compared the herbal combination to an antibiotic in treatment of bronchitis and urinary tract infections. It proved very effective.

Another study compared it to antibiotics in 536 people with sinusitis, 634 with bronchitis and 479 with urinary tract infections (UTIs). Again it showed the natural product worked just as well as the drug.

It may help prevent infection. A study of 219 women and men with UTIs began with all patients symptom free and divided into a dose daily or placebo for three months. A reduction of 50% urinary tract infections was observed over control.

Horseradish modulates adaptive response in human lymphocytes induced by zeocin, an antibiotic. Adding the herb decreased DNA damage by drug by more than 50%. Hudecova A et al. *Neoplasma* 2012 59:1.

Horseradish contains organic germanium, which confers significant anti-cancer protection. Natural germanium, also known as germanium sesquioxide, has been shown to induce interferon gamma, enhance natural killer cell activity, inhibit tumour and metastatic growth, and is non-toxic.

Considerable misinformation in a 1987 scientific paper has led to confusion and dis-interest in this very promising element. One recent case of terminal lung cancer treated successfully with 7 grams daily of organic germanium showed complete remission in 42 months. Mainwaring et al, *Chest* 2000 117. See *Ganoderma applanatum* in my book *The Fungal Pharmacy: The Complete Guide to Medicinal Mushrooms and Lichens of North America*.

The dried leaves can be poulticed after soaking in warm water and inserted vaginally for itching, odors or vaginitis associated with poor pelvic circulation.

CAUTION- When injections of peroxidase were given to cats, it raised their blood pressure. Please do not experiment with your pet cat.

Avoid horseradish if you are taking cholinergic drugs like Mestinon, Prostigmin or Urecholine; or if you suffer from low thyroid function. Like other mustard family members, thiocyanate and isothiocyanate are goitergens that interfere with thyroid hormone production and utilization.

NOTE- Tests for fecal blood use the guaiac slide test, in which alpha guaiaconic acid turns blue when exposed to blood. Horseradish and other mustard family plants may produce peroxidase in stool and give false positive. Use a three-day washout before tests to prevent mis-diagnosis. Diabetic tests using Clinistix may false positive.

HOMEOPATHY

Cochlearia armoracia-Aromoracia sativa (Horseradish) specifically affects the frontal bone and sinus, as well as salivary glands.

It is useful when thinking is difficult, or there is anxiety and the patient is driven to despair by pain.

A pressing, boring pain, as if the frontal bone would fall out is experienced. At times, a violent headache with vomiting can occur, or impaired hearing.

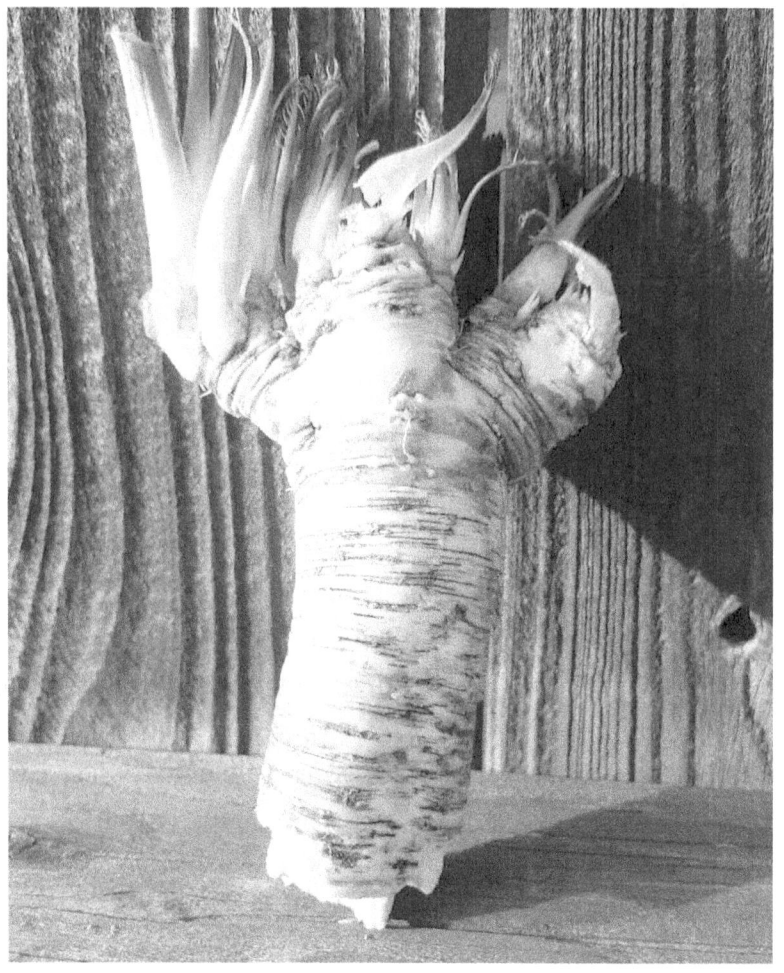

FRESHLY HARVESTED ROOT

The eyes are sore and scrofulous, with inflammation, bleariness and cataract formation. The eyes also tear easily and continually.

In the stomach, there is pain toward the back, with pressure on the dorsal vertebrae. Belching and cramping with violent cramps from the stomach goes through the back and down the sacrum.

The lungs have a dry, hacking laryngeal cough, worse lying down and in the evening. Throat is hoarse, with mucus asthma, and edema of lungs.

There is a cutting, burning pain before during and after frequent urination.

DOSE- First to third attenuation. The mother tincture is prepared from the whole fresh plant including root while in flower.

ESSENTIAL OIL

Distillation of the root yields about 0.5% of a volatile oil that is very hot and pungent.

It contains sinigrin, similar to that in white mustard. In the presence of water and the influence of peroxidase, this produces allyl mustard oil.

A study by Kienholz et al, *Arzneim Forsch* 1961:10 found that at levels attainable in human urine after taking the essential oil, it was shown to kill bacteria that cause urinary tract infections.

It helps control chalkbrood disease caused by *Ascosphaera apis*. Kloucek P et al, *Nat Prod Commun* 2012 7(2).

FLOWER ESSENCES

Horseradish flower essence wakens people out of their doldrums. There may be boredom, lethargy, depression or hysteria. Alertness and clarity of thought develop. Use in shock: creates mental clarity.   **PEGASUS**

Horseradish flower essence is useful in situations where a person feels "stuck", especially when the idea of moving forward evokes a fear that results in inertia.   **UNKNOWN**

In some cases, obsessive thinking patterns can develop, or a depression sets in where one feels separated from one's true self or from one's real mission and goals in life. Children who tend to be timid and lack confidence can benefit from this essence.

Use the essence for animals who become depressed and inactive due to owners feeling or expressing "bad temper" during stressful times. It is helpful for animals who tend to have poor circulation, slow digestion or colds.   **DALTON**

PERSONALITY TRAITS

As Horse Chestnut typifies the Germanic nature, Horseradish may be said to typify the British. This person picture is one of leathery and inactive stomach linings, maybe from too much alcohol.

Think of the bygone Victorian era and you have a picture of Horseradish; pragmatic, dogmatic, and pragmatic were the codes of behaviour, with rigid public moral principles, and Lord-knows-what private repressions and inhibitions. Emotions were out! To cry (even to laugh at the wrong moment!) were social disasters indicative of "poor breeding". Stiff upper lips were part of the required facial expression. Grimness of visage matched rigidity of principles and stereotyped behaviour.

"The British love their dogs and train their children", was a Shavian comment.

This narrow rigid cod of behaviour and emotional deprivation produced the inescapable effect of all life's experiences in the body as well as in the mind.

Its controlled attitudes led not only to suppression of the emotions, but to suppression of those organs and systems related to emotional "feeding".

A life deprived of an emotional range of experience, will eventually cause hypo-function of body assimilation systems.

Paucity of emotional feeding, plus unimaginative, overcooked, physical feeding produce in them the grayish eyed person, whose grim philosophy "Life wasn't meant to be easy!", is reflected in hypo-activity of the gastro-intestinal tract.

The diets of there people, like their lives, become plainer and plainer.

The positive Horseradish person knows that emotional stimulation and digestive stimulation run hand in hand.

Those who are comfortable to laugh, cry, and feel, need no "sauce" to digest their raw foods, or their fresh fruit. Life's more raw experiences are well digested too, with active and positive elimination of these from the character as well as from the bowels.   **DOROTHY HALL**

RECIPES

TINCTURE- 6-12 drops. Fresh root tincture is made with 1:3 at 60% alcohol.

FRESH JUICE- One tbsp 2-3 times daily. A slice of the fresh root can be gently sucked for sinus congestion and colds.

KIDNEY TEA- Take one ounce of fresh horseradish root, one-half oz. of crushed mustard seed, and one pint of boiling water. Soak for 4 hours, and strain. Take 3 Tablespoons three times daily.

CAUTION- Horseradish should be avoided by those with stomach, or duodenal ulcers, severe kidney disease, or hypothyroidism. It is speculated that antacids may be antagonized.

SAUCE- There are numerous versions of horseradish sauce. But basically, take the root, wash it, and let it dry. Grate three tablespoons of root and add one quarter teaspoon mustard powder and three tablespoons of thick cream. Mix well.

Or mix the grated root with double the amount of whipped cream and then frozen for a condiment with cold salmon.

Or, you can grate the roots and add just enough white wine vinegar to cover, salt and little honey. Use as desired. Never store in silver, which blackens the sauce.

A good ratio is for every cup of grated root add one half cup vinegar and ¼ tsp salt. Never serve in silver.

VINEGAR- add one ounce of freshly grated root to one pint of wine vinegar. Use 1-2 teaspoons in water for sinusitis, catarrh, poor circulation or as a male tonic.

Cider vinegar causes discoloration. The addition of cream extended life to several months rather than days. Refrigeration also helps.

THROAT SYRUP- Grated horseradish, honey and water make an acceptable remedy for throat soreness and hoarseness. It combines well with elecampane, licorice root or mallow.

An un-cooked syrup can be made by covering fresh root with double the amount of honey. After one week syrup will form on top, but leave it for up to one month.

Use one teaspoon three times daily for bronchitis, sore throat, anemia, arthritis and liver deficiency.

SKIN LOTION- for acne, blemishes, discoloration of any type. Take four ounces of freshly scraped horseradish root, four ounces of vegetable glycerine and combine in one quart of buttermilk. Leave overnight, shake well, and strain. Bottle and store cold.

After washing face, apply lotion and when tingling wipe off and go to bed. Repeat as needed.

POULTICE- Horseradish root can be finely grated and applied as a counter-irritant poultice for colds, sinusitis, headaches, strained muscles, and neuralgia. Like mustard, care must be taken to avoid blistering skin.

For sinusitis, the poultice is applied to the upper neck region for 2-5 minutes. After removing, wipe with vegetable oil.

Horseradish poultices can also be useful in chronic cystitis, indwelling catheters, and irritable bladder.

PROPAGATION- An efficient method for production of plantlets from Horseradish hairy root was developed and presented fully in the *Journal of Fermentation and Bioengineering* 1995 79:5. It shows how hairy root fragments were obtained by fragmentation in a blender after growth. Thirty seconds gave the best results, and with the addition of NAA at one milligram per litre prior to blending, also resulted in the highest number of plantlets.

A more traditional transplant procedure is a small piece of plant root with a crown bud, dug up and replanted in fall.

Roots increase in diameter more than depth. High quality market roots come from small lateral roots gathered when the plant crown is lifted, and then replanted. Lifting is best when leaves are ten inches long and again in six weeks.

HARVESTING- Dig up in fall after leaves have died down. On a large scale, use a potato digger with small modification. Some root pieces are left behind, so there is no need to replant. Large root need to be cut before they dry rock hard. Temperatures for drying should not exceed 35 degrees Celsius.

ABOUT THE AUTHOR

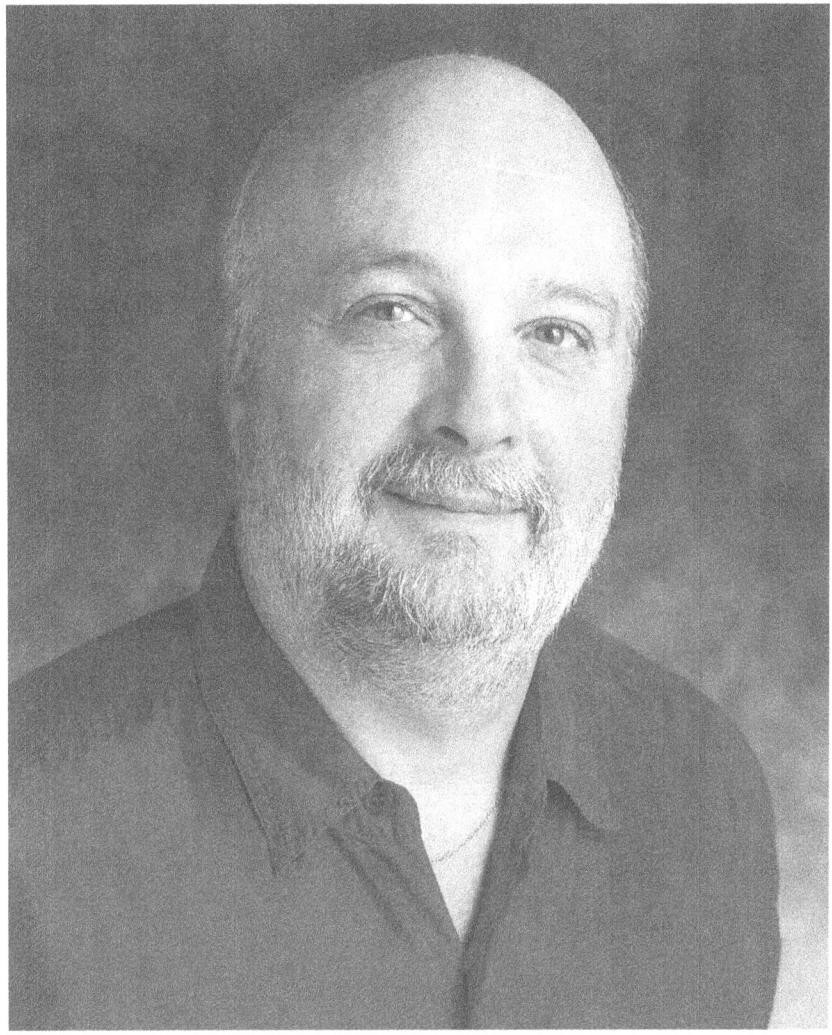

Robert Dale Rogers has been an herbalist for over forty-five years. He has a Bachelor of Science from the University of Alberta, where he is an assistant clinical professor in Family Medicine. He teaches plant medicine, including herbology and flower essences in the Earth Spirit Medicine Program at the Northern Star College of Mystical Studies in Edmonton, Alberta, Canada.

Robert is past chair of the Alberta Natural Health Agricultural Network and Community Health Council of Capital Health. He is a Fellow of the International College of Nutrition, past chair of the medicinal mushroom committee of the North American Mycological Association and on the editorial board of the International Journal of Medicinal Mushrooms. He writes occasional article for Fungi magazine.

Robert co-hosts The Alberta Herb Gathering held every second year (www.albertaherbgathering.com)

He lives on Millcreek Ravine in Edmonton with his beautiful and talented wife, Laurie Szott–Rogers and out of control cat Ceres.

You can email him at scents@telusplanet.net
or visit
www.selfhealdistributing.com

BIBLIOGRAPHY

Abbe, Elfriede, *The Fern Herbal,* Cornell University Press, Ithaca, 1981

Acorn, J. Bugs of Alberta, Lone Pine Publishing, Edmonton, AB, 2000.

Adams, J. *Les Plantes Medicinales.* Bulletin 23, Agriculture Canada. 1916

Adams, Jean. *Insect Potpourri, Adventures in Entomology.* Sandhill Crane Press, FL. 1992

Aggarwal, Bharat. Healing Spices. Sterling Pub. New York 2011.

Albert-Puleo, Michael. *Economic Botany, 32, Jan-Mar, 1978.*

Allaby, Michael. *Temperate Forests.* Facts on File. New York. 1999.

Allen, D & Hatfield, G. *Medicinal Plants in Folk Tradition.* Timber Press, Portland. 2004

Allen,E, Morrison,D, &Wallis,G. *Common Tree Diseases of B.C. Canada Forest Service,* '96

Allende, Isabel. *Aphrodite- A Memoir of the Senses.* Harper Flamingo. New York. 1998.

Alstat, Ed. *Electic Dispensatory of Botanical Therapeutics.* Ecl Med. Oregon. 1989.

Anderson, Anne, *Some Native Herbal Remedies,* Pub 8A, Devonian Botanical Gardens 1980

_____*Plants in Cree.* Duval House Pub. Edmonton AB 2000.

Anderson, C.&Tischer,T. *Poinsettias, the December Flower,* Waters Edge Press, CA, 1997

Andoh, Anthony. *The Science & Romance of Selected Herbs used in Medicine and Religious Ceremony.* North Scale Institute. San Francisco. 1986.

Andre, Alestine & Fehr, Alan. *Gwich'in Ethnobotany.* Gwich'in Social and Cultural Institute, Box 46, Tsiigehtchie, NWT, X0E 0B0, fax 1867-953-3820.

Andrews, Tamra. Nectar and Ambrosia. ABC-CLIO Box 1911 Santa Barbara CA. 2000.

Andrews, Ted. *Animal Speak- The Spiritual and Magical Powers,* Llewellyn. Minn. 1996.

_____*Animal Wise,* DragonHawk, Jackson, TN, 1999.

Antol, Marie. *The Incredible Secrets of Mustard.* Avery Pub. New York. 1999.

Aronson J K Ed. Meyler's Side Effects of Herbal Medicines. Elsevier Amsterdam. 2009.

Arrowsmith, Nancy. Essential Herbal Wisdom. Llewellyn Pub. Woodbury, Minn. 2009.

Arsdall, Anne Van. *Medieval Herbal Remedies.* Routledge, New York. 2002.

Arvigo & Balick, *Rainforest Remedies,* Lotus Press, Twin Lakes, WI. 1993

Arvigo & Epstein. *Rainforest Home Remedies,* Harper SanFrancisco, 2001.

Assiniwi, Bernard. *La Medecine des Indiens d' Amerique,* Guerin Literature, 1988

Atal C.K. & Kapur B. *Cultivation and Utilization of Medicinal Plants,* Jammu-Tawi, 1982

Attenborough, David. *The Private Life of Plants.* Princeton U Press. Princeton NJ 1995.

Ausubel, K. *Seeds of Change The Living Treasure.* HarperSanFrancisco, 1994.

Aversano, Laura. *The Divine Nature of Plants.* Swan•Raven & Co. Columbus, NC, 2002.

Ayensu, Edward,S. *Medicinal Plants of the West Indies,* Reference Publications, 1981

Baïracli Levy, Juliette *Herbal Handbook for Farm and Stable,* Faber&Faber, London, 1952

Baker, Phil. The Dedalus Book of Absinthe. Dedalus 2001.

Barl, Branka et al, *Saskatchewan Herb Database,* U. of Sask. Saskatoon, 1996.

Barlow, Max. *From the Shepherd's Purse.* 1990

Barnes J, Anderson L, &Phillipson J. *Herbal Medicines, A guide for healthcare professionals.* Pharmaceutical Press, London, 2002.

Barnett, Robert A. *Tonics,* Harper Collins, New York, N.Y. 1997

Bartram, Thomas. *Bartram's Encyl. of Herbal Medicine,* Robinson Pub. London, 1998.

Bascom, Angella. *Incorporating Herbal Medicine into Clinical Practice.* F. Davis Co. 2002

Beals, Katherine, M. *Flower Lore and Legend,* Henry Holt, 1917

Beers, Susan-Jane. *Jamu The ancient Indonesian Art of Herbal Healing,* Periplus, 2001.

Belcourt, Christi. Medicines to Help Us. Gabriel Dumont Instit. Saskatoon, SK 2007.

Béliveau, R & Gingras,D. *Foods That Fight Cancer.* McClelland & Stewart Toronto. 2006.

Belsinger S & Dille C. *Cooking with Herbs.* CBI- Van Nostrand Reinhold, N.Y. 1984.

Benjamin, D.R. *Mushrooms: Poisons and Panaceas.* WH Freeman, San Francisco, 1995.

Bennet, Doug & Tiner, Tim. *Up North.* Reed Books Canada. Markham, Ont. 1993.

_____*Up North Again.* McClelland and Stewart. Toronto, 1997.

Bennet, J & Rowley S. *Uqalurait An Oral History of Nunavut.* McGill Queens, Mont. 2004

Benyus, Janine. *Biomimicry Innovation Inspired by Nature.* William Morrow. 1997.

Berenbaum,May R. *Buzzwords, A Scientists Muses on Sex, Bugs and Rock N Roll,* Joseph Henry Press, Washington, D.C. 2000.

_____*Bugs in the System.* Helix Books, Addison-Wesley Pub. 1995.

Beresford-Kroeger, Diana. The Global Forest. Viking Penguin. 2010.

_____Arboretum Borealis. U Michigan Press. 2010.

Berliocchi,Luigi. *The Orchid in Lore and Legend.* Timber Press, Portland Oregon, 2000.

Berlund B & Bolsby C. *The Edible Wild* Pagurian Press, Toronto, Ont. 1971.

Berkowsky, Bruce. *Mount Julius Flower Remedies. Mt. Vernon Washington, 1986*

Bermejo, J & Leon,J. *Neglected Crops-1492 ...* FAO Series 26, United Nations, Rome, 1994.

Bernhardt, P. *The Rose's Kiss, A Natural History of Flowers* . Island Press, Covelo CA 1999

Bianchi, Ivo. *Geriatrics and Homotoxicology.* Aurelia-Verlag GmbH, Baden Baden, 1994.

Bianchini, F. *The Complete Book of Health Plants.* Crescent Books, New York, 1975.

Biship, Carol. *The Book of Home Remedies &Herbal Cures,* Jonathan-James, Toronto, 1979.

Bisset, Norman G. *Herbal Drugs and Phytopharmaceuticals.* 2nd Ed. CRC Press, 2001.

Blackburn, Thomas. *December's Child: A Book of Chumash Oral Narratives* , U of California Press, Berkeley, 1975.

Blanchan, Neltje. *Nature's Garden.* Doubleday, Page&Co. New York, 1900.

Bland, John. *Forests of Liliput.* Prentice Hall, Englewood Cliffs, New Jersey, 1971.

Bliss, Anne. *Rocky Mountain Dye Plants.* Juniper House, Boulder, Colorado, 1976

Blouin, Glen. *Weeds of the Woods.* Goose Lane, Fredericton, New Brunswick 1992.

_____*An Eclectic Guide to Trees, east of the Rockies.* Boston Mills, 2001.

Boas, F. *Ethnology of the Kwakiutl.* Bureau of Am. Ethnology, 35th annual report, 1921.

Boericke, Wm. *Materia Medica with Repetory.* B. Jain Publishers. 1976

Boik, John. *Natural Compunds in Cancer Therapy.* Oregon Med Press, Princeton,Minn 2001

Boland, Bridget. *Gardener's Magic &Other Old Wives' Lore.* The Bodley Head, London, 77.

Bolton, Brett L. *The Secret Powers of Plants.* Berkley Pub Co. New York. 1974.

Bolton, J.L. *Alfalfa, Botany, Cultivation &Utilization.* Interscience Pub, New York, 1962.

Bone, Kerry. *A Clinical Guide to Blending Liquid Herbs.* Churchill Livingstone. 2003

Borrel, Marie. *Healing Plants.* Cassell & Co. Wellington House, London. 2001.

Bouchardon, Patrice. *The Healing Energies of Trees.* Journey Editions, Boston, 1999.

Bossenmaier, Eugene. *Mushrooms of the Boreal Forest.* U. of Saskatchewan Press, 1997

Boulos, Loutfy. *Medicinal Plants of North Africa,* Reference Pub. Algonac, Mich. 1983

Bowles, E. Joy. *The Chemistry of Aromatherapeutic Oils.* Allen & Unwin, Crow's Nest, Australia, 2003.

Bowman, Daria. *Hydrangeas.* Friedman/Fairfax Pub. New York. 1999.

Bradley, Peter. British Herbal Compendium Vol 2 Brit Herb Med Assoc. Bournemouth 2006.

Brahmachari, Goutam Ed. Natural Products, Alpha Sci Int Ltd. Oxford UK 2009.

Brandeis, Gayle. *Fruitflesh.* Harper Collins, San Francisco. 2002.

Brennan, M. *Complete Holistic Care & Healing for Horses.* Trafalgar Sq. Pub. VT. 2001.

Bringhurst, Robert. *A Story as Sharp as a Knife.* Douglas&Mc Intyre Vancouver, 1999.

Brinker, Francis N.D. *Herb Contraindications and Drug Interactions* .Third Edition Eclectic Medical Publications, Sandy, Oregon, 2001

_____*The Toxicology of Botanical Medicines,* revised 2ⁿᵈ. Eclectic Med, Oregon, 1996.

_____*Eclectic Dispensatory of Botanical Therapeutics,* Vol 2, Ecl. Med . Oregon, 1995.

Brodo, Irwin & Sharnoff. *Lichens of North America.* Yale University Press, 2001.

Brown, Deni. *Encyclopedia of Herbs and Their Uses.* Reader's Digest Press, Que. 1995.

Bruneton, J *Pharmacognosy, Phtyochemistry, Medicinal Plants,* Lavoisier Pub. Paris, 1995

_____*Toxic Plants Dangerous to Humans and Animals.* Editions TEC&Doc, Paris, '99.

Brunschwig, Hieronymus. *Book of Distillation.* Johnson Reprint Co No. 79. New York, 1971.

Brynaherb Essences 29, Kells Meend Berry Hill, Gloucestershire GL16 7AD

Bubar, Carol et al. *Weeds of the Prairies.* Alberta Agriculture Pub. Edmonton, 2000.

Buchanan, Carol. *Brothers Crow, Sister Corn.* Ten Speed Press, Berkeley, 1997.

Buckle, Jane. *Clinical Aromatherapy. 2ⁿᵈ ed.* Churchill Livingstone, Toronto, 2003.

Buhner, Stephen H. *Sacred and Herbal Healing Beers,* Siris Books, Boulder, Co, 1998

_____*Sacred Plant Medicine.* Robert Rinehart, Boulder, Co. 1996.

_____Herbal Antibiotics. Storey Books, Vermont, 1999.

_____*The Lost Language of Plants.* Chelsea Green Pub. White River, Vt. 2002

_____Secret Teachings of Plants. Bear & Co. Rochester, Vt. 2004.

_____The Natural Testosterone Plan. Healing Arts Press, Rochester VT. 2007

Burbridge, Joan. *Wildflowers of the Southern Interior of B.C.* U. of B.C. Press, 1989.

Burger, W. Flowers- *How they changed the world. Prometheus Books.* Amherst NY 2006.

Burgess, Isla. *Weeds Heal.* Viriditas Pub Group. Cambridge NZ 1998.

Burlando, Bruno et al, Herbal Principles in Cosmetics. CRC Press Boca Raton 2010.

Caius, Rev. Fr. Jean F., *The Medicinal and Poisonous Plants of India,* Scientific Pub, 1986.

Cameron, Elizabeth. *A Floral ABC.* John Wiley and Sons. Toronto. 1980.

Carpenter D. Snr Pub. *Nursing Herbal Medicine Handbook,* Springhouse Corp. 2001.

Carpinella, Maria et al. Novel Therapeutic Agents from Plants. Sci Pub. Enfield NJ 2009.

Carr, Emily. *Wild Flowers.* Royal BC Museum, Victoria, B.C, 2006

Carroll, Roisin. *The Crane Bag Celtic Tree Ogam Oils* , Feasibility Pub. Dublin

Carter, Bernard F. *The Floral Birthday Book.* Bloomsbury Books, London. 1990.

Casselman, Bill. *Canadian Garden Words.* Little, Brown & Co. Toronto, 1997.

Castleman, Michael. *The Healing Herbs.* Bantam Books. 1995.

Castro, Miranda. *The Complete Homeopathy Handbook.* MacMillan, 1990

Catty, Suzanne. *Hydrosols the next Aromatherapy,* Healing Arts Press, Vermont, 2001.

Cavers, Paul ed, *The* Biology *of Canadian Weeds* 62-83,Ag Institute of Canada, Ottawa, 1995

_____84-102 Ag Inst. of Canada, Ottawa, 2000.

_____103-129 Ag Inst. of Canada, Ottawa 2005

Ceres. *Herbal Teas for Health and Healing.* Healing Arts Press, Rochester, Vermont, 1984.

Chan, K, and Cheung L. *Interactions between Chincese Herbal Medicinal Products and Orthodox Drugs.* Harwood Academic Publishers, Canada, 2000.

Chandler, F. *Herbs-Everyday Reference for Health Professionals,* Can. Pharm Assoc. 2000

Chang & But. *Pharmacology &Applications of Chinese Materia Medica,* World Scientific, 86

Chang Chao-liang et al, *Vegetables as Medicine,* Pelanduk Pub, Malaysia, 1999.

Chappell, P. Emotional Healing with Homeopathy. North Atlantic Books. Berkeley, 2003.

Charissa's Cauldron. www.charissacauldron.com

Chase, Pamela & Pawlik, J. *Newcastle Trees for Healing* , Newcastle Pub. Van Nuys,1991

Chatroux, Sylvia. *Botanica Poetica*. Poetica Press 2004 1-877-POETICA.

_____*Materica Poetica*. Poetica Press 1998.

Chen, John K & Chen, Tina T. Chinese Medical Herbology & Pharmacology. Art of Medicine Press, City of Industry, CA 2004.

Chevalllier, Andrew. *The Encyclopedia of Medicinal Plants*. Reader's Digest, 1996.

Chishti, Hakim. *The Traditional Healer*, Healing Arts Press, Vermont,1988.

Christchurch Flower Essences. www.christchurchfloweressences.com

Clark, Ella E. *Indian Legends of Canada*. McClelland & Stewart. Toronto, 1960.

Coats, Peter. *Flowers in History*. Weidenfeld and Nicolson, London. 1970.

Coffey, Timothy.*The History and Folklore of North American Wildflowers*, Houghton-Mifflin, 1993.

Cohen, Kenneth. *Honoring the Medicine*. Random House, Toronto. 2003.

Conrad, Chris, *Hemp for Health*, Healing Arts Press, Rochester, Vermont, 1997.

Cook, Wm.H. *The Physio-Medical Dispensatory*. 1869. Reprinted by Eclectic Medical Publications, Portland, Oregon, 1985.

_____A compendium of the new Materia medica together with additional descriptions of some old remedies. Wm. Cook Publisher, Chicago, 1896.

Cooper, J.C. *Dictionary of Symbolic & Mythological Animals,* Thorsons, London, 1992.

Cormack, R.G.H. *Wild Flowers of Alberta*. Hurtig Publishers, 1977

Coupland, Francois. *The Encyclopedia of Edible Plants of N. America*. Keats Pub. 1998.

Cousin, Pierre J. *Eat Well, Be Well*. Thorsons, London. 2001.

Cowan, Eliot. *Plant Spirit Medicine*. Swan Raven & Co. Box 726 Newberg, Oregon, 1995.

Cowan, Thomas. The Fourfold Path to Healing. New Trends Pub. Washington DC 2007.

Crane, Eva. *Honey- A Comprhensive Survey* , Heinemann Pub. London 1975.

Craydon D. & Bellows W. Floral Acupuncture. The Crossing Press Berkeley CA 2005.

Creekmore, H. *Daffodils are Dangerous*. Walker and Co. New York. 1966.

Crow, Tis Mal. *Native Plants, Native Healing*. Native Voices Book Pub. Box 99 Summertown, Tennessee, 2001 1-888-260-8458.

Crowell, Robert L. *The Lore & Legends of Flowers*. Thomas Crowell, New York, 1982.

Crowfoot & Baldensperger. *From Cedar to Hyssop*. Sheldon Press, London, 1932.

Cruden, Loren. Medicine Grove. Destiny Books. Inner Traditions Vermont. 1997.

Cummings, S. and Ullman, Dana. *Everyone's Guide to Homeopathic Medicines,* St. Martins

Cupp, Melanie. *Toxicology and Clinical Pharmacology of Herbal Products*. Humana P. 1999

Curtin, LSM. *Healing Herbs of the Upper Rio Grande*. SouthWest Museum, Los Angeles 1965

Cutler & Cutler Eds. Biologically Active Natural Products: Agrochemicals, CRC Press 1999.

Dai Yin-fang&Liu Cheng-jun. *Fruit As Medicine*. Rams Skull Press, Kuranda, Aust. 1987

Dalton, David. Stars of the Meadow. Lindisfarne Books. Great Barrington, Mass. 2006.

D'Amelio Sr. Frank. *Botanicals A Phytocosmetic Desk Reference* CRC Press, Boca Raton, 99

Darby,Wm et al. *Food: The Gift of Osiris,* Vol 1. Academic Press, San Francisco, 1977

Darwin, Tess. The Scots Herbal, the Plant Lore of Scotland. Birlinn Ltd, Edinburgh 2008

Davidow, Joie. *Infusions of Healing, A Treasury of Mexican-American Herbal Remedies,* Fireside Books, New York, 1999.

Davis,W. *El Gringo, New Mexico and Her People*. Harpers, New York, 1857.

Demargaux, N. *Phytotherapy*. Herbal Health Publishers Ltd. 1989

De Bairacli Levy, Juliette. *Herbal Handbook for Farm and Stable*, Faber and Faber 1952

Deer Lame, J & Erdoes, R. *Lame Deer Seeker of Visions*. Washington Sq Press, 1976.

Deer, Thea Summer. Wisdom of the Plant Devas. Bear&Company Vermont 2011.

Delta Gardens Flower Essences. www.deltagardens.com

De Smet et al. *Adverse Effects of Herbal Drugs*. Springer-Verlag, Berlin. 1997.

Der Marderosian, Ara & Liberti L. *Natural Product Medicine,* George Stickley Co, Philadel.

DeRios, Marlene D. *Hallucinogens: Cross Cultural Perspectives*. U. New Mexico Press, 1984

DeSmet, P. et al. *Adverse Effects of Herbal Drugs. vol 2* Springer-Verlag

Devi, Lila. The Essential Flower Essence Handbook. Crystal Clarity Pub. Nevada City 2007.

Dewey, Laurel. *Plant Power- revised.* Safe Goods/New Century Pub, Markham Ont, 2001.

Dewick, Paul M. *Medicinal Natural Products.*3rd Ed John Wiley and Sons, West Sussex, 2009.

Diederichsen, Axel. *Coriander.* Int. Plant Genetic Resources Institute. Rome, Italy. 1996.

Dixon, Bernard.*Power Unseen, How Microbes Rule the World*. W.H. Freeman, Oxford, 1994

Dow, Elaine. *Simples and Worts*. Historical Presentations, Topsfield, MA. 1982.

Duke, James. *Handbook of Medicinal Herbs*. CRC Press, Boca Raton, Florida, 1985

_____*Handbook of Edible Weeds*. CRC Press. 1992

_____*The Green Pharmacy,* Rodale Press, Emmaus, Pennsylvania, 1997.

_____*The Green Pharmacy Herbal Handbook,* Rodale Press, 2000.

_____*Anti-aging Prescriptions*. Rodale Press. 2001.

Dumas, Anne. Book of Plants and Symbols. English Ed. Octopus Pub. London 2004.

Dymock,Wm. *Pharmacographia Indica, Vol 2*, Kegan Paul, Trench, Trubner and Co. 1891

Earle, Liz. *Vital Oils*, Ebury Press, London, 1991.

Eason, Cassandra. Fabulous Creatures, Mythical Monsters… Greenwood Press, CT. 2008.

Eastman, John. *The Book of Swamp and Bog...* Stackpole Books, Mechanicsburg, Penn, 1995

Ebadi, M. *Pharmacodynamic Basis of Herbal Medicine,* CRC Press, Boca Raton. 2002.

Eckey, E.W. *Vegetable Fats and Oils,* Rheingold Publishing Co, New York, 1954.

Eclare, Melanie. *Flower Spirit Cards*. Quadrille Publishing, London, England, 2004.

Edwards, Lawrence. *The Vortex of Life*. Floris Books. Edinburgh 2nd Ed. 2006.

Eisner T et al. *Secret Weapons*. Belknap Press, Harvard U Press. Cambridge & London 2005.

Ellingwood F. *American Materia Medica,* Eclectic Med. Pub. Portand, Oregon, reprint, 1983

Elliot, Douglas B. *Roots* . Chatham Press, Old Greenwich Conneticut.

Ellis, Hattie. *Sweetness & Light*. Hodder and Stoughton, London, 2004.

Erdoes & Ortiz. *American Indian Myths and Legends,* Pantethon Books, New York, 1984.

Erichsen-Brown,Charlotte. *Use of Plants for the Past 500 Years,* Breezy Creeks Press, 1979

_____*Medicinal and Other Uses of North American Plants,* General Pub, 1979.

Erickson, David, Wai Kit Nip *Food uses of whole oil and protein seeds,* Amer. Oil Chemists Society, 1989.

Eskin, N. A. Michael, Tamir, S. *Dictionary of Nutraceuticals and Functional Foods*. CRC Press, 2006.

Etkin, Nina. Edible Medicines, An Ethnopharmacology of Food. U Arizona Press. 2006.

Evans, W.C. *Trease and Evans' Pharmacognosy*. WB Saunders Co. Toronto, 2000.

Fang Jing Pei, Dr. *Natural Remedies from the Chinese Cupboard*. Weatherhill, 1998.

Farmer-Knowles,Helen. *The Healing Garden*. Sterling Publishing, New York, 1998.

Fielder, Mildred. *Plant Medicne and Folklore,* Winchester Press, New York, 1975.

Felter, Harvery and Lloyd, John. *King's American Dispensatory* . 1898. Reprinted by Eclectic Medical
        Publications, Portland Oregon, 1983.

Ferguson, Gary. *Spirits of the Wild*. Clarkson Potter/Random New York, 1996.

Fernie, W.T. Dr. *Old Fashioned Herbal Remedies*. Coles Pub. Toronto, 1980. Reprint.

Fingerman M. et al editors. *Bioremediation of Aquatic and Terresrial Ecosytems*. Sci Pub. Enfield NH 2005.

Fischer-Rizzi, S. *Complete Aromatherapy Handbook,* Sterling Pub. New York. 1990.

_____*The Complete Incense Book,* Sterling Pub. New York. 1998.

_____*Medicine of the Earth,* Rudra Press, Portland, Oregon, 1996

Florey, H.W. et al. Antibiotics vol 1. Oxford University Press. London 1949.

Ford, Gillian. *Plant Names Explained.* Friends of the Devonian Botanic Garden, #16, 1984

Foster, Steven. *Herbal Renaissance,* Gibbs Smith Pub. Salt Lake City

_____& Yue Chongxi. *Herbal Emissaries,* Healing Arts Press, Vermont, 1992

_____& Johnson R. *Desk Reference to Nature's Medicine.* Nat Geographic. Washington, D.C.

Fox, H. M. Gardening with Herbs. Macmillan Pub. New York 1933.

Freeman, D. & Mongeau D. Nettles and More…Vol One. Self published 2nd printing 2009.

Freeman, Lyn. *Mosby's Complementary & Alternative Medicine.*3rd Ed. Mosby Elsevier 2009

Friedman, Sara Ann, *Celebrating the Wild Mushroom,* Dodd, Mead & Co. New York, 1986

Friend, Tim. The Third Domain: the Untold Story of Archaea. Joseph Henry Press. 2007.

Fugh-Berman, Adriane. *The 5-minute Herb &Dietary Supplement Consult.* Lippincott Williams &Wilkins, Philadelphia 2003.

Gaertner, Erika. *Reap without Sowing.* General Store Publishing, Burnstown, Ont. 1995

Galun, Margalith. *Handbook of Lichenology,* CRC Press, 1988

Garran, Thomas. *Western herbs according to Traditional Chinese Medicine.* Healing Arts Press. 2008.

Garrett, J.T. *The Cherokee Herbal.* Bear&Company, Rochester, Vermont. 2003.

Genders, Roy. *Floral Scents of the World* . St. Martin's Press, London, 1977

Geuter, *Herbs in Nutrition.* Bio-Dynamic Agricultural Assoc. London. 1978.

Gildemeister, E. *The Volatile Oils.* John Wiley and Sons, New York. 1916

Gifford, Jane. The Wisdom of Trees. Sterling Pub. New York 2000.

Gill S. & Sullivan I. *Dictionary of Native American Mythology.* Oxford U Press 1992.

Gilmore, M.R. Uses of Plants by Indians of the Missouri river region. 33rd Annual Report Bureau American Ethnology, 1911-12, Washington D.C. 1919.

Gladstar R & Hirsch P. *Planting the Future.* Healing Arts Press, Rochester, Vt. 2000.

Gladstar, Rosemary. *Family Herbal.* Storey Books, North Adams, Mass. 2001.

Glasby, J.S. *Dictionary of Plants Containing Secondary Metabolites,* Taylor & Francis, London 1991.

Godfrey, A & Saunders P. Principles and Practices of Naturopathic Botanical Medicine, Vol 1, CCNM Press Toronto ON 2010.

Goodrick-Clarke, Clare. Alchemical Medicine for the 21st Century. Healing Arts Press. 2010.

Gordon, David G. *The Compleat Cockroach.* Ten Speed Press, Berkeley, CA. 1996.

Gordon, Lesley. The Mystery and Magic of Trees & Flowers. Grange Books. London 1993.

Gottesfeld, Leslie M. Johnson. *Plants, Land and People, A Study of Wet'suwet'en Ethnobotany.*U of A, 1993.

Grae, Ida. *Nature's Colors, Dyes From Plants.* Macmillan Pub. New York, 1974.

Graham, Frances K. *Plant lore of an Alaskan Island.* Alaska Northwest Pub. 1985

Grandparents of the Forest flower essences. www.grandparentsoftheforest.com

Grange, Michael etal, *Handbook of Plants with Pest Control Properties,* J. Wiley& Son 1988

Gray, Bev. The Boreal Herbal. Wild Food & Medicine Plants of the North. Aroma Borealis Press 2011

Green, James. *The Male Herbal* . Crossing Press, Freedom, California, 1991.

_____*The Herbal Medicine-Maker's Handbook.* Crossing Press, Freedom CA 2000

Green, Jonathan. *Consuming Passions.* Sphere Books, London, 1985.

Grey Wolf. *Earth Signs,* Raincoast Books, Vancouver, B.C. 1998.

Grieve, M. *A Modern Herbal.* Jonathan Cape. 1931

Griffiths, Deirdre. *Elk Island National Park.* U. of Alberta Press, 1979.

Grigson, Geoffrey. *A Herbal of All Sorts*. Phoenix House, London

Grimaud, Baptiste,Paul. *TAROT DES FLEURS*, France Cartes, France 1989

Grimshaw, John. *The Gardener's Atlas*. Firefly Books, Willowdale, Ont. 2002.

Grohmann,Gerbert. *The Plant Vol 2*, Bio-Dynamic Farming & Gardening Assoc. 1989.

Gruenwald et al, Ed. PDR for Herbal Medicines. 4ᵗʰ Ed. Thomson Pub. 2007.

Guillet, Alma. *Make Friends of Trees and Shrubs*. Doubleday & Co. New York, 1962.

Gumbel, Dietrich. *Principles of Holistic Skin Therapy with Herb Essences*. Haug Pub. Heidelberg 1986.

Gurudas. *The Spiritual Properties of Herbs* , Cassandra Press, 1988

_____*Flower Essences and Vibrational Healing*, Cassandra Press, 1983

Hageneder, Fred. The Spirit of Trees. Continuum. NY and London. 2005.

Hale, Mason. *The Biology of Lichens*. Edward Arnold Pub. London, 1967.

Hall, Dorothy. *Creating Your Herbal Profile* , Keats, 1988

Hallworth, B & Chinnappa CC. *Plants of the Kananaskis Country* U of A Press 1997.

Hanchuk, Rena. *The Word and Wax*. Can Inst of Ukrainian Studies Press, Edmonton, 1999.

Hanson, J, & Morrison D. *Of Kinkajous, Capybaras, Horned Beetles...*Harper Collins, NY '91

Harbourne & Baxter. *The Handbook of Natural Flavonoids Vol 1&2*. John Wiley & Sons, 1999

_____*Phytochemical Dictionary*. Taylor & Francis 1993.

Harrington, Geri. *Growing Your Own Chinese Vegetables*, MacMillan, N.Y. 1978.

Harrington, H.D. *Edible Native Plants of the Rocky Mtns*. U. of New Mexico Press, 1967.

Harris, Ben C. *Eat the Weeds*, Keats Pub. New Cannan, Conneticut 1973.

_____*Make Use of Your Garden Plants*. General Pub. New York. 1978.

Harris, Marjorie. *Botanica North America*. Harper Collins, New York, 2003.

Harrison, Nora. *Flower Remedy Rhymes* , self published, England, 1990.

Hart, Jeff. *Montana Native Plants and Early Peoples*, Montana Historical Society Press. '92

_____The Ethnobotany of the Northern Cheyenne Indians of Montana. Journal of Ethnopharmacology 1981 4.

Hartung, Tammi. *Growing 101 Herbs That Heal*. Storey Books, Pownal, Vt. 2000.

Hartwell, Jonathan, *Plants Used Against Cancer*. Quarterman Pub. 1982

Hartzell, Jr. H. *The Yew Tree A Thousand Whispers*. Hulogosi, Box 1188, Eugene, OR 1991.

Harvey, C & Cochrane A. *The Healing Spirit of Plants*. Godsfield Press, Sterling Pr N.Y. 1999

Harvey Clare. The New Encyclopedia of Flower Remedies. Watkins Pub. London 2007.

Hatfield, Gabrielle. *Encyclopedia of Folk Medicine*. ABC CLIO Santa Barbara. 2004.

Haughton, Claire. *Green Immigrants*. Harcourt Brace Jovanovich. New York and London.

Hawksworth, Frank & Wiens, D. Dwarf Mistletoes, Ag Handbook 709, USDA, Wash, DC, '96

Health Canada, Native Foods and Nutrition. Medical Services Branch, 1995.

Heatherington, M. and Steck,W. *Natural Chemicals from Northern Prairie Plants,* Ag West Biotech Publishers, Saskatoon, Canada. 1997.

Heilmeyer, Marina. The Language of Flowers-Symbols & Myths. Prestel Pub. Munich 2001.

Heinerman, John. *Encyclopedia of Nuts, Berries and Seeds*, Parker Publishing, 1995.

_____*Encyclopedia of Healing Herbs & Spices*. Parker Pub. N.Y. 1996.

Heinrich, Bernd. *Winter World The Ingenuity of animal survival*. HarperCollins. NY 2003.

Heinrich, Clark. *Magic Mushrooms in Religion and Alchemy*. Park St. Press, VT. 2002.

Heiser, Charles B. Jr. *Of Plants and People*. U. of Oklahoma Press, 1985.

Hellson, John C, *Ethnobotany of the Blackfoot Indians* No. 19, National Museums of Canada, Ottawa 1974.

Henderson, Robert K. *The Neighborhood Forager*. Key Porter Books, Toronto, 2000.

Hendrickson, Robert. *Encycl of Word and Phrase Origins*. Facts on File Inc. NewYork, 1997.

Hendry, G. *Natural Food Colorants* , Blackie and Son, Glasgow Scotland, 1992.

Henry, J. David. *Canada's Boreal Forest.* Smithsonian Institute. 2002.

Hilarion. *Wildflowers, Their Occult Gifts.* Marcus Books, Queensville, Ont. 1982.

Hobbs, Christopher. *Usnea : The Herbal Antibiotic.* Botanica Press. 1986.

_____*Medicinal Mushrooms*, Botanica Press, Santa Cruz, 1995.

Hoffman, David. *The Holistic Herbal.* Findhorn Press, 1983.

_____*Welsh Herbal Medicine.* Abercastle Publications, Dyfed, 1978.

_____*Medical Herbalism.* Healing Arts Press, Rochester, VT, 2003.

Hole, Lois. *Favorite Trees and Shrubs.* Lone Pine Pub. Edmonton Alta. 1997.

_____*Perennial Favorites.* Lone Pine Pub. 1995.

Holm, LeRoy G. *World Weeds,* John Wiley and Sons, 1997.

Holmes, Peter. *The Energetics of Western Herbs, Vol 1 and 2,* Artemis Press, 1989.

_____*Jade Remedies, Vol 1 and 2,* Snow Lotus Press, Boulder 1996.

Hopman, Ellen. *A Druid's Herbal,* Destiny Books, Rochester, Vermont. 1995.

Howarth, D& Kahlee Keane. *Wild Medicines of the Prairies* Self Published, 1995.

_____*Native Medecines* Self Published , 1995

Hozeski, Bruce. *Hildegard's Healing Plants.* Beacon Press. Boston, Mass. 2001.

Hsu, Hong-Yen. *Oriental Materia Medica,* Keats Publishing,Connecticut, 1986.

Huang, Kee Chang. *The Pharmacolocy of Chinese Herbs.* 2nd Edition, CRC Press, 1999.

Hu-Nan. *A Barefoot Doctor's Manual.* Running Press, Philadelphia, 1977.

Hudson, James B. *Antiviral Compounds from Plants,* CRC Press, Florida, 1990

Hudson, Rick. *A Field Guide to Gold, Gemstone and Mineral Sites.* Orca Pub, Victoria, 1999

Hurley, Judith. *The Good Herb* Wm. Morrow and Co. New York, 1995.

Hutchens, Alma. *Indian Herbology of North America.* Merco. 1969

Ingram, Cass. *Supermarket Remedies.* Knowledge House, Buffalo Grove, Ill. 1998.

Injoynow essences.

Inkpen W & Van Eyk, R. *Guide to the Common Native Trees and Shrubs of Alberta,* Government of Alberta, Environmental Protection, 1995.

James & Keeler, *Poisonous Plants- 3rd Int. Symposium,* Iowa State U. Press, 1992.

Jason, Dan & Nancy. *Some Useful Wild Plants,* Talon Books, Vancouver, 1972.

Jiao Shu-De. *Ten Lectures on the Use of Medicinals.* Paradigm Pub. Brookline, Mass. 2003.

Johnson, Kershaw, MacKinnon & Pojar *Plants of the Western Boreal Forest and Aspen Parkland,* Lone Pine Press, Edmonton, Alberta 1995.

Johnson, L. *Tending the Earth A Gardener's Manifesto.* Penguin Books, Toronto, 2002.

Johnson, Leslie. Journal of Ethnobotany and Ethnomedicine. 2006 2:29.

_____*Health, Wholeness & the Land: Gitksan Traditional Plant Use and Healing.* U of Alberta 1997.

Jones, Alison. *Larousse Dictionary of World Folklore.* Larousse, New York, 1995.

Jones, Pamela. *Just Weed, History, Myths and Uses.* Prentice Hall Press, Toronto, 1991.

Kamm, Minnie W. *Old Time Herbs for Northern Gardens* Little Brown & Co. 1938.

Kane, Charles W. Herbal Medicine of the American Southwest. Lincoln Town Press. 2007.

_____Herbal Medicine: trends and traditions. Lincoln Town Press 2009.

Kapoor, L.D. *CRC Handbook of Ayurvedic Medicinal Plants,* CRC Press, Boca Raton, 1990.

Kari, Priscilla. *Tanaina Plantlore.* National Park Service, Alaska Region 1987.

Kaur, Sat Dharam. *The Complete Natural Medicine Guide to Breast Cancer.* Robert Rose Inc Toronto, 2003.

Kavash E, Barrie & Barr K, *American Indian Healing Arts.* Bantam Books, Toronto 1999.

_____*The Medicine Wheel Garden.* Bantam Books, N.Y. 2002.

Kay, Margarita Artschwager. *Healing with Plants in the American and Mexican West,* The University of Arizona Press, Tucson. 1996

Kays, S & Nottingham S. Biology and Chemistry of Jerusalem Artichoke. CRC Press 2008.

Keane, Kahlee & Howarth,D. *The Standing People.* Saskatoon, Saskatchewan. 2003.

Kee Chang Huang, *The Pharmacology of Chinese Herbs,* 2nd Edition, CRC Press, 1999.

Kemp, Cynthia. *Cactus and Company.* Desert Alchemy, Tucson, Arizona, 1993.

Kenner D &Requena Y. *Botanical Medicine:* .Paradigm Pub. Brookline, Mass, 1996.

Kerik, Joan. *Living with the Land:Use of Plants by the Native People of Alberta,* Alberta Culture, Circulating Exhibits Program, National Museums of Canada Fund, 1981.

Kershaw, Linda. Edible & Medicinal Plants of the Rockies, Lone Pine, Edmonton 2000.

_____*Alberta Wayside Wildflowers.* Lone Pine, Edmonton, 2003.

_____*Saskatchewan Wayside Wildflowers.* Lone Pine, Edmonton, 2003.

_____*Manitoba Wayside Wildflowers.* Lone Pine, Edmonton, 2003.

Kershaw, L. et al. *Rare Vascular Plants of Alberta.* U. of Alberta Press, Edmonton, 2001.

Kershaw, MacKinnon & Pojar. *Plants of the Rocky Mountains.* Lone Pine, Edmonton 1998.

Keys, John. D. *Chinese Herbs,* Charles E. Tuttle Co. 1976.

Kimmerer,Robin. *Gathering Moss.* Oregon State University Press, Corvallis, 2003.

Kindscher, Kelly. *Medicnal Wild Plants of the Prairies.* Univ. Press of Kansas. 1987.

King, Francis X. *Rudolf Steiner and Holistic Medicine.* Rider & Co. England, 1986.

Klein, Carol. Plant Personalities. Timber Press, Portland, Oregon. 2005.

Klein, Richard. *The Green World.* 2nd edition. Harper Collins, 1987.

Kloss, Jethro. *Back to Eden.* Woodbridge Press Pub.Co. Santa Barbara, Ca. 1975.

Knab, Sophie H. *Polish Herbs, Flowers and Folk Medicine.* Hippocrene Books, N.Y. 1999.

Knowles, Hugh. *Woody Ornamentals for the Prairies.* U. of Alberta , 1995.

Knudtson,P & Suzuki D. Wisdom of the Elders. Greystone Books. Vancouver BC 2006.

Kraft, K & Hobbs C. *Pocket Guide to Herbal Medicine.* Thieme, N.Y. 2004.

Kranich, Ernst M. Planetary Influences Upon Plants. Bio-Dynamic Lit. Wyoming RI 1984.

Krymow, V. Healing Plants of the Bible. Wild Goose Pub. Glasgow, UK 2002.

Kuhnlein, Harriet and Turner, Nancy. *Traditional Plant Foods of Canadian Indigenous Peoples.* Gordon and Breach Science Publishers. 1991.

Kuijt, Job. *The Biology of Parasitic Flowering Plants,* U. of California Press, 1969

Kunkele, U. & Lohmeyer, T. *Herbs for Healthy Living.* Parragon Pub. Bath UK 2007.

Lacey, Laurie. *Micmac Medicines Remedies and Recollections.* Nimbus Pub. Halifax, 1993.

Lahring, Heinjo. *Water and Wetland Plants of the Prairie Provinces,* Can Plains Research Center, U. of Regina, 2003

Lambert, Grant. *Falling Leaf Essences.* Healing Arts Press, Rochester Vermont, 2002.

Lamont, SM. *The Fisherman Lake Slave and their environment: a story of floral and faunal resources.* Master's thesis. U. of Saskatchewan, Saskatoon, 1977.

Langenheim, Jean. *Medicinal Plant Resins.* Timber Press Portland Oregon 2003.

Larsen,Henning. *An Old Icelandic Medical Miscellany,* Norske Akademi, Oslo, Norway '31

Lavabre, Marcel. *Aromatherapy Workbook.* Healing Arts Press, Vermont. 1990.

Lawless, Julia, *The Encyclopedia of Essential Oils* , Element Books, 1992.

LeClaire,N &Cardinal,G. *Alberta Elders' Cree Dictionary,* U of Alberta Press, 1998.

Leduc, M.A. *The Explorers Guide to Boreal Forest Plants,* Hwy Book Shop, Cobalt, Ont. 1997

Leighton, Anna L. *Wild Plant Use by the Woods Cree (NIHITHAWAK) of East-Central Saskatchewan* . Paper no. 101, National Museums of Canada, Ottawa, 1985

Lepore, Donald. *The Ultimate Healing System.* Woodland Books, Provo, Utah, 1988.

Le Strange, Richard, *A History of Herbal Plants.* Arco Pub. New York. 1977.

Leung, Albert. *Chinese Herbal Remedies.* Universe Books, New York, 1984.

Leung & Foster, *Encyclopedia of Common Natural Ingredients,* J. Wiley&Sons, N.Y. 1996.

Levey,M. *The Medical Formulary or Aqrabadhin of Al-Kindi* U of Wisconsin Press, 1966

Leyel, C.F. *Elixirs of Life,* Faber and Faber, London.1948

Li, Thomas. *Medicinal Plants, Culture, Utilization & Phytopharmacology.* Technomic Publishing, Lancaster, Pennsylvania, 2000.

Li, Thomas. *Chinese and related North American Herbs.* CRC Press, Boca Raton, 2002.

Libster, Martha. *Delmar's Integrative Herb Guide for Nurses.* Delmar, 2002.

Lininger et al. *The Natural Pharmacy.* Healthnotes, Prima Pub. Rocklin Ca, 1999.

L'Orange Darlena, *Herbal Healing Secrets of the Orient.* Prentice Hall, New Jersey, 1998.

Lock, Carolyn. *Country Colours.* Nova Scotia Museum. 1981

Lovejoy, Sharon. *Sunflower Houses.* Workman Pub Co. New York 2001.

Lu, Henry. *Using Foods to Stay Young,* Sterling Press, New York, 1996.

_____*Chinese Natural Cures.* Black Dog & Leventhal Pub. New York, 1994

Luetjohann, Sylvia. *The Healing Power of Black Cumin.* Lotus Light, Twin Lakes, WI, 1998

Lyle, Katie Letcher. *The Wild Berry Book,* NorthWord Press, Minocqua, WI, 1994.

Mabey, Richard. *Plantcraft.* Universe Books. 1978.

MacKinnon, Pojar, Coupe. *Plants of Northern British Columbia.* Lone Pine Press, 1992.

Mailhebiau, Philippe. *Portraits in Oils.* C.W. Daniel Company, Essex, England, 1995.

Malmud, René. *The Amazon Problem,* trans by M. Stein, Spring Pub. Dallas TX, 1980.

Maloof, Joan. *Teaching the Trees, Lessons from the Forest.* U Georgia Pr, Athena GA. 2005.

Manandhar, N.P. *Plants and People of Nepal.* Timber Press, Portland, Oregon, 2002.

Maple, Eric. *The Secret Lore of Plants and Flowers.* Robert Hale Ltd. London 1980.

March, Kathryn & Andrew. *The Wild Plant Companion.* Meridian Hill Pub. 1986.

Marles, Robin. *The Ethnobotany of the Chipewyan of Northern Saskatchewan,* 1984. Thesis.

_____et al. *Aboriginal Plant Use in Canada's Northwest Boreal Forest.* UBC Press, Vancouver, and Natural Resources Canada, 2000

McBride, L.R. *Practical Folk Medicine of Hawaii.* Petroglyph Press, Hilo,Hawaii, 1975.

McCune B. & Geiser L. *Macrolichens of the Pacific Northwest.* Oregon State U. Press, 1997

McFarland, Phoenix. *The Complete Book of Magical Names.* Llewellyn Pub. St Paul 1996

McGrath, Judy. *Dyes from Lichens and Plants.* Van Nostrand Rheinhold, 1977.

McGuffin, Nancy. *Spectrum: dye plants of Ontario.* Burr House Spinner, Richmond Hill '86

Mc Intyre, Anne. *The Complete Woman's Herbal,* Henry Holt, New York, 1995.

Mears, R & Hillman,G. Wild Food. Hodder and Stoughton

MELODY. *Love is in the Earth, A Kaleidoscope of Crystals.* Earth Love Pub. Col. 1995.

Mercatante, A. S. The Facts on File Encyclopedia of World Mythology. New York 1988

Merriam, C. Hart. *Dawn of the World, Weird Tales of Mewan Indians.* Arthur H. Clark, Cleveland, 1910

Meyer, George et al. *Folk Medicine and Herbal Healing,* Charles Thomas, Springfield, 1981

Meyerowitz,Steve. *Sprout It!* The Sprout House, Box 1100,Great Barrington, MA, 1993.

Meyers, Edward C. *Basic Bush Survival,* Hancock House, Surrey, B.C. 1997.

Miller, L &Murray,W. *Herbal Medicinals A Clinician's Guide.* Hawthorn Press, N.Y. 1998.

Miller, Sandra. Editor Echinacea- Medicinal and Aromatic Plants. CRC Press, 2004.

Mills S. & Bone,K. *Principles and Practice of Phytotherapy.* Churchill Livingstone, 2000.

_____*The Essential Guide to Herbal Safety.* Churchill Livingstone, 2005.

Mills, Simon. *Out of the Earth.* Viking Penquin Books, Toronto. 1991.

Millsbaugh, Charles. *American Medicinal Plants,* Dover Pub. New York, 1974

Milne, Courtney. *Visions of the Goddess*, Penguin Studio, Toronto, 1998

Minnis & Elisens. *Biodiversity and Native America.* U. Oklahoma Press, 2000.

Mitchel, Jr. Wm. *Plant Medicine in Practice.* Churchill Livingstone, St. Louis, 2003.

Moerman, Daniel, *Medicinal Plants of Native America.* U of Michigan No. 19, 1986

Mohammed, G. *Catnip & Kerosene Grass* Candlenut Books, Sault Ste. Marie, Ont, 2002.

Montgomery, Pam. *Plant Spirit Healing.* Bear and Company, Rochester, VT 2008.

Moore, Michael. *Los Remedios.* Red Crane Books, 1990

_____*Medicinal Plants of the Desert and Canyon West.* Museum of New Mexico Press 1989

_____*Medicinal Plants of the Mountain West,* Museum of New Mexico Press '79

_____Med Plants of the Mountain West. Revised, expanded. 2003

_____*Medicinal Plants of the Pacific West,* Red Crane Books, 1993

More, Daphne. *The Bee Book,* Universe Books, New York, 1976.

Morelli, I. et al. *Selected Medicinal Plants.* University of Pisa. FAO 53/1

Morton, Julia. *Major Medicinal Plants .* Charles Thomas, Springfield, Illinois 1977

_____*Atlas of Medicinal Plants of Middle America, Bahamas to Yucatan.* 1981

Moss, E.H. *Flora of Alberta.* University of Toronto Press. 1983

Mother, The. *Flowers and their Messages.* Sri Aurobindo Ashram Trust, India 1979.

Mourning Dove. Coyote Stories. Caxton Press Caldwell Idaho. 1933.

Mowrey, Daniel. *The Scientific Validation of Herbal Medicine.* Cormorant Books, 1986.

Mucz, Michael. *Baba's Kitchen Medicines.* U of Alberta Press, Edmonton, 2012.

Mulders, Evelyn. *Western Herbs for Eastern Meridian & 5 Element Theory. Self publ. 2006.*

Mulligan, G editor *The biology of Canadian Weeds,* 1-32 Pub. 1693 Ag Canada 1979

_____33-61 Pub. 1765 Ag Canada 1984

Murphy, Cristine Editor, *Practical Home Care Medicine,* Lantern Books, New York, 2001

Murray, Michael. *The Pill Book Guide to Natural Medicines.* Bantam Books, April, 2002.

_____& Pizzorno, J. The condensed Encycl of Healing Foods. Pocket Books NY 2005.

Naegele, Thomas A. *Edible and Medicinal Plants of the Great Lakes Region,* Wilderness Adventure Books, Davisburg, Michigan. 1996.

Naiman, Ingrid. *Cancer Salves, A Botanical Approach to Treatment.* N. Atlantic Books, 99.

Nesse R & Williams G. *Why We Get Sick.* Vintage Books/Random House, New York, 1996.

Neuwinger H.D. *African Traditional Medicine.* Medpharm Sci. Pub. Stuttgart 2000.

_____African Ethnobotany, Poisons and Drugs. Chapman & Hall, London 1996.

Newcombe C.F. unpub notes on Haida plants. Dept of Anthro. Am Mus Nat Hist. NY 1897

_____unpublished papers. Prov Archives B.C. Victoria. 1898-1913.

Nicander. *The Poems and Poetical Fragments.* Cambridge U. Press, New York, 1953.

Norman,Howard. *Northern Tales.* Pantheon Books, New York, 1990.

Northcote, Rosalind. *The Book of Herbs.* John Lane: The Bodley Head, London, 1912.

Null, Gary. *The Clinician's Handbook of Natural Healing.* Kensington Books, N.Y. 1997.

Olive, Barbara. *The Flower Healer.* Cico Books, London and New York. 2007.

Ollsin, Don. *Herbal Healing Journey-Playful Workbook.* Aquiline Comm, Victoria,BC 1998.

Ootoova I. et al. *Interviewing Inuit Elders, Perspectives on Traditional Health.* Vol 5, Nunavut Arctic College, Box 600, Iqaluit, Nunavut X0Z 0H0.

Page, George. *Inside the Animal Mind.* Doubleday, New York, 1999.

Pallasdowney, Rhonda. *The Complete Book of Flower Essences.* New World Library, 2002.

Pappalardo, Joe. Sunflowers (the secret history). The Overlook Press. Woodstock NY 2008.

Parish, Coupé & Lloyd. *Plants of S. Interior British Columbia.* Lone Pine Edmonton 1996

Park, Willard Z. *Ethnographic Notes on the Norhern Paiute of Western Nevada, 1933-40* compiled by Catherine Fowler, U. of Utah, Salt Lake City, 1989.

Parvati, J. *Hygieia, A Woman's Herbal.* Freestone Collective. 1978

Paturi, Felix *Nature, Mother of Invention.* Harper and Row Pub. New York. 1976.

Peirce,Andrea. *Practical Guide to Natural Medicines.* Stonesong Press. 1999.

Pelikan, W. Healing Plants. Mercury Press, Spring Valley NY 1997.

Pellowski, Anne. *Hidden Stories in Plants.* MacMillan Pub. New York. 1990.

Penoel,Daniel & Franchomme, P. *L'Aromatherapie Exactement* , Roger Jollois, France, 1990

Peneol, Daniel. *Medecine Aromatique, Medecine Planetaire.* Roger Jollois France 1991.

_____& Peneol, Rose-Marie. *Natural Home Health Care Using Essential Oils.* Osmobiose Pub. 1998.

People of 'Ksan, The. *Gathering What the Great Nature Provided.* Douglas & Mc Intyre. Vancouver, B.C. 1980.

Peters, Josephine & Ortiz B. After the First Full Moon in April. Left Coast Press. Walnut Creek CA, 2010.

Pettitt,Sabina. Energy Medicine, Healing from the Kingdoms of Nature, Pacific Essences, Box 8317, Victoria, B.C. V8W 3R9 Canada, 1999

Phaneuf, Holly. Herbs Demystified. Marlowe and Company, New York. 2005

Pielou, E.C. *The Naturalist's Guide to the Arctic.* U. of Chicago Press. 1994.

Pieroni, A & Price L. Eating and Healing, Trad Food as Medicine. Haworth Press. N.Y. 2006.

Pfeiffer E. *The Earth's Face and Human Destiny,* Rodale Press, Emmaus, Pa. 1947.

Plotkin, Mark. *Medicine Quest.* Viking Penguin Books, New York, 2000.

Pojar, J & MacKinnon, A. *Plants of Coastal British Columbia* Lone Pine Edmonton 1994.

Pollock, L. With Faith and Physic: the life of a tudor gentlewoman. Collins & Brown,1993.

Polya, Gideon. *Biochemical Targets of Plant Bioactive Comp.* CRC Press, Boca Raton 2003

Pond, Barbara, *A Sampler of Wayside Herbs,* Chatham Press, Riverside, Conn.

Pressor, Arthur, *Pharmacist's Guide to Medicinal Herbs,* Smart Pub. Petaluma, CA,2000

Price, Len & Shirley. *Understanding Hydrolats.* Churchill Livingstone, Toronto, 2004.

_____Aromatherapy for Health Professionals. Churchill Livingstone 1995.

Purvis, William. *Lichens.* Smithsonian Institution Press. Washington D.C. 2000

Quin, Frederick F. *The Flora Homoeopathica.* B. Jain Pub. New Delhi, India. 1997.

Radin, Paul. *The Winnebago Tribe,* Bur of Am Ethnology, Smithsonian Inst. 37th. 1923.

Rätsch, C. *Plants of Love, The History of Aphrodisiacs.* Ten Speed Press, Berkeley,1997.

_____The Dictionary of Sacred & Magical Plants. ABC-CLIO St Barbara 1992.

_____The Encyclopedia of Psychoactive Plants. Park St Press. 2005.

Raven Essences. www.ravenessences.com

Ravenworks flower essences. www.ravenworksministries.weebly.com

Reaume, Tom. 620 Wild Plants of North America. Nature Manitoba. Canadian Plains Research Center, U of Regina, U of Toronto Press. 2009.

Reckeweg, Hans-Heinrich, *Materia Medica, Vol 1. Aurelia-Verlag GmbH, Baden Baden* 1996.

Reich, Lee. *Uncommon Fruits Worthy of Attention,* Addison-Wesley Pub. 1991.

Reid, Daniel, *A handbook of Chinese Healing Herbs,* Shambala, Boston, 1995

Rhode, David. Native Plants of Southern Nevada. U of Utah Press. 2002.

Richards B & Kanecko A. *Japanese Plants- Know Them &Use Them.* Shufunotomo, Tokyo 1995

Richardson, David. *The Vanishing Lichens.* David and Charles, Vancouver, BC, 1975

Riddle, John M. *Eve's Herbs.* Harvard U Press. Cambridge Mass. 1997.

_____Goddesses, Elixirs and Witches. Palgrave MacMillan. England 2010.

Rister, Robert. *Healing Without Medication.* Basic Health Pub. N. Bergen, N.J. 2003.

Roberts, Jonathan. *The Origins of Fruit and Vegetables.* Universe Pub. New York. 2001.

Robicsek, F. *The Smoking God: Tobacco....*Norman: U. of Oklahoma Press, 1978.

Robinson, Peggy. *Profiles of Northwest Plants.* Far West Book Service. Portland, OR 1979

Rogers, Dilwyn. *Edible, Medicinal, Useful & Poisonous Wild Plants of the Northern Great Plains —South Dakota Region.* Buechel Memorial Lakota Museum, St. Francis,SD, 1980.

Rogers, Pattiann. *Firekeeper:New & Selected Poems.* Milkweed Editions, 1994.

Rogers, Robert Dale. *Sundew Moonwort Vols-1-7, self-published.* Edmonton 1995-present.

_____Rogers' Herbal Manual. Karamat Wilderness Ways, Edmonton, 2000.

_____& Capital Health, Herbal Drug Interactions. Mediscript Comm. 2003.

_____The Fungal Pharmacy, The Complete Guide to Medicinal Mushrooms and Lichens of North America, North Atlantic Books 2011.

Rombi, Max. *Phytotherapy.* Herbal Health Publishers. U.K. 1990.

Rosengarten,Jr. F. *The Book of Edible Nuts.* Walker and Co. New York. 1984.

Ross, Gary. *Nature's Guide to Healing.* Freedom Press, Topanga, Ca. 2000.

Ross, Ivan. *Medicinal Plants of the World.* Vol 1 Humana Press, Totowa, New Jersey. 1999.

_____ Vol 2 Humana Press, Totowa, N. J. 2002.

Rotella, Rev. Alexis. *The Essence of Flowers,* Jade Mountain Press, N.J. 1991.

Royer F. & Dickinson R. *Plants of Alberta.* Lone Pine Pub. Edmonton, AB. 2007.

Rudginsky, Marlene *The Flower Speaks.* U.S. Games Systems, Stamford, Conn. 1999.

Rupp, Rebecca. *Red Oaks and Black Birches* , Storey Comm. Garden Way Publishing. 1990

Russell, Sharman Apt. *Anatomy of a Rose.* Perseus Pub. Cambridge, Mass. 2001.

_____An Obsession with Butterflies. Perseus Publishing 2003.

Ryan, J et al, *Traditional Dene Medicine.* Lac La Martre NWT, 1993.

Ryden, Hope. *Wildflowers around the year.* Clarion Books, New York. 2001.

Ryrie, Charlie. Garden Folklore That Works. Reader's Digest. Pleasantville, NY 2001.

Sagadic O. & Ozcan M. *Food Control* 2003 14.

Salmon, Wm. *Botanologia: The English Herbal.* London: I. Dawkes, 1710.

Sandberg & Corrigan. *Natural Remedies, their origins and uses.* Taylor & Francis 2001.

Sanders, Jack. *The Secrets of Wildflowers.* The Lyons Press, Guilford, CT, 2003.

Sapolsky, Robert. *The Trouble with Testosterone.* Scribner, New York. 1997.

Sauer, Johann Christopher, Compendious Herbal-see Weaver below.

Savage, Candace. Bees, Nature's Little Wonders. Greystone Books. Vancouver 2008.

Schalkwijk-Barendsen, Helene. *Mushrooms of Western Canada* . Lone Pine Pub. 1991.

Schar, Douglas. *The Backyard Medicine Chest.* Elliott&Clark Pub. Washington, DC. 1995.

Scheffer, Mechthild, *Bach Flower Therapy, Theory and Practice,* Healing Arts Press, 1988

Schenk, George. *Moss Gardening.* Timber Press, Portland Oregon. 1997.

Schnaubelt, Kurt. *Medical Aromatherapy.* Frog Ltd. Berkeley CA. 1999.

Schneider, Anny. *Wild Medicinal Plants.* Key Porter Books, Toronto. 2002.

Schnell, Donald. *Carnivorous Plants.* 2nd Ed. Timber Press, Portland, Oregon, 2002.

Schofield, Janice. *Discovering Wild Plants.* Alaska Northwest Books. 1989.

_____*Nettles.* Keats Publishing, New Canaan, Conneticut, 1998.

Schulman, Robert. *Solve It With Supplements.* Rodale Press. New York. 2007.

Shapiro, R & Rapkins J. Awakening to the Plant Kingdom, Cassandra Press 1991.

Shauenberg, Paul and Paris. *Guide to Medicinal Plants.* Keats Publishing, 1977.

Shook, Edward Dr. *Advanced Treatise on Herbology* . Reprint Health Research.

Shosteck,Robert. *Flowers and Plants*. Quadrangle/The New York Times Book Co. 1974.

Siegfried, EV. Masters Thesis, Ethnobotany of the Northern Cree of Wabasca/Desmarais. U of Calgary, Alberta. 1994.

Silverman, Maida. *A City Herbal*. David R. Godine , 1990.

Silvertown, Jonathan. An Orchard Invisible. U of Chicago Press. 2009.

Simonot, Danielle. *Bio-Manufacturing in Saskatchewan-* Assessment of the Manufacturing Potential of Select Saskatchewan Plants, Sask. Nutraceutical Network, Saskatoon, 2000

Simpson, Brenan, M. *Flowers At My Feet,* Hancock House, Surrey, B.C. 1996.

Sionneau, P. *An Introduction to the Use of Processed Chinese Medicinals.* Blue Poppy Press, Second Printing 2003, Translated by Bob Flaws.

Smagghe, Guy Ed. Ecdysone: Structures and Functions. Springer Sci 2009.

Small, E & Catling, P. *Canadian Medicinal Crops,* NRC Research Press, Ottawa 1999.

Small, Ernest. *Culinary Herbs, Second Ed.* NRC Research Press, Ottawa, 2006.

_____*Medicinal Herbs,* NRC Research Press, Ottawa, 2000.

_____Top 100 Food Plants. NRC Press, Ottawa. 2009.

Smith, Andrew. *Strangers in the Garden, the Secret Lives of Our Favorite Flowers.*McClelland & Stewart 2004.

Smith, Annie Lorrain. *Lichens,* Cambridge at the University Press, 1921.

Smith, Harlan, *Ethnobotany of the Gitksan Indians of B.C.* Edited by B. Compton, B. Rigsby, and M.L. Tarpent, Mercury Series, Can Ethno Service, Paper 132, Can Mus of Civil. 1997.

Smith, Huron H. Manataka American Indian Council. www.manataka.org.

Snell, Alma Hogan. A Taste of Heritage. Crow Indian Recipes and Herbal Medicines. University of Nebraska Press 2006.

Soule, Deb. *The Roots of Healing, A Woman's Book of Herbs.* Citadel Press, 1995.

Spencer, Kate. *The Magic of Green Buckwheat ,*Richard Clay, England, 1987.

Spinella, Marcello. *The Psychopharmacology of Herbal Medicine.* MIT Press, 2001.

Steedman, E.V. *The Ethnobotany of the Thompson Indians of British Columbia.* 1930.

Stein, Sara. *My Weeds, A Gardener's Botany.* Harper and Row, 1988.

Stern, Gai. *Australian Weeds.* Harper and Row, Australia 1986

Stern Wm. *Stern's Dictionary of Plant Names for Gardeners.* Cassell Pub, London, 1972

Stewart, Hilary. *CEDAR.* Douglas & Mc Intyre. Vancouver/Toronto, 1984.

Storl, Wolf D. Healing Lyme Disease Naturally. NorthAtlantic Books, Berkeley, CA 2010.

Strehlow,W & Hertzka,G. *Hildegard of Bingen's Medicine* Bear & Co. Santa Fe 1988

Stuart, David. *Dangerous Garden.* Harvard University Press, Cambridge, Mass. 2004

Sturdivant L.&Blakley,T. *Medicinal Herbs in the Garden, Field and Marketplace* Bootstrap Guide, San Juan Naturals, Friday Harbor,WA, 1999.

Sumner, Judith. *The Natural History of Medicinal Plants.* Timber Press, Oregon, 2000.

Sun Bear & Wabun, *The Medicine Wheel* Prentice Hall, NJ 1980.

Swanton, J.R. *Haida Texts and Myths.* Bureau Am Ethnol, Bull #29. Smithsonian Inst. Washington, D.C. 1905.

_____*Bureau of Am Ethno 26th Ann Report.* Smithsonian Inst. Washington, 1908.

Szczeklik, Andrzej. Kore: On Sickness, the Sick and the Search for the Soul of Medicine. Counterpoint Berkeley 2012.

Tainter, D& Grenis A, *Spices and Seasonings ,* VCH Pubishers, New York, 1993.

Talalaj,S.& Czechowicz,A S. *Herbal Remedies,* Hill of Content Press, Melbourne, 1989

Taylor, Wm &Farnsworth,N. The Vinca Alkaloids, Marcel Dekker, New York, 1973.

Teeguarden, Ron. *The Ancient Wisdom of the Chinese Tonic Herbs.* Warner Bros. 1998.

Telesco, Patricia. *The Victorian Flower Oracle,* Llewellyn Pub. St. Paul 1994

Temple, Robert. *The Genius of China*. Simon and Schuster. New York. 1986.

Thompson, Gerry, *Astral Sex to Zen Teabags*. Findhorn Press, 1994.

Thoreau, Henry David. *Wild Fruits*. W. W. Norton & Co. New York, 2000.

Throop, Priscilla. *Hildegard von Bingen's Physica*. Healing Arts Press, Vt. 1998.

Tick, Edward. *The Practice of Dream Healing*. Quest Books Wheaton, Illinois, 2001.

Tierra, Michael. *The Way of Herbs- revised Pocket Rooks*, New York, 1998.

Tigner, Daniel. *Canadian Forest Tree Essences*, self published,1998. ISBN 0968365809

Tilford, Gregory. *Edible and Medicinal Plants of the West*. Mountain Press, Missoula 1997.

Timbrook, Jan. Chumash Ethnobotany. St. Barbara Mus, Heyday Books, Berkeley Ca 2007.

Traill, E.C. *Studies of Plant Life in Canada*. A. S. Woodburn, Ottawa, 1885.

Traill, C. P. *The Backwoods of Canada*. McClelland and Stewart. Toronto. 1846.

Tobyn, G., Denham, A., Whitelegg, M. The Western Herbal Tradition. 2000 years of medicinal herbal knowledge. Churchill Livingstone Toronto 2011.

Toop, Edgar W & Williams, Sara. *Perennials for the Prairies*. U of A&Saskatchewan. 1991.

Treben, Maria. *Health Through God's Pharmacy*. Wilhelm Ennsthaler. 1982.

Tresidder, Jack. Symbols and Their Meaning. Friedman/Fairfax Pub. 2007.

Tucker A. & DeBaggio,T. *The Big Book of Herbs*. Interweave Press. Loveland CO. 2000.

_____The Encylcopedia of Herbs. Timber Press, Portland. 2009.

Turkington, Carol. *The Home Health Guide to Poisons and Antidotes*, Facts on File 1994

Turner, Nancy J. *Food Plants of Interior First Peoples*. UBC Press, Vancouver, 1997.

_____*Food Plants of Coastal First Peoples*. UBC Press, Vancouver, 1995.

_____*Plant Technology of First Peoples in B.C.* UBC Press, Vancouver, 1998.

_____et al. *Thompson Ethnobotany*. Memoir #3, Royal B.C. Museum, 1996.

_____*Plants of Haida Gwaii*. Sononis Press, Winlaw, B.C. 2004.

_____The Earth's Blanket. Douglas & Mc Intyre. Vancouver. 2005.

Turner, N & von Aderkas, P. Common Poisonous Plants and Mushrooms. Timber Press 2009

Turner, W.B. *Fungal Metabolites,* Academic Press, London and New York, 1971.

Twitchell, Paul. *Herbs The Magic Healers*. Eckankar, Box 3100 Menlo Park, CA, 1986.

Vermeulen, Nico. *Encyclopedia of Herbs*. Whitecap Books, Vancouver B.C. 1998.

Viereck, Eleanor, G. *Alaska's Wilderness Medicines*. Alaska Northwest Pub. 1987

Vitt, Marsh and Bovey, *Mosses, Lichens, and Ferns,* Lone Pine Press, 1988.

Vogel, A. *Swiss Nature Doctor*. A. Vogel, Switzerland. 1952

_____*Nature-Your Guide to Healthy Living*. Verlag A. Vogel, Teufen, Switzerland 1986.

Vogel, Virgil. *American Indian Medicine,* U. of Oklahoma Press, Norman, 1970

Vortex Essences (Mt. Shasta Essences) www.vortexessences.com

Walker, Barbara. *The Woman's Dictionary of Symbols&Sacred Objects*. Csstle Books, 1988.

Walker, Marilyn. Wild Plants of Eastern Canada. Nimbus Pub. Halifax NS. 2008.

Ward, Bobby J. The Plant Hunter's Garden. Timber Press, Portland. 2004.

Ward-Harris, Joan.*More Than Meets the Eye, The Life and Lore of Western Wildflowers* Oxford University Press, Toronto, 1983

Watanabe & Shibuya. *Pharmacological Research on Traditional Herbal Medicines*. Harwood Academic Publishers, 1999.

Watt, John, and Breyer-Brandwijk, Maria *The Medicinal and Poisonous Plants of Southern and Eastern Africa* . E and S. Livingstone. Edinburgh and London. 1962.

Watts, Donald. Elsevier's Dictionary of Plant Lore. Elsevier. 2007.

Waugh, F.W. *Iroquois Foods and Food Preparation* #12 Anthropological Series, Ottawa. 1916. Reprinted by Iroqrafts, RR #2, Ohsweken, Ontario N0A 1M0, 1991.

Weaver, Wm. *100 Vegetables & Where They Came From.* Workman Pub. New York, 2000.

_____*Sauer's Herbal Cures America's First Book of Botanic Healing 1762-1778,* Routledge, New York, 2001.

Weed, Susan. *Menopausal Years, The Wise Woman Way.* Ash Tree Pub. Woodstock NY, 1992

Weigle, Marta. *Spiders and Spinsters.* U. of New Mexico Press, Albuquerque, 1982.

Weiner, M. *The People's Herbal, A family guide.* Putnam Publishing, New York, 1984.

Weiss, Rudolf. *Herbal Medicine.* Beaconsfield Publishers, 1988.

_____*Herbal Medicine* 2nd Edition. Thieme, Stuttgart, New York, 2000.

Wells, Diana.*100 Flowers and How They Got Their Names,* Algonquin Books, Chapel Hill,97

Westcott, Frank. *The Beaver Nature's Master Builder.* Hounslow Press, Willowdale, ON '89.

Westrich, LoLo, *California Herbal Remedies,* Gulf Pub Co. Houston, TX, 1989.

Wetzel, Suzanne et al. Bioproducts from Canada's Forests. Springer Netherlands 2006.

WHO monographs on selected medicinal plants, vol 1, 1999; vol 2, 2002.

White, Ian. *Australian Bush Flower Essences.* Bantam Books, 1991

White, Florence. *Flowers as Food* . Jonathan Cape. 1934

Whitmont, Edward. *Psyche and Substance.* North Atlantic Books. 1980

Wilkinson, Kathleen. *Trees and Shrubs of Alberta.* Lone Pine Books, Edmonton 1990.

_____*Wildflowers of Alberta.* U of A/Lone Pine Books, Edmonton 1999.

Williams, Jude. *Nature's Gentle Cures.* Sterling Publishing. New York. 1997.

Williamson, Darcy. 130 Medicinal Plant Monographs of the NW. self pub. E-book. 2011.

Williamson, E. *Major Herbs of Ayurveda.* Churchill Livingstone, Elsevier Science, 2002.

FLOWER ESSENCE RESOURCES

Aditi Himalaya Flower Essences, 15,Jaybharat Society, 3rd Road, Khar (W), Bombay 400 052, India.

Alaskan Flower Essence Project, P.O. Box. 1369, Homer, Alaska USA 99603-1369. www.alaskanessences.com.

Australian Bush Flower Essences. Australia. www.ausflowers.com.au.

Bach- Healing Herbs English Flower Essences- in Canada by Self Heal Distributing, Box 95008, Whyte Postal Outlet, Edmonton, AB T6E 0E5, 1800-593-5956 or www.selfhealdistributing.com Also www.healingherbs.co.uk or www.fesflowers.com

Bailey Flower Essences, 8 Neslon Road, Ilkley, West Yorkshire England, LS298HN. www.flowervr.com

Bloesem Remedies. Netherlands. www.bloesem-remedies.com

BrynaHerb Essences. www.brynaherbessences.uk

Canadian Forest Essences, PO Box 29128,1996 W. Broadway, Vancouver, BC V6J 1Z0

Canadian Forest Tree Essences. Ottawa. www.essences.ca. 613-725-9764.

Choming Flower Essences. www.mkprojects.com

Clear Path Essences. www.clearpathessences.com

Dancing Light Orchid Essences. Fairbanks, Alaska. www.orchidessences.com

Desert Alchemy, PO Box 44189, Tucson, Arizona, USA 85733. www.desert-alchemy.com.

Deva Flower Essences BP3 38880, Autrans, France. www.lab-deva.com

Eastern Flower Herbal Essences. julied@hfx.eastlink.ca.

Falling Leaf Essences. Box 78, Kallista, Victoria 3791, Australia. www.advancedalchemy.com.au.

Findhorn Flower Essences, Morayshire, Scotland IV36 0TY. www.findhornessences.com

Florais des Minas, Rua Albita, 194-Sala 408, Cruziero, CEP 30310-160,BH, MG, BRAZIL

FlorAlive˚, Brent Davis. Contact info@floralive.com

FES Flower Essence Society, PO Box 1769, Nevada City, California, USA, 95959. www.fesflowers.com Canadian Distributor- Self Heal Distributing, Box 95008, Whyte Postal Outlet, Edmonton, AB T6E 0E5 – www.selfhealdistributing.com

Green Hope Farm Flower Essences, PO Box 125, Meriden, New Hampshire USA 03770

Green Man Tree Essences. www.greenmantrees.demon.co.uk.

Habundia Flower Essences. c/o Peter Aziz. PO Box 90, Totnes, Devon, England TQ11 0YG.

Harebell Remedies. Scotland. ellie@harebellremedies.co.uk.

Hawaiian Gaia Flower Essences. www.gaiaessences.com

High Sierra Flower Essences. PO. Box 4275 Truclee, CA 96160. holly.hsb@highoctavehealing.com

Horus Flower Essences- horus@floweressences.de.

Hummingbird Remedies, PO Box 50161, Eugene, Oregon, USA 97405

Icelandic Flower Essences. www.kristbjorb.is.

Jade Mountain Flower Essences, Box 125, Mountain Lakes, New Jersey USA 07046-0125

Korte Phi. www.PHIessences.com

Light Heart Essences. England. www.lightheartessences.co.uk.

Light Mountain Flower Essences, Michael A. Vertolli, 1-800-667-HERB.

Living Essences of Australia, Box 355, Scarborough, 6019, Perth, Australia. www.livingessences.com.au

Living Flower Essences, www.livingfloweressences.com . Rhonda Pallasdowney.

Master's Flower Essences, 14618 Tyler Foote Rd Nevada City, California, USA, 95959. www.masteressences.com

Miriana fortem Flower Essences. www.mirianaflowers.com and info@miraflowers.com.

NaturaSacredplay, PO Box 32, Buckhorn, New Mexico, 88025, (505-535-2255).

New Millenium Flower Essences of New Zealand. info@nmessences.com.

New Zealand New Perception Flower Essences, PO Box 60-127,Titirangi, Auckland 7, NZ

Pacific Essences, Box 8317, Victoria, B.C. V8W 3R9. www.pacificessences.com.

Pegasus Products, PO Box 228, Boulder, Colorado, USA 80306-0228. 1-800- 527-6104.

Perelandra, Box 3603, Warrenton, VA. 22186. www.perelandra-ltd.com

Petite Fleur Essence, 8524 Whispering Creek Trail, Fort Worth, Texas, USA 76134. www.aromahealthtexas.com

Prairie Deva Flower Essences, Box 95008, Whyte Postal Outlet, Edmonton, AB T6E 0E5 1-(780) 433-7882. www.selfhealdistributing.com

Ravenworks- joni@ravenworksministries.org

Running Fox Farm PO Box 381,Worthington, Maryland USA 01098

Star Peruvian Flower Essences. Santa Barbara. www.starfloweressences.com

Stars of the Meadow, David Dalton, Lindisfarne Books, Mass. 2006.

Sun Essences. Norfolk, England. www.sunessence.co.uk

Sweetwater Sanctuary Essences. www.plantspirithealing.com

Tree Frog Farm Flower Essences. www.treefrogfarm.com

Whole Energy Essences, PO Box 285, Concord, Mass. 01742

Wild Rose Essences. www.wildrose.com

Woodland Essence, PO Box 206, Cold Brook, New York, USA 13324.

www.ingramcontent.com/pod-product-compliance
Lightning Source LLC
Chambersburg PA
CBHW081107170526
45165CB00008B/2357